Controlled Drug Delivery

DRUGS AND THE PHARMACEUTICAL SCIENCES

A Series of Textbooks and Monographs

Edited by

James Swarbrick

School of Pharmacy

University of North Carolina

Chapel Hill, North Carolina

Volume 1. PHARMACOKINETICS, *Milo Gibaldi and Donald Perrier* (out of print)

Volume 2. GOOD MANUFACTURING PRACTICES FOR PHARMACEUTICALS: A PLAN FOR TOTAL QUALITY CONTROL, *Sidney H. Willig, Murray M. Tuckerman, and William S. Hitchings IV* (out of print)

Volume 3. MICROENCAPSULATION, *edited by J. R. Nixon*

Volume 4. DRUG METABOLISM: CHEMICAL AND BIOCHEMICAL ASPECTS, *Bernard Testa and Peter Jenner*

Volume 5. NEW DRUGS: DISCOVERY AND DEVELOPMENT, *edited by Alan A. Rubin*

Volume 6. SUSTAINED AND CONTROLLED RELEASE DRUG DELIVERY SYSTEMS, *edited by Joseph R. Robinson*

Volume 7. MODERN PHARMACEUTICS, *edited by Gilbert S. Banker and Christopher T. Rhodes*

Volume 8. PRESCRIPTION DRUGS IN SHORT SUPPLY: CASE HISTORIES, *Michael A. Schwartz*

Volume 9. ACTIVATED CHARCOAL: ANTIDOTAL AND OTHER MEDICAL USES, *David O. Cooney*

Volume 10. CONCEPTS IN DRUG METABOLISM (in two parts), *edited by Peter Jenner and Bernard Testa*

Volume 11. PHARMACEUTICAL ANALYSIS: MODERN METHODS (in two parts), *edited by James W. Munson*

Volume 12. TECHNIQUES OF SOLUBILIZATION OF DRUGS, *edited by Samuel H. Yalkowsky*

Volume 13. ORPHAN DRUGS, *edited by Fred E. Karch*

Volume 14. NOVEL DRUG DELIVERY SYSTEMS: FUNDAMENTALS, DEVELOPMENTAL CONCEPTS, BIOMEDICAL ASSESSMENTS, *edited by Yie W. Chien*

Volume 15. PHARMACOKINETICS, Second Edition, Revised and Expanded, *Milo Gibaldi and Donald Perrier*

Volume 16. GOOD MANUFACTURING PRACTICES FOR PHARMACEUTICALS: A PLAN FOR TOTAL QUALITY CONTROL, Second Edition, Revised and Expanded, *Sidney H. Willig, Murray M. Tuckerman, and William S. Hitchings IV*

Volume 17. FORMULATION OF VETERINARY DOSAGE FORMS, *edited by Jack Blodinger*

Volume 18. DERMATOLOGICAL FORMULATIONS: PERCUTANEOUS ABSORPTION, *Brian W. Barry*

Volume 19. THE CLINICAL RESEARCH PROCESS IN THE PHARMACEUTICAL INDUSTRY, *edited by Gary M. Matoren*

Volume 20. MICROENCAPSULATION AND RELATED DRUG PROCESSES, *Patrick B. Deasy*

Volume 21. DRUGS AND NUTRIENTS: THE INTERACTIVE EFFECTS, *edited by Daphne A. Roe and T. Colin Campbell*

Volume 22. BIOTECHNOLOGY OF INDUSTRIAL ANTIBIOTICS, *Erick J. Vandamme*

Volume 23. PHARMACEUTICAL PROCESS VALIDATION, *edited by Bernard T. Loftus and Robert A. Nash*

Volume.24. ANTICANCER AND INTERFERON AGENTS: SYNTHESIS AND PROPERTIES, *edited by Raphael M. Ottenbrite and George B. Butler*

Volume 25. PHARMACEUTICAL STATISTICS: PRACTICAL AND CLINICAL APPLICATIONS, *Sanford Bolton*

Volume 26. DRUG DYNAMICS FOR ANALYTICAL, CLINICAL, AND BIOLOGICAL CHEMISTS, *Benjamin J. Gudzinowicz, Burrows T. Younkin, Jr., and Michael J. Gudzinowicz*

Volume 27. MODERN ANALYSIS OF ANTIBIOTICS, *edited by Adorjan Aszalos*

Volume 28. SOLUBILITY AND RELATED PROPERTIES, *Kenneth C. James*

Volume 29. CONTROLLED DRUG DELIVERY: FUNDAMENTALS AND APPLICATIONS, Second Edition, Revised and Expanded, *Joseph R. Robinson and Vincent H. L. Lee*

Other Volumes in Preparation

Controlled Drug Delivery

Fundamentals and Applications

SECOND EDITION,
REVISED AND EXPANDED

Edited by

Joseph R. Robinson
SCHOOL OF PHARMACY
UNIVERSITY OF WISCONSIN
MADISON, WISCONSIN

Vincent H. L. Lee
SCHOOL OF PHARMACY
UNIVERSITY OF SOUTHERN CALIFORNIA
LOS ANGELES, CALIFORNIA

MARCEL DEKKER, INC. New York and Basel

Library of Congress Cataloging-in-Publication Data

Controlled drug delivery.

(Drugs and the pharmaceutical sciences ; v. 29)
Rev. ed. of: Sustained and controlled release drug delivery systems / edited by Joseph R. Robinson. c1978.
Includes bibliographies and indexes.
1. Drugs--Controlled release. 2. Drugs--Dosage forms. I. Robinson, Joseph R. II. Lee, Vincent H. L. III. Sustained and controlled release drug delivery systems. IV. Series. [DNLM: 1. Delayed--Action Preparations. 2. Dosage Forms. W1 DR893B v.29 / QV 785 C7595]
RS201.C64C65 1987 615'.191 86-29108

ISBN 0-8247-7588-0

MARCEL DEKKER, INC.
270 Madison Avenue, New York, New York 10016

Current printing (last digit):
10 9 8 7 6 5 4 3

PRINTED IN THE UNITED STATES OF AMERICA

In memory of our fathers,
and to our mothers

Preface to the Second Edition

Controlled drug delivery is the phasing of drug administration to the needs of a condition at hand so that an optimal amount of drug is used to cure or control the condition in a minimum time. Research in controlled drug delivery during the past decade has led to increasingly sophisticated means to sustain drug delivery. It has also stimulated greater awareness among the pharmaceutical industry, the regulatory agencies, the health care profession, and the public at large of the therapeutic advantages of controlled drug delivery systems. Presently, the majority of these systems are based on synthetic polymers of some sort that differ in the degree of erodibility, swellability, and sensitivity to the biological environment in which they are placed. These polymers have been used to fabricate systems such as microcapsules and nanoparticles for implantation, hydrogels for oral and parenteral drug delivery, the osmotic pump for oral drug delivery, and patches for transdermal drug delivery. Clearly, in order to fully utilize the potential of polymers in the broad area of drug delivery, it is necessary to understand their fundamental physical, chemical, and biological properties.

When the first edition of this text was written a decade ago, liposomes were considered by many to be the answer to drug delivery optimization in virtually all routes of drug administration. Research since then has revealed that liposomes in particular and microparticulate carriers in general would probably have their greatest impact in targeting drugs for diseases affecting the reticuloendothelial system, to which these carriers are directed, as well as for diseases involving blood cells in the systemic circulation, to which these carriers are confined.

The frustrations associated with targeting drugs to specific sites in the body using systems such as liposomes have led to research to seek alternative carriers, such as insulin, that are biological in nature and capable of exiting the circulation by virtue of their ability to cross endothelial barriers via endocytosis and transcytosis. Parallel research has focused on other biological carriers such as monoclonal antibodies and certain glycoproteins that can recognize specific determinants at their target cells. While these approaches are still at their early stages of development and their role in controlled drug delivery is therefore still uncertain, it is clear that the area of controlled drug delivery is increasingly being based on molecular biology.

The area of controlled drug delivery is also becoming broader in scope in terms of routes of administration. Traditionally, controlled drug delivery systems were developed primarily for the oral route and, to some extent, for the parenteral route. Recently, there has been an explosion in research on drug delivery via the skin, due primarily to the success of several transdermal devices in sustaining drug delivery to the systemic circulation. Meanwhile, a better understanding of the potential therapeutic role of biologically active peptides and of their susceptibility to inactivation in the gastrointestinal tract has stimulated research in delivering these substances systemically via the nasal, buccal, rectal, and vaginal routes, the so-called unconventional routes. In the short term, there will be a need to fabricate systems perhaps more sophisticated than those now available to deliver peptides via these routes as well as parenteral routes. In the long term, it will be necessary to understand the biochemistry and cell biology of these uncoventional routes, since these may affect drug delivery system design. At the same time, there will be a need to seek means to deliver these peptides orally. This would require an enormous leap in our understanding of gross physiology and cellular physiology, as well as of immunology of the digestive system. Research has already begun in this area as exemplified by the bioadhesion approach, whose initial aim is to prolong the residence time of drugs in the gastrointestinal tract.

With this background in mind, we have organized the book into three parts. Part I deals with the fundamentals of controlled drug delivery. These include biological considerations of selected routes of drug administration (Chapter 1), theory of mass transfer (Chapter 2), fundamentals of polymer science (Chapter 3), use of polymers in controlled drug release (Chapter 4), pharmacokinetic/pharmacodynamic basis of controlled drug delivery (Chapter 5), bioavailability assessment and dosing considerations of controlled drug delivery systems (Chapter 6), and regulatory assessment of such systems (Chapter 7). Part II deals with the design and fabrication of technology-based controlled release drug delivery systems. These include novel chemical approaches (Chapter 8), oral products (Chapter 9), parenteral products (Chapter 10), implantable systems (Chapter 11), and transdermal systems (Chapter 12). Finally, Part III deals with several biochemical and molecular biology approaches to controlled drug delivery. These include microparticulate drug carriers (Chapter 13), selective endocytosis of macromolecular drug carriers (Chapter 14), and antibodies (Chapter 15).

With the possible exception of Chapters 6, 9, 10, and 11, this edition of the text is not a mere updating of the first edition. Rather, it is a companion to the first edition. It is the work of an interdisciplinary panel of scientists, reflecting the nature of controlled drug delivery research today and certainly in the foreseeable future. In reviewing the manuscripts, we recognized some overlaps among a few chapters but chose to retain these overlaps since they were viewed from a subtly different perspective by the respective authors. Thus, we consider these overlaps a strength rather than a weakness of this book.

As stated in the preface of the first edition, this book will fulfill our expectations if it creates further interest in the area of controlled as well as targeted drug delivery, provides a framework by which the pharmaceutical scientists can begin assessing the candidacy of a specific drug for controlled and targeted release, and serves as a plan of attack in formulating an appropriate drug delivery system.

Joseph R. Robinson
Vincent H. L. Lee

Preface to the First Edition

Great strides have been made in the management of diseases through the intervention of drugs over the past 50 years, as judged by the introduction and success of immunizing agents, antibiotics, steroids, tranquilizers, and many other drugs. These accomplishments in drug development have not been matched by a similar growth in the area of drug delivery. Clearly, unless a drug can be delivered to its target area at a rate and concentration that both minimize side effects and maximize therapeutic effects, the drug will not be maximally beneficial to the patient and, in the extreme, an otherwise useful drug may be discarded.

For accessible target tissues it is possible to directly titrate the patient on the basis of biological response, and temporal administration of drug in these situations is straightforward. However, the reality of the situation is that the desired target tissue, when identified, is usually well removed from the site of administration so that drug placement becomes difficult, especially when control over the time course of therapy is desired. Adding to the complexity of drug localization at the target tissue is the problem of drug behavior in the dosage form and body proper, as well as reliance on the patient to administer drug in the correct amount at the right time.

Over the years there has been available a variety of drug modifications and dosage forms with which we have attempted to control the time course and specificity of drugs in the body; these have been identified by various names, such as "prodrug," "controlled release," "sustained release," "prolonged release," and "timed release." In each of these types of drug delivery there has been some degree of control over the temporal pattern of drug placement in the target tissue. However, a maximization of therapy has generally not been achieved. To maximize drug utilization, it is necessary to deliver drug to the target tissue in the correct amount at the proper time to elicit the desired response. Moreover, drug delivery must be continued at a rate such that the condition in question is cured or controlled in a minimum time with the fewest side effects. Thus, an appropriate definition of controlled drug release is as follows: It is the phasing of drug administration to the needs of the condition at hand so that an optimal amount of drug is used to cure or control the condition in a minimum time. In some situations this might mean that drug is delivered more promptly for short periods of time and in other cases it would mean prolongation of drug levels. In the latter category we employ the terms "sustained release" and "prolonged release" interchangeably; this designates only one aspect of controlled release, namely, to produce protracted levels of drug in the body. Actually, controlled drug delivery is the desired effect of all drug delivery systems, and all presently fabricated sustained and prolonged drug delivery systems provide some degree of control, albeit incomplete. Thus, whereas second-generation sustained release products have made significant advances over their first-generation counterparts, none of the commercially available systems presently on the market is in truth a controlled drug delivery system; some are just better than others.

The present text was designed to fulfill a perceived need to provide a comprehensive picture of the sustained release drug product area. Admittedly, there are numerous review articles, chapters, and a few texts devoted to one or more topics in the sustained release drug or chemical area, but a current and comprehensive treatment appears to be lacking.

To accomplish this task, I have organized the book in the following manner. The principal chapters describing the various physical, chemical, and bioengineering approaches to the preparation of sustained release drug products are Chapters 3, 4, 6, and 7. The various physiological, drug-related, and formulation constraints on the design of these products are described in Chapters 1 and 2, the early part of Chapter 3, and Chapter 5. Chapters 1, 2, and 3 focus primarily on the physiological and drug-related constraints, and Chapter 5 deals with parenteral drug and formulation biocompatibility considerations. Thus, the first seven chapters provide a description of the problems and potential approaches of sustained release drug product preparation. I have elected to place those chapters with modest amounts of mathematics at the end of the text. Thus, Chapter 8 deals with pharmacokinetic considerations in the design of sustained release drug products, and Chapter 9 describes the very important area of dosing considerations.

The text will fulfill my expectations if it creates interest in the area of controlled drug delivery, provides a framework by means of which the pharmaceutical scientist can begin to assess a specific drug as to its candidacy for a sustained release system, and serves as a plan of attack in formulating an appropriate drug delivery system. Thus, the book is aimed at those interested in understanding the principles of sustained and controlled drug delivery systems.

Joseph R. Robinson

Contents

Part III
BIOCHEMICAL AND MOLECULAR BIOLOGY APPROACHES TO CONTROLLED DRUG DELIVERY

Contributors

William H. Barr, Pharm.D., Ph.D. Department of Pharmacy and Pharmaceutics, Virginia Commonwealth University/Medical College of Virginia, Richmond, Virginia

Meir Bialer, Ph.D.* Pharmacodynamics Department, Medical Research Division, American Cyanamid Corporation, Pearl River, New York

Nicholas Bodor, Ph.D. Department of Medicinal Chemistry, College of Pharmacy, University of Florida, Gainesville, Florida

Ronald R. Burnette, Ph.D., Pharm.D., M.S. School of Pharmacy, University of Wisconsin, Madison, Wisconsin

Yie W. Chien, Ph.D. Controlled Drug Delivery Research Center, College of Pharmacy, Rutgers—The State University of New Jersey, Piscataway, New Jersey

Michael R. Dobrinska, Ph.D. Department of Drug Metabolism, Merck Sharp & Dohme Research Laboratories, West Point, Pennsylvania

---

**Current affiliation*: Department of Pharmacy, School of Pharmacy, The Hebrew University of Jerusalem, Jerusalem, Israel

Ruth Duncan, B.Sc., Ph.D. Department of Biological Sciences, University of Keele, Keele, Staffordshire, England

Gary E. Goodman, M.S., M.D. Tumor Institute, Swedish Hospital Medical Center, Seattle, Washington

Jorge Heller, Ph.D. Polymer Sciences Department, SRI International, Menlo Park, California

Ingegerd Hellström, M.D. ONCOGEN, Seattle, Washington

Karl Erik Hellström, M.D. ONCOGEN, Seattle, Washington

Ho-Wah Hui, Ph.D.* School of Pharmacy, University of Wisconsin, Madison, Wisconsin

Rudy L. Juliano, Ph.D. Department of Pharmacology, University of Texas Medical School, Houston, Texas

Vincent H. L. Lee, Ph.D. Department of Pharmaceutics, School of Pharmacy, University of Southern California, Los Angeles, California

Sau-Hung S. Leung, M.S. School of Pharmacy, University of Wisconsin, Madison, Wisconsin

Vincent H. K. Li, M.S. School of Pharmacy, University of Wisconsin, Madison, Wisconsin

Thorsteinn Loftsson, M.S., Ph.D.† Department of Medicinal Chemistry, College of Pharmacy, University of Florida, Gainesville, Florida

Joseph R. Robinson, Ph.D. School of Pharmacy, University of Wisconsin, Madison, Wisconsin

B. Michael Silber, Ph.D. Pharmacodynamics Department, Medical Research Division, American Cyanamid Company, Pearl River, New York

---

**Current affiliation*: Pharmaceutical Products Division, Abbott Laboratories, North Chicago, Illinois
†*Current affiliation*: Department of Pharmacy, University of Iceland, Rekjavik, Iceland

Jerome Philip Skelly, Ph.D. Division of Biopharmaceutics, Center for Drugs and Biologics, Food and Drug Administration, Rockville, Maryland

Peter G. Welling, Ph.D., D.Sc. Department of Pharmacokinetics and Drug Metabolism, Warner–Lambert/Parke–Davis Pharmaceutical Research Division, Ann Arbor, Michigan

Avraham Yacobi, Ph.D. Pharmacodynamics Department, Medical Research Division, American Cyanamid Company, Pearl River, New York

Controlled Drug Delivery

I

Fundamentals of Controlled Release Drug Delivery

1

Influence of Drug Properties and Routes of Drug Administration on the Design of Sustained and Controlled Release Systems

VINCENT H. K. LI and JOSEPH R. ROBINSON / University of Wisconsin, Madison, Wisconsin

VINCENT H. L. LEE / University of Southern California, Los Angeles, California

I. INTRODUCTION

In recent years, considerable attention has been focused on the development of new drug delivery systems. This is evidenced by the spate of books [1–8] and review articles [9–18] published on this subject. There are a number of reasons for the intense interest in new systems. First, recognition of the possibility of repatenting successful drugs by applying the concepts and techniques of controlled release drug delivery systems, coupled with the increasing expense in bringing new drug entities to market, has encouraged the development of new drug delivery systems. Second, new systems are needed to deliver the novel, genetically engineered pharmaceuticals, i.e., peptides and proteins, to their sites of action without incurring significant immunogenicity or biological inactivation. Third, treating enzyme deficient diseases and cancer therapies can be improved by better targeting. Finally, therapeutic efficacy and safety of drugs, administered by conventional methods, can be improved by more precise spatial and temporal placement within the body, thereby reducing both the size and number of doses.

If one were to conceptualize the ideal drug delivery system, two prerequisites would come to mind. First, it should deliver drug at a rate dictated by the needs of the body over the period of treatment. This may necessitate delivery at a constant rate for drugs that have a clear relationship between steady state plasma levels and the resultant therapeutic response, or at a variable rate for drugs which need either a series of peaks and valleys or act on a rhythmn. Second, it should channel the active entity solely to the site of action. This may necessitate delivery to specific receptors, as in the case of H_1 and H_2 antagonists, localization to tumor cells, as required by most cancer treatments, or to specific areas of the body as for arthritis or gout. At present, no available drug delivery systems can achieve all these lofty goals. Conventional dosage forms, including prolonged-release dosage forms, are unable to control either the rate or site of action. While rate-controlled release drug delivery systems are capable of delivering a drug at some predetermined rate either systemically or locally for a specific period of time, they do so with virtually no control over the fate of the drug once it enters the body. Targeted drug delivery systems, on the other hand, while capable of achieving site specific delivery, are usually unable to control the release kinetics of drug in a predictable manner. To date, their usefulness is limited to systemic administration.

This chapter will describe those factors influencing the design of sustained/controlled drug delivery systems with particular emphasis on limitations imposed by the intrinsic physicochemical and biological properties of a drug candidate and by the route of administration.

II. TERMINOLOGY

Before initiating a discussion of sustained and controlled release dosage forms, it is necessary to provide a short explanation of terminology used because there is considerable confusion in this area. The general consensus is that controlled release denotes systems which can provide some control, whether this be of a temporal or spatial nature, or both, of drug release in the body. In other words, the system attempts to control drug concentrations in the target tissue or cells. Thus, prolonged release or sustained release systems, which only prolong therapeutic blood or tissue levels of the drug for an extended period of time, cannot be considered as controlled release systems by this definition. They are distinguished from rate-controlled drug delivery systems, which are able to specify the release rate and duration *in vivo* precisely, on the basis of simple *in vitro* tests [15]. Drug targeting, on the other hand, can be considered as a form of controlled release in that it exercises spatial control of drug release within the body. Since rate-controlled release and drug targeting represent totally separate delivery approaches, they will be discussed separately in this chapter.

In general, controlled delivery attempts to:

1. *Sustain drug action at a predetermined rate* by maintaining a relatively constant, effective drug level in the body with

concomitant minimization of undesirable side effects associated with a sawtooth kinetic pattern

2. *Localize drug action* by spatial placement of a controlled release system (usually rate-controlled) adjacent to or in the diseased tissue or organ
3. *Target drug action* by using carriers or chemical derivatization to deliver drugs to a particular "target" cell type

In practice, very few of the applied systems embrace all of these actions. In most cases, the release system creates constant concentration of drug within the body over an extended period of time. The assumption is that there is a steady state drug levels in plasma and in target tissues or cells are correlated. Ideally, it is desirable to place the drug at the target, be it a tissue, a population of cells, or receptors, leaving the rest of the body drug free. Obviously, this would be quite difficult, especially if the target is sheltered from systemic circulation by various barriers. For example, drug targeting to the brain via systemic administration is severely limited by selectivity of the blood-brain barrier.

In order to maintain a constant drug level in either plasma or target tissue, release rate from the controlled release system should be equal to the elimination rate from plasma or target tissue. The most conventional method to achieve a constant plasma level is the use of intravenuous infusion. However, this would be inconvenient for most therapeutic situations so that other noninvasive routes, such as the oral or transdermal route, are preferred.

Various designations such as "smart" [19], "targeted" [20], "intelligent" [15], "novel" [6], and "therapeutic" [21], have been given to controlled release systems. Therapeutic systems have also been used interchangeably with rate-controlled release systems. These usually operate on an advanced engineering system-control approach, consisting of a logic element with or without a sensor. Three types of therapeutic systems are available, namely, passive preprogrammed, active preprogrammed, and active self-programmed [22]. Most rate-controlled release systems fall in the category of passive preprogrammed, in which the release rate is predetermined and is irresponsive to the external biological environment. Examples of active preprogrammed are few and include most metered insulin pumps, whose release rate can be altered by a source external to the body [23]. The active, self-programmed therapeutic systems modulate release rate of the drug in response to information, registered by a sensor, on the changing biological environment such as blood sugar level in diabetes [24]. In our view, the term therapeutic system, while helpful for marketing purposes, is inappropriate as a substitute for controlled release systems since non-controlled release systems are therapeutic systems also.

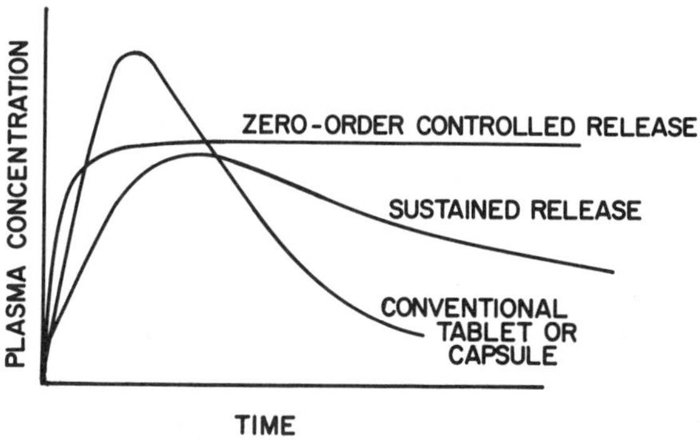

Fig. 1 Plasma drug concentration-profiles for conventional tablet or capsule formulation, a sustained release formulation, and a zero-order controlled release formulation.

Figure 1 shows comparative blood drug level profiles obtained from administration of conventional, controlled as well as prolonged release dosage forms. Thus, the conventional tablet or capsule provides only a single and transient burst of drug. As long as the amount of drug is above the minimum effective concentration, a pharmacological response is observed. Problems occur when the therapeutic range is very narrow or when the peak is greater than the upper limit of this range. Indeed, one of the main purposes of controlled release is to improve safety and minimize side effects of the drug by reducing fluctuations in drug level. Prolonged-release dosage forms also reduce fluctuations in plasma drug levels by slowing down the absorption rate due to slower drug release rate. In many cases, this is achieved by intermittently releasing a small burst of drug over a prolonged period of time as in the case of repeat-action dosage forms.

III. RATIONALE OF SUSTAINED/CONTROLLED DRUG DELIVERY

The basic rationale for controlled drug delivery is to alter the pharmacokinetics and pharmacodynamics of pharmacologically active moieties by using novel drug delivery systems or by modifying the molecular structure and/or physiological parameters inherent in a selected route of administration. It is desirable that the duration of drug action become more a design property of a rate-controlled dosage form, and less, or not at all, a property of the drug molecule's inherent kinetic properties. Thus, optimal design of controlled release systems necessitates a thorough understanding of the pharmacokinetics and pharmacodynamics of the drug.

As mentioned earlier, the primary objectives of controlled drug delivery are to ensure safety and to improve efficacy of drugs as well as patient compliance. This is achieved by better control of plasma drug levels and less frequent dosing. For conventional dosage forms, only the dose (D) and dosing interval (τ) can vary and, for each drug, there exists a therapeutic window of plasma concentration, below which, therapeutic effect is insufficient, and above which undesirable or toxic side effects are elicited. As an index of this window, the therapeutic index TI can be used. This is often defined as the ratio of median lethal dose (LD_{50}) to median effective dose (ED_{50}). Alternatively, it can be defined as the ratio of maximum drug concentration (C^*_{max}) in blood that can be tolerated to the minimum concentration (C^*_{min}) needed to produce an acceptable therapeutic response. Table 1 lists the therapeutic indices of a variety of drugs in plasma in humans.

For drugs whose disposition show pronounced linear, one-compartment characteristics, Theeuwes and Bayne [25] have demonstrated the following relationship between dosing interval (τ) and therapeutic index (TI). Thus,

$$\tau < t_{1/2}(\ln \text{TI})/\ln 2 \tag{1}$$

where $t_{1/2}$ is the half-life. Since the therapeutic index for most drugs is around 2, it will be necessary to dose the patients at intervals shorter than the half-life. Such inconvenient regimens often result in reduced compliance and inadequate treatment. For drugs with pronounced multicompartmental characteristics, a better estimate of the dosing interval may be obtained by replacing $t_{1/2}$ with 0.693* (MRT), where MRT is the mean residence time. In such cases, the drug must be given even more frequently than suggested by Eq. (1).

In general, the dosing interval may be increased either by modifying the drug molecule to decrease the rate of elimination (k_{el}) or by modifying the release rate of a dosage form to decrease the rate of absorption (k_a). Both approaches seek to decrease fluctuations in plasma levels during multiple dosing, allowing the dosing interval to increase without either overdosing or underdosing. When attempting to extend the dosing interval by decreasing the rate of absorption, the formulator will be confronted with the physiological constraint of a finite residence time at the absorption site. For example, an effective absorption time for orally administered drugs is about 9–12 hr. If the rate of absorption decreases too much, some of the unabsorbed drug will pass into the large intestine, where absorption is slower and more variable and where bacterial degradation of the drug may occur. Thus, drugs with half-lives of 6 hr or less and

Table 1. Usual Ranges of Therapeutic Serum Concentrations and Terminal Half-Lives in Humans

Drug substance	Therapeutic serum concentrations[a] (C^*_{min} to C^*_{max})	Terminal half-lives[b]
Digitoxin	14–30 μg/liter	6.3–11.3 days
Digoxin	0.9–2 μg/liter	1.4–2.2 days
Lidocaine	1.5–5 mg/liter	1.2–1.7 hr
Lithium	0.5–1.3 mEq	14.2–24.1 hr
Nortriptyline	50–140 μg/liter	18.2–35.0 hr
Phenytoin	10–20 mg/liter	18.7–27.6 hr
Procainamide	4–8 mg/liter	2.5–4.7 hr
Propranolol	20–50 μg/liter	1.1–9.9 hr
Quinidine	2–5 mg/liter	3.0–16.0 hr
Salicylates	150–300 mg/liter	2.9–22 hr
Theophylline	10–20 mg/liter	5.3–8.3 hr

[a]Data were obtained from Koch-Weser [26].
[b]Data were obtained from Pagliaro and Benet [27].

possessing therapeutic indices less than 3 must be given no less frequently than every 12 hr [28]. Unless gastrointestinal transit time can be lengthened, once-daily oral dosing may prove to be difficult to achieve for drugs with such extremely short half-lives [28]. For other routes of administration, where residence time is less of a problem, dosing intervals can be lengthened to months or even years. For example, implants containing contraceptives may be effective for a year or two.

In summary, only when the rate-limiting step resides in the drug delivery system, and not in physiological constraints, can control over drug administration be achieved.

IV. FACTORS INFLUENCING THE DESIGN AND PERFORMANCE OF SUSTAINED/CONTROLLED RELEASE PRODUCTS

To establish criteria for the design of controlled release products, a number of variables must be considered.

1. *Drug properties*: The physiochemical properties of a drug, including stability, solubility, partitioning characteristics, charge, and protein binding propensity, play a dominant role in the design and performance of controlled release systems.
2. *Route of drug delivery*: The area of the body in which drugs will be applied or administered can be restrictive on the basis of technological achievement of a suitable controlled release mechanism or device. At times, the drug delivery system, in certain routes of administration, can exert a negative influence on drug efficacy, particularly during chronic administration, and hence other routes of administration should be considered. Performance of the controlled release systems may also be influenced by physiological constraints imposed by the particular route, such as first-pass metabolism, GI motility, blood supply, and sequestration of small foreign particles by the liver and spleen.
3. *Target sites*: In order to minimize unwanted side effects, it is desirable to maximize the fraction of applied dose reaching the target organ or tissue. This can be partially achieved by local administration or by the use of carriers. However, the absorptive surfaces of most routes are impermeable to macromolecules or other targeted delivery systems, thereby necessitating either intravascular or intraarterial administration.
4. *Acute or chronic therapy*: Consideration of whether one expects to achieve cure or control of a condition and the expected length of drug therapy are important factors in designing controlled release systems. Attempts to generate a one year contraceptive implant presents significantly different problems in design than does an antibiotic for acute infection. Moreover, long term toxicity of rate-controlled drug delivery systems is usually different from that of conventional dosage forms [29].
5. *The disease*: Pathological changes during the course of a disease can play a significant role in the design of a suitable drug delivery system. For example, in attempting to design an ocular controlled-release product for an external inflammation, the time course of changes in protein content in ocular fluids and in the integrity of the ocular barriers would have to taken into consideration. Sometimes, one can take advantage of the unique manifestations of the disease state. For example, the higher plasminogen activator levels in some tumor cells can lead to preferential bioconversion of peptidyl prodrugs in these cells [30–32]. Similarly, the higher tyrosinase level in melanoma cells has been demonstrated to allow targeting to and preferential bioconversion of 2,4-dihydroxphenylalanine in them [33].

6. *The patient*: Whether the patient is ambulatory or bedridden, young or old, obese or gaunt, etc., can influence the design of a controlled release product. An implant or intramuscular injection of a drug to a bedridden patient with little muscle movement may perform in a manner significantly different from that of an ambulatory patient. Some of these factors represent individual patient variation and cannot be controlled by the research scientist while others must be considered. For example, single unit controlled release products are particularly prone to intra- and inter-subject variation because of variabilities in individual GI motility [34].

While all of these variables are important in the design of controlled and targeted release delivery systems, our discussion will center on drug properties and routes of administration as they relate to controlled release drug delivery in general. In particular, this chapter is concerned with increasing the visibility of some of the detrimental or prohibitive factors in the design of controlled release system. The release mechanism and the applicability of the various approaches (physical, chemical, and biological) used in the design of individual controlled release system will be discussed in Chapters 8–15.

To establish a basis for discussion of the influence of drug properties and the route of administration on sustained/controlled release product design, it is worthwhile focusing on:

1. Behavior of the drug in its delivery system
2. Behavior of the drug and its delivery system in the body

The first of these two elements is concerned with the ways in which drug properties can influence release characteristics from its delivery system. For conventional drug delivery systems, the rate-limiting step in drug availability is usually absorption of drug across a biological membrane such as the gastrointestinal wall (Scheme 1). In a sustained/controlled release product, one aims for release of drug

$$(\text{Drug})_{\text{Dosage form}} \xrightarrow{\text{Drug release}} (\text{Drug})_{\text{Solution at absorption site}} \xrightarrow{\text{Absorption}} (\text{Drug})_{\text{Target area}} \xrightarrow{\text{Elimination}}$$

Scheme 1

from the dosage form as the rate-limiting step instead. Thus, drug availability is controlled by the kinetics of drug release rather than absorption. Consequently, the associated rate constant(s) for drug release from the dosage form are smaller than the absorption rate constant and kinetically the process appears as shown in Scheme 2.

$$(\text{Drug})_{\text{Dosage form}} \xrightarrow{\text{Drug release}} (\text{Drug})_{\text{Target area}} \dashrightarrow \text{Elimination}$$

Scheme 2

To control drug release one can employ a variety of approaches, such as dissolution, diffusion, swelling, osmotic pressure, complexation, ion-exchange, and magnetic field, each of these will be amplified on in subsequent chapters. The interplay between physiochemical properties of a drug and characteristics of its delivery system determines the temporal release pattern that is observed.

The second element, behavior of the drug and its delivery system in the body, is extremely complex, involving the fate of drug during transit to the target area as well as its fate while in the biophase. Availability of drug to its target will depend on its pharmacokinetics as well as that of its carrier. In the case of drug targeting, the carrier is used to alter the pharmacokinetics of drug in the body. The influence of physiological constraints on the fate of the delivery system in the body is usually negative, for example, oral absorption is usually limited by GI transit time of the delivery system.

From the previous discussion, it is clear that the formulation and performance of sustained/controlled release dosage forms have roots in the physicochemical properties of the drug and its carrier. The pharmacokinetics and pharmacodynamics, to a large extent, are derived functions of the intrinsic properties of the drug. Thus, development and assessment of a sustained/controlled drug delivery system requires a rather complete knowledge of the intrinsic properties of a drug and the ways in which it can influence the design of sustained/controlled release systems. Oftentimes, undesirable physiochemical and biological properties can be altered by suitable chemical modification, by use of a carrier, or perhaps can be altered by suitable chemical modification, by use of a carrier, or perhaps by administration via another route. The first approach will be discussed in Chapter 9, while the other two approaches will be briefly discussed in this chapter and further amplified upon in subsequent chapters.

V. PHYSICOCHEMICAL PROPERTIES OF A DRUG INFLUENCING DRUG PRODUCT DESIGN AND PERFORMANCE

The performance of a drug in its release pattern from the dosage form as well as in the body proper is a function of its properties.

These properties can at times prohibit/restrict placement of the drug in a sustained/controlled release form, restrict the route of drug administration, and significantly modify performance for one reason or another. Most of the time these properties are restrictive rather than prohibitive, making sustained/controlled release product design more difficult. For the purpose of this discussion, it is convenient to describe the properties of a drug as being either physiochemical or biological. Obviously, there is no clear distinction between these two since the biological properties of a drug are a function of its physicochemical properties. By our definition, physiochemical properties are those that can be determined from *in vitro* experiments. Biological properties will be those that result from typical pharmacokinetic studies on the absorption, distribution, metabolism, and excretion (ADME) characteristics of a drug as well as those resulting from pharmacological studies.

A. Aqueous Solubility

Since drugs must be in solution before they can be absorbed, compounds with very low aqueous solubility usually suffer oral bioavailability problems because of limited gastrointestinal transit time of the undissolved drug particles and limited solubility at the absorption site. Unfortunately, for many compounds, the site of maximum absorption will also be the area in which the drug is least soluble. For example, tetracycline dissolves to a greater extent in the stomach than in the intestine, although it is best absorbed in the intestine [35]. Such drugs may be poor candidates for sustained/controlled release systems, unless the system is capable of retaining the drug in the stomach and gradually releasing it to the small intestine or unless the solubility is made higher and independent of the external environment by encapsulating the drug with an acid (if the drug is a weak base) or a base (if the drug is a weak acid) in a membrane system. Examples of other drugs which are limited in absorption by their dissolution rate are digoxin [36], warfarin [37], griseofulvin [38], and salicylamide [39]. Although the action of a drug can be prolonged by making it less soluble, this may occur at the expense of inconsistent and incomplete bioavailability.

The choice of mechanism for oral sustained/controlled release systems is limited by aqueous solubility of the drug. Diffusional systems will be poor choices for slightly soluble drugs since the driving force for diffusion, the concentration in aqueous solution, will be low. In contrast, such drugs may be effectively incorporated in matrix systems.

In selecting polymer coatings for sustained/controlled systems, the dissolution rate of a drug must be considered. Some antiobiotics and high molecular weight drugs may have reasonably good to excellent aqueous solubility, but very slow dissolution rates. On the positive side, the slow dissolution rate of such compounds can be utilized to achieve sustained/controlled drug release by incorporation in a matrix system. On the negative side, dissolution-limited bioavailability may occur.

Aqueous solubility also limits the loading efficiency of drugs into a variety of carriers such as liposomes, erythrocytes, and other microparticles. Most water-soluble drugs tend to leak out from such carriers readily.

B. Partition Coefficient and Molecular Size

Partition coefficient and molecular size influence not only the permeation of a drug across biological membranes, but also diffusion across or through a rate-controlling membrane or matrix. Following administration, the drug must traverse a variety of membranes to gain access to the target area. Drugs with extremely high partition coefficient (i.e., very oil-soluble) readily penetrate the membranes but are unable to proceed further, while drugs with excessive aqueous solubility, i.e., low oil/water partition coefficients cannot penetrate the membranes. A balance in the partition coefficient is needed to give an optimum flux for permeation through the biological and rate-controlling membranes. Hansch and Dunn [40] as well as Fujita et al. [41] have shown that, for many body tissues, such as the gastrointestinal tract, skin, and blood-aqueous barrier of the eye, the optimum *n*-octanol/water partition coefficient at which maximum flux occurs is approximately 1000.

The ability of a drug to diffuse through membranes, its so called diffusivity, is related to its molecular size by the following equation:

$$\text{Log } D = -s_V \log V + k_V = -s_M \log M + k_M$$

where D is diffusivity, M is molecular weight, V is molecular volume, and s_V, s_M, k_V, and k_M are constants in a particular medium. In general, the denser the medium, the smaller the diffusivity. For drugs of intermediate molecular weight (150–400), diffusivities through flexible polymers are typically of the order of 10^{-8} cm^2 sec^{-1}.

C. Drug Stability

The stability of a drug in the environment to which it is exposed is another physicochemical factor to be considered in the design of sustained/controlled release systems. Drugs that are unstable in the stomach can be placed in a slowly soluble form or have their release delayed until they reach the small intestine. However, such a strategy would be detrimental for drugs that either are unstable in the small intestine or undergo extensive gut-wall metabolism, as evidenced by decreased bioavailability when these drugs are administered from a sustained release dosage form [42, 43]. To achieve better bioavailability and controlled release of drugs that are unstable in the small intestine, a different route of administration should be chosen. Controlled release of nitroglycerin is a good example. On the positive side, the presence of metabolizing enzymes at the site of administration or along the pathway to the target area can sometimes be utilized in controlled drug delivery. Chapter 8 will describe some of these approaches.

D. Protein Binding

It is well known that many drugs bind to plasma proteins with a concomitant influence on the duration of drug action [44–48]. Since blood proteins are for the most part recirculated and not eliminated, drug protein binding can serve as a depot for drug producing a prolonged release profile, especially if a high degree of drug-binding occurs. This aspect of prolonged drug activity has been described in the literature [49]. There are, however, other drug-protein interactions that have a bearing on drug performance. Levine [50] has shown that quaternary ammonium compounds bind to mucin in the GI tract. Drugs bound to mucin may increase absorption, if the bound drug act as a depot. However, if degradation and/or washing of the drug further down the GI tract occurs, binding of drug to mucin may result in a reduction of free drug available for absorption. The issue of drug and vehicle interaction with the mucin layer and its influence on extent and duration of drug absorption has been reviewed [51].

VI. BIOLOGICAL FACTORS INFLUENCING DESIGN AND PERFORMANCE OF SUSTAINED/CONTROLLED RELEASE PRODUCTS

The design of a sustained/controlled release product should be based on a comprehensive picture of drug disposition. This would entail a complete examination of the ADME characteristics of a drug following multiple dosing. Unfortunately, an imcomplete picture of a drug's disposition is usually the case and decisions are generally made on this basis. The biological parameters that form the basis of controlled release product design will be described in Chapters 5 and 6.

Every pharmacokinetic property and biological response parameter has a useful range for the design of sustained/controlled release products, outside of which sustained/controlled release product design becomes difficult or impossible. Presumably, with unlimited technological capability and strategic placement of a drug in the body, all of these limitations could be circumvented but this capability is usually not available and thus constraints are generally imposed. In the following discussion, it is assumed that the level of drug in blood or body tissue parallels biological activity of the drug.

A. Absorption

To maintain constant blood or tissue level of drug, it must be uniformly released from the controlled release system and then uniformly absorbed. It would be desirable to have the released dose completely absorbed as well but this is not a prohibitive consideration. Usually, the rate-limiting step in drug delivery from a controlled release product is release from the dosage form rather than absorption. Thus, rapid drug absorption, relative to drug release from a dosage form, is expected but this is not always the case. In addition, variation in both the extent and rate of drug absorption can occur, particularly with orally administered drugs.

The fraction of drug absorbed from a single noncontrolled dose of drug can sometimes be quite low for a variety of reasons, such as drug degradation due to solvolysis or metabolism, binding of drugs to proteins, physical loss, or perhaps site- or dose-dependent absorption. Nevertheless, as long as the drug is uniformly absorbed, albeit incomplete, a successful controlled release product can be generated. As stated earlier it is preferable, but not essential, to have the drug completely absorbed. The development of the controlled release ocular system, Ocusert[R], is an excellent illustration of dealing with this problem. Pilocarpine is usually absorbed across the cornea to the extent of about 1% from an applied dose, the extensive loss due to drainage and absorption into nontarget tissues [52,53]. However, despite the low fraction of dose absorbed, a controlled release product was prepared that in fact significantly improved the low bioavailability problem and was able to maintain a constant level of drug in the target tissues for extended periods of time [54].

When considering orally administered drugs, significant loss prior to appearance in the systemic circulation can occur through hydrolytic degradation in the contents of the GI tract [55], metabolism by the intestinal flora [56], and metabolism during its transit across the GI wall [57]. Metabolism at the site of administration is a potential problem for all routes of administration, as is hydrolytic degradation. However, some routes, such as the GI tract, possess a relatively rich supply of metabolizing enzymes whereas other, such as the precorneal portion of the eye, have few. Hydrolytic and metabolic reactions are usually first order in drug concentrations, but fortunately degradation is primarily restricted to drugs in solution, and thus drugs in the solid state or in solid dosage forms are protected from degradation. Indeed, placement of a labile drug in a sustained or controlled release drug delivery system can sometimes improve the fraction of dose absorbed. The extent of this protection, hence improved bioavailability, is at times difficult to predict a priori and thus it is sometimes necessary to rely on empirical manipulations of the release rate after obtaining blood or tissue drug levels with a prototype controlled release system.

If the drug were erratically absorbed, as might occur in a route of administration with variable absorptive surface, such as the GI tract, design of a controlled release product would be more difficult or prohibitive. With respect to the oral route, it is well known that the absorptive character of the different segments of the GI tract varies [58], which in turn can influence the amount and rate of absorption for certain drugs. The oral anticoagulant dicumarol [59], the quaternary ammonium compounds hexamethonium and decamethonium [60], and the aminoglycosides such as gentamicin and kanamycin [61] are examples of such drugs. Similarly, drugs absorbed by specialized transport processes and drugs at special sites of the GI tract are also poor candidates for controlled release products. Riboflavin is absorbed by an active transport process, a process which is saturable [62], and is preferentially absorbed in the upper part of the GI tract [63]. Consequently, unless this drug can be localized at the absorptive site one expects a gradation in absorption for this drug but this is not necessarily prohibitive. Indeed, riboflavin has been formulated in various sustained release multivitamin preparations. However, Morrison et al. [63] found that such preparations provided no demonstrable advantages over conventional preparations.

Iron is another drug which is not uniformly well absorbed along the length of the GI tract. The greatest uptake of drug occurs at the upper part of the duodenum with significantly reduced absorptive capacity in the lower segment of the intestine [64–66]. Middleton et al. [67] found that iron given in divided doses, a situation analogous to a sustained release product, was only 68% as available as the same amount of drug taken as a single dose. Sustained release iron products have been evaluated by several investigators and the results are equivocal. Crosland-Taylor et al. [68] found that absorption of iron from sustained release tablets was extremely variable. Bothwell et al. [69] reported that the amount of iron absorbed from Spansules^{R} was a function of the rate at which drug was released; significant reduction in the amount of iron absorbed occurred in the Spansules^{R} with slow release rates. On the other hand, Baird et al. [70] found that iron formulated in a wax matrix sustained release product was as well absorbed as conventional ferrous sulfate tablets. Indeed, Webster [71], Callender [72], and Bentley and Jacobs [73] detected no significant differences in the elevation of hemoglobin levels in iron-deficient anemic patients taking the sustained release Gradumet^{R} and nonsustained release ferrous sulfate products. These studies, together with others [74–76], leave in doubt the appropriateness of some commercially available sustained release iron preparations. Nevertheless, they indicate that the selection of sustaining mechanisms has an important bearing on ultimate biological response.

When considering the problem of variable absorption rates, it is necessary to cite intramuscular injections as a route of administration with significant difficulties in this regard. Aside from the large individual variation with this route of administration, due to muscle mobility, water content, tissue integrity, etc., there is the additional problem of tissue insult upon initial injection and further changes in the tissue from repeated injection, all of which can change the release and absorption pattern of a drug.

A more prohibitive aspect of the absorption process via the oral route is the magnitude of the absorption rate constant. For single nonsustained doses, a minimum absorption rate constant of 0.25 hr^{-1} to 0.35 hr^{-1} is necessary for 95% of the administered dose to be absorbed, assuming that the GI transit time is between 10 and 12 hr. To formulate drugs at the lower limit of absorption rate constants into controlled or sustained release systems, the desired rate constant of release from the dosage form would have to be even lower, resulting in decreased bioavailability. As the GI transit time is finite, a suitable controlled release system, giving a high fraction of dose absorbed, can be difficult to design. In addition, the rate constant of release based on absorption considerations may be very different from that based on biological half-life considerations so that a compromise is achieved generating less than ideal release rates. In essence, oral drugs which are slowly absorbed are poor candidates for sustained dosage forms primarily because drug availability is limited by GI transit time. An example of a slowly absorbed drug is iron. Other problems relative to the design of a sustained release iron dosage form have already been described.

B. Distribution

The distribution of drugs into tissues can be an important factor in the overall drug elimination kinetics since it not only lowers the concentration of circulating drug but it also can be rate limiting in its equilibration with blood and extracellular fluid. One aspect of this distribution is binding of drug to tissues and proteins in blood. An extensive discussion of this phenomenon can be found in a series of papers by Kruger-Thiemer et al. [77–81]. In general, the bound portion of a drug can be considered inactive and unable to cross membranes. At high binding one sees prolonged drug action.

The apparent volume of distribution of a drug is frequently used to describe the magnitude of distribution, including binding, within the body. Conceptually, this pharmacokinetic parameter can be viewed as a proportionality constant relating plasma or serum *concentration* of drug to total *amount* of drug in the body. Since rate processes are driven by concentration and not amount, it is this quantity in which we are interested. Physiological interpretation of the apparent volume of distribution is difficult in the one-compartment kinetic system and even more difficult in cases where multicompartment kinetics are operative. Indeed, in the absence of definitive studies, it should probably be treated as a proportionality constant or "fudge factor" rather than a specific physiological parameter. Unlike drugs that follow one-compartment kinetics, those with multicompartment kinetics usually do not equilibrate with various tissues instantaneously. Consequently, the apparent volume of distribution assumes different values depending on the time course of drug disposition. Thus, one has to be cautious in interpreting the numerical values of apparent volumes of distribution in the literature.

For design of sustained/controlled release products one would like to have as much information on drug disposition as possible but, in reality, decisions are usually based on only a few pharmacokinetic parameters, one of which is the apparent volume of distribution. The apparent volume of distribution influences the concentration and amount of drug either circulating in the blood or in target tissues. It can also influence the elimination kinetics of a drug. Unfortunately, the influence is frequently not a predictable one because of difficulties in interpreting apparent volume of distribution. Nevertheless, the magnitude of apparent volume of distribution can be used as a guide for additional studies and for some a priori comments concerning drug dosing and hence the need for a prolonged release system. These a priori comments are made in conjunction with consideration of other pharmacokinetic parameters, such as amount of drug in the various compartments and elimination constants for removal of drug from these compartments.

The total apparent volume of distribution for a drug at steady state can be calculated from Eqs. (2–4):

$$V_d ss = [(k_{12} + k_{21})/k_{21}]V_p \tag{2}$$

$$V_d extrap = [(\alpha - \beta)/k_{21} - \beta)]V_p \tag{3}$$

$$V_d area = V_d ss + [(k_{el} - \beta)/k_{21}]V_p \tag{4}$$

where $V_d ss$, $V_d extrap.$, and $V_d area$ are apparent volumes of distribution at steady state—$V_d extrap$, is that obtained by the extrapolation method, $V_d area$ is that obtained by the area method, V_p is the volume of the central compartment, α is the fast disposition constant, β is the slow disposition constant, k_{el} is the constant for elimination of drug from the central compartment, k_{12} is the constant for distribution of drug from the central to peripheral compartment, and

k_{21} is that from the peripheral to central compartment. Riegelman et al. [82] demonstrated that the best estimate of total drug volume at steady state is $V_d$ss, while $V_d$extrap. and $V_d$area tend to overestimate this parameter.

While $V_d$ss can be used to correctly estimate amount of drug in the body when amount of drug in the peripheral compartment is at a maximum, it tends to underestimate or overestimate amount of drug in the body at other times during the time course of drug disposition. This observation has been elaborated upon by Gibaldi et al. [83], who proposed the use of $V_d$area instead of $V_d$ss to estimate amount of drug in the body.

To avoid ambiguity inherent in apparent volume of distribution as an estimator of amount of drug in the body, and noting that the same parameter does not differentiate relative distribution of drug in two or more compartments, one can use the T/P ratio as defined in Eq. (5) to describe relative amount of drug in the central and peripheral compartments at steady state. Provided amount of drug in the central compartment (P) is known, the amount of drug in the peripheral compartment (T) and hence total amount of drug in the body can be calculated:

$$T/P = k_{12}/(k_{21} - \beta) \tag{5}$$

where k_{12}, k_{21}, and β are as defined previously. Note that one cannot infer from the T/P ratio the physical state of the drug, such as the extent of binding, in the two compartments. The model merely assumes that distribution between the two compartments is controlled by two first-order constants, k_{12} and k_{21}. Moreover, it implies that the amount of drug transferred to the tissues increases proportionally with dose without limit. In view of this shortcoming of the model, DiSanto and Wagner [84] proposed a nonlinear model to describe disposition kinetics of drugs in tissues.

From the preceding discussion it can be seen that the distribution characteristics of a drug can be described by the volume of distribution at steady state and the T/P ratio. However, one should be aware of the fundamental difference between the two parameters; namely, $V_d$ss estimates the *extent* of distribution in the body, while the T/P ratio estimates the *relative distribution* of drug between compartments. One cannot predict a priori the magnitude of volume of distribution at steady state from the T/P ratio, and vice versa. Indeed, Table 2 shows that the two parameters behave independently of each other. As examples, the T/P ratio for procainamide is about 10 times that for pentobarbital although the $V_d$ss for both drugs is about the same. Similarly, while the T/P ratio for procainamide is larger than that for digoxin, the volume of distribution at steady state of procainamide is less than that of digoxin.

Table 2 Relationship Between Apparent Volume of Distribution at Steady State (V_dss) and T/P Ratio

Drug	T/P	V_dss (liters)	Ref.
Amoxicillin	1.04	22	91
Cefazolin	2.20	9	92
Diazepam	2.85	130	93
Digoxin	4.31	500	94
Furosemide	0.96	5	95
Meperidine	2.04	289	96
Metolazone	2.71	113	97
Pentobarbital	1.30	63	98
Pivampicillin	1.16	13	99
Procainamide	14.35	62	100
Sulfisoxazole	0.60	11	101
Theophylline	0.97	40	102
Tobramycin	1.78	34	103,104
Tolbutamide	0.27	24	105
Trimethoprim	1.24	12	106

Presently, there are insufficient data to allow one to gauge the relative importance of the two parameters in terms of contribution to approximating drug distribution characteristics. Presumably one can use volume of distribution at steady state as a starting point. Noting that the 95% confidence interval on the average value for volume of distribution of drugs at steady state is about 35 ± 1 liters, volumes of distribution exceeding total body water volume (about 50 liters in a 70-kg man) would suggest extensive tissue accumulation and/or binding of drugs. Table 3 lists some examples of such drugs. Provided that drug elimination is rate-limited by the release of drug from tissue binding sites and that drug is released from the tissues to give concentrations exceeding the threshold level or within the therapeutic range, one can probably assume that such drugs are inherently sustained. Naturally, in the absence of information on binding constants and extent of binding, one should be cautious in asserting

Table 3 Examples of Drugs with Apparent Volumes of Distribution Larger Than Total Body Water Volume (52 liters)

Drug	V_d^{ss} (liters)	$t^a_{1/2,\beta}$ (hr)	TBC[b] (ml/min)	Ref.
Chlorphentermine	213	40	62	107
Clindamycin	83	2.8	342	108,109
Diazepam	130	30.8	49	93
Digoxin	500	34	170	94
Lidocain		120	1.8	110
Meperidine		289	3.2	96
Metolazone		113	19.8	66,97
Ouabain	1430	24–74	230–690	111
Pentobarbital		63	22	98
Phenytoin		54	21.3	112,113
Practolol		151		114
Procainamide	62	2.7	265	100
Propranolol		182	3.3	115,116
Quinidine		146	7.2	117,118
Tetracycline	100	9.6	120	119,120

[a]Terminal long-linear half-life.
[b]Total body clearance = $V_d^{ss}\,(0.693/t_{1/2,\beta})$.

the above assumption. As shown in Table 3, the β half-lives ($t_{1/2,\beta}$) of lidocaine and metolazone differ by a factor of 10 although they have similar volumes of distribution at steady state. A similar pattern is observed in the pairs quinidine-diazepam, pentobarbital-procainamide, and chlorphentermine-propranolol. It follows that V_d^{ss} and $t_{1/2,\beta}$ are not related linearly. A possible solution to this dilemma is to use total body clearance at steady state as defined in Eq. (6) to gauge the importance of tissue binding in drug elimination kinetics.

$$\text{Total body clearance at steady state} = V_d^{ss}\,(0.693/t_{1/2,\beta}) \qquad (6)$$

Consider the lidocaine-metolazone example in this light. Lidocaine with a clearance of 820 ml/min probably experiences less tissue binding than metolazone with a clearance of 66 ml/min and hence would be cleared from the body at a faster rate. Furthermore, from the standpoint of need for sustained drug delivery, lidocaine would be a more likely candidate than metolazone.

Presently, while it is recognized that the disposition of many drugs follows multicompartment kinetics, dose calculations for sustained release products are based primarily on one-compartment kinetic considerations. Whether such an approach represents a good approximation to the more complex multicompartment kinetics situation has yet to be proven. Nevertheless, it should be pointed out that implicit in such an approach is the assumption that tissue distribution in the additional compartments has minimal influence on dose considerations. According to this approach, for a given therapeutic concentration of drug, the dose would be similar for drugs with similar volumes of distribution. This assumption hold only when the relative distribution of the two drugs between compartments is similar. The error introduced would be especially pronounced in the extreme case where the active sites of the two drugs reside in different compartments. In order to minimize this error, one may have to incorporate the T/P ratio into sustaining dose considerations for drugs exhibiting multicompartment kinetics.

In summary, no conclusion can be made on the relative importance of volume of distribution at steady state and the T/P ratio in estimating the distribution characteristics of a drug. Undoubtedly, both parameters contribute to this aspect of drug disposition. Perhaps mention should be made of the use of T/P ratio in conjunction with total body clearance at steady state to gain further insight into drug disposition. Table 4 gives an example of how this can be done.

C. Metabolism

Metabolism of a drug can either inactivate an active drug or convert an inactive drug to an active metabolite. Metabolic alteration of a drug can occur in a variety of tissues, some of which are richer in enzymes than others. For example, the organ most responsible for metabolism is the liver and thus the greatest metabolic conversion occurs after a drug has been absorbed into the general circulation. Clearly, for optimal bioavailability, the route of drug administration may be dictated by the drug's metabolic pattern.

Metabolism of a drug will be reflected in the elimination constant of a drug or by the appearance of metabolite. It is possible to incorporate this pharmacokinetic property into the design of a controlled release product, provided that the rate and extent of metabolism are predictable and that the rate constant(s) for the process are not too large. Undoubtedly, complex metabolic patterns would make the design much more difficult, particularly when biological activity is wholely or partly due to a metabolite, as is the case in

Table 4 Use of T/P Ratio and Total Body Clearance at Steady State to Estimate Drug Disposition Characteristics

T/P ratio[a]	Total body clearance[b]	Disposition characteristics[c]
High	High	Little and/or weak tissue binding
High	Low	Extensive and/or strong tissue binding; possible extensive and/or strong plasma protein binding
Low	Low	Strong tissue binding; extensive and/or strong plasma protein binding
Low	High	Little or weak plasma protein binding

[a]Average T/P ratio is 1.
[b]Average total body clearance at steady state is about 80 ml/min.
[c]Assume that elimination of drug occurs primarily in the central compartment.

isosorbide 2,5-dinitrate [85]. There are, however, two areas of concern relative to metabolism that significantly restrict sustained release product design. First, if a drug, upon chronic administration, is capable of either inducing or inhibiting enzyme synthesis, it will be a poor candidate for a sustained release product because of the difficulty of maintaining uniform blood levels of drug. Second, if there is a variable blood level of drug through either intestinal (or other tissue) metabolism or through a first-pass effect, this also will make preparation of a sustained release product difficult. Since most of these processes are saturable, the fraction of drug lost would be dose-dependent and one would anticipate a significant reduction in bioavailability if a drug is slowly released over a period of time.

There are some excellent examples of these metabolic drug problems in the literature. Hydralazine is metabolized by the intestinal wall and/or the liver during absorption, although it is well absorbed [86]. In contrast, bromocriptine is incompletely absorbed, the poor bioavailability of which is further reduced by first pass metabolism in the liver resulting in an absolute bioavailability of only 6% [87]. Likewise, only 23–30% of an orally administered dose of levopoda reaches the systemic circulation as intact drug [88] and the plasma level after an oral dose is about 20% of that after an intravenous dose [89]. Abrams [89] stated that the orally administered dose of the drug was completely absorbed and attributed the reduction in bioavailability to metabolism of the drug during its first pass through the liver. In addition, Sandler et al. [90,91] reported that levodopa was metabolized by gut microbial flora, thus constituting an additional route of loss of drug prior to absorption. The metabolism of levodopa by the gut flora was shown to occur mostly in the portion of the GI tract distal to the duodenum [91]. This would significantly reduce the amount of drug available for absorption from oral sustained release products, since a substantial portion of the dose released past the duodenum would be lost. This may be one of the reasons for the findings of Woods et al. [92] and Curzon et al. [93] that as far as duration of action was concerned, Brocadopa Temtabs (a sustained release levodopa product) provided no advantage over the standard form of levodopa.

Perrier and Gibaldi [94] predicted that due to a first-pass effect, a maximum of about 41% of an oral dose of propoxyphene would reach the systemic circulation, provided the entire dose was released, absorbed, and not metabolized during its transit through the intestinal wall. Their experimental results indicated that only 18% of a 65-mg dose, 28% of a 130-mg dose, and 33% of a 195-mg dose reached the systemic circulation, implying that bioavailability was dose dependent. Provided that this dose-dependent bioavailability could be predicted, a sustained release delivery system could be generated although it makes the sustained dosage form candidacy of propoxyphene less desirable.

Dose-dependent bioavailability behavior has also been demonstrated for salicylamide [57,95,96], which is metabolized during its passage through the intestinal wall. Barr and Riegelman [57,95] showed that as much as 60% of the drug administered in a small dose that appeared in blood was in the glucuronide form. Johansson et al. [97] obtained similar results with alprenolol. They showed that the metabolism of drug during its passage through the intestinal wall was more complete when it was administered in a sustained release form than in conventional tablets. However, these investigators claimed that this increase in drug loss was not enough to render sustained release tablets unsuitable. This would be in accord with our expectation that as long as the extent of metabolism is constant, albeit extensive, a suitable sustained release product can be generated. It does, however, suggest that some manipulation of the dosage form release rate may be needed to accommodate this metabolism. Wagner et al. have derived an equation to calculate variation of systemic availability with input rate [98].

One final example centers on nitroglycerin. The effectiveness of the oral route of administering nitroglycerin as opposed to the sublingual route was the focus of several studies and reviews [99–109] and a conflicting picture emerged. Historically, the argument against the oral route of administration is that nitroglycerin is extensively metabolized during its first pass through the liver [99,100], but recently this has been challenged [109]. Nonetheless, Friend et al. [101] found that nitroglycerin in doses of 2 mg orally four times daily exerted no observable effect in angina pectoris, an effect that was indistinguishable from that of a placebo. Similarly, Bogaert et al. [102] detected no significant fall in blood pressure after oral administration of nitroglycerin despite high plasma levels of the drug. No explanation was offered for this observation. Other studies [103–107], in contrast, indicated that nitroglycerin was absorbed from the GI tract in sufficient quantities to bring about peripheral vasodilation. Since sustained release nitroglycerin products are available on the market, one can assume improved performance against angina attacks for these systems. Indeed, Turner [103] and others [104–106,110, 111] found that sustained release products gave a duration of action longer than oral nonsustained tablets. This observation is not incompatible with the view that nitroglycerin is extensively metabolized during first pass through the liver, as long as metabolism is constant. However, it is incompatible with reports on lack of biological activity via the oral route. The role of prolonged act on nitroglycerin products in angina pectoris therapy will be evaluated subsequently from the standpoint of therapeutic need.

Based on the few examples just cited, controlled release systems for drugs which are extensively metabolized is possible as long as the rate of metabolism is not too great nor metabolism variable with the oral and other routes. It is reasonable to assume that a controlled release product can be made as long as the metabolism remains predictable.

D. Duration of Action

The biological half-life and hence duration of action of a drug obviously play a major role in the process of considering a drug for controlled release. Factors influencing the biological half-life of a drug include its elimination, metabolism, and distribution patterns. Dittert [112] has stated that most drugs have half-lives of elimination in the range of 1–20 hr. Drugs with short half-lives require frequent dosing on order to minimize fluctuations in blood levels accompanying conventional oral dosage regimens [113]. Therefore, controlled release dosage forms would appear very desirable for such drugs. At present, the lower limit of the biological half-life needed for controlled release products has not been defined. Basic pharmacokinetic principles (Chapter 5) suggest that for a given steady-state drug concentration, the zero-order rate of release of a drug from its dosage form is directly proportional to its rate of elimination. Thus, for a drug with a very short half-life, the desired rate of release will be quite large. For a modest duration of time over which the drug is to be released, this large rate of release in turn will lead to a prohibitively large dose, so that the upper limit imposed on the size of the tablet, capsule, or other dosage form may be exceeded. Table 5

Table 5 Ratio of Sustaining Dose to Immediate Release Dose, Φ_m/Φ_i, as a Function of $t_{1/2}$ and Intended Duration of Release[a]

$t_{1/2}$ (hr)	Td = 6 hr	Td = 8 hr	Td = 12 hr
1	4.6	5.54	8.32
2	2.08	2.77	4.16
3	1.39	1.85	2.77
4	1.04	1.39	2.08
5	0.83	1.11	1.66
6	0.69	0.92	1.39
7	0.59	0.79	1.19
8	0.52	0.69	1.04
9	0.46	0.62	0.92
10	0.42	0.55	0.83

[a]Based on a one-compartment open model.

shows the ratio of sustaining dose Φ_m to immediate release dose Φ_i as a function of the biological half-life of drug and intended duration of release T_d. Table 6 lists the maximum size D of the controlled release dosage unit. Table 7 lists some examples of drugs with extremely short half-lives.

To date, the numerical value of biological half-life which makes a drug a good candidate for controlled release has not been established. Heimlich et al. [114] quoted a value of about 4 hr. For a drug with such a half-life, the ratio of sustaining dose to immediate release dose is approximately 2 if the duration of intended release is 12 hr (Table 5). Moreover, for this duration of intended release, it would be possible to formulate a controlled release dose unit of 1 g even if the immediate release dose (minimum effective dose) is 325 mg (Table 6). Considering this criterion alone, propranolol ($t_{1/2}$ = 4 hr) [120,121], propoxyphene ($t_{1/2}$ = 3 hr) [122], and procainamide ($t_{1/2}$ = 3 hr) [123] would be borderline candidates for prolonged release products. As an illustration, Koch-Weser et al. [124,125] suggested that dose of procainamide must be administered every 3 hr to prevent fluctuations of plasma level by more than 50%. Sustained release formulations of procainamide are available and have been shown

Table 6 Maximum Value of the Ratio of Sustaining to Immediate Release Dose, Φ_m/Φ_i, as a Function of Initial Dose D_i and Size of the Sustained Release Unit D[a]

	$(\Phi_m/\Phi_i)max$[b]		
D_i (mg)	D = 1000 mg	D = 500 mg	D = 250 mg
5	199	99	49
10	99	49	24
25	99	19	9
50	19	9	4
75	12.3	5.7	2.3
100	9	4	1.5
125	7	3	1
250	3	1	0
325	2	0.5	–
500	1	–	–
1000	–	–	–

[a]Based on a one-compartment open model.
[b]$(\Phi_m/\Phi_i)_{max} = D/D_i - 1$.

Table 7 Examples of Drugs with Extremely Short Half-Lives

Drug	Half-life (min)	Ref.
Ampicillin	100	115
Cephalexin	54	116
Cloxacillin	90	115
Furosemide	29.5	117
Levodopa	45	89
Penicillin G	45	118
Propylthiouracil	63	119

to be capable of either maintaining therapeutic plasma level or minimizing the fluctuations in plasma level over an 8-hr period [123,126, 127]. In essence, assuming a duration of release of 6, 8, or 12 hr, drugs with half-lives between 4 and 6 hr and whose minimum effective doses are in the range of 125–325 mg will impose little problem insofar as dose size is concerned.

It should be pointed out that the duration of action of many drugs, such as monoamine oxidase inhibitors [128] and corticosteroids [129, 130], is longer than that suggested by their biological half-lives. As a case in point, it is the persistence of antiinflammatory effects of corticosteroids that forms the basis for alternate-day dosing schedule and this is unrelated to the biological half-life as shown in Table 8. This dosage regimen has the additional advantage of minimizing adrenal suppression side effects frequently associated with chronic corticosteroid therapy [131]. Thus, it is probably justified to assume that sustained release corticosteroids are unnecessary from the standpoint of therapy, undesirable from the point of view of side effects [132], and unphysiological from that of the diurnal variations in cortisol secretions [133,134]. In fact, sustained release formulations of prednisolone sodium phosphate and methylprednisolone have been shown to be equally effective as conventional tablets, offering no advantages over the latter [135,136].

Similarly, there is little reason to prepare sustained release formulations for drugs with long biological half-lives. Nelson [137] has indicated that if there are no appreciable differences in effectiveness when a drug is given as a single large dose per day or in several smaller doses throughout the day, the therapeutic need for a prolonged action dosage form would be doubtful. Phenylbutazone is such a drug. Due to extensive protein binding, its rate of metabolism is relatively slow, resulting in a biological half-life of about 72 hr [139]. Para-aminosalicylic acid [140] and the phenothiazines [141] belong to the same category as phenylbutazone. Examples of other drugs with long biological half-lives are shown in Table 9. Surprisingly, sustained release products for drugs with intrinsically long biological half-lives are available. As expected, little or not therapeutic advantages have been demonstrated in these products over

Table 8 Biological Half-Life and Duration of Antiinflammatory Effects of Selected Corticosteroids

Drug	Half-life (hr)	Duration (hr)	Ref.
Methylprednisolone	3.3	24–36	138
Prednisone	1.0	36	131

Table 9 Examples of Drugs with Long Biological Half-Lives

Drug	Half-life	Ref.
Bishydroxycoumarin	27 hr	151
Chlordiazepoxide	15 hr	152
Chlorphentermine	41 hr	153
Chlorpropamide	36 hr	154,155
Diazepam	54 hr	156
	20 hr	157
Ethchlorvynol	24 hr	158
Digitoxin	5–7 days	159
	28 days	160
Digoxin	34 hr	159,161
Guanethidine	9–10 days	162
Meprobamate	11.3 hr	163
Phenytoin	22 hr	164
Warfarin	52 hr	165

conventional tablets or capsules. Notable examples are meprobamate [142], amitripyline [143–145], and phenothiazines [146–150].

E. Side Effects

It is believed that for some drugs, the incidence of side effects is a function of plasma concentrations [166]. Theoretically, the incidence of side effects can be minimized by controlling the concentration at which the drug exists in plasma at any given time, and hence controlled release formulations appear to offer a solution to this problem. Nau et al. [167] and Sikic et al. [168] demonstrated that the toxic effects of valproic acid and bleomycin, respectively, were ameliorated upon administering these drugs as a constant infusion than as a bolus. Eckstein et al. [169] reported that Brocadopa Temtabs, a controlled release form of levodopa, lowered the incidence of drug-induced dyskinesis, and the patients in the study seemed to be able to tolerate a larger daily dose of the drug. On the other hand, a sustained release product of prednisolone produced adrenocortical suppression to a degree indistinguishable from that produced by the same dose given in conventional tablets [135]. Moreover, an attempt to reduce the incidence of drowsiness due to chlorpheniramine maleate by dispensing the drug in a porous matrix was unsuccessful [170]. Thus, the success or failure of these specific products to minimize side effects would appear to be related to the type and success of preparing a controlled release product.

The technique of controlled release has been more widely used to lower the incidence of GI side effects than that of systemic side effects and appears to produce more satisfactory results. Drugs that are prone to cause gastric irritation include aspirin [171], ferrous sulfate [172], potassium chloride [173], nitrofurantoin, and several others. It is postulated that by slowing the rate at which these drugs are released, the likelihood of GI irritation would be reduced due to a smaller amount of drug exposed to the GI mucosa at any given time [174]. Such is the case with sustained release ferrous sulfate products [71,74,76] and an aminophylline sustained release preparation [175]. In contrast, two cases of gastric bleeding following the ingestion of Bayer's Timed-Release Aspirin were reported [176]. The extent of gastric bleeding relative to that due to conventional aspirin tablets was not quantitated, however. Nevertheless, this observation suggests that controlled release preparations are not foolproof against GI side effects.

One of the common complaints of oral potassium therapy is gastric irritation associated with its use [176]. To circumvent this problem, enteric coated tablets are usually prepared, but this has led to another problem, namely, intestinal erosion and stenosis due to a high local concentration of potassium ions released in the intestine [177–181]. Placement of potassium chloride in a controlled release system, such as a wax matrix (Slow-K), programmed to release its contents over 4–6 hr appears to be a satisfactory solution [182–185]. Moreover, it has been shown that such tablets are as bioavailable as their nonsustained counterparts [184]. Utilizing the same principles as Slow-K, a sustained release form of sodium chloride (Slow-Na) has been formulated. The incidence of side effects such as nausea and vomiting is claimed to be less than that in a tablet or capsule [186,187], and the formulation has been used to treat and to prevent acute and chronic deficiency in athletes and in patients on maintenance sodium therapy. In summary, it would appear that drug properties can induce local and systemic side effects which can often be circumvented by placement in a suitable controlled release system. The specific controlled release mechanism employed depends on the drug property inducing side effects.

F. Margin of Safety

Among the indices used to describe the margin of safety of a drug [188–190], the therapeutic index as defined in Eq. (7) is the most widely used:

$$\text{Therapeutic index} = \text{Median toxic dose/median effective dose} = TD_{50}/ED_{50} \quad (7)$$

However, this ratio provides no information on (a) the nature of the distribution of toxicity and effectiveness, (b) the size of doses producing therapeutic and toxic effects, and (c) plasma or serum drug concentrations corresponding to toxic and therapeutic levels. Consequently, it can only be used as a crude estimate of the relative safety of a drug. As might be expected and as illustrated in Table 10, there is wide variation in the therapeutic index for various drugs. In general, the larger the ratio, the safer is the drug; in particular, a drug is considered to be relatively safe if its therapeutic index exceeds 10 [190]. However, since the definition of therapeutic index is relative rather than absolute, the toxic and therapeutic effects have to be clearly defined. Decisions on margin of safety of a drug perhaps can be better made on the basis of its therapeutic index in combination with the range of plasma concentration within which the drug is considered to be therapeutically safe and effective. This approach has been very valuable as a therapeutic guide in monitoring drug therapy, especially for drugs with narrow therapeutic indices and a narrow range of therapeutic concentration, such as the cardiac glycosides and antiarrhythmic (Table 11) [26,113].

In designing controlled or sustained release systems for drugs with narrow therapeutic indices, it is imperative that the drug release pattern be precise so that the plasma concentration achieved is within the therapeutically safe and effective range. However, a precise release pattern by itself is not sufficient to ensure attainment of such

Table 10 Therapeutic Indices of Selected Drugs

Drug	Therapeutic index	Ref.
Aprobarbital	5.3	191
Chlorpheniramine	1400	192
Digitoxin	1.5–2.0	193
Diphenhydramine	2300	192
Penicillin	>100	193
Phenobarbital	2.6	191
Tripelennamine	19,000	192

Table 11 Examples of Drugs with Narrow Ranges of Therapeutic Plasma Concentration at Steady State

Drug	Range of therapeutic concentration
Digoxin	0.02–2 μg/liter
Digitoxin	14–30 μg/liter
Lidocaine	1.5–4 mg/liter
Lithium	0.5–1.3 mEq/liter
Phenytoin	10–20 μg/liter
Procainamide	4–8 mg/liter
Propranolol	20–50 μg/ml
Quinidine	2–5 mg/liter
Theophylline	10–16 μg/ml

Source: Refs. 26,113.

plasma levels. There are other factors, such as patient variability and the very important drug accumulation upon multiple dosing factors (Chapter 6), that can potentially alter plasma drug level. Considering all these factors it is obvious that the design of sustained release system for drugs with narrow therapeutic indices can be difficult. Nevertheless, it is conceivable that an unfavorable therapeutic index can be overcome by suitable manipulation of prolongation mechamisms. Indeed, it is the same narrow therapeutic index that makes it desirable to precisely control drug concentration.

G. Role of Disease State

Strictly speaking, disease state and circadian rhythm are not drug properties. However, in a few instances they are equally important as drug properties in considering a drug for controlled release. Indeed, it is not unusual for a disease state to act as a stimulus for development of a controlled release drug delivery system. A case in point is rheumatoid arthritis, for which aspirin is still the drug of choice [194]. Normally, aspirin would not be considered to be a likely candidate for sustained release because its biological half-life is 6 hr [195]. However, a sustained release product would be advantageous to maintain therapeutic concentrations, particularly throughout the night, thus alleviating morning stiffness [196]. Note that a limitation to formulating a sustained release aspirin preparation is the size of a dose, which necessitates the taking of two sustained release tablets to obtain the desired degree and duration of relief. The results of several studies indicated that sustained release aspirin tablets in the proper dosage provided and maintained blood levels at therapeutic concentration over 8–10 hr, a duration that was about twice as long as that provided by nonsustained release tablets [196–198].

Among the therapeutic armamentarium in peptic ulcer management are belladonna alkaloids and synthetic anticholinergics. Although the usefulness of this class of drugs in this disease state is controversial [199], they are sometimes prescribed as adjuncts to therapy by virtue of their ability to decrease gastric secretion of acid and pepsin induced by vagal stimulation [200]. Since belladonna alkaloids are relatively short-acting [201], a sustained release dosage form may be helpful to exercise continuous control on gastric acid and pepsin secretion. Burness [202] and Resse et al. [201 found that sustained release belladonna preparations employing the Spansule[R] principle appeared to maintain therapeutic plasma concentrations of alkaloids from 8 to 12 hr, but they did not measure gastric acid and pepsin output. Kasich [203] as well as Alp and Grant [204] reported similar findings with hexocyclium. In contrast, Bachrach [43] found that the prolonged acting forms Antrenyl Prolonged[R], Prantal Repetabs[R], Banthine Prolonged[R], and Probanthine Prolonged[R] did not sufficiently extend the duration of action of drug and he attributed this observation to the design of the products concerned.

Angina pectoris is another disease state that probably would be benefited by sustained release medications. In spite of the dispute over the efficacy of nitroglycerin when administered by the oral route, sustained release nitroglycerin preparations are available. Similar to the situation with the orally administered nonsustained products, there are conflicting reports on the value of sustained release nitroglycerin products in controlling the symptoms of angina pectoris. One reason that may account for this confusion is the high incidence of placebo response to prophylaxis of angina pain [205]. The findings of Russek et al. [107] and Pilkington and Purves [104] supported the argument that a sustained release ntiroglycerin preparation was of questionable value in conferring propylaxis to those patients suffering from the typical short attacks of angina pectoris. They based their conclusions on the findings of studies employing sustained release ntiroglycerin preparations containing from 6 to 10 times the dose normally used sublingually. However, Winsor et al. [105], Hirshleifer [106], Turner [103], Wendkos and Meshulam [110], and Preti et al. [111] obtained results contrary to those of Russek and Pilkington. They found that the sustained release nitroglycerin preparations used in their studies not only reduced the incidence and severity of angina attacks but also lowered the nitroglycerin requirements. Kamil and Klinger [206] as well as Feinblatt and Ferguson [207] reported similar findings with pentaerythritol tetranitrate, another drug used in angina pectoris. The conflicting nature of the above reports suggests that additional studies are warranted to establish the role of sustained release preparations as a prophylactic aid in angina pectoris. Perhaps the acute and fleeting nature of angina attacks [205], the large placebo effect [205], and the development of tolerance with chronic administration of long-acting oral nitrate preparations [208] should be major consideration in the design and interpretation of such studies. An interesting statement on the need for prolonged action forms of nitrates in the prophylactic treatment of angina pectoris was made by Wilson [209]. He noted that prophylaxis carries with it the danger of obscuring the warning symptoms of pain, eventually leading to over-exertion with potentially harmful results.

H. Role of Circadian Rhythm

Several biological processes and disease states have been shown to be influenced by circadian rhythm [210]. As examples, acute myocardial insufficiency occurs most commonly around 4:00 a.m. [211] and epileptic seizures have the highest incidence in the morning [212]. Liver enzyme activity [248], blood pressure [213,214], and intraocular pressure [215] also follow a circadian rhythm. As a result, the response to certain drugs also follows a circadian rhythm. These include digitalis glycosides, diuretics, and psychoactive drugs such as the amphetamines, barbiturates, carbamazepine, ethyl alcohol, and chlordiazepoxide [211,212,216–218].

The disease of asthma follows a circadian rhythm, with most of the attacks occuring before bedtime [219]. This observation is postulated to be related to a low cortisol level at that time [211]. It was found that the highest cortisol level occurred between 12 midnight and 4:00 a.m. [211]. Like many other diurnal variations, this variation in cortisol levels makes the design of a controlled release dosage form much more difficult. Foremost among the limitations is GI transit time. Methylprednisolone has been made available in a prolonged action product (Medrol MeduleR). In one study [219], such a product was shown to produce the same duration of relief of rheumatoid arthritis as the same dose administered as a conventional tablet.

Although circadian variations of corticosteroid levels is well known, there is some uncertainty as to whether diurnal variations in glucose and insulin levels exist. Jarrett and Keen [220] reported that in diabetics, the diurnal variation in glucose appeared not to exist, or when it did, it was to a lesser extent. Prior to the reports of Jarrett and Keen [220], Hayner et al. [221], Freinkel et al. [222], and Faiman and Morrhouse [223] obtained results opposite to those of the former investigators, that is, a diurnal variation in blood glucose existed in the diabetic but not in the normal subject, with blood glucose levels significantly higher in the morning than in the afternoon. Freinkel et al. [222] also found that, in normal subjects, insulin level was higher in the morning than in the afternoon. Rigas et al. [224] postulated that insulin synthesis and storage proceeded to a greater extent during the night than during the day, thus accounting for Freinkel's observations on diurnal variation in insulin levels. Theoretically, once diurnal variations in blood glucose and/or insulin are established, controlled release oral hypoglycemic products could be designed to release their contents in accordance with circadian rhythm. However, the fluctuation in blood glucose levels in diabetics is not controlled solely by diurnal variations but also by such variables as diet and exercise [225]. Conceivably, the net result of interaction of these two influences is to diminish the importance of circadian rhythm in dosage form design.

Perhaps the classes of drugs that would benefit the most from incorporation of circadian rhythm into their dosing regimen are the chemotherapeutic agents and peptide hormones. That the timing of chemotherapy is possible in conferring greater specificity is based on the assumption that, unlike malignant tissues, normal tissues are under more stringent circadian control. Hrushesky [226] demonstrated that during the course of treatment of ovarian cancer patients with a combination of adriamycin and cisplatin, administration of adriamycin in the morning and cisplatin in the evening caused fewer complications than a regimen in which the order of dosing of these drugs was reversed. The secretion of neuropeptides and peptide hormones like LHRH, parathyroid hormone, and growth hormone is also under circadian control [227]. Thus, the treatment of conditions by a number of these substances, notably LHRH [228–230], parathyroid hormone [231], and triiodothyronine [232] has been found to benefit more from intermittent, periodic administration than from constant infusion, in part because a constant tissue level of these substances may lead to down regulation of their receptors [233–237]. The net effect of circadian regulation of these substances is to make the design of a controlled release system for such substances more challenging, as exemplified by a prototype delivery device programmed to release melatonin, a pineal gland hormone, in a periodic fashion [238].

VII. SELECTED ROUTES OF DRUG ADMINISTRATION

The route of administration has a significant impact on the therapeutic outcomes of a drug [239,240]. In controlled and sustained drug delivery system design, the parenteral and oral routes have received by far the most attention, although transdermal route is gaining attention recently. At the same time, advances in biotechnology have made possible an increasing number of peptides and proteins which, by virtue of the biophysical and biochemical properties, have made specific demands on the route of delivery as well as on the design of delivery systems. Thus, routes which were of minor importance as ports of drug delivery in the past have assumed added importance in peptide and protein delivery. These include the buccal, rectal, nasal, pulmonary, vaginal, intrauterinal, and ocular routes. The purpose of this section is to present an overview of the physiological constraints inherent in each of the routes mentioned above.

A. Parenteral

Strictly speaking, parenteral products are all systems administered outside of the GI tract. However, parenteral routes are more commonly restricted to injectables such as subcutaneous, intramuscular, intraperitoneal, intrathecal, and intraventricular sites.

1. *Intravenous/Intraarterial*

The intravenous route is attractive because drugs are placed directly into the blood with the associated potential to give an immediate biological response. However, sustaining blood concentrations of drugs given by intravenous injection poses a considerably challenge. Although continuous intravenous infusion can be tailored to maintain a constant and sustained drug level within a therapeutic concentration range during the entire treatment period, such a mode of drug administration necessitates continuous hospitalization during treatment and requires frequent drug level monitoring.

There are several reasons for the lack of commercial sustained release intravenous products. Aside from the irretrievable nature of such injected drugs, there are the issues of biocompatibility and limitations on the size of injected drugs. Thus, wishing to avoid blockage of small capillaries requires that only very small particles be employed as physical systems for intravenous injections. However, the reticuloendothelial system, consisting primarily of liver, spleen, lung, and bone marrow, sequesters "foreign" substances out of the blood stream rapidly, thus making it difficult to sustain drugs via this route.

Numerous attempts to provide either prolongation of drug release or spatial placement of drug, a very desirable attribute for cancer chemotherapy, have been made. Each appears to suffer from one or more deficiencies. Thus, loaded red blood cells, where a drug is placed within a red blood cell, offers a number of attractive features, the most notable being biocompatability and a duration akin to the half-life of a red blood cell, i.e., 30 days. However, such factors as loading capacity of red blood cells for drug, damage to the cell during drug loading resulting in sequestration by the reticuloendothelial system, and lack of control of drug release from the red blood cell have reduced the therapeutic utility of such systems for controlled drug delivery. Liposomes and other particulate systems suffer from similar shortcomings, which will be discussed in Chapter 13.

In general, depot-type parenteral controlled drug release formulations duplicate the benefits of continuous intravenous infusion without its potential discomfort. Various techniques have been used [241–245], including viscous vehicles, suspension, sparingly soluble derivatives and biodegradable microspheres. Biodegradable microspheres are particularly attractive because labile drugs such as peptides and proteins are protected by and released at a controlled, efficacous rate for desired periods of time from this delivery system. These microspheres can also be utilized to direct drugs to certain organs through capillary blockade [243,246]. Its success depends on the size of the microspheres used and on the mode of administration (intravenous or intraarterial). Microspheres with a diameter exceeding 25 μm upon intraarterial administration can be entrapped temporarily in the first capillary bed encountered. In contrast, microspheres greater than 7 μm in diameter when given intravenously will be trapped in the lungs by mechanical filtration, while smaller ones will be cleared by the reticuloendothelial system [247]. The key to a reproducible degree of occlusion for a given dose appears to be due to lack of a tendency of microspheres to aggregate. However, the use of blockage incurs the risk of irreversible cellular damage. The brain can only tolerate a few minutes of anoxia, in comparison to the majority of organs which can tolerate a 20–40-min "shutdown."

2. *Intramuscular/Subcutaneous*

Next to oral administration, injection into subcutaneous or muscular tissues is the most commonly used and acceptable route of drug administration. These routes of administration are most useful either when the disease state or the pharmacokinetic properties of a drug preclude oral dosing, or prolonged drug action is desired. The latter can be achieved in a number of ways [241,248], including reduction of aqueous solubility, gelling of the oily vehicle, use of biodegradable systems, implants, or a combination of these. All of these approaches aim to decrease the release rate of a drug from its dosage form and will be discussed further in Chapter 10. A major factor that needs to be considered during development of biodegradable systems and implants is biocompatibility of the polymers. Release rate from implants may decrease with time when a fibrous envelope is formed around the system as a result of bioincompatibility [249]. In addition, for biodegradable systems as exemplified by poly(ortho esters), it is imperative that breakdown products of the polymer be nontoxic [250].

In general, drugs are assumed to be absorbed at the same rate when given intramuscularly and subcutaneously and the sites are often considered bioequivalent [251,252]. However, subtle differences between these two modalities of drug administration do exist. The vascularity in the subcutaneous tissue is poorer than that of muscle tissue [253] and thus may lead to slower absorption unless there is compensation with an increase in surface area. Moreover, lymphatic vessels of subcutaneous tissue are mainly found in the connective tissue, whereas those of the muscular tissue usually exist where facial planes enter muscles [253].

Unlike intravenous injections, subcutaneous and intramuscular injections require an absorption step before a drug reaches the systemic circulation. However, since absorption from subcutaneous and muscle tissue does not involve passage through an epithelial layer and the tissues are well supplied with capillary and lymphatic vessels, absorption from these routes is usually faster relative to the oral route. Depending on its physicochemical properties, the rate-limiting step in drug absorption from aqueous solution may be either drug diffusion in the connective tissue [254,255] or blood flow through and around the injection site [247,256–260]. Therefore, any factor that influences the above two parameters should influence the absorption rate. For example, vasoconstrictors such as epinephrine reduce the subcutaneous absorption of a number of drugs, whereas hyaluronidase which digests connective tissues markedly increases drug absorption from both muscle and subcutaneous tissues [254]. Probably due to differences in blood flow, absorption is most rapid following injections into the deltoid muscle and least so when injected into the gluteal muscle [247]. In contrast, the absorption rate of drugs administered intramuscularly does not seem to be affected by the water content of connective tissues [254].

Recently, intramuscular and subcutaneous absorption from aqueous solutions [259–265], oil solutions [251,266], and aqueous suspensions [267,268] has been examined. Absorption from aqueous and oil solutions follows first-order kinetics. Absorption rate decreases with increasing volume, probably because of mechanical compression of the adjacent capillary bed and because of a smaller area-to-volume ratio [257]. Moreover, absorption rate was found to be inversely related to molecular size for water soluble compounds and directly proportional to partition coefficient for lipophilic compounds [258]. Low molecular weight compounds are readily absorbed via the capillaries, while high molecular weight compounds appear to be absorbed primarily via lymphatic vessels [255]. Inclusion of adjuvants such as serum albumin was found to increase subcutaneous absorption of high molecular weight compounds, but the mechanism is unknown [269].

For oil solutions, absorption rate depends on partitioning between the oil and the aqueous medium in the connective tissue, with little dependence on viscosity. Clearance of oily vehicles following intramuscular and subcutaneous injections has been studied in albino rabbits [270]. It was found to be independent of the injection site. However, clearance was mainly via capillary vessels whereas clearance via lymphatic uptake or phagocytosis by cells was found to be insignificant. In the case of suspensions, the absorption rate increases with decreasing particle size, probably due to an increase in lateral spread of the particles in the connective tissue [267,268]. Phagocytosis appears unimportant except for exceedingly fine drug particles.

B. Oral

The oral route is by far the most popular route of drug administration. Nevertheless, current knowledge on mechanisms of drug absorption, GI transit and the microenvironment of the GI tract is still incomplete. In addition, oral administration is also beset with inherent physiological constraints such as chemical degradation in the stomach, gastric empyting, intestinal motility, mucosal surface area, specific absorption sites, and metabolic degradation during passage through the mucosa and subsequently the liver. Adding to these constraints is the commonly substantial intra- and intersubject variability associated with some of these factors. Generally, these factors cannot be controlled and hence severely limit the design of oral drug delivery systems.

The duration of a drug after oral administration is mainly a function of drug-releated properties such as rate of absorption and clearance as well as residence time of the delivery system at the absorption site. Most sustained release drug delivery systems developed thus far are aimed at slowing the apparent absorption rate by reducing drug release rate from the dosage form. However, these systems will have only limited utility in oral controlled administration of drugs unless they can remain in the vicinity of the absorption site for the life time of drug delivery.

The residence time of most sustained/controlled release dosage forms is primarily determined by gastric emptying and intestinal motility. Gastric emptying is influenced by factors such as autonomic and hormonal activity, and volume, composition, viscosity, osmolality, pH, caloric value, temperature of stomach contents as well as by many drugs [271]. The human/canine stomach behaves differently in the fed and fasted states [272]. During the fed state, fluids and solid particles smaller than 2 mm are discharged together whereas solid particles larger than 2 mm, including pellets and tablets are retained until arrival of the next phase III of the migrating motor complex (MMC) [273]. In the fasted state, gastric emptying patterns of fluids depend on the volume administered. A lag phase is commonly observed for volumes of fluid less than 100 ml. The onset of discharge depends on the phase activity of the stomach, and fluid is discharged before the suspended particles. In contrast, large volumes of fluids (>200 ml) are discharged immediately, as in the fed state, and the square root of volume vs. times or an exponential relationship is usually observed.

Motility of the small intestine during digestion consists mainly of segmental contractions, whose purpose is to mix its contents. Distal propulsion also occurs, but its mechanism is unknown [272]. Distal propulsion in fasted state occurs mainly in phase III of the MMC.

Liquids are spread out over the entire small intestine quite quickly following ingestion. It has been found that the transit of liquids and solids are similar in the small intestine, so that differences in their GI transit time are primarily due to differences in gastric emptying time. Studies in humans have shown a surprising consistency of small intestinal motility in that, irrespective of dosage form, it takes approximately three hours for substances to traverse the small intestine. The methodology of studying GI transit has been summarized by Hoffman et al. [272].

It is generally assumed that the desirable site of absorption is the proximal and mid small intestine, the transit time of most delivery systems in which is only 2–3 hr long [272]. Consequently, a sustained release formulation of about 12-hr duration or longer can only be achieved by slowing gastric emptying. Several approaches have been proposed for prolongation of GI transit time. These include flotation tablets and capsules (U.S. patent #4,140,755), unfolding of stratified medicated sheet (BE patent #867,692), bioadhesive polymers [274,275], certain fatty acids [276], and certain drugs such as propantheline. However, the use of drugs is generally considered undesirable because of potential side effects.

An important issue relative to oral controlled release products is the animal species that is used during the design phase of these systems. Although our understanding of the anatomical and physiological aspects of all animals is rudimentary, there are certain species which seem to be preferred. The beagle dog is a frequently utilized animal for this purpose, in spite of marked differences in its transit time and GI pH relative to human subjects. Transit time of dosage forms in the dog is only two-thirds of that in humans, analogous to that in a young child, aged 1–3. This can be an important consideration for those systems that require drug absorption for an extended time. Thus, for such systems, dogs will show incomplete absorption. The second issue is GI pH. Some workers have found (a) a higher pH in the stomach as compared to humans and (b) an acid pH extending over a larger segment of the small intestine of the beagle dog. As an alternative animal species to obviate this pH problem some pharmaceutical firms routinely employ the cynomolgus monkey as well as rodents. Here, a word of caution regarding the use of rodents as test animals is in order. The rat has a portion of its stomach in keratinized form with unknown stomach emptying of oral controlled release dosage forms. Moreover, both the rat and the rabbit eat their own feces, thereby rendering the composition of stomach contents and the associated influence of this composition on drug release and stomach emptying somewhat uncertain.

In summary, because of limited residence time and possible existence of an absorption window for some drug, control of GI transit time and site-specific release through specific binding of the drug delivery system to the absorption site are attractive approaches to controlled oral administration. With some exceptions, targeting of drugs is not the primary concern for most orally administered drugs. Rather, the aim is to increase the amount of drug delivered to, with concommitant prolongation in, the general circulation. For this reason, most systems employed are of the sustained release type. In cases where systems are used to target a drug, the site of absorption rather than the site of action is targetted. The assumption is that by increasing drug concentration at the absorption site, the amount of drug reaching the site of action will increase correspondingly. This is exemplified by colon drug delivery [277–279].

C. Buccal/Sublingual

Drugs can be absorbed from the oral cavity through the oral mucosa either sublingually (under the tongue) or buccally (between the cheek and gingiva). In general, rapid absorption from these routes is observed because of the thin mucous membrane and rich blood supply. For highly hydrophilic drugs ($\log P < 2$), which also suffer from extensive presystemic elimination and require a rapid onset of action, sublingual or buccal administration may offer advantages over oral administration. After absorption, drug is transported through the deep lingual vein or facial vein which then drains into the general circulation via the jugular vein. Thus, the buccal and sublingual routes can be used to bypass hepatic "first-pass" elimination. Lymphatic uptake of drug also occurs, but is less common [280].

Drug absorption into the oral mucosa is mainly via passive diffusion into the lipoidal membrane [281–283]. Compounds with favorable oil-to-water partition coefficients are readily absorbed through the oral mucosa. Since the mean pH of saliva is 6.0, adequate absorption through the oral mucosa occurs if the pK_a is greater than 2 for an acid or less than 10 for a base. An oil-water partition coefficient range of 40–2000 is considered optimal for drugs to be absorbed sublingually [284,285]. Compounds administered by either the buccal or sublingual routes include steroids, barbiturates, papain, trypsin, and streptokinase-streptodornase [282]. Besides transcellular diffusion, there is evidence that water-soluble molecules with a molecular volume of less than 80 cm^3/mole cross primarily through membrane pores and large water-soluble molecules pass paracellularly [285]. Regardless of polarity, large molecules are poorly absorbed [286, 287].

Conventional buccal and sublingual dosage forms are typically short acting because of limited contact time between the dosage form and the oral mucosa. Since sublingual administration of drugs interferes with eating, drinking, and talking, this route is generally considered unsuitable for prolonged administration. On the other hand, the duration of buccal drug administration can be prolonged with saliva-activated adhesive troches without the problems of sublingual administration [288]. Unfortunately, the buccal nitroglycerin adhesive troche has yet to be met with commercial success [289].

D. Rectal

The rectal route is commonly used as an alternative when oral administration is inconvenient because of inability to swallow or because of gastrointestinal side effects such as nausea, vomiting and irritation. More important, rectal drug administration has the advantage of minimizing or avoiding hepatic first pass metabolism [290,291]. For instance, the rectal bioavailability of lidocaine in man is 65%, as compared to an oral bioavailability of 30% [291].

The human rectum is about 15–20 cm long. In the resting state the rectum does not have any active motility. Normally the rectum is empty and contains only 2–3 ml of inert mucous fluid (pH 7–8) which has no enzymatic activity or buffering capacity. There are no villi or micrivilli on the rectal mucosa and thus, a very limited surface area (200–400 cm^2) is available for absorption. The internal volume of the rectum depends on the pressure exerted on the rectum by the surrounding organs. This pressure, together with motility, affects spreading of a dosage form.

Both blood and lymphatic vessels are abundant in the submucosal region of the rectal wall. The upper veins drain into the portal circulation, while the lower and middle veins drain directly into the inferior vena cava. However, there are extensive anastomoses among these veins, so that a clear-cut anatomical differentiation cannot be made. Nevertheless, systemic bioavailability seems to depend on the site of absorption in the rectum [292], rectal motility [293], as well as animal species [291].

In general, absorption occurs at a slower rate and to a lesser extent than after oral drug administration with a particular dose [294]. Drug absorption from the rectum is assumed to occur by mechanisms similar to those operating in other parts of the GI tract, i.e., passive diffusion [295,296]. For poorly water-soluble drugs, the rectal absorption rate is determined by the release surface area rather than by drug concentration in the dosage form. Absorption from aqueous and alcoholic solutions is in general much faster than that from suppository, which is often very much dependent on the particle size of the active ingredient as well as on the nature of the suppository base, surfactants and other addditives [294–298].

Recently, some non-surfactant adjuvants, such as the salicylates, have been found to enhance rectal absorption of water-soluble drugs [298–301] and high molecular weight drugs like insulin, heparin, and gastrin [302–304]. Some peptides, such as *N*-acyl derivatives of collagen peptide [305], have also been found to exert a self-enhancing effect [306]. Apparently, a high local concentration and/or simultaneous absorption of the adjuvants are required to alter membrane permeability, thereby assuring rapid drug absorption in the rectum [300,304]. Membrane permeability enhancement by non-steroidal anti-inflammatory drugs is reversible [307] whereas that by surfactant adjuvants and chelating agents is not [308].

Design of rectal controlled release drug delivery systems is likely to be limited by some inherent problems of the rectal area, including interruption of absorption by defecation and, in certain parts of the world, lack of patient acceptance of this route. Only a limited number of compounds given rectally have been shown as effective as when given orally [309]. Thus, this route may serve as an alternative pathway to oral administration for compounds that undergo extensive first-pass metabolism or for high molecular weight/enzymatically sensitive compounds such as insulin and heparin.

E. Nasal

For many years, the nasal route was used primarily for local action on the nasal mucosa. Despite its use in systemic delivery of desmopressin and vasopressin, its use as an alternate route for poorly absorbed oral drugs seems to have been ignored until recently. A variety of drugs including propranolol [310], testosterone [311], naloxone [312], buprenorphrine [312], ergotamine tartrate [313], clofilium tosylate [314], cromolyn sodium [315], meclizine [316], as well as endogenous hormones such as luteinizing-hormone-releasing hormone [317], tetracosactrin [318], oxytocin [319], ACTH [320], insulin [321–324], and enkephalins [325], have been shown to be absorbed nasally in animals and humans. By virtue of relatively rapid drug absorption, possible bypassing of presystemic clearance, and relative ease of administration, delivery of drugs by the nasal route offers an attractive alternative for administering systemically active drugs.

The anatomy of the nasal cavity is described in detail elsewhere [326,327]. The thickness and vascularity of the mucous membrane lining the nasal cavity depends on location. The mucous membrane is thickest and most vascular in the upper regions and over the septum, whereas it is very thin on the floor of the nasal cavity and in the sinuses. The surface area of the nasal cavity is increased by the sinuses, where most drug absorption occurs [328]. The absorptive surface area is further increased by the microvilli in the mucous membrane. The vascular bed of the nasal mucosa provides rapid absorption with little metabolizing capacity. The pH of nasal mucosal surface is reported to be around 7.4 [328].

Dosage forms must deposit and remain in the nasal cavity sufficiently long for effective absorption to occur. Aerosol and particulate dosage forms should contain particles greater than 4 μm to minimize their passage into the lung [329], where mucociliary clearance will remove most particulate materials. However, before nasal delivery can be a viable alternative route for systemic drug absorption, it will be necessary to have a better understanding of how to control particle deposition within the nasal cavity reproducibly, how drug and particle interact with mucus, and how certain disease states of the nasal mucosa may affect the rate and extent of drug absorption.

F. Pulmonary

Delivery of medication to the respiratory tract for localized therapy of respiratory diseases is commonly accomplished via the airways because of their enormous surface area and accessibility [330]. The respiratory tract consists of a nasopharyngeal region, a tracheobronchial region, and lungs (bronchioles and alveoli). The diameter of the dichotomous branchings of the bronchial tree decreases in the distal parts of the respiratory tract, with a simultaneous increase in total cross-sectional area and the total surface area [331]. Thus, the flow in the central airway is rapid and turbulent, whereas flow in the peripheral airways is smooth and laminar [332]. The total surface area of alveoli in an adult is about 35 m^2 during expiration and about 100 m^2 during deep inspiration [333]. Thus, most solute exchange takes place at the alveolar level.

For purposes of discussion of the deposition and clearance of inhaled aerosols, the airways can be divided into three functional regions [334] (Fig. 2):

1. Nasopharyngeal region—cavity to entrance of trachea
2. Tracheobronchial region—trachea to terminal bronchioles
3. Pulmonary region—bronchioles to alveoli, no ciliated cells

In general, prediction of the site of deposition of an aerosolized drug is difficult because airway sizes and anatomy differ from person to person and appear to be influenced by pathological changes.

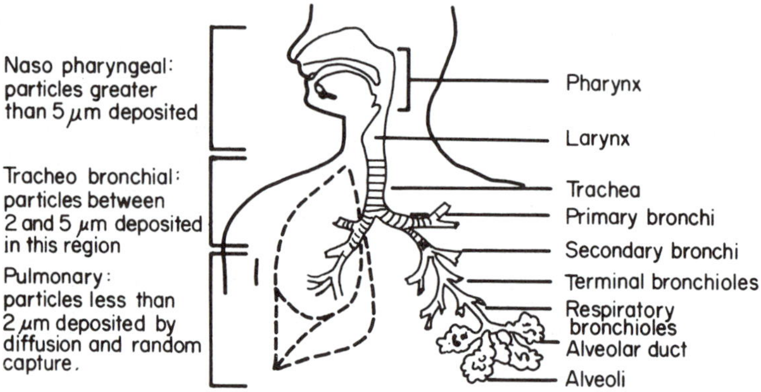

Fig. 2 Disposition of particles in various regions of the respiratory tree.

Moreover, alterations in regional ventilation that result from lung disease can influence the site at which a drug is deposited [335–337]. Deposition of aerosolized particles is mediated by a variety of mechanisms, depending on particle size, shape, density, charge and hygroscopicity [338,339]. The geometry of the airways and physiological factors such as breathing patterns, air flow dynamics in the respiratory tract, and variations of the relative humidity and temperature inside the airways also influence deposition. The influence of particle size on aerosol deposition is depicted in Figure 3 [340].

Therapeutic aerosols are typically polydispersed with sizes ranging from 1 to 10 μm (341). These particles are small enough to be carried down the respiratory tract with inspired air [342]. Large particles (>5 μm) are usually deposited via inertial impaction on the upper airways, where air velocity is high [341]. Pathological changes usually increase the inertial impact by narrowing the airways [339,341]. Moderate size particles (1–5 μm) can sediment out of the air stream under the force of gravity. Deposition by sedimentation occurs predominantly in the lower levels of the airways, where air velocity is low [341]. Thus, peripheral deposition of aerosols is maximized by inhaling slowly, followed by a period of breath holding [339]. For submicron particles, diffusion becomes important. All particles smaller than about 10 μm in diameter are deposited to some extent in the pulmonary region of the lung upon inhalation, while deposition of particles smaller than 0.01 μm is usually negligible because of diffusional deposition in the nasopharyneal and tracheobronchial regions. Thus, the efficiency of deposition of intermediate size particles [0.02–1.0 μm] is less compared to larger and smaller sizes.

Particulate material deposited in the respiratory tract may eventually be cleared by mucociliary action and/or the lymphatic system and/or may be transferred to the blood [340,343] (Fig. 4). The physiocochemical characteristics of aerosols, site of deposition, and respiratory physiology are important determinants of clearance. Soluble deposited particles, on the other hand, are cleared via absorption into the blood stream. Clearance of insoluble particles deposited on the ciliated regions of the respiratory tract is mainly via mucociliary transport [335,342,343], whereas those deposited on the non-ciliated surfaces of the pulmonary region may be phagocytized by macrophages [344,345] or may leak into the interstitium [346], which may then be translocated to a lymph node [347]. The mechanisms of deposition and clearance are summarized in Table 12.

Once the aerosolized drug particles deposit on the alveolar surface, they must cross the alveolar-capillary barrier before reaching the systemic circulation. Both alveolar epithelium and pulmonary capillary endothelium are continuous, but the former has more tight junctions than the latter [348–350]. Physiological measurements give an equivalent pore radius of 8–10 Å for alveolar epithelium and 20–200 Å for capillary endothelium [351,352]. Thus, the alveolar epithelium has a much lower permeability to liquids and solutes than the pulmonary endothelium. Of special interest is the large number of pinocytotic, lamellar vesicles, many of which discharge their content

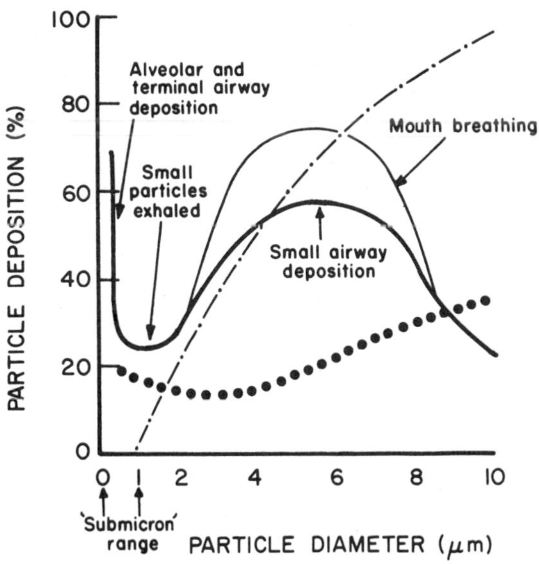

Fig. 3 Effect of particle size on deposition of particles in various regions of the respiratory tree. The curves indicate the proportion of total material of any particle size likely to deposit upon an internal surface: _._._, nasal compartment; ...., tracheobronchial compartment; _____, pulmonary compartment. (From Ref. 340.)

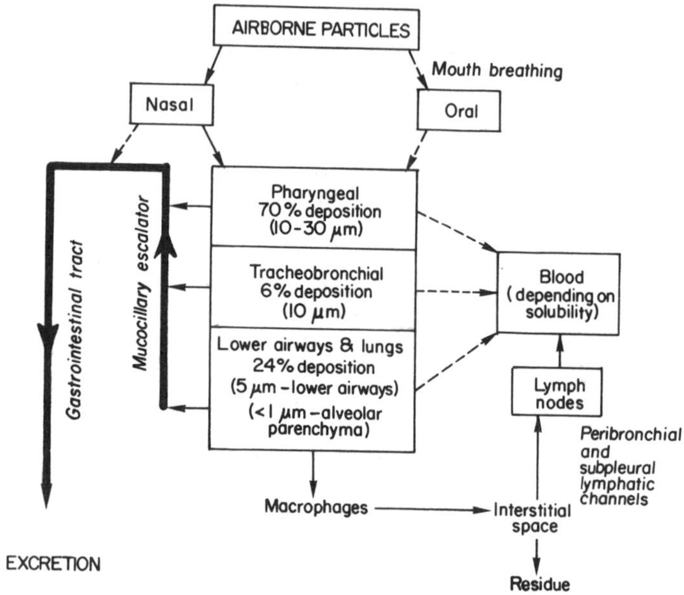

Fig. 4 The ultimate distribution of particulate material inhaled and deposited in airways and lungs, as affected by lung clearance mechanisms. The figures in individual compartments represent the proportions that are typically likely to be deposited of an inhalable dust of uniform particle size distribution. Solid arrows indicate major routes, and dotted arrows indicate minor routes of particle distribution. (From Ref. 340.)

Table 12 Deposition and Clearance of Inhaled Aerosols

Region	Deposition	Clearance
Nasopharyngeal	Impaction	Mucociliary
	Diffusion	Sneezing
	Interception	Blowing
	Attraction	Dissolution
Tracheobronchial	Impaction	Mucociliary
	Diffusion	Coughing
	Settling	Dissolution
	Interception	
	Attraction	
Pulmonary	Diffusion	Dissolution
	Settling	Phagocytes
	Attraction	Lymph flow
	Interception	

into the capillary lumen [353,354]. These vesicles contain enzymes for metabolism of adenine nucleotide and angiotensin I [354]. The basal lamina subtending the cellular layers offer a substantial barrier to the penetration of large molecules [355].

In general, drug absorption from the lung is considerably faster than from the intestine [356]. However, the nature of drug transport from the pulmonary epithelium to blood is poorly understood. Results to date reveal that, the absorption rate of small lipophilic molecules is related to the oil/water partition coefficient [357], whereas the absorption rate of some organic cations and anions as well as neutral, hydrophilic saccharide molecules appears to be related to molecular size, suggesting diffusion through aqueous membrane pores [357]. While large hydrophilic molecules such as aminoglycoside antibiotics are poorly absorbed [357], others such as phenol red [358] and cromolyn sodium [359] appear to be better absorbed when compared to oral absorption. However, this is primarily the result of a saturable carrier-type transport process in the pulmonary epithelium [358,359].

For drugs used for local treatment of pulmonary disorders, it is desirable that the drug exert a local effect with minimal systemic absorption [360,361]. Successful use of inhaled corticosteroids in the treatment of asthma with minimal systemic side effects was due to metabolism of the drug prior to entry into the circulation [362]. It appears that presystemic metabolism of drugs delivered by the intrabronchial route may differ quantitatively from their metabolism following systemic administration [363,364]. Besides metabolism, the lung can also bind and accumulate drugs, especially basic drugs. This binding is mostly reversible [365] and can prolong duration of the drug in the body.

In summary, the efficiency of delivery of drugs via the airways is relatively poor in man. As much as 90% of the instilled dose may impact in the mouth and pharynx or be swallowed without ever reaching the lung. Thus, success of pulmonary delivery will depend on a number of factors. First, drugs used in aerosols must be quite poent but with negligible systemic side-effects. Second, the drug must be able to gain access to its target site. Third, drug must bind to tissue components thereby providing a high local concentration for prolonged periods. Finally, better aerosol delivery from nebulizers is needed to enhance the amount of drug reaching the lung. Nevertheless, controlled delivery of drugs to the respiratory area is useful mainly for localized treatment of inflammation or cancer. It is unlikely that this route will supplant the oral or intravenous routes to achieve systemic effects.

G. Vaginal

Intravaginal controlled release drug administration of steroidal compounds or spermicidal agents is aimed at obtaining contraception for prolonged periods with minimal systemic side effects. In general, most steroids are readily absorbed so that their bioavailability after intravaginal administration is higher than from oral administration because of a reduced first-pass metabolism [366,367]. Recently, the vaginal route has also been investigated for peptide and protein drug delivery [368,369].

The human vagina is a fibromuscular tube 4 to 6 in. long, directed upward and backward, extending from the vulva to the lower part of the uterine cervix. It is in the form of a collapsed tube under normal conditions. The vagina is drained by a rich plexus, which empties into internal iliac veins [370]. Blood supply to the vagina is via uterine and pedendal arteries, which arise from the iliac artery.

The vagina consists of three principal layers: an outer fibrous layer, a middle muscular layer, and the epithelial layer. The epithelial layer consists of lamina propria and a surface epithelium [370], which is composed of noncornified, stratifeid squamous cells. The vaginal epithelium is essentially devoid of glands, but its surface is kept moist by a cervical secretion, whose composition and volume varies with age, stage of menstrual cycle, and degree of sexual excitement [371]. After puberty, the pH of vaginal fluid varies between 4 and 5 depending on the stage of the cycle and location [372]. Cells of the superficial mucosal layer contain a high level of glycogen, which is metabolized to lactic acid ($pK_a = 3.79$) in the vaginal canal to maintain the vaginal pH on the acidic side. The pH is lowest around the anterior fornix and highest around the cervix.

Higuchi et al. have developed an in situ method to study vaginal abosrption in the rabbit [373] and monkey [374]. The absorption rates of a series of unbranched aliphatic alcohols from methanol to octanol in the rabbit vagina were found to be first-order and increased with increasing chain length [375]. The barrier of absorption appears to consist of an aqueous diffusion layer in contact with the membrane, which in turn is composed of parallel lipoidal and aqueous pore pathways [376]. For drugs with high membrane permeability, vaginal absorption is determined by permeability of the aqueous diffusion layer; whereas for drugs with low membrane permeability, such as testosterone and hydrocortisone, vaginal absorption is determined by membrane permeability. Similar results were obtained with alcohols in the monkey [374] and 1-alkanoic acids in the rabbit [376]. No correlation between vaginal membrane permeability and menstrual cycle was found in the monkey [377]. However, at ovulation, the monkey's vaginal permeability is several-fold lower than that of the noncyclic rabbit [378].

Two major types of intravaginal controlled release systems are available: vaginal rings [379–386] and microcapsules [387–390]. The rationale for vaginal ring steroid-releasing systems is based on the observation that steroids readily penetrate the vaginal mucosa [391] and that the vagina can accomodate foreign bodies of reasonable size with minimal discofort for an extended period of time. There are two common types of vaginal rings: homogeneous [380] and shell [385]. Burst effect of drug release on insertion and a declining release rate after extended wear are commonly observed with homogenous rings. Shell rings apparently minimize the burst effect and are able to maintain a steady drug release rate. For most vaginal rings, the rate of vaginal drug absorption shortly after insertion is controlled by either an aqueous hydrodynamic diffusion layer or by the vaginal wall. At later times, the rate of vaginal absorption is determined by the drug release rate from the ring [392].

Reported problems associated with the use of vaginal rings are: erosion of the vaginal wall, ring expulsion, interference with coitus, unpleasant ring odor, and difficulty with storage and sanitation [393]. These problems are usually the major causes for discontinued use of vaginal rings and, because of these problems, vaginal rings have received only moderate acceptance.

A potential intravaginal contraceptive system free of most of the aforementioned problems is the biodegradable microsphere. The rationale for its development is that inert particles have been demonstrated to be able to migrate from the vagina across the cervix into the fallopian tube or the perimetrial lining of the uterus without causing erosion of the vaginal wall by virtue of its small size [294,295].

Microspheres for intracervical administration have also received attention. Small doses of progesterone can be released locally to alter the structure of the cervical mucus so as to interfere with sperm migration [396]. In addition, a medicated intracervical system has been tested [397]. The rationale for its development is that contractility is less severe in the lower segment of the uterus, especially the cervix. This system still incurs the problems of expulsion and possibility of infection and does not offer enough advantages over existing intravaginal or intrauterinal systems to be worth pursuing.

H. Intrauterine

The effectiveness of nonmedicated intrauterine devices (IUDs) is primarily dependent on the relationship of the device morphology (size, shape, and area) to uterine geometry [398]. The human uterus is a pear-shaped, muscular structure, about 3 in. in length and about 2 in. wide, consisting of a body, fundus, isthmus, and cervix. Its wall has three layers: an external peritoneal layer (perimetrium), a middle muscular layer (myometrium), and an inner mucous membrane (endometrium). This organ undergoes dynamic changes in the size and shape of its various segments during different phases of the menstrual cycle [399]. Lack of structural adaptability and unfavorable geometry of the device may lead to clinical complications such as expulsion, bleeding, infection, perforation, and pain. It appears that the mode of action of nonmedicated systems originates promptly in the uterus, disappears rapidly, is not affected by menstruation and does not interfere with the normal estrogen-progesterone balance [400].

The objectives in the development of medicated IUDs are to enhance their contraceptive effectiveness with concomitant reduction in pain and bleeding. These objectives are achieved by using small devices and the incorporation of antifertility agents such as steroids and/or antifibrinolytic agents-proteinase inhibitors such as aminocaproic acid, tranexamic acid and aprotonin, and/or antiprostaglandins.

Since the contraceptive action of the medicated device lies mainly with the antifertility agent itself but not with the structural features of the device, the geometry and size should be designed for minimal clinical complications. The T or 7 configurations came closest to the ideals set forth above [401]. The major contraceptive agents employed in medicated IUD's include copper, progresterone and levonorgestrel. The most extensively studied IUD's have been Progestasert^{R} and Cu-7^{R}.

The concept of continuous intrauterine administration of progesterone is based on these observations: (a) local effect of progesterone on the uterus might reduce the incidence of expulsion and bleeding provoked by the inert device, (b) the estrogenic component of oral contraceptives is not essential for contraception, and (c) progestin-only mini-pills provide adequate contraception, possibly by preventing blastocyte implantation without inhibiting ovulation. The Progestasert^{R} system is a T-shaped progesterone-containing drug delivery system enclosed by a rate-limiting membrane. It releases 65 μg/day for a period of 1 year.

Cu-7^{R} is a polypropylene 7-shaped device with 89 mg of copper wire surrounding the vertical arm, giving a surface area of 200 mm^2 of copper, which is released at 9.87 μg/day for up to 40 months. The exact mechanism by which copper works as a contraceptive agent is unclear. Copper is known to be cytotoxic if present in sufficiently high concentrations [402]. It interferes with implantation of the fetus in rats [403], enhances the spermatocidal and spermatodepressive action of the IUD [404], and inhibits the binding of estrogen and progesterone to their receptors [404].

Levonorgestrel-releasing IUDs have also been studied clinically. Since levonorgestrel is effective at concentrations lower than those required with progesterone, the system can have a life time of about 7 years. Furthermore, it is believed that levonorgestrel offers a balance of estrogenic and progestational activity, which may lessen intermenstrual bleeding [405].

Future research in intrauterine controlled drug administration will depend on increased understanding of reproductive physiology so that contraception can be achieved by interference with pertinent reproductive processes at the right time with minimal side effects. Future research will most likely focus on minimizing intermenstrual bleeding and pain, searching for longer duration systems as well as self-regulating drug delivery systems. An example of a self-regulating system may be one that utilizes human chorionic antibodies as a sensor, so that drug delivery will occur only when an egg has undergone fertilization, but not at other times [406].

I. Transdermal

The skin is one of the most extensive and readily accessible organs of the human body. It covers an area of about 2 m^2 and at any point in time is in contact with about one-third of all blood circulating through the body [407]. Skin consists of three tissue layers: epidermis, dermis, and hypodermis (subcutaneous tissue). The rate-limiting step in percutaneous absorption of most drugs appears to be passage through the stratum corneum [408–414]. The pathway of drug movement through this layer is believed to be mainly transcellular, although the paracellular pathway may become important for small molecular weight compounds [408]. In addition to being a diffusion barrier, the stratum corneum also serves as a reservoir for compounds such as corticosteroids, griseofulvin and many other drugs. While drugs are carried away by the capillary network upon reaching the subcutaneous tissue, there is evidence that certain drugs such as thyroxin, β-methoxypsoralen, estradiol and corticosteroids, remain in this layer for an extended period of time [415–417]. Such localization of drugs may prove desirable for exerting local effects in deeper tissues of the skin or for prolonged release of drugs.

In the past, topically applied dermatological drugs were used for localized treatment of skin diseases only. Recently, due to a better understanding of the anatomy and physiology of the skin as well as a more thorough understanding of percutaneous absorption, the limited permeability of human skin has also been utilized for systemic drug administration.

There are several advantages to the transdermal route provided the drug is absorbed in sufficient quantity to exert a systemic effect. Thus, it is possible to:

1. Avoid hepatic "first-pass" metabolism and gastrointestinal incompatibility of drugs
2. Provide controlled administration for drugs with narrow therapeutic indices, thereby reducing side effects or inadequate dosing
3. Allow utilization of drugs with short biological half-lives
4. Enhance therapeutic efficacy

5. Reduce frequency of dosing
6. Improve patient compliance
7. Permit relatively abrupt termination of drug effect by removal of the patch from the skin surface

These advantages aside, systemic drug absorption from ointments or creams is commonly unpredictable, partly because of variability in skin permeation and partly because of the difficulty in delivering a dose reliably. The use of rate-controlled tranddermal drug delivery systems appears to minimize these two problems. However, because of the relatively low permeability of skin by most drugs, these systems are only applicable for highly potent drugs which permeate the skin rapidly, which cause no irritation to the skin, and which are relatively stable to enzymes present in the epidermis. The additional requirement is that the drug delivery system rather than the skin acts as the rate-limiting step in the overall transport process [418]. Drugs such as scopolamine [419], nitroglycerin [420,421], and clonidine [422] have been administered in this fashion.

The low skin permeability of most drugs necessitates the use of penetration enhancers such as dimethyl sulfoxide [423], urea [424], and, more recently, Azone^{R} [425,526]. One of the major difficulties associated with penetration enhancers is lack of specificity. This, coupled with a lack of understanding of their mechanism of action, limits the rational design and use of penetration enhancers.

Occlusion has been shown to enhance drug absorption across the skin. It appears to do so partly by increasing hydration of the stratum corneum and partly by raising the temperature of the skin surface. However, the contribution of changes in blood flow due to this treatment is still unclear [412].

Ion-pair formation between a carrier molecule and an anionic drug has been proposed to enhance penetration [427]. This approach takes advantage of the pH gradient that exists across the stratum corneum and the hydrophilic nature of the viable epidermis. Another approach to improve penetration of poorly absorbed molecules is the use of prodrugs [428–430]. In this case, the metabolic activity of the skin is used to transform prodrugs to active drugs. With a better understanding of metabolizing enzymes in the skin, the use of prodrugs can be an attractive approach. Theoretical considerations suggest that this is a useful approach in enhancing drug permeation [431,432].

One factor that has not been extensively studied is the influence of pathological states in skin permeability. Bronaugh and Stewart [316], Scott et al. [433], as well as Flynn et al. [434], have conducted studies on drug absorption through abnormal and damaged skin. A better understanding of percutaneous absorption through diseased skin is needed for effective treatment of cutaneous diseases.

J. Ocular

For treatment of many disease affecting the external eye and anterior segment of the eye, topical instillation is preferred over systemic administration because a high drug concentration at the absorbing membrane can be obtained, thereby maximizing drug delivery to the affected tissues while minimizing systemic side effects. However, topical application of drugs to the eye is impeded significantly by efficient ocular physiological protective mechanisms, such as drainage, tear turnover, limited permeability of corneal membranes to most drugs, and aqueous humor turnover. Typically, drug from an instilled aqueous solution is essentially eliminated from the precorneal area within 1–2 min of application [435], so that less than 3% of an applied dose penetrates into the aqueous humor following topical instillation of an aqueous solution [436]. The duration of drug action is, therefore, brief, and frequent dosing is needed.

The duration of drug action in the eye can be extended by two approaches: (a) reducing drainage through the use of viscosity-enhancing agents, suspensions, emulsions, ointments, erodible and nonerodible matrices [437] and (b) improving corneal drug penetration through the use of ionophores [438], ion-pairs [439], liposomes [440], and prodrugs [441]. For low viscosity solutions, the improvement in ocular bioavailability is usually modest [442–444]. Suspensions and emulsions suffer from the same problem as low viscosity solutions in that the contact time, though lengthened, is still relatively brief. Moreover, in the case of suspensions, the solid particles must dissolve slow enough to offer an advantage over a saturated solution [455]. The release rate of drug is usually rapid from swollen hydrophilic matrices such as soft contact lenses. Release rate from lipophilic ointments can be slower, but these systems suffer from the problem of blurring vision thus reducing their use to night time medication. The use of ion-pair and ionophores is limited to a small group of drugs and their improvement is still considered moderate [438,439]. Liposomes appear to be able to enhance the absorption of large, hydrophilic molecules [446–450] and may prove to be useful in delivering macromolecules such as peptides and proteins. Their usefulness in delivering lipophilic molecules seems to depend on the way the drugs are incorporated into the liposomes [446,447,450]. The use of liposomes in ocular drug delivery has been reviewed [440].

Prodrugs can be used to improve ocular bioavailability by enhancing corneal penetration, protecting the parent compound from metabolism, or decreasing its elimination. Recently, the first ophthalmic prodrug, dipivalyl epinephrine, was marketed under the trade name Propine[R]. With improved corneal penetration characteristics, a much lower dose of epinephrine is needed, thereby reducing side-effects. Via a different mechanism to affect ocular drug absorption, systems such as Ocusert[R] [451] and erodible matrices [452], which provide controlled drug delivery to the conjunctival sac, are able to reduce fluctuations commonly observed with pulse-entry systems, thereby allowing the use of drugs with very short biological half-lives. Moreover, systems such as Ocusert[R] do optimize precorneal delivery of drug. Unfortunately, patient acceptance of these systems is unsatisfactory partly because they are easily expelled during sleep.

In summary, the currently available ocular drug delivery systems are far from ideal. Future research should be directed toward controlled delivery to the absorbing surface with minimization of nonproductive loss. Since eye-drops are the most acceptable dosage form, it appears that the ideal dosage form should be of low viscosity but reside near the absorbing surface for an extended period of time and release its drug in a controlled manner.

VIII. DRUG TARGETING

The objective of drug targeting is to achieve a desired pharmacological response at a selected site without undesirable interactions at other sites. This is especially important in cancer chemotherapy and enzyme replacement treatment. At present, drug targeting is achieved by one of two approaches. The first approach involves chemical modification of the parent compound to a derivative which is activated only at the target site [453,454]. The second approach utilizes carriers such as liposomes [455,456], microspheres [457], nanoparticles [458], antibodies [459–461], cellular carriers (erythrocytes and lymphocytes) [462,463], and macromolecules [464,465] to direct the drug to its site of action.

There are a variety of strategies to modify the chemical structure of drug molecules, the most common being the prodrug approach and the most sophisticated being the chemical delivery system approach (Chapter 8). A prodrug is an inactive chemical derivative of a parent compound that is activated predictably *in vivo* to the active drug species, but, with few exceptions [466], it cannot achieve site-specific delivery [467]. In contrast, a chemical delivery system involves transformation of the active drug by synthetic means into an inactive derivative which, when placed in the body, will undergo several predictable enzymatic transformations principally at its site of action. This approach has proven to be successful in local delivery of drugs to the eye, brain and testes [454,468].

Because of impermeability of the GI tract to most macromolecules and instability of the drug-carrier complex in the hostile environment of the GI tract, administration of large drug-carrier complexes is restricted to intravenous or intraarterial injections or to direct injection into the target tissue such as a tumor. At present, the major obstacle of drug targeting using macromolecular and particulate carriers is rapid sequestration of intravascularly administered drug carriers by mononuclear phagocytes of the reticuloendothelial system (RES) [469-470]. Because of rapid clearance, only a small fraction of the injected carrier untimately reaches the target, if at all. The approaches have been attempted to alleviate this problem. The first involves blocking the RES prior to administering the drug carrier [471,472]. However, paralysis of the RES is undesirable especially in cancer patients. Without the first-line defense mechanism of the RES against infectious agents, these cancer patients will be at risk to infections.

A second approach is to impart specificity to the drug carrier by coupling specific ligands onto its external surface. These include desialylated fetulin [427], erthyrocyte membrane glycoproteins [473, 474], heat aggregated immunoglobulins [475], monoclonal antibodies [460], and native immunoglobulins [476]. So far, none of these strategies has proven to be successful due to difficulties in preserving the recognition ability *in vivo* and avoiding triggering any immunological response.

Another obstacle in targeting particulate drug carriers is the vascular system itself. This subject has been carefully reviewed by Poste [477] as well as by Poznansky and Juliano [478]. In order for a drug carrier to be able to recognize the target, it must first extravasate. The vascular endothelium of most tissues and organs, being continuous with an effective pore diameter of 2 nm, is essentially impermeable to molecular assemblages such as liposomes (0.025–5.0 μm) and nanoparticles (<1 μm). Significant extravasation of the structures in this size range is only possible at those sites with a discontinuous endothelium, notably in the sinusoids of the liver and spleen, where the effective pore diameter is approximately 100 nm. Thus, most particulate matter is confined to the general circulation.

On the positive side, impermeability of the capillary endothelial lining may be a useful property under certain conditions: (a) confinement of drug within a physiological compartment, (b) use of particles whose direction or release characteristics are under external control, and (c) drug delivery to the lung, liver and spleen.

Two forms of external control have been explored. Liposomes can be made from lipids with release characteristics which are a function of a temperature gradient [479] due to either local inflammation or localized heating via collimated radiation. Drug is released from circulating liposomes as they pass through the target region [480]. Another approach involves the use of microspheres of denatured albumin [457] and, more recently, Sephadex^{R} [481] containing ferromagnetic particles. The microspheres are restricted at the microvascular level under the influence of a directed external field. Enhanced drug delivery to the target, in theory, can be achieved by this approach.

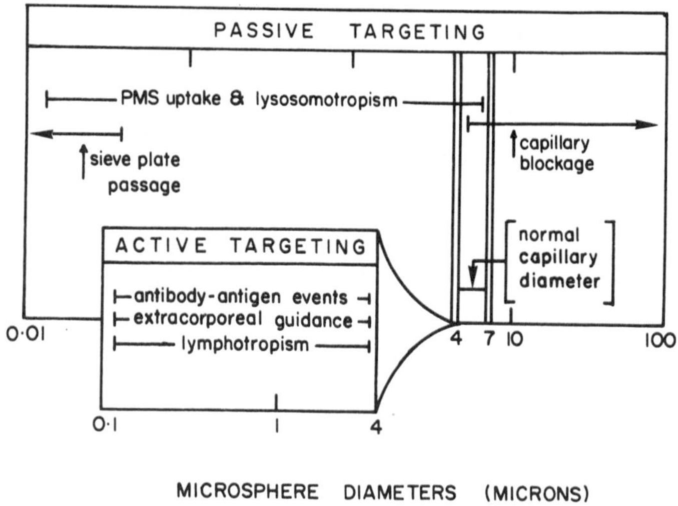

Fig. 5 Strategies in achieving drug targeting. (From Ref. 483.)

Microspheres have also been used for passive targeting to organs such as the liver, spleen, lung and kidney (Fig. 5) [482,483]. Intravenous injection of particles between 7 and 12 μm leads to mechanical filtration by the lungs, whereas particles between 2 and 12 μm leads to their blockage in the first capillary bed encountered. Such blockage can lead to first-order targeting of, for example, the liver and kidney, and second-order targeting to tumor-bearing organs [484].

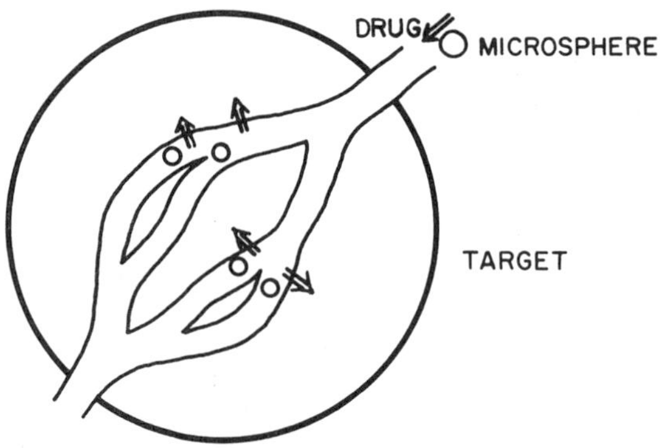

Fig. 6 Method of chemoembolism to achieve drug targeting.

This latter effect is probably due to a qualitative and quantitative difference in the capillary networks of the tumor compared to those of the host organ [485].

Recently, intraarterial injection of biodegradable microspheres was used to produce a tumor chemoembolism in cancer chemotherapy [486–488]. Figure 6 gives the rationale behind this use. A mixture of drug and starch microspheres (about 40 μm) were injected together. The large size of microspheres caused temporary blockage of the tumor-bearing organ's arteriole, thereby increasing absorption time of the drug by the tumor organ. However, obstruction of the feeder vessels of a tumor using microsphres by themselves could also bring about tumor regression [489].

In addition to the difficulties encountered by carriers to extravasate, drug targeting by carriers also suffers from such problems as stability of the carrier on storage and *in vivo*, drug loading, immunogenicity, and degradability. Consequently, except for passive targeting to the reticuloendothelial system of the liver and spleen, the concept of systemic drug targeting via carriers and biological recognization has met with little success. It is clear that, for successful targeting, a better understanding of diseases and the biology of the body at a cellular and molecular level is needed.

IX. CONCLUSIONS

In the past decade, the number of new drug entities appearing on the market yearly has declined and pharmaceutical manufacturers for a variety of reasons have a renewed interest in improving existing dosage forms and developing more sophisticated drug delivery systems, including those employing the principles of sustained/controlled drug release. The need for a sustained/controlled release preparation often arises: (a) as a result of undesirable drug properties, such as short biological half-life, local irritation, extensive metabolism, and narrow therapeutic index, (b) perhaps through the nature of the disease state, or (c) for patient compliance reasons. Most important of all is the need to improve the efficacy and safety of drug through proper temporal and/or spatial control of drug release.

In considering a drug for this mode of drug delivery, certain criteria have to be examined and evaluated. These are the physicochemical, pharmacokinetic and pharmacodynamic characteristics of the drug. With each drug property there is a range of values that lends itself to the design of sustained/controlled release products, and outside this range the design becomes more difficult or, in the extreme, prohibitive. Extremes of aqueous solubility, oil/water partition coefficients, binding, extensive metabolism/degradation of the drug during transit from the point of drug delivery to the target area, and narrow therapeutic index are some of the limiting factors in formulating an effective sustained release product. Paradoxically, all these limitations are precisely the reasons why controlled release drug delivery is desirable. Furthermore, advances in biotechnology have brought about peptides and proteins which, by virture of their chemical and biological properties, demand special systems for their delivery. Theoretically, each of these limitations can be overcome and successful controlled drug delivery can be accomplished by using physical, chemical, biological, and biomedical engineering approaches, alone or in combination, as described in subsequent chapters.

Throughout this chapter, an attempt has been made to delineate the influence of drug properties on the design of sustained/controlled release drug delivery system. Information on the physicochemical properties of a new or existing drug is usually relatively abundant. In addition, with the increase in application of pharmacokinetic analysis, there is a steady growth in the volume of information on the biological parameters of drug action, such as absorption rate constant, biological half-life and volume of distribution, which may also be available to the formulator. When examining animal and clinical data in the literature, th formulator must take into consideration conflicting information which is not uncommon due to differences in experimental design and compartmental analysis of the data. Obviously, many of these uncertainties have to be resolved in the course of evaluating a drug for sustained/controlled drug delivery. Moreover, for some drugs, the various biological parameters behave differently in a single dose vs. a multiple dose situation or in a single dose vs. a continuous infusion situation [490]. Consequently, multiple dose and perhaps continuous infusion studies are a necessary prerequisite in terms of evaluation. Thus, each drug must be evaluated for its potential as a sustained/controlled release product by examining the complete profile for that drug, being cognizant of the limiting and restraining aspects of drug properties.

In this chapter, we have also tried to emphasize the importance of routes other than oral for systemic drug administration. Although the oral route is preferred for the majority of drugs, it is beset with numerous potential problems such as possible degradation, first-pass metabolism, and variable and limited residence time. The transdermal route has proved to be effective for controlled delivery of certain drugs. The nasal route is potentially useful to deliver drugs include peptides and proteins which undergo extensive first-pass metabolism. The rectal route offers a longer residence time than the nasal and buccal routes and may allow controlled release of drugs for a day or two. Replacement of the defecated unit with a new unit may permit controlled release for extended periods of time. The parenteral route is currently the preferred route to achieve drug targeting since other routes are commonly impermeable to drug carrier complexes. Even this route is beset with the problem of inability of the drug-carrier complex to traverse the capillary endothelium before reaching its target in extravascular tissues. Thus, drug targeting has met with little success except in the case of direct injection into the target tissues. As a result, placement of the controlled release system in the vicinity of the target tissue becomes the alternative. This modality does improve therapeutic drug efficacy allowing the use of a lower initial dose and less frequent dosing. Ideally, in order to avoid undesirable side effects, drug candidates for local treatment should possess limited permeability or are prone to immediate inactivation after exerting their local actions.

In the final analysis, a complete knowledge and understanding of the behavior of a drug and the limitation of a particular route of administration, as well as judicious selection of the approach, is indispensable to the process of designing a useful controlled release product. It is the usual case that the desired temporal pattern of release, i.e., a constant tissue drug level, is not achieved. In addition, it has to be realized that, without exception, sustained and/or controlled drug release products on the market today do not maximize drug utilization. These products commonly do not take into account changes in drug need during the course of treatment due to circadian rhythm, changes in the pathological state, patient variation, etc. Thus, the term, controlled drug delivery, is used in a rather loose sense. Nevertheless, these types of products are a significant improvement over their nonsustained counterparts in terms of temporal drug level control and patient compliance. The challenge of drug delivery is the recognition of how far away we usually are from maximization of drug therapy and the substantial changes that are yet to be made in the area of controlled drug delivery.

REFERENCES

1. V. F. Smolen and L. A. Ball (eds.), *Controlled Drug Bioavailability*, Vols. 1 and 2, John Wiley, New York, 1984.
2. R. I. Langer and D. L. Wise (eds.), *Medical Applications of Controlled Release*, Vols. 1 and 2, CRC Press, Florida, 1984.
3. S. D. Bruck (ed.), *Controlled Drug Delivery*, Vols. 1 and 2, CRC Press, Florida, 1984.
4. R. L. Juliano, (ed.), *Drug Delivery Systems*, Oxford, New York, 1980.
5. J. M. Anderson and S. W. Kim (ed.), *Recent Advances in Drug Delivery Systems*, Plenum, New York, 1984.
6. Y. W. Chien, *Novel Drug Delivery Systems: Fundamentals, Developmental Concepts and Biomedical Assessments*, Marcel Dekker, New York, 1982.

7. T. J. Roseman and S. Z. Mansdorf (ed.), *Controlled Release Delivery Systems*, Marcel Dekker, New York, 1983.
8. A. F. Kydonienus (ed.), *Controlled Release Technologies: Methods, Theory and Applications*, Vols. 1 and 2, CRC Press, Florida, 1980.
9. P. Goldman, Rate-controlled drug delivery, *N. Engl. J. Med. 307*, 286 (1982).
10. W. A. Check, New drugs and drug-delivery systems in the year 2000, *Am J. Hosp. Pharm. 41*, 1536 (1984).
11. N. L. Henderson, Recent advances in drug delivery system technology, In, *Annual Reports in Medicinal Chemistry*, Vol. 18 (H. J. Hess, ed.), Academic Press, New York, 1983.
12. A. Zaffaroni, Systems for controlled drug delivery, *Med. Res. Rev. 1*, 373 (1981).
13. H. A. Struyker Boudier, Rate-controlled drug delivery: Pharmacological, therapeutic and industrial perspectives, *Trends Pharmacol. Sci. 3*, 162 (1982).
14. S. K. Chandrasekaran, F. Theeuwes, and S. I. Yum, The design of controlled drug delivery systems. In, *Drug Design* (E. J. Ariens, ed.), Vol. 8, Academic Press, New York, 1979, pp. 133–167.
15. O. Vaizoglu and P. Speiser, Intelligent drug delivery systems, *Trends Pharmacol. Sci. 3*, 28 (1982).
16. J. Urquhart, Rate-controlled drug dosage, *Drugs 23*, 207 (1982).
17. L. R. Beck and V. Z. Pope, Controlled-release delivery systems for hormones: a review of their properties and current therapeutic use, *Drugs 27*, 528 (1984).
18. R. A. Siegel and R. Langer, Controlled release of polypeptides and other macromolecules, *Pharm. Res. 1*, 2 (1984).
19. Y. W. Chien and J. R. Robinson, "Smart" drug-delivery systems, *J. Parenter. Sci. Technol. 36*, 231 (1982).
20. E. P. Goldberg (ed.), *Targeted Drugs*, Wiley, New York, 1983.
21. K. Heilman, *Therapeutic Systems*, 2nd ed., George Thieme Verlag, Stuttgurst, 1984.
22. G. S. Banker, Pharmaceutical applications of controlled release: on overview of the past, present, and future. In, *Medical Applications of Controlled Release* (R. S. Langer and D. L. Wise, ed.), CRC Press, Florida, 1984, pp. 1–34.
23. M. V. Sefton, D. G. Allen, V. Horvath, and W. Zingg, Insulin delivery at variable rates. In, *Recent Advances in Drug Delivery* (J. M. Anderson and S. W. Kim, eds.), Plenum Press, New York, 1984, pp. 349–365.
24. T. A. Horbett, B. D. Ratner, J. Kost, and M. Singh, A bioresponsive membrane for insulin delivery. In, *Recent Advances in Drug Delivery* (J. M. Anderson and S. W. Kim, eds.), Plenum Press, New York, 1984, pp. 209–220.

25. F. Theeuwes and W. Bayne, Dosage form index an objective criterion for evaluation of controlled-release drug delivery systems, *J. Pharm. Sci. 66*, 1388 (1977).
26. J. Koch-Weser, Serum drug concentrations as therapeutic guides, *N. Engl. J. Med. 287*, 227 (1972).
27. L. A. Pagliaro and L. Z. Benet, Critical compilation of terminal half-lives, percent excreted unchanged, and changes of half-life in renal and hepatic dysfunctions for studies in humans with references, *J. Pharmacokin. Biopharm. 3*, 333 (1975).
28. M. Gibaldi and P. J. McNamara, Steady-state concentrations of drugs with short half-lives when administered in oral sustained release formulations, *Int. J. Pharm. 2*, 167 (1979).
29. J. Fara and J. Urquhart, The value of infusion and injection regimens in assessing efficacy and toxicity of drugs, *Trends Pharmacol. Sci., 5*, 21 (1984).
30. P. L. Carl, P. K. Chakravarty, J. A. Katzenellenbogen, and M. J. Weber, Protease-activated "produrg" for cancer chemotherapy, *Proc. Natl. Acad. Sci. USA 77*, 2224 (1980).
31. P. K. Chakravarty, P. L. Carl, M. J. Weber, and J. A. Katzenellenbogen, Plasmin-activated prodrugs for cancer chemotherapy. 1. Synthesis and biological activity of peptidylacivicin and peptidylphenylenediamine mustard, *J. Med. Chem. 26*, 633 (1983).
32. P. K. Chakravarty, P. L. Carl, M. J. Weber, and J. A. Katzenellenbogen, Plasmin-activated prodrugs for cancer chemotherapy. 2. Synthesis and biological activity of peptidyl derivatives of doxorubicin, *J. Med. Chem., 26*, 638 (1983).
33. M. E. Morrison, M. J. Yagi, and G. Cohen, In vitro studies of 2,4-dihydroxyphenylalanine, a prodrug targeted against maligant melanoma cells, *Proc. Natl. Acad. Sci. USA 82*, 6020 (1985).
34. S. S. Davis, J. G. Hardy, M. J. Taylor, D. R. Whaley, and C. J. Wilson, The effect of food on the gastrointestinal transit of pellets and osmotic device (Osmet), *Int. J. Pharm. 21*, 331 (1984).
35. W. H. Barr, J. Adir, and L. Garrettson, Decrease of tetracycline absorption in man by sodium bicarbonate, *Clin. Pharmacol. Ther. 12*, 799 (1971).
36. V. Manninen, K. Ojala, and P. Reisell, New formulation of digoxin, *Lancet 2*, 922 (1972).
37. J. G. Wagner, P. G. Welling, K. O. Lee, and J. E. Walker, In vivo and in vitro availability of commercial warfarin tablets, *J. Pharm. Sci. 60*, 666 (1971).
38. B. Katchen and S. Symchowicz, Correlation of dissolution rate and griseofulvin absorption in man, *J. Pharm. Sci. 56*, 1108 (1967).

39. T. R. Bates, D. A. Lambert, and W. H. Jones, Correlation between the rate of dissolution and absorption of salicylamide from tablet and suspension dosage forms, *J. Pharm. Sci. 58*, 1468 (1969).
40. C. Hansch and W. J. Dunn, II, Linear relationships between lipophilic character and biological activity of drugs, *J. Pharm. Sci. 61*, 1 (1972).
41. T. Fujita, J. Iwasa, and A. Hansch, A substituent constant, π, derived from partition coefficients, *J. Am Chem. Soc. 86*, 5175 (1964).
42. B. Keerman, K. Hellstrom, and A. Rosen, Metabolism of propantheline in man, *Clin. Pharm. Ther. 13*, 212 (1972).
43. W. H. Bachrach, Anticholinergic drugs, *Am. J. Digest. Dis. 3*, 743 (1958).
44. B. K. Martin, Potential effects of the plasma proteins on drug distribution, *Nature 207*, 274 (1965).
45. J-P. Tillement, G. Houin, R. Zini, S. Urien, B. Albengres, The binding of drugs to blood plasma macromolecules, *Recent Adv. Drug Res. 13*, 59 (1984).
46. L. D. De Leve and K. M. Piasky, Clinical significance of plasma binding of basic drugs, *Trends Pharmacol Sci. 3*, 283 (1981).
47. M. Rowland, Protein binding and drug clearance, *Clin. Pharmacokin. 9*, (Suppl. 1), 10 (1984).
48. J. J. Mackichan, Pharmacokinetic consequences of drug displacement from blood and tissue proteins, *Clin. Pharmacokin. 9*, (Suppl.), 32 (1984).
49. B. K. Martin, Kinetics of elimination of drugs possessing high affinity for the plasma proteins, *Nature 207*, 959 (1965).
50. R. R. Levine, The influence of the intraluminal intestinal milieu on absorption of an organic cationic and anionic agent, *J. Pharmacol. Exp. Ther. 131*, 328 (1961).
51. K. Park, S. L. Cooper, and J. R. Robinson, Bioadhesive hydrogels. In, *Hydrogels in Medicine and Pharmacy* (N. Peppas, ed.), Vol. 2, CRC Press, Boca Raton (in press).
52. S. S. Chrai, T. F. Patton, A. Mehta, and J. R. Robinson, Lacrimal and instilled fluid dynamics in rabbit eyes, *J. Pharm. Sci., 62*, 1112 (1973).
53. V. H. L. Lee and J. R. Robinson, Mechanistic and quantitative evaluation of precorneal pilocarpine disposition in albino rabbits, *J. Pharm. Sci. 68*, 673 (1979).
54. H. A. Quigley, I. P. Pollack, and T. S. Harbin, Jr., Pilocarpine Ocuserts: long-term clinical trials and selected pharmacodynamics, *Arch. Ophthalmol. 93*, 771 (1975).
55. E. R. Garrett, Drug systems affecting availability and reliability of response, *J. Am. Pharm. Assoc. NS9*, 110 (1969).
56. R. R. Sheline, Metabolism of foreign compounds by gastrointestinal microorganisms, *Pharmacol. Rev. 25*, 451 (1973).

57. W. H. Barr and S. Riegelman, Intestinal drug absorption and metabolism. I. Comparison of methods and models to study physiological factors of in vitro and in vivo intestinal absorption, *J. Pharm. Sci. 59*, 154 (1970).
58. C. C. Booth, Sites of absorption in the small intestine. *Fed. Proc., 26*, 1583 (1967).
59. M. Weiner, S. Shapiro, J. Axelrod, J. Cooper, and B. Brodie, The physiological disposition of dicumarol in man, *J. Pharmacol. Exp. Ther. 99*, 409 (1950).
60. R. M. Levine, M. R. Blair, and B. B. Clark, Factors influencing the intestinal absorption of certain mono-quarternary anticholinergic compounds with special reference to benzomethamine, *J. Pharmacol. Exp. Ther. 114*, 78 (1955).
61. L. Weinstein, Antibiotics. IV. Miscellaneous antimicrobial, antifungal, and antiviral agents. In, *The Pharmacological Basis of Therapeutics* (L. S. Goodman and A. Gilman, eds.), 4th Ed., Macmilan, New York, 1970, p. 1269.
62. G. Levy and W. J. Jusko, Factors affecting the absorption of riboflavin in man, *J. Pharm. Sci. 55*, 285 (1966).
63. A. B. Morrison, C. B. Perusse, and J. A. Campbell, Physiologic availability and in vitro release of riboflavin in sustained-release vitamin preparations, *N. Engl. J. Med. 263*, 115 (1960).
64. E. B. Brown, Jr. and B. W. Justus, In vitro absorption of radioiron by everted pouches of rat intestine, *Am. J. Physiol. 194*, 319 (1958).
65. R. E. Reed, Iron deficiency anemia "refractory" to oral iron, *Missouri Med. 66*, 120 (1969).
66. C. E. Blezek, J. L. Lach, and J. K. Guillory, Some dissolution aspects of ferrous sulfate tablets, *Am. J. Hosp. Pharm. 27*, 533 (1970).
67. E. J. Middleton, E. Nagy, and A. B. Morrison, Studies on the absorption of orally administered iron from sustained-release preparations, *N. Engl. J. Med. 274*, 136 (1966).
68. P. Crosland-Taylor, D. H. Keeling, and B. W. Cromie, Trial of slow-release tablets of ferrous sulfate, *Curr. Ther. Res. 7*, 244 (1965).
69. T. H. Bothwell, G. Pirzio-Biroli, and C. A. Finch, Iron absorption. I. Factors influencing absorption, *J. Lab. Clin. Med. 51*, 24 (1958).
70. I. M. Baird, R. L. Walters, and D. R. Sutton, Absorption of slow-release iron and effects of ascorbic acid in normal subjects and after partial gastrectomy, *Br. Med. J. 4*, 505 (1974).
71. J. J. Webster, Treatment of iron deficiency anemia in patients with iron intolerance: clinical evaluation of controlled-release form of ferrous sulfate, *Curr. Ther. Res. 4*, 130 (1962).
72. S. T. Callender, Quick and slow-release iron: a double-blind trial with a single daily dose regimen, *Br. Med. J. 4*, 531 (1969).

73. D. P. Bentley and A. Jacobs, Accumulation of storage iron in patients treated for iron-deficiency anemia, *Br. Med. J. 2*, 64 (1975).
74. G. J. Mouratoff and R. C. Batterman, Serum iron absorption tests of sustained-release form of oral iron, *J. New Drugs 1*, 157 (1961).
75. T. P. Stevenson, Therapeutic assay of sustained-release form of oral iron, *Curr. Ther. Res. 4*, 107 (1962).
76. L. B. Posner and F. Wilson, Evaluation of sustained-release molybdenized ferrous sulfate in iron-deficiency anemia of pregnancy, *J. New Drugs 3*, 155 (1963).
77. E. Krüger-Thiemer, W. Diller, L. Dettli, P. Bunger, and J. Seydel, Demonstration des Einflusses der Eiweissbindung und der Ionisation duf die Pharmackokinetick am kombinierten gaskinetischen Modell nach van't Hoff and Langmuir, *Antibiot. Chemother. 12*, 171 (1964).
78. E. Krüger-Thiemer and P. Bunger, The role of therapeutic regimen in dosage design. Part I, *Chemotherapia 10*, 61 (1965–1966).
79. E. Krüger-Thiemer and P. Bunger, The role of therapeutic regimen in dosage design. Part II, *Chemotherapia 10*, 129 (1965–1966).
80. E. Krüger-Thiemer, P. Bunger, L. Kettli, P. Spring, and E. Wempe, Dosage regimen calculation of chemotherapeutic agents. Part III. Sulfasymazine, *Chemotherapia 10*, 325 (1965–1966).
81. E. Krüger-Thiemer, W. Diller, and P. Bunger, Pharmacokinetic models regarding protein binding of drugs. In, *Antimicrobial Agents and Chemotherapy—1965* (G. L. Hobby, ed.), American Society of Microbiology, Ann Arbor, Mi., 1966, pp. 183–191.
82. S. Riegelman, J. C. K. Loo, and M. Rowland, Shortcomings in pharmacokinetic analysis by conceiving the body to exhibit properties of a single compartment, *J. Pharm. Sci. 57*, 117 (1968).
83. M. Gibaldi, R. Nagashima and G. Levy, Relationship between drug concentration in plasma or serum and amount of drug in the body, *J. Pharm. Sci. 58*, 193 (1969).
84. A. R. DiSanto and J. G. Wagner, Potential erroneous assignment of nonlinear data to the classical linear two-compartment open model, *J. Pharm. Sci. 61*, 552 (1972).
85. T. Taylor, L. F. Chasseaud, R. Major, E. Doyle, and A. Darragh, Isosorbide 5-mononitrate pharmacokinetics in humans, *Biopharm. Drug Disp. 2*, 255 (1981).
86. M. M. Reidenberg, D. Drayer, A. L. DeMarco, and C. T. Bello, Hydralazine elimination in man, *Clin. Pharmacol, Ther. 14*, 970 (1973).
87. H. F. Schran, F. L. S. Tse and S. I. Bhuta, Pharmacokinetics and pharmacodynamics of bromocriptine in the rat, *Biopharm. Drug Disp. 6*, 301 (1985).

88. C. B. Coutinho, H. E. Spiegel, S. A. Kaplan, M. Yu, R. P. Chroistian, J. J. Carbone, J. Symington, J. A. Cheripko, M. Lewis, A. Tonchen, and T. Crews, Kinetics of absorption and excretion of levodopa in dogs, *J. Pharm. Sci. 60,* 1014 (1971).
89. W. B. Abrams, C. B. Coutinho, A. S. Leon, and H. E. Spiegel, Absorption and metabolism of levodopa, *JAMA 218,* 1912 (1971).
90. M. Sandler, F. Karoum, and C. R. J. Ruthven, M-hydroxyphenylacetic acid formation from L-dopa in man: Suppression by neomycin, *Science 166,* 1417 (1969).
91. M. Sandler, C. R. J. Ruthven, B. L. Goodwin, K. R. Hunter, and G. M. Stern, Variation of levodopa metabolism with gastrointestinal absorption site, *Lancet 1,* 238 (1974).
92. A. C. Woods, G. A. Glaubiger, and T. N. Chase, Sustained-release levodopa, *Lancet 1,* 1391 (1973).
93. G. Curzon, J. Friedel, L. Grier, C. D. Marsden, J. D. Parkes, M. Shipley, and K. J. Zilkha, Sustained-release levodopa, *Lancet 1,* 781 (1973).
94. D. Perrier and M. Gibaldi, Influence of first-pass effect on the systemic availability of propoxyphene, *J. Clin. Pharmacol. 12,* 449 (1972).
95. W. H. Barr and S. Riegelman, Intestinal drug absorption and metabolism. II. Kinetic aspects of intestinal glucuronide conjugation, *J. Pharm. Sci. 59,* 164 (1970).
96. G. Levy and J. J. Matsuzawa, Pharmacokinetics of salicylamide in man, *J. Pharmacol. Exp. Ther. 156,* 285 (1967).
97. R. Johansson, C. G. Regardh, and J. Sjogren, Absorption of alprenolol in man from tablets with different rates of release, *Acta. Pharm. Suec. 8,* 59 (1971).
98. J. G. Wagner, E. J. Antal, A. T. Elvin, W. R. Gillespie, E. A. Pratt, and K. S. Albert, Theoretical decrease in systemic availability with decrease in input rate at steady-state for first-pass drugs, *Biopharm. Drug Disp. 6,* 341 (1985).
99. E. M. Johnson, Jr., A. B. Hrkey, D. J. Blehm, and P. Needleman, Clearance and metabolism of organic nitrates, *J. Pharmacol. Exp. Ther. 182,* 56 (1972).
100. P. Needleman, S. Lang, and E. M. Johnson, Jr., Organic nitrates: Relationship between biotransformation and rational angina pectoris therapy, *J. Pharmacol. Exp. Ther. 181,* 489 (1972).
101. D. G. Friend, J. P. O'Hare, and H. D. Levine, Action of triethanolamine trinitrate in angina pectoris, *Am. Heart J. 48,* 775 (1954).
102. M. G. Bogaert, M. T. Rosseel, and A. F. deSchaepdryver, The metabolic fate of nitroglycerin (Trinitrin) in relation to its vascular effects, *Eur. J. Pharmacol. 12,* 224 (1970).
103. R. A. Turner, Absorption of nitroglycerin from the alimentary tract of the rabbit, *J. Pharm. Sci. 54,* 464 (1965).

104. I. R. E. Pilkington and J. J. Purves, Long acting glyceryl trinitrate in angina pectoris of out-patients, *Br. Med. J. 1*, 38 (1960).
105. T. Winsor, H. Kaye, and B. Mills, Hemodynamic response of oral long-acting nitrates: evidence of gastrointestinal absorption, *Chest 62*, 407 (1972).
106. I. Hirshleifer, Peripheral hemodynamic effects of oral controlled-release nitroglycerin (Nitrong) in man, *Curr. Ther. Res. 15*, 158 (1973).
107. H. I. Russek, B. L. Zohman, A. E. Drumm, W. Weingarten, and V. J. Dorset, Long acting coronary vasodilator drugs: Metamine, Paveril, Nitroglyn, and Peritrate, *Circulation 12*, 169 (1955).
108. W. Modell, Clinical pharmacology of antianginal drugs, *Clin. Pharmacol. Ther. 3*, 97 (1962).
109. S. H. Curry and S. M. Aburawi, Analysis, disposition and pharmacokinetics of nitroglycerin, *Biopharm. Drug Disp. 6*, 235 (1985).
110. M. H. Wendkos and N. Meshulam, Comparative effects of placebo and sustained-release nitroglycerin in angina subjects, *J. Clin. Pharmacol. 13*, 160 (1973).
111. M. Preti, G. Abbondati, and C. Carpi, Protective action of a sustained release form of nitroglycerin in an infarct experimentally induced by isoproterenol in the rat, *Boll. Chim. Farm. 108*, 576 (1969).
112. L. W. Dittert, Pharmacokinetic considerations in clinical drug trials, *Drug Intell. Clin. Pharm. 8*, 222 (1974).
113. P. J. Niebertgall, E. T. Sugita, and R. L. Schnaare, Potential dangers of common drug dosing regimen, *Am. J. Hosp. Pharm. 31*, 53 (1974).
114. K. R. Heimlich, D. R. MacDonnell, T. L. Flanagan, P. D. O'Brien, Evaluation of a sustained-release form of phenylpropanolamine hydrochloride by urinary excretion studies, *J. Pharm. Sci. 50*, 232 (1961).
115. F. O'Grady, W. R. L. Brown, H. Gaya, and I. P. MacKintosh, Antibiotic levels on continuous intravenous infusion, *Lancet 2*, 209 (1971).
116. H. S. Brown, S. M. Caiola, F. M. Eckel, D. C. McCleod, C. C. Pulliam, and H. B. Woodhall, Cephalexin, *Drug Intell. Clin. Pharm. 5*, 134 (1971).
117. R. E. Cutler, Pharmacokinetics of furosemide in normal subjects and functionally anephric patients, *Clin. Pharmacol. Ther. 16*, 588 (1974).
118. J. Kampmann, J. M. Hansen, K. Siersbaek-Nielsen, and H. Laursen, Effects of some drugs on penicillin half-life in blood, *Clin. Pharmacol. Ther. 13*, 516 (1972).

119. D. Schuppany, S. Riegelman, B. von Lehmann, A. Pilbrandt, and C. Becker, Preliminary pharmacokinetics studies of propylthiouracil in humans, *J. Pharmacokinet. Biopharm. 1*, 307 (1973).
120. D. G. Shand and R. E. Rangno, The disposition of propranolol. I. Elimination during oral absorption in man, *Pharmacology 7*, 159 (1972).
121. G. H. Evans, A. S. Nies, and D. G. Shand, The disposition of propranolol. III. Decreased half-life and volume of distribution as a result of plasma binding in man, monkey, dog and rat, *J. Pharmacol. Exp. Ther. 186*, 114 (1973).
122. K. Verebely and C. E. Inturrisi, Disposition of propoxyphene in man after a single oral dose, *Clin. Pharmacol. Ther. 15*, 302 (1974).
123. L. Graffner, G. Johansson, and J. Sjogren, Pharmacokinetics of procainamide intravenously and orally as conventional and slow-release tablets, *Clin. Pharmacol. Ther. 17*, 414 (1975).
124. J. Koch-Weser, S. W. Klein, L. L. Foo-Canto, J. A. Kaster, and R. W. DeSantis, Antiarrhythmic prophylaxis with procainamide in acute myocardial infarction, *N. Engl. J. Med. 281*, 1253 (1969).
125. J. Koch-Wester and S. W. Klein, Procainamide dosage schedules, plasma concentrations and clinical effects, *JAMA 215*, 1454 (1971).
126. R. Ruosteenoja, P. Torsti, and A. Sothmann, Experiences on a sustained-release procainamide preparation, *Curr. Ther. Res. 15*, 707 (1973).
127. E. Karlsson, Plasma levels of procainamide after administration of conventional and sustained-release tablets, *Eur. J. Clin. Pharmacol. 6*, 245 (1973).
128. R. J. Levine and A. Sjoerdsma, Estimation of monoamine oxidase activity in man: techniques and applications, *Ann. NY Acad. Sci. 107*, 966 (1963).
129. J. C. Harter, W. J. Reddy, and G. W. Thorn, Studies on an intermittent corticosteroid dosage regimen, *N. Engl. J. Med. 269*, 591 (1963).
130. C. J. Falliers, H. Chai, L. Molk, H. Bane, and R. R. de A. Cardoso, Pulmonary and adrenal effects of alternate-day corticosteroid therapy, *J. Allergy Clin. Immunol. 49*, 156 (1972).
131. M. E. Jacobson, The rationale of alternate-day corticosteroid therapy, *Postgrad Med. 49*, 181 (1971).
132. J. G. Wagner, O. W. Carpenter, and E. J. Collins, Sustained action oral medication. I. A quantitative study of prednisolone in man, in the dog, and in vitro, *J. Pharmacol. Exp. Ther. 129*, 101 (1960).
133. C. J. Migeon, F. K. Tyler, J. P. Mahoney, A. A. Florentin, H. Castle, E. L. Bliss, and L. T. Samuels, The diurnal variation

of plasma levels and urinary excretion of 17-hydroxycorticosteroids in normal subjects, night workers and blind subjects, *J. Clin. Endocrinol. Metab. 16*, 622 (1956).

134. R. E. Peterson, Metabolism of adrenocorticosteroids in man, *Ann. NY Acad. Sci. 82*, 846 (1959).

135. P. F. D'Arcy, J. P. Griffin, J. S. Jenkins, W. F. Kirk, and A. W. C. Peacock, Sustained-release formulation of prednisolone administered orally to man, *J. Pharm. Sci. 60*, 1028 (1971).

136. I. I. Lubowe, Sustained-release oral methylprednisolone in dermatology: a clinical evaluation, *Curr. Ther. Res. 4*, 111 (1962).

137. E. Nelson, Pharmaceuticals for prolonged action, *Clin. Pharmacol. Ther. 4*, 283 (1963).

138. G. W. Thorn, R. E. Fuisz, and R. C. Fuisz, *Steroid Therapy: A Clinical Update for the 1970s*, Medcom, New York, 1971.

139. J. J. Burns, R. K. Rose, T. Chenkin, A. Goldman, A. Schulert, and B. B. Rodie, The physiological disposition of phenylbutazone (Butazolidin) in man and a method for its elimination in biological material, *J. Pharmacol. Exp. Ther. 109*, 346 (1953).

140. D. T. Carr and A. G. Karlson, Optimal dosage regimens of antituberculosis drugs, *Am. Rev. Respir. Dis. 84*, 90 (1961).

141. F. J. Roberts, Single daily dose treatment of psychiatric patients with phenothiazine derivatives, *J. Ment. Sci. 107*, 104 (1961).

142. L. E. Hollister, Studies of delayed-action medication. I. Meprobamate administered as conventional tablets and as two delayed action capsules, *N. Engl. J. Med. 266*, 281 (1962).

143. I. Haides, Single daily dose of a new form of amitriptyline in depressive illness, *Br. J. Psychiatry 120*, 521 (1972).

144. Anon., Two new antidepressive preparation, *Drug Ther. Bull. 9*, 99 (1971).

145. J. R. Gomez and G. Gomez, Depression in general practice: comparison between thrice daily amitriptyline tablets and a single sustained-release capsule at night, *Br. J. Clin. Pract. 26*, 33 (1972).

146. L. E. Hollister, S. H. Curry, J. E. Doerr, and S. L. Kanter, Studies of delayed-action medication. V. Plasma levels and urinary excretion of four different dosage form of chlorpromazine, *Clin. Pharmacol. Ther. 11*, 49 (1970).

147. T. J. Mellinger, Serum concentrations of thioridazine after different oral medication form, *Am. J. Psychiatry 121*, 1119 (1965).

148. L. E. Hollister, Studies of prolonged-action medication. II. Two phenothiazine tranquilizers (thiroidazine and chlorpromazine) administered as coated tablets and prolonged-action preparations, *Curr. Ther. Res. 4*, 471 (1962).

149. M. Hruska, B. Morris, and J. J. Hsu, Therapeutic effects of different modes of chlorpromazine administration, *Dis. Nerv. Syst. 27*, 522 (1966).
150. C. Bartlett, Comparison of thioridazine tablets to chlorpromazine spansules in the maintenance care of chronic schizophrenics, *Curr. Ther. Res. 13*, 100 (1971).
151. H. M. Solomon and J. J. Schrogie, The anticoagulant response to bishydroxycoumarin. I. The role of individual variation, *Clin. Pharmacol. Ther. 8*, 66 (1967).
152. M. A. Schwartz, E. Postma, and Z. Gaunt, Biological half-life of chlordiazepoxide and its metabolite, demoxepam, in man, *J. Pharm. Sci. 60*, 1500 (1971).
153. H. W. Jun and E. J. Triggs, Blood levels of chlorphentermine in man, *J. Pharm. Sci. 59*, 206 (1970).
154. J. A. Taylor, Pharmacokinetics and biotransformation of chlorpropamide in man, *Clin. Pharmacol. Ther. 13*, 710 (1972).
155. B. Pepitpierre, L. Perrin, M. Rudhardt, A. Herreru, and J. Fabre, Behavior of chlorpropamide in renal insufficiency and under the effect of associated drug therapy, *Int. J. Clin. Pharmacol. Ther. Toxicol. 6*, 120 (1972).
156. L. Hillestad, T. Hansen, and M. Melsom, Diazepam metabolism in normal man. 2. Serum concentration and clinical effect after oral administration and cumulation, *Clin. Pharmacol. Ther. 16*, 485 (1974).
157. U. Klotz, G. R. Avant, A. Hoyumpa, S. Schanker, and G. R. Wilkinson, Effects of age and liver disease in the disposition and elimination of diazepam in adult man, *J. Clin. Invest. 55*, 247 (1975).
158. L. M. Cummins, Y. C. Martin, and E. E. Scherfling, Serum and urine levels of ethchlorvynol in man, *J. Pharm. Sci. 60*, 261 (1971).
159. J. E. Doherty, Digitalis glycosides pharmacokinetics and their clinical implications, *Ann. Intern. Med. 79*, 299 (1973).
160. L. Storstein, Studies on digitalis. 1. Renal excretion of digitoxin and its cardioactive metabolites, *Clin. Pharmacol. Ther. 16*, 14 (1974).
161. J. E. Doherty, W. H. Perkins, and G. K. Mitchell, Tritiated digoxin studies in human subjects, *Arch. Intern. Med. 108*, 531 (1961).
162. C. McMartin, R. K. Rondel, J. Vinter, B. R. Allan, P. M. Humberstone, A. W. D. Leisman, G. Sandler, and J. L. Thirkettle, The fate of guanethidine in two hypertensive patients, *Clin. Pharmacol. Ther. 11*, 423 (1970).
163. L. E. Hollister and G. Levy, Kinetics of meprobamate elimination in humans, *Chemotherapia 9*, 20 (1964).
164. K. Arnold, Rate of decline of dipheylhydantoin in human plasma, *Clin. Pharmacol. Ther. 11*, 121 (1970).

165. M. C. MacDonald, D. S. Robinson, D. Sylvester, and J. J. Jeffe, The effects of chloral betaine and glutethimide administration on warfarin plasma levels and hypoprothrombinemic response in man, *Clin. Pharmacol. Ther. 10*, 80 (1969).
166. J. G. Wagner, Aspects of pharmacokinetics and biopharmaceutics in relation to drug activity, *Am. J. Pharm. 141*, 5 (1969).
167. H. Nau, R. Zierer, H. Spielmann, D. Neubert, and C. Gansau, A new model for embryotoxicity testing: tetratogenicity and pharmacokinetics of valproic acid following constant-rate administration in the mouse using human therapeutic drug and metabolite concentrations, *Life Sci. 29*, 2803 (1981).
168. B. I. Sikic, J. M. Colins, E. G. Mimnaugh, and T. E. Gram, Improved therapeutic index of bleomycin when adminsitered by continuous infusion in mice, *Cancer Treat. Rep. 62*, 2011 (1978).
169. B. Eckstein, K. Shaw, and G. Stern, Sustained-release levodopa in Parkinsonism, *Lancet 1*, 431 (1973).
170. B. W. McGuiness and J. B. Parkin, New long-acting formulation of chlorpheniramine maleate in hay fever, *Br. J. Clin. Pract. 25*, 139 (1971).
171. G. Levy and B. A. Hayes, Physicochemical basis of the buffered acetylsalicylic acid controversy, *N. Engl. J. Med. 262*, 1053 (1960).
172. V. Herbert, Drugs effective in iron-deficiency and other hypochronic anemias. In, *The Pharmacological Basis of Therapeutics* (L. S. Goodman and A. Gilman, eds.), 4th ed., Macmillan, New York, 1970, p. 1045.
173. AMA Department of Drugs, *AMA Drug Evaluations*, 2nd ed., American Medical Association, Chicago, 1973, p. 183.
174. C. Boroda, R. B. Miller, S. T. Leslie, E. G. Nicol, and I. Thomson, Comparison of the bioavailability of aminophylline in a conventional base and in a continuous release base, *J. Clin. Pharmacol. 13*, 383 (1973).
175. J. R. Hoon, Bleeding gastritis induced by long-term release aspirin, *JAMA 229*, 841 (1974).
176. E. Jacobs and J. Pringot, Gastric ulcers due to the intake of potassium chloride, *Am. J. Digest. Dis. 18*, 289 (1973).
177. D. R. Baker, W. H. Schrader, and C. R. Hitchcock, Small-bowel ulceration apparently associated with thiazide and potassium therapy, *JAMA 190*, 586 (1964).
178. L. Gee, B. Berg, T. G. Tong, and C. Becker, Enteric-coated potassium supplements, *JAMA 228*, 975 (1974).
179. J. M. Jefferson and P. Aukland, Enteric-coated potassium chloride: A continuous hazard, *Br. Med. J. 1*, 456 (1974).
180. W. Hasker and J. McCaffrey, Ulceration of a Meckel's diverticulum due to a potassium chloride tablet, *Med. J. Aust. 2*, 261 (1972).

181. B. L. Phillips, Potassium-induced bowel ulceration, *Br. J. Clin. Pract. 28*, 143 (1974).
182. W. H. Thomas, Measurement of dissolution rates of potassium chloride from various slow release potassium chloride tablets using a specific ion electrode, *J. Pharm. Pharmacol. 25*, 27 (1973).
183. E. L. Tarpley, Controlled-release potassium supplementation, *Curr. Ther. Res. 16*, 734 (1974).
184. C. Graffner and J. Sjogren, Potassium absorption from sustained-release tablets, *Acta Pharm. Suec. 8*, 13 (1971).
185. T. J. McKenna, J. F. Donohoe, J. J. Healy, B. Canning, and F. P. Muldowney, Potassium-sparing agents during diuretic therapy in hypertension, *Br. Med. J. 2*, 739 (1971).
186. E. M. Clarkson, Slow sodium: an oral slowly released sodium chloride preparation, *Br. Med. J. 3*, 604 (1971).
187. Anon., Slow Na, *Drug Ther. Bull, 9*, 98 (1971).
188. M. A. Schneiderman, M. H. Myers, Y. S. Sathe, and P. Kofsky, Toxicity, the therapeutic index and the ranking of drugs, *Science 144*, 1212 (1964).
189. O. Jardetzky, On the quantitative evaluation of pharmacologic agents, *J. New Drugs 6*, 203 (1966).
190. T. Rudy, personal communication, 1976.
191. J. H. Gaddum, Pharmacology, Oxford University Press, New York, 1953.
192. C. A. Winter, A study of comparative antihistaminic activity of six compounds, *J. Pharmacol. Exp. Ther. 90*, 224 (1947).
193. J. C. Krantz, Jr., C. J. Carr, and B. N. La Du, Jr., *The Medical Principles of Medical Practice*, 7th ed., William & Wilkins, Baltimore, 1969, p. 28.
194. B. S. Katcher, Rheumatoid arthritis, *J. Am. Pharm. Assoc. NS12*, 383 (1972).
195. E. H. Wiseman, Plasma salicylate concentrations following chronic administration of aspirin as conventional and sustained-release tablets, *Curr. Ther. Res. 11*, 681 (1969).
196. J. B. Dick-Smith, Pilot trial of sustained-release aspirin (Bi-Prin), *Med. J. Aust. 1*, 18 (1970).
197. E. H. Wiseman and N. J. Federici, Development of a sustained-release aspirin tablet, *J. Pharm. Sci. 57*, 1535 (1968).
198. M. S. Vora, Z. J. Zimmer, and P. V. Maney, Sustained-release aspirin tablet using an insoluble matrix, *J. Pharm. Sci. 53*, 487 (1964).
199. S. C. Harvey, Gastric antacids and digestants. In, *The Pharmacological Basis of Therapuetics* (L. S. Goodman and A. Gilman, eds.), 4th ed., Macmillan, New York, 1965, p. 1013.
200. W. A. Sodeman, Jr., N. A. Augur, and H. M. Pollard, Physiology and pharmacology of belladonna therapy in antipeptic disease, *Med. Clin. North Am. 53*, 1379 (1969).

201. D. R. Reese, S. M. Free, J. V. Swintosky, and M. I. Grossman, The effect of dosage forms on the duration and continuity of belladonna alkaloids, *Am. J. Dig. Dis. 4*, 220 (1958).
202. H. Burness, Clinical evaluation of a sustained-release belladonna preparation, *Am. J. Dig. Dis. 22*, 111 (1955).
203. A. M. Kasich, Relief of nocturnal pain in duodenal ulcer, *Am. J. Gastroenterol. 33*, 66 (1960).
204. M. H. Alp and A. K. Grant, Effect of sustained-release hexocyclium tablets on gastric acid secretion, *Med. J. Aust. 1*, 337 (1969).
205. R. A. Kerr, Angina pectoris, *J. Am. Pharm. Assoc. NS12*, 178 (1972).
206. M. Kamil and I. Klinger, Timed disintegration capsules of pentaerythritol tetranitrate in a selected angina group, *NY State J. Med. 59*, 3398 (1959).
207. T. M. Feinblatt and E. A. Ferguson, Timed-disintegration capsules: a further study. An in vivo roentgenographic study, blood level study and relief of angina pain with pentaerythritol tetranitrate, *N. Engl. J. Med. 256*, 331 (1957).
208. J. L. Schelling and L. Lasagna, A study of cross-tolerance to circulatory effects of organic nitrates, *Clin. Pharmacol. Ther. 8*, 256 (1967).
209. A. Wilson, The modification of the duration of drug action, *J. Pharm. Pharmacol. 11*, 446 (1959).
210. J. S. Takahashi and M. Zatz, Regulation of circadian rhythmicity, *Science 217* 1104 (1982).
211. J. A. Martinex-O'Gerrall, Circadian rhythms, *J. Occup. Med. 10*, 305 (1968).
212. G. G. Luce, *Biological Rhythms in Psychiatry and Medicine*, National Institute of Mental Health, Bethesda, Md, 1970.
213. C. E. Brush and R. Fayerweather, Observations on the changes in blood pressure during normal sleep, *Am. J. Physiol.* 5, 199 (1901).
214. H. Brooks and J. H. Carroll, Clinical study of the effects of sleep and rest blood pressure, *Arch Intern. Med. 10*, 97 (1912).
215. T. Aimoto, B. H. Rohde, G. C. Y. Chiou, and J. K. Lauber, N-Acetyltransferase activity and melatonin level in the eyes of glaucomtous chickens, *J. Ocular Pharmacol. 1*, 149 (1985).
216. E. Marte and F. Halberg, Circadian susceptibility in relation to administration of pharmacologic agents, *Fed. Proc. 20*, 305 (1961).
217. E. Haus and F. Halberg, 24-hour rhythm in susceptibility of C Mice to a toxic dose of ethanol, *J. Appl. Physiol. 14*, 878 (1959).
218. P. J. Wedlund and R. H. Levy, Time-dependent kinetics VII: Effect of diurnal oscillations on the time course of carbamazepine

autoinduction in the rhesus monkey, *J. Pharm. Sci. 72*, 905 (1983).
219. E. L. Dubois and D. C. Adler, Single daily dose oral administration of corticosteroids in rheumatic disorders: An analysis of its advantages, efficacy and side effects, *Curr. Ther. Res.* 5, 43 (1963).
220. R. J. Jarrett and H. Keen, Diurnal variation of oral glucose tolerance: a possible pointer to the evolution of diabetes mellitus, *Br. Med. J. 2*, 341 (1969).
221. N. S. Hayner, M. D. Kjelsberg, F. H. Epstein, and T. Francis, Carbohydrate tolerance and diabetes in a total community, Tecumseh, Michigan. I. Effects of age, sex and test conditions on one-hour glucose tolerance in adults, *Diabetes 14*, 413 (1965).
222. N. Freinkel, M. Mager, and L. Vinnick, Cyclicity in the interrelationships between plasma insulin and glucose during starvation in normal young men, *J. Lab. Clin. Med. 17*, 171 (1968).
223. C. Faiman and J. A. Morrhouse, Diurnal variation in the levels of glucose and related substances in healthy and diabetic subjects during starvation, *Clin. Sci. 32*, 111 (1967).
224. A. N. Rigas, A. H. Bittles, D. R. Hadden, and D. A. D. Montgomery, Circadian variation of glucose, insulin and free fatty acids during long-term use of oral hypoglycemic agents in diabetes mellitus, *Br. Med. J. 4*, 25 (1968).
225. M. A. Kimble, Diabetes, *J. Am. Pharm. Assoc. NS14*, 80 (1974).
226. W. J. M. Hruschesky, Circadian timing of cancer chemotherapy, *Science 228*, 73 (1985).
227. S. A. Nicholson, T. E. Adrian, A. J. Bacarese-Hamilton, B. Gillham, M. T. Jones, and S. R. Bloom, 24-Hour variation in content and release of hypothalamic neuropeptides in the rat, *Reg. Peptides 7*, 385 (1983).
228. G. Leyendecker, T. Struve, and E. J. Plotz, Induction of ovulation with chronic intermittent (pulsatile) administration of LH-RH in women with hypothalamic and hyperprolactinemic amenorrhea, *Arch. Gynecol. 229*, 117 (1980).
229. W. F. Crowley Jr. and J. W. McArthur, Stimulation of the normal menstrual cycle in Kallman's syndrome by pulsatile administration of luteinizing hormone-releasing hormone (LHRH), *J. Clin. Endocrinol. Metab. 51*, 173 (1980).
230. G. Leyendecker, L. Wildt and M. Hansmann, Pregnacies following chronic intermittent (pulsatile) administration of Gn-RH by means of a portable pump ("Zyklomat")—A new approach to the treatment of infertility in hypothalamic amenorrhea, *J. Clin. Endocrinol. Metab. 51*, 1214 (1980).
231. C. S. Tam, J. N. M. Heersche, T. M. Murray, and J. A. Parsons, Parathyroid hormone stimulates the bone apposition rate

independently of its resorptive action: Differential effects of intermittent and continuous administration, *Endocrinology 110*, 506 (1982).
232. A. Soll, C. R. Kahn, D. M. Neville, Jr. and J. Roth, Insulin receptor deficiency in genetic and acquired obesity, *J. Clin. Invest. 56*, 779 (1975).
233. J. R. Gavin, J. Roth, D. M. Neville, P. deMeyts, and D. N. Buell, Insulin dependent regulation of insulin receptor concentrations: a direct demonstration in cell culture, *Proc. Natl. Acad. Sci. USA 71*, 84 (1974).
234. A. J. W. Hsuen, H. L. Dufau, and K. J. Catt, Regulation of luteinzing hormone receptors in testicular cells by gonadotropin, *Biochem. Biophys. Res. Commun. 72*, 1145, 1976.
235. M. A. Lesniak and J. Roth, Regulation of receptor concentration by homologous hormone. Effect of human growth hormone on its receptor in IM-9 lymphocytes, *J. Biol. Chem. 251*, 3720 (1976).
236. P. M. Hinkle and A. H. Tashjian, Jr., Thyrotropin-releasing hormone regulates the number of its own receptors in the GH_3 strain of pituitary cells in culture, *Biochemistry 14*, 3845 (1975).
237. P. E. Belchetz, T. M. Plant, Y. Nakai, E. J. Keogh, and E. Knobil, Hypophyseal responses to continuous and intermittent delivery of hypothalamic gonadotropin-releasing hormone, *Science 202*, 631 (1978).
238. H. J. Lynch, R. W. Rivest, and R. J. Wurtman, Artificial induction of melatonin rhythms by programmed microinfusion, *Neuroendocrinology 31*, 106 (1980).
239. J. V. Moore, Dose-response curves after in vivo experimental chemotherapy: influence of route of administration on biological outcomes, *Cancer Chemother. Pharmacol. 15*, 91 (1985).
240. L. Z. Benet, Effect of route of administration and distribution on drug action, *J. Pharmacok. Biopharm. 6*, 559 (1978).
241. Y. W. Chien, Long-acting parenteral drug formulations, *J. Parenteral Sci. Technol. 35*, 106 (1981).
242. G. F. J. Russell, Starch microspheres drug delivery systems, *Pharm., Int. 3*, 260 (1983).
243. S. S. Davis, Colloids as drug delivery systems, *Pharm. Technol. 5*, 71 (1981).
244. T. R. Tice and D. R. Cowar, Biodegradable controlled-release parenteral systems, *Pharm. Technol. 8*, 25 (1984).
245. Y. Morimoto, K. Sugibayashi and M. Akimoto, Magnetic guidance of ferrocolloid-entrapped emulsion for site-specific drug delivery, *Chem. Pharm. Bull. 31*, 279 (1983).
246. M. A. Davis and T. A. Taube, Pulmonary perfusion imaging: acute toxicity and safety factors as a function of particle size, *J. Nucl. Med. 19*, 1209 (1978).

247. E. F. Evans, J. D. Proctor, M. Fratkin, J. Velandia, and A. J. Wasserman, Blood flow in muscle groups and drugs absorption, *Clin. Pharmacol. Ther. 17*, 44 (1975).
248. A. T. Florence and W. R. Vezin, Prolongation of the action of intramuscular formulations of phenothiazines. In, *Optimization of Drug Delivery*, Alfred Benzon Symposium 17 (H. Bundguaard, A. B. Hansen, and H. Kofod, eds.), Munksgaard Copenhagen, 1982, pp. 93–113.
249. M. Ermini, F. Carpino, M. Russo and G. Benagiano, Studies on sustained contraceptive effects with subcutaneous polydimethylsiloxane implants, *Acta Endocrinol. 73*, 360 (1973).
250. S. L. Sendelbeck and C. L. Girdis, Disposition of a ^{14}C-labeled bioerodible polyorthoester and its hydrolysis products, 4-hydroxybutyrate and cis,trans-1,4-bis(hydroxymethyl)cyclohexane, in rats, *Drug Metab. Disp. 13*, 291 (1985).
251. K. Hirano, T. Ichihashi and H. Yamada, Studies on the absorption of practically water-insoluble drugs following injection. V. Subcutaneous absorption in rats from solutions in water immiscible oils, *J. Pharm. Sci. 71*, 495 (1982).
252. M. Pfeffer, R. D. Smyth, K. A. Pittman, and P. A. Nardella, Pharmacokinetics of subcutaneous and intramuscular butorphenol in dogs, *J. Pharm. Sci. 69*, 801 (1980).
253. D. I. Abramson, *Blood Vessels and Lymphatics*, Academic Press, New York, 1962, p. 520.
254. J. Schou, Subcutaneous and intramuscular injection of drugs. In, *Concepts in Biochemical Pharmacology*, Part 1 (B. B. Brodie and J. R. Gillette, eds.), Springer-Verlag, Heidelberg, 1971, pp. 47–66.
255. B. E. Ballard, Biopharmaceutical considerations in subcutaneous and intramuscular drug administration, *J. Pharm. Sci. 57*, 357 (1967).
256. A. E. Jorgensen and J. Schou, The local effect of cholinergic agents and cholinesterase inhibition on the clearance of surcose from muscles, *Acta. Pharmacol. (Kbh) 23*, 205 (1965).
257. G. F. Warner, E. L. Dobson, N. Pace, M. E. Johnson, and C. R. Finney, Studies of human peripheral blood flow: the effect of injection volume on the intramuscular radiosodium clearance rate, *Circulation 8*, 732 (1953).
258. R. B. Sund and J. Schou, The determination of absorption rates from rat muscles: an experimental approach to kinetic descriptions, *Acta Pharmacol. Toxicol. 21*, 313 (1964).
259. K. Kakemi, H. Sezaki, K. Okumura and S. Ashida, Absorption and excretion of drugs XXXIX. The absorption of isonicotinic acid derivatives from the skeletal muscle of the rats, *Chem. Pharm. Bull. 17*, 1332 (1969).

260. K. Kakemi, H. Sezaki, K. Okumura, C. Takada and S. Furusawa, Absorption of drugs from the skeletal muscle of the rats (2), *Chem. Pharm. Bull. 19*, 2058 (1971).
261. K. Kakemi, H. Sezaki, K. Okumura, H. Kobayashi and S. Furusawa, Absorption of drugs from the skeletal muscle of the rats (3). Effect of water-soluble adjuvants and vehicles on the intramuscular absorption, *Chem. Pharm. Bull. 20*, 443 (1972).
262. K. Okumura, H. Sezaki, and K. Kakemi, Absorption of drugs from the skeletal muscle of the rats (4). Absorption of cationic drugs from the muscle, *Chem. Pharm. Bull. 20*, 1607 (1972).
263. H. Kobayashi, T. Nishimura, K. Okumura, S. Muranishi, and H. Sezaki, Effect of polysorbates on absorption rates of water-soluble, micelle-free drugs administered intramuscularly in the rat, *J. Pharm. Sci. 63*, 580 (1974).
264. R. H. Levy and M. Rowland, Absorption kinetics of a series of local anesthetics from rat subcutaneous tissue. I, *J. Pharmacokin. Biopharm. 2*, 313 (1974).
265. R. H. Levy and M. Rowland, Absorption kinetics of a series of local anesthetics from rat subcutaneous tissue. II. Effects of vasodilators, *J. Pharmacokin. Biopharm. 2*, 337 (1974).
266. K. Hirano, T. Ichihashi and H. Yamada, Studies on the absorption of practically water-insoluble drugs following injection. I. Intramuscular absorption from water-immiscible oil solutions in rats, *Chem. Pharm. Bull. 29*, 519 (1981).
267. K. Hirano, T. Ichihashi and H. Yamada, Studies on the absorption of practically water-insoluble drugs following injection. II. Intramuscular absorption from aqueous suspensions in rats, *Chem. Pharm. Bull. 29*, 817 (1981).
268. K. Hirano, T. Ichihashi and H. Yamada, Studies on the absorption of practically water-insoluble drugs following injection. VI. Subcutaneous absorption from aqueous suspensions in rats, *J. Pharm. Sci. 71*, 500 (1982).
269. V. Bocci, Evaluation of routes of administration of interferon in cancer: A review and a proposal, *Cancer Drug Delivery 1*, 337 (1984).
270. J. R. Howard and J. Hadgraft, The clearance of oily vehicles following intramuscular injections in rabbits, *Int. J. Pharm. 16*, 31 (1983).
271. W. S. Nimmo, Drugs, diseases and altered gastric empyting, *Clin. Pharmacokin. 1*, 189 (1976).
272. A. F. Hoffman, J. H. Dressman, C. F. Code, K. F. Witztum, Controlled entry of orally administered drugs: physiological considerations, *Drug Dev. Ind. Pharm. 9*, 1077 (1983).
273. I. L. MacGregor, P. Martin, and J. H. Meyer, Gastric emptying of solid food in normal man and after subtotal gastrectomy and truncal vagotomy with pyloroplasty, *Gastroenterology 72*, 206 (1977).

274. H. S. Ch'ng, H. Park, P. Kelly and J. R. Robinson, Bioadhesive polymers as platforms for oral controlled drug delivery II: Synthesis and evaluation of swelling, water-insoluble bioadhesive polymers, *J. Pharm. Sci. 73*, 399 (1985).
275. M. A. Longer, H. S. Ch'ng, and J. R. Robinson, Bioadhesive polymers as platforms for oral controlled drug delivery III: Oral delivery of chlorothiazide using a bioadhesive polymer, *J. Pharm. Sci. 74*, 406 (1985).
276. R. Groning and G. Heun, Oral dosage forms with controlled gastrointestinal transit, *Drug Dev. Ind. Pharm. 10*, 527 (1984).
277. M. J. Dew, P. J. Hughes, M. G. Lee, B. K. Evans and J. Rhodes, An oral preparation to release drugs in the human colon, *Br. J. Clin. Pharmacol. 14*, 405 (1982).
278. C. Bogentoft, C. Eskilsson, U. E. Jonsson, P. O. Lagerstrom, K. Lovgren and L. Rosen, Delivery of drugs to the colon by means of a new encapsulated oral dosage form, *Acta Pharm. Seu 20*, 311 (1983).
279. D. R. Friend and G. W. Chang, A colon specific drug-delivery system based on drug glycides and the glycosidases of colon bacteria, *J. Med. Chem. 27*, 261 (1984).
280. M. Gibaldi and J. L. Kanig, Absorption of drugs through the oral mucosa, *J. Oral Ther. Pharmac. 1*, 440 (1965).
281. N. F. H. Ho and W. I. Higuchi, Quantitative interpretation of in vivo buccal absorption of alkonoic acids by the physical model approach, *J. Pharm. Sci. 60*, 537 (1971).
282. I. A. Siegel, Effect of chemical structure on nonelectrolyte penetration of oral mucosa, *J. Invest. Dermatol. 76*, 137 (1981).
283. I. A. Siegel, Permeability of the oral mucosa. In, *The Structure and Function of Oral Mucosa* (J. Meyer, C. A. Squier, and S. J. Gerson, eds.), Pergamon Press, Oxford, 1984, pp. 95–108.
284. R. P. Walton, Absorption of drugs through the oral mucosa. III. Fat-water solubility coefficient of alkaloids, *Proc. Soc. Exp. Biol. Med. 32*, 1488 (1935).
285. I. A. Segel, K. T. Izutsu and E. Watson, Mechanisms of nonelectrolyte penetration across dog and rabbit oral mucosa, *Arch. Oral Biol. 26*, 357 (1981).
286. A. C. Moffat, Absorption of drugs through the oral mucosa. In, *Topics in Medicinal Chemistry*, Vol. 4, John Wiley & Sons, New York, 1971, pp. 1–26.
287. A. H. Beckett and R. D. Hossie, Buccal absorption of drugs. In, *Handbook of Experimental Pharmacology*, Vol. 28, Part I (B. B. Brodie and J. R. Gillete, eds.), Springer-Verlag, Heidelberg, 1971, pp. 25–46.
288. S. S. Davis, P. B. Daly, J. W. Kennerley, M. Frier, J. G. Hardy and C. G. Wilson, Design and evaluation of sustained

release formulations for oral and buccal administration, *Adv. Pharmacother.* *1*, 17 (1982).
289. J. Abrams, Nitrate delivery systems in perspectives, a decade of progress, *Am. J. Med.* *75*, 38 (1984).
290. A. B. de Boer, L. G. J. Leede and D. D. Breimer, Rectal drug administration: partial avoidance of hepatic first-pass elimination, *Pharm. Int.* *3*, 267 (1982).
291. W. A. Ritschel, H. Elconin, G. J. Alcorn, and D. D. Denson, First-pass elimination of lidocaine in the rabbit after peroral and rectal route of administration, *Biopharm. Drug Disp.* *6*, 281 (1985).
292. L. G. J. Leede, A. G. de Boer, C. D. Feijen and D. D. Breimer, Site specific rectal drug administration in man with an osmotic system: influence on "first-pass" elimination of lidocaine, *Pharm. Res.* *1*, 129 (1984).
293. J. J. Tukker, D. J. de Blaey and G. A. Charbon, Rectal motility and bioavailability, *Pharm. Res.* *1*, 173 (1984).
294. F. Moolenaar and A. J. M. Schoonen, Biopharmaceutics of the rectal administration of drugs, *Pharm. Int.* *1*, 144 (1980).
295. N. Senoir, Rectal administration of drugs. In, *Advances in Pharmaceutical Sciences*, Vol. 4, Academic Press, London, 1974, pp. 363–435.
296. C. J. de Blaey and J. Polderman, Rationales in the design of rectal and vaginal delivery forms of drugs. In, *Drug Design*, Vol. 9 (E. J. Ariens, ed.), Academic Press, New York, 1980, pp. 237–266.
297. K. Morimoto, Y. Iwamoto, T. Katashima, T. Takeeda, Y. Nakamoto, and K. Morisaka, Absorption and bioavailability of diclofenac after rectal administration of diclofenac-Na gel preparation in rat and man, *Pharm. Res.*, *2*, 166 (1985).
298. T. Nishihata, J. Rytting and T. Higuchi, Enhanced rectal absorption of theophylline, lidocaine, cefnetazole and levodopa by several adjuvants, *J. Pharm. Sci.* *71*, 865 (1982).
299. T. Nishihata, J. Rytting and T. Higuchi, Effect of salicylate on rectal absorption of lidocaine, levodopa and cefmetazole in rats, *J. Pharm. Sci.* *71*, 869 (1982).
300. T. Nishihata, J. Rytting, T. Higuchi, L. Caldwell and S. J. Selk, Enhancement of rectal absorption of water-soluble antibiotics in dogs, *Int. J. Pharm.* *21*, 239 (1984).
301. T. Nishihata, K. Yasiu, M. Yamazaki and A. Kamada, Effect of adjuvants on the rectal uptake of bleomycin in rats, *J. Pharm. Dyn.* *7*, 278 (1984).
302. T. Nishihata, J. Rytting, T. Higuchi and L. Caldwell, Enhanced rectal absorption of insulin and heparin in rats in the presence of non-surfactant adjuvants, *J. Pharm. Pharmacol.* *33*, 334 (1981).

303. T. Nishihata, G. Liversidge and T. Higuchi, Effect of aprotinin on rectal delivery of insulin, *J. Pharm. Pharmacol. 35*, 616 (1983).

304. T. Nishihata, J. Rytting, L. Caldwell, S. Yoshioka and T. Higuchi, Adjuvant effect on rectal absorption. In, *Optimization of Drug Delivery*, Alfred Benzon Symposium 17 (H. Bundgaard, A. B. Hansen, and H. Kofod, eds.), Munksgaard, Copenhagen, 1982, pp. 17–34.

305. N. Yata, W. M. Wu, R. Yamajo, T. Murkami, Y. Higashi, and T. Higuchi, Enhanced rectal absorption of sodium ampicillin by N-acyl derivatives of collagen peptide in rabbits and rats, *J. Pharm. Sci. 74*, 1058 (1985).

306. T. Nishihata, C. S. Lee, M. Yamamoto, J. Rytting, and T. Higuchi, The effects of salicylate on the rectal absorption of phenylalanine and some peptides, and the effects of these peptides on the rectal absorption of cefoxitin and cefmetazole, *J. Pharm. Sci. 73*, 1326 (1984).

307. K. Nakanishi, A. Ogata, M. Masada and T. Nadai, Effect of non-steroidal anti-inflammatory drugs on the rectal mucosa, *Chem. Pharm. Bull. 32*, 1956 (1983).

308. K. Nakanishi, M. Masada and T. Nadai, Effect of pharmaceutical adjuvants on the rectal permeability of drugs III. Effect of repeated administration and recovery of the permeability, *Chem. Pharm. Bull. 31*, 4161 (1983).

309. A. G. de Boer, F. Moolenenaar, L. G. J. de Leede and D. D. Breimer, Rectal drug administration: clinical pharmacokinetic consideration, *Clin. Pharmacokin. 7*, 285 (1982).

310. A. Hussain, S. Hirai, R. Bawarshi, Nasal absorption of propanolol in rats, *J. Pharm. Sci. 73*, 1300 (1984).

311. A. Hussain, S. Hirai, and C. H. Huang, Nasal absorption of testosterone in rats, *J. Pharm. Sci. 73*, 1300 (1984).

312. A. Hussain, R. Kimura, C. H. Huang and T. Kashihara, Nasal absorption of naloxone and buprenorphine in rats, *Int. J. Pharm. 21*, 233 (1984).

313. A. Hussain, R. Kimura, C. H. Huang and R. Mustafa, Nasal absorption of ergotamine tartrate in rats, *Int. J. Pharm. 21*, 289 (1984).

314. K. S. E. Su, K. M. Campanale and C. L. Gries, Nasal drug delivery system of a quarternary ammonium compound: clofilium tosylate, *J. Pharm. Sci. 73*, 1251 (1984).

315. A. N. Fisher, K. Brown, S. S. Davis, G. D. Parr, and D. A. Smith, The nasal absorption of sodium cromoglycate in the albino rabbit, *J. Pharm. Pharmacol. 37*, 38 (1985).

316. R. L. Bronaugh and R. F. Stewart, Methods for in vitro percutaneous absorption studies V: Permeation through damaged skin, *J. Pharm. Sci. 74*, 1062 (1985).

317. D. L. London, W. R. Butt, S. S. Lynch, J. C. Marshall, S. Owusu, W. R. Robinson and J. M. Stephenson, Hormal response to intranasal luteinizing hormone, *J. Clin. Endocrinol.* *37*, 829 (1973).
318. J. Keenan and M. A. Chamberlain, Nasal mucosal absorption of tetracosactrin as indicated by a rise in plasma fluorogenic corticosteroids, *Br. Med. J.* *4*, 407 (1969).
319. K. Muller and M. Osler, Induction of labor, a comparison of intravenous, intranasal and transbuccal oxytocin, *Acta Obstet. Gynecol. Scand.* *46*, 59 (1967).
320. G. Bauman, A. Walser, P. A. Desaulles, F. J. A. Paesi and L. Geller, Corticotropic action of an intranasally applied synthetic ACTH derivative, *J. Clin. Endocrinol.* *42*, 60 (1976).
321. S. Hirai, T. Ikenaga and T. Matsuzawa, Nasal absorption of insulin in dogs, *Diabetes* *27*, 296 (1978).
322. S. Hirai, T. Yashiki and H. Mima, Effect of surfactants on the nasal absorption of insulin in rats, *Int. J. Pharm.* *9*, 165 (1981).
323. T. Nagai, Y. Nishimoto, N. Nambu, Y. Suzuki and K. Sekine, Powder dosage form of insulin for nasal administration, *J. Controlled Release* *1*, 15 (1984).
324. K. Morimoto, K. Morisaka and A. Kamada, Enhancement of nasal absorption of insulin and calcitonin using polyacrylic acid gel, *J. Pharm. Pharmacol.* *37*, 134 (1985).
325. K. S. E. Su, K. M. Campanale, L. G. Mendelsohn and C. L. Gries, Nasal delivery of polypeptides I: Nasal absorption of enkephalins in rats, *J. Pharm. Sci.* *74*, 394 (1985).
326. D. F. Proctor and G. K. Adams III, Physiology and pharmacology of nasal function and mucus secretion, *Pharmacol. Ther.*, Part B, *2*, 493 (1976).
327. G. D. Parr, Nasal delivery of drugs, *Pharm. Int.* *4*, 202 (1983).
328. S. Hirai, T. Yashiki, T. Matsuzawa and H. Mima, Absorption of drugs from the nasal mucosa of rat, *Int. J. Pharm.* *7*, 317 (1981).
329. O. G. Rabbe, H. C. Yeh, G. J. Newton, R. F. Phalen and D. J. Velasquez, In, *Inhaled Particles IV*, Part 1, British Occupational Hygiene Society, Edinburgh, 1977, p. 13.
330. J. W. Paterson, A. J. Woolcock and G. M. Shenfield, State of art: bronchodilator drugs, *Am. Rev. Respir. Dis.* *120*, 1149 (1979).
331. K. Horsfield, Structure of the tracheobronchial tree. In, *Scientific Foundations of Respiratory Medicine* (J. G. Scadding and G. Cummings, eds.), W. B. Saunders, Philadelphia, 1981, pp. 54–70.
332. W. D. Fenn and H. Rahn, *Handbook of Physiology: Respiration*, American Physiology Society, Washington, DC, 1973.
333. H. Von Hayek, *The Human Lung*, Hafer, New York, 1960.

334. P. E. Morrow, Task group of lung dynamics: Disposition and retention models for internal dosimetry of the human respiratory tract, *Health Phys. 12*, 173 (1966).
335. M. B. Dolovich, J. Sanchis, C. Rossman and M. T. Newhouse, Aerosol penetrance: a sensitive index of peripheral airway obstruction, *J. Appl. Physiol. 40*, 468 (1976).
336. S. P. Newman, F. Moren, D. Pavia, F. Little and S. W. Clarke, Deposition of pressurized suspension aerosols inhaled through extension devices, *Am. Rev. Respir. Dis. 124*, 317 (1981).
337. K. F. Lampe, Influence of disease on pharmacokinetic parameters of inhaled substances. In, *Modeling of Inhalation Exposure to Vapors: Uptake, Distribution, and Elimination*, Vol. II (V. Fiserova-Bergerova, ed.), CRC Press, Florida, 1983, pp. 157–164.
338. J. D. Brain and P. A. Valberg, Deposition of aerosols in the respiratory tract, *Am. Rev. Respir. Dis. 120*, 1325 (1979).
339. J. Heyder, Mechanism of aerosol particle deposition, *Chest 80*, 820 (1981).
340. R. Hicks, Pulmonary fibrosis: allergies, dust diseases and drugs, *Pharm. Int. 5*, 304 (1984).
341. D. F. Proctor, I. Andersen and G. Linquist, Clearance of inhaled particles from the human nose, *Arch. Intern. Med. 131*, 132 (1973).
342. R. E. Albert, M. Lippmann, J. Spiegelman, C. Strehlow, W. Briscoe, P. Wolfson, and N. Nelson, The clearance of radioactive particles from the human lungs. In, *Inhaled Particles and Vapors II* (C. N. Davies, ed.), Pergamon Press, Oxford, 1967, pp. 361.
343. C. W. LaBelle and H. Brieger, Patterns and mechanisms in the elimination of dust from the lung. In, *Inhaled Particles and Vapors* (C. N. Davies, ed.), Pergamon Press, Oxford, 1961, pp. 356.
344. F. F. Hahn, G. J. Newton, and Pl L. Bryant, In vitro phagocytosis of respirable-sized monodisperse particles by alveolar macrophages. In, *Pulmonary Macrophage and Epithelial Cells*, CONF-760927, U.S. Department of Commerce, Springfield, VA, 1977, pp. 424.
345. F. J. Strecker, Tissue reactions in rat lungs after dust inhalaation with special regard to bronchial dust elimination and to the penetration of dust into the lung interstices and lymphatic nodes. In, *Inhaled Particles and Vapors II* (C. N. Davies, ed.), Pergamon Press, Oxford, 1967, pp. 141.
346. J. M. Lauweryns and J. H. Baert, Alveolar clearance and the role of the pulmonary lymphatics, *Am. Rev. Respir. Dis. 115*, 627 (1977).

347. E. A. B. Brown, The localization, metabolism, and the effects of drugs and toxicants in lung, *Drug Metab. Rev. 3*, 33 (1974).
348. M. Simonescu, Ultrastructural organization of the alveolar-capillary unit, In, *Metabolic Activities and the Lung*, Ciba Foundation Symposium No. 78 (J. Vane, ed.), Amsterdam, 1980, pp. 11-26.
349. E. E. Schneeberger, Structural basis for some permeability properties of the air-blood barrier, *Fed. Proc. Fed. Am. Soc. Exp. Biol. 37*, 2471 (1978).
350. O. D. Wangensteen, L. E. Wittmers, Jr., and J. A. Johnson, Permeability of the mammalian blood-gas barrier and its components, *Am. J. Physiol. 216*, 719 (1969).
351. E. Taylor and K. A. Gaar, Jr., Estimation of equivalent pore radii of pulmonary capillary and alveolar membranes, *Am. J. Physiol. 218*, 1133 (1970).
352. J. Gil, Organization of microcirculation in the lung, *Ann. Rev. Physiol. 42*, 177 (1980).
353. S. L. Schwartz, Interaction of nicotine and other amines with the endocytic and exocytic functions and macrophages, *Fed. Proc. 35*, 85 (1976).
354. U. Smith and J. W. Ryan, An electron microscopic study of the vascular endothelium as a site for bradykinin and ATP activation in rat lung, In, *Advances in Experimental Medical Biology*, Vol. 8 (N. Back, F. Sicuteri, and M. R. Silva, eds.), 1970, pp. 249-262.
355. R. Effros, Small solutes and water. In, *Lung Biology in Health and Disease*, Vol. 7 (N. C. Staub, ed.), Marcel Dekker, New York, 1978, pp. 183-222.
356. S. J. Eunaad, L. S. Schanker, Absorption of drugs from the rat lung, *Am. J. Physiol. 223*, 1227 (1972).
357. L. S. Schanker and M. J. Less, Lung pH and pulmonary absorption of nonvolatile drugs in the rat, *Drug. Metab. Dispos. 5*, 174 (1977).
358. S. J. Enna and L. S. Schanker, Phenol red absorption from the rat lum: evidence of carrier transport, *Life Sci. 12*, 231 (1973).
359. T. H. Gardiner and L. S. Schanker, Absorption of disodium cromoglycate from the rat lung: Evidence of carrier transport, *Xenobiotica 4*, 725 (1974).
360. K. R. Chapman, A. C. Braude and A. S. Rebuck, Anticholinergic therapy in asthma and chronic bronchitis, *Hosp. Formulary 17*, 686 (1982).
361. J. Hartiala, P. Uotila and W. Nienstedt, Absorption and metabolism of intratracheally instilled cortisol and beclamethasone dipropionate in the isolated perfused rat lung, *Med. Biol. 57*, 294 (1979).

362. P. A. Routledge and D. G. Shand, Presystemic drug elimination, *Ann. Rev. Pharmacol. 19*, 447 (1979).
363. R. H. Briant, E. W. Blackwell, F. M. Williams, D. S. Davies and C. T. Dollery, The metabolism of sympathomimetic bronchodilator drugs by the isolated perfused dog lung, *Xenobiotica 3*, 787 (1973).
364. Y. S. Bakhle, First-pass metabolism of endogenous and exogenous substrates by lung. In, *Presystemic Drug Elimination* (C. F. George and D. G. Shand, ed.), Butterworth Scientific, London, 1982, pp. 147–172.
365. T. E. Pickett, T. C. Orton and M. W. Anderson, A study of the dynamics of imipramine accumulation in the isolated perfused rabbit lung, *Drug Metab. Dispos. 3*, 389 (1975).
366. D. P. Benziger and J. Edelson, Absorption from the vagina, *Drug Metab. Rev. 14*, 137 (1983).
367. D. J. Black and M. E. Orme, Interindividual variability in oral contraceptive disposition, *TIPS 5*, 480 (1984).
368. H. Okada, I. Yamazaki, Y. Ogawa, S. Hirai, T. Yashiki, and H. Mima, Vaginal absorption of a potent luteinizing hormone-releasing hormone analog (leuprolide) in rats I: Absorption by various routes and absorption enhancement, *J. Pharm. Sci. 71*, 1367 (1982).
369. H. Okada, I. Yamazaki, T. Yashiki, and H. Mima, Vaginal absorption of a potent luteinizing hormone-releasing hormone analogue (leuprolide) in rats II: Mechanism of absorption enhancement with organic acids, *J. Pharm. Sci. 72*, 75 (1983).
370. M. H. Burgos and C. E. Roig de Vargas-linares. In, *The Human Vagina* (E. S. E. Hafez and T. N. Evans, ed.), Elsevier/North Holland Biomedical Press, Amsterdam, 1978, pp. 63–69.
371. C. E. Flowers, Jr., L. R. Beck, and W. H. Wilborn, The contraceptive aspects of the anatomy, morphology, and physiology of the vagina. In, *Vaginal Contraception* (G. I. Zatuchni, A. J. Sobreero, J. J. Speidel and J. J. Sciarra, eds.), Harper and Row, Hagerstown, 1979, pp. 13–22.
372. R. E. Trussell and R. F. MacDougal, Vaginal acidity (in vivo glass electrode measurement) in late pregnancy and its relation to the vaginal flora, *Am. J. Obstet. Gynecol. 39*, 77 (1940).
373. T. Yotsuyanagi, A. Molokhia, S. Hwang, N. F. H. Ho, G. L. Flynn and W. I. Higuchi, System approach to vaginal delivery of drugs I: Development of in situ vaginal drug absorption procedure, *J. Pharm. Sci. 64*, 71 (1975).
374. E. Owada, C. R. Behl, S. S. Hwang, L. Suhardja, G. L. Flynn, and W. I. Higuchi, Vaginal drug absorption in rhesus monkeys I: Development of methodology, *J. Pharm. Sci. 66*, 216 (1977).

375. S. Hwang, E. Owada, T. Yotsuyanagi, L. Suhardja, G. L. Flynn, and W. I. Higuchi, Systems approach to vaginal delivery of drugs II: In situ vaginal absorption of unbranched aliphatic alcohols, *J. Pharm. Sci. 65*, 1574 (1976).
376. S. Hwang, E. Owada, L. Suhardja, N. F. H. Ho, G. L. Flynn, and W. I. Higuchi, Systems approach to vaginal delivery of drugs V: In situ vaginal absorption of 1-alkanoic acids, *J. Pharm. Sci. 66*, 781 (1977).
377. C. R. Behl, System approach to the study of vaginal drug absorption in rhesus monkey, Ph.D. Thesis, University of Michigan, Ann Arbor, 1979.
378. G. L. Flynn, N. F. H. Ho, S. Hwang, E. Owada, A. Molokhla, C. R. Behl, W. I. Higuchi, T. Yotsuyanagi, Y. Shah, and J. Park, Interfacing matrix release and membrane absorption—analysis of steroid absorption from a vaginal device in the rabbit doe. In, *Controlled Release Polymeric formulations* (D. R. Paul and F. W. Harris, eds.), *Am. Chem. Soc.*, Washington, D.C., 1976, p. 87.
379. D. R. Mishell, Jr., M. Talas, A. F. Parlow and D. L. Moyer, Contraception by means of a Silastic vaginal ring impregnated with medroxyprogesterone acetate, *Am. J. Obstet. Gynecol. 107*, 100 (1970).
380. D. R. Mishell, Jr., M. Lumkin, S. Stone, Inhibition of ovulation with cyclic use of progestrone-impregnated intravaginal devices, *Am. J. Obstet. Gynecol. 113*, 927 (1972).
381. M. R. Henzl, D. R. Mishell, Jr., J. G. Velazquez, and W. E. Leitch, Basic studies for prolonged progestogen administration by vaginal devices, *Am. J. Obstet. Gynecol. 117*, 101 (1973).
382. N. H. Lauersen and K. H. Wilson, The abortifacient effects of a newly developed vaginal silastic device impregnated with an 0.5% concentration of 15(5)-15-methyl-prostaglandin-F2(alpha)-methyl ester in the first trimester, *Contraception 13*, 697 (1976).
383. A. Victor and D. B. Johnson, Contraceptive rings: self-administered treatment governed bleeding, *Contraception 16*, 137 (1977).
384. D. R. Mishell, Jr., D. E. Moore, I. Roy, P. F. Brenner, and M. A. Page, Clinical performance and endocrine profiles with contraceptive vaginal rings containing a combination of estradiol and d-norgestrel, *Am. J. Obstet. Gynecol. 130*, 55 (1978).
385. T. M. Jackanicz, Levonorgestrel and estradiol release from an improved contraceptive vaginal ring, *Contraception 24*, 323 (1981).
386. E. Diczfalusy and B-M. Landgren, Some pharmacokinetic and pharmacodynamic properties of vaginal delivery systems that release small amounts of progestogens at a near zero-order rate. In, *Long-Acting Contraceptive Delivery Systems* (G. I.

Zatuchni, A. J. Sobrero, J. J. Speidel and J. J. Sciarra, eds.), Harper and Row, Hagerstown, 1984, pp. 213–227.

387. E. S. Nuwayser, D. L. Williams, P. M. Meier, T. C. Wu, S. F. Merchant, and J. H. Kerrigan, A microcapsule system for drug delivery. In, *Proceedings of Drug Delivery Systems* (H. L. Gabelnick, ed.), U.S. Department of Health, Education, and Welfare, Bethesda, Maryland, 1976, pp. 193–251.

388. D. L. Gardner, A. J. Patnaus and D. L. Fink, Steroid release from microcapsules. In, *Proceedings of Drug Delivery Systems* (H. L. Gabelnick, ed.), U.S. Department of Health, Education, and Welfare, Bethesda, Maryland, 1976, pp. 193–251.

389. D. L. Gardner, D. J. Fink, and C. R. Hassler, Potential delivery of contraceptive agents to the female reproductive tract. In, *Controlled Release of Pesticides and Pharmaceuticals* (D. H. Lewis, ed.), Plenum Press, New York, 1981, pp. 99–109.

390. G. A. Digenis, M. Jay, R. M. Beihn, T. R. Tice, and L. R. Beck, External scintigraphy in the study of long-acting contraceptive delivery systems. In, *Long-Acting Contraceptive Delivery Systems* (G. I. Zatuchni, A. J. Sobrero, J. J. Speidel, and J. J. Sciarra, eds.), Harper and Row, Hagerstown, 1984, pp. 241–245.

391. A. Victor, Vaginal absorption of contraceptive steroids. In, *Long-Acting Contraceptive Delivery Systems* (G. I. Zatuchni, A. J. Sobrero, J. J. Speidel and J. J. Sciarra, eds.), Harper and Row, Hagerstown, 1984, pp. 241–245.

392. Y. W. Chien, S. Y. Mares, J. Berg, S. Huber, H. J. Lambert, and K. F. King, Controlled drug release from polymeric delivery devices III: In vitro-in vivo correlation for intravaginal release of ethynodiol diacetate from silicone devices in rabbits, *J. Pharm. Sci. 64*, 1776 (1975).

393. I. Sivin, D. R. Mishell, Jr., A. Victor, S. Diaz, F. A. Sanchez, N. C. Nielsen, O. Akinla, T. Pyorala, E. Coutinho, A. Faundes, S. Roy, P. Brenner, T. Ahren, M. Pavez, V. Brache, O. F. Giwa-Osagie, M. O. Fason, B. Zausner-Guelman, E. Darze, J. C. Silva, J. Diaz, T. M. Jackanicz, J. Stern, and H. Nash, A multicenter study of levonorgestrel-estradiol contraceptive vaginal rings. II. Subjective and objective measure of effects, *Contraception 24*, 359 (1981).

394. G. E. Egli, and M. Newton, The transport of carbon particles in the human female reproductive tract, *Fertil. Steril. 12*, 151 (1961).

395. D. H. de Boer, Transport of particulate matter through the human female genital tract, *J. Reprod. Fertil. 28*, 295 (1972).

396. N. S. Mason, D. V. S. Gupta, D. W. Keller, R. S. Youngquist, and R. S. Sparks, Microencapsulation of progestrone for contraception by intracervical injection. In, *Biomedical*

Applications of Microencapsulation (F. Lim, ed.), CRC Press, Florida, 1984, pp. 76–84.
397. P. Lahteenmaki, H. Kurunmaki, T. Luukkainen, P. O. A. Lahteenmaki, K. Ratsula, J. Toivonen, Development of intracervical steroid-releasing system. In, *Long-Acting Contraceptive Delivery Systems* (G. I. Zatuchni, A. J. Sobrero, J. J. Speidel, and J. J. Sciarra, eds.), Harper and Row, Hagerstown, MD, 1984, pp. 595–600.
398. H. M. Hasson, Morphologic features affecting IUD performance. In, *IUD Technology* (E. S. E. Hafez and W. A. A. Van Os, eds.), G. K. Hall Medical Publishers, Boston, 1980, pp. 13–19.
399. O. Puroinen and H. L. Kaihola, Uterine size measured by ultrasound during the menstrual cycle, *Acta Obstet. Gynecol. Scand. 54*, 247 (1975).
400. H. Tatum, Clinical aspects of intrauterine contraception: Circumspection 1976. In, *Modern Trends in Infertility and Conception Control* (E. Wallach and R. Kempers, eds.), Williams and Wilkins, Baltimore, 1979, p. 333.
401. H. J. Tatum, Intrauterine contraception, *Am. J. Obstet. Gynecol. 112*, 1000 (1972).
402. C. C. Chang and H. J. Tatum, Effects of intrauterine copper wire on resorption of fetuses in rats, *Contraception 11*, 79 (1975).
403. F. Hefnawi, O. Kandil, G. Askalani, I. Serour, K. Zaki, F. Nasr, M. Mousa, Mode of action of the copper IUD: effect on endometrium copper and cervical mucus sperm migration. In, *Analysis of Intrauterine Contraception* (F. Hefnawi and S. Segal, eds.), North-Holland Publishing Co., Amsterdam, 1975, p. 459.
404. T. Tamaya, Y. Nakata, Y. Ohno, S. Nioka, N. Furuta, and H. Okada, The mechanism of action of the copper intrauterine device, *Fertil. Steril. 27*, 767 (1976).
405. B. Pharriss and C. Mitchell, Values of steroidal intrauterine contraception for developing countries, *J. Steroid Biochem. 11*, 469 (1979).
406. J. J. Sciarra, A. Scommengna and G. I. Zatuchi, Research and new developments in interuterine contraception. In, *IUD Technology* (E. S. E. Hafez and A. J. M. Audebert, eds.), MTP Press, Lancaster, 1982, pp. 165–174.
407. G. F. Odland, Structure of the skin. In, *Biochemistry and Physiology of the Skin* (L. A. Goldsmith, ed.), Oxford University Press, New York, 1983, pp. 3–63.
408. R. Scheuplein, Mechanisms of percutaneous absorption II: Transient diffusion and the relative importance of various routes of skin penetration, *J. Invest. Dermatol. 45*, 334 (1967).
409. R. J. Scheuplein, Mechanism of percutaneous absorption, *J. Invest. Dermatol. 48*, 79 (1967).

410. W. J. Albery and J. Hadgraft, Percutaneous absorption: *In vivo* experiments, *J. Pharm. Pharmacol. 31*, 140 (1979).
411. T. Higuchi, Physical chemical analysis of the percutaneous absorption process from creams and ointments, *J. Soc. Cosmet. Chem. 11*, 85 (1960).
412. A. M. Kligman, A biological brief on percutaneous absorption, *Drug Develop. Ind. Pharm. 9*, 521 (1983).
413. J. Hadgraft, Percutaneous absorption: possibilities and problems, *Int. J. Pharm. 16*, 255 (1983).
414. R. J. Scheuplein and I. H. Blank, Permeability of the skin, *Physiol. Rev. 51*, 702 (1971).
415. R. H. Guy and H. I. Maibach, Drug delivery to local subcutaneous structures following topical administration, *J. Pharm. Sci. 72*, 1375 (1983).
416. J. Wepierre and J-P. Marty, Percutaneous absorption of drugs, *Trends Pharmacol. Sci. 1*, 23 (1979).
417. J. Wepierre, Facteurs physiques et physiologiques intervenant dans l'absorption percutanee des medicaments. In, *Actualités Pharmacologiques*, 31e serie, Masson, Paris, 1979, pp. 170–202.
418. J. E. Shaw, Development of transdermal therapeutic systems, *Drug Dev. Ind. Pharm. 9*, 579 (1983).
419. S. K. Chandrasedaran, Controlled release of scopolamine for prophylaxis of motion sickeness, *Drug Dev. Ind. Pharm. 9*, 627 (1983).
420. W. R. Good, Transderm[R]-Nitro controlled delivery of nitroglycerin via the transdermal route, *Drug Dev. Ind. Pharm. 9*, 647 (1983).
421. A. Karim, Transdermal absorption: a unique opportunity for a constant delivery of nitroglycerin, *Drug Dev. Ind. Pharm. 9*, 671 (1983).
422. J. E. Shaw, Pharmacokinetics of nitroglycerin and clonidine delivered by the transdermal route, *Am. Heart J. 108*, 217 (1984).
423. D. L. Sekura and J. Scala, The percutaneous absorption of alkylmethyl sulfoxide, *Adv. Biol. Skin 12*, 257 (1972).
424. R. J. Folkman and H. I. Maibach, Percutaneous penetration of hydrocortisone with urea, *Arch. Dermatol. 109*, 58 (1974).
425. R. E. Stoughton, Enhanced percutaneous penetration with 1-dodecylazacycloheptan-2-one (Azone), *Arch. Dermatol. 118*, 474 (1982).
426. R. E. Stoughton and W. O. McClure, Azone[R]: A new nontoxic enhancer of cutaneous penetration, *Drug Dev. Ind. Pharm. 9*, 725 (1983).
427. N. Baker and J. Hadgraft, Faciliated percutaneous absorption: a model system, *Int. J. Pharm. 8*, 193 (1981).

428. N. Bodor, J. Zupan, and S. Selk, Improved delivery through biological membranes VII. Dermal delivery of cromoglycic acid (cromolyn) via its prodrugs, *Int. J. Pharm. 7*, 63 (1980).
429. C. D. Yu, J. L. Fox, N. F. H. Ho, and W. I. Higuchi, Physical model of evaluation of topical prodrug delivery-simultaneous transport and bioconversion of vidarabine-5'-valerate II: Parameter determinations, *J. Pharm. Sci. 68*, 1341 (1979).
430. C. D. Yu, J. L. Fox, N. F. H. Ho, and W. I. Higuchi, Physical model evaluation of topical prodrug delivery-simultaneous transport and bioconversion of vidarabine-5'-valerate II: parameter determinations, *J. Pharm. Sci. 86*, 1347 (1979).
431. J. Hadgraft, Theoretical aspects of metabolism in the epidermis, *Int. J. Pharm. 4*, 229 (1980).
432. R. H. Guy and J. Hadgraft, Percutaneous metabolism with saturable enzyme kinetics, *Int. J. Pharm. 11*, 187 (1982).
433. R. C. Scott and P. H. Dugard, A potential model for studying absorption through abnormal stratum corneum, *J. Pharm. Pharmacol. 34*, 35 (1982).
434. C. R. Behl, E. E. Linn, G. L. Flynn, N. F. H. Ho, W. I. Higuchi, and C. L. Pierson, Permeation of skin and eschar by antiseptics II: influence of controlled burns on the permeation of phenol, *J. Pharm. Sci. 72*, 397 (1983).
435. J. H. Trueblood, R. M. Rossomondo, W. H. Carlton and L. A. Wilson, Corneal contact times of ophthalmic vehicles. Evaluation by microscintigraphy, *Arch. Ophthalmol. 93*, 127 (1975).
436. H. Benson, Permeability of the cornea to topically applied drugs, *Arch. Ophthalmol. 91*, 313 (1974).
437. J. W. Shell, Ophthalmic drug delivery systems, *Surv. Ophthalmol. 29*, 117 (1984).
438. A. Mitra, Passive and facilitated transport of pilocarpine across the corneal membrane of the rabbit, Ph.D. Thesis, University of Kansas, 1983.
439. E. Tomlinson, S. S. Davis, O. Olejnik, and C. G. Wilson, Altered ocular disposition of sodium cromoglycate upon ion-pair and complex coacervate formation with dodecylbenzyldimethylammonium chloride, *J. Pharm. Pharmacol. 31*, 749 (1981).
440. V. H. L. Lee, P. T. Urrea, R. E. Smith and D. J. Schanzlin, Ocular drug bioavailability from topically applied liposomes, *Surv. Ophthalmol. 29*, 335 (1985).
441. C. P. Wei, J. A. Anderson, and I. Leopold, Ocular absorption and metabolism of topically applied epinephrine and a dipivalyl ester of epinephrine. *Invest. Ophthalmol. Vis. Sci. 17*, 315 (1978).
442. S. S. Chrai and J. R. Robinson, Ocular evaluation of methylcellulose vehicle in albino rabbits, *J. Pharm. Sci. 63*, 1218 (1974).

443. T. F. Patton and J. R. Robinson, Ocular evaluation of polyvinyl alcohol, *J. Pharm. Sci. 64*, 1312 (1975).
444. C. A. Alder, D. M. Maurice and M. E. Patterson, The effect of viscosity of the vehicle on the penetration of fluorescein into the human eye, *Exp. Eye. Res. 11*, 34 (1971).
445. H. W. Hui and J. R. Robinson, Effect of particle dissolution rate on ocular drug bioavailability, *J. Pharm. Sci. 75*, 280 (1986).
446. R. E. Stratford, D. C. Yang, M. A. Redell and V. H. L. Lee, Effects of topically applied liposomes on disposition of epinephrine and insulin in the albino rabbit eye, *Int. J. Pharm. 13*, 263 (1983).
447. R. E. Stratford, D. C. Yang, M. A. Redell and V. H. L. Lee, Ocular distribution of liposome-encapsulated epinephrine and inulin in the albino rabbit, *Curr. Eye. Res. 2*, 377 (1983).
448. G. Smolin, M. Okumoto, S. Feiler, D. Condon, Idoxuridine-liposome therapy for herpes simplex keratitis, *Am. J. Ophthalmol. 91*, 220 (1981).
449. H. E. Schaeffer and D. L. Krohn, Liposomes in topical drug delivery, *Invest. Ophthalmol. Vis. Sci. 22*, 220 (1982).
450. M. Barza, J. Baum, F. Szoka, Pharmacokinetics of subconjunctival liposome-encapsulated gentamicin in normal rabbit eyes, *Invest. Ophthalmol. Vis. Sci. 25*, 486 (1984).
451. J. W. Shell and R. W. Baker, Diffusion systems for controlled release of drugs to the eye, *Ann. Ophthalmol. 6*, 1037 (1974).
452. R. C. Capozza, L. Sendelbeck, W. J. Balkenhol, Preparation and evaluation of a bioerodible naltrexone delivery system. In, *Polymeric Delivery Systems*: Midland Macromolecular Monographs, Vol. 5, Gordon and Breach, New York, 1978, pp. 59–73.
453. H. Bundgaard, Drug targeting: Prodrugs. In, *Topics in Pharmaceutical Sciences 1983* (D. D. Breimer and P. Speiser, eds.), Elsevier Science Publishers, 1983, pp. 329–343.
454. N. Bodor, Novel approaches to the design of safer drugs: soft drugs and site-specific chemical delivery systems, *Adv. Drug Res. 13*, 255 (1984).
455. C. R. Alving, Delivery of liposome-encapsulated drugs to macrophages, *Pharmac. Ther. 22*, 407 (1983).
456. C. A. Hunt, H. Kinada, M. Raeder-Shikorr, K. Hirano, J. Nakamura, R. Abra, and H. Screier, Liposomes, Are they effective drug carriers? In, *Topics in Pharmaceutical Sciences 1983* (D. D. Breimer and P. Speiser, eds.), Elsevier Science Publishers, 1983, pp. 257–263.
457. K. J. Widder and A. E. Senyei, Magnetic microspheres: A vehicle for selective targeting of drugs, *Pharmac. Ther. 20*, 377 (1983).

458. P. Couvreur, B. Kante, L. Grislain, M. Roland, and P. Speiser, Toxicity of polyalkylcyanoacrylate nanoparticles II: Doxorubicin-loaded nanoparticles. *J. Pharm. Sci. 71*, 790 (1982).
459. D. C. Edwards, Targeting potential and antibody conjugates, *Pharmac. Ther. 23*, 147 (1983).
460. R. B. Bankert, Development and use of monoclonal antibodies in the treatment of cancer, *Cancer Drug Delivery, 1*, 251 (1984).
461. R. Obrist, Monoclonal antibodies as drug carriers in oncology, *Trends Pharmacol. Sci., 4*, 375 (1983).
462. U. Zimmermann, Cellular drug-carrier systems and their possible targeting. In, *Targeting of Drugs* (E. P. Goldberg, ed.), John Wiley & Sons, 1983, pp. 153–200.
463. D. A. Lewis and H. O. Alpar, Therapeutic possibilities of drugs encapsulated in erythrocytes, *Int. J. Pharm. 22*, 137 (1984).
464. M. J. Poznansky, Enzyme-protein conjugates: new possibilities for enzyme therapy, *Pharmac. Ther. 21*, 53 (1983).
465. L. Gros, H. Ringsdorf, and H. Schupp, Polymeric antitumor agents on a molecular and on a cellular level, *Agnew. Chem. Int. Engl. 20*, 305 (1981).
466. D. P. Worth, J. N. Harvey, J. Brown, and M. R. Lee, C-*L*-glutamyl-*L*-dopa is a dopamine pro-drug, relatively specific for the kidney in normal subjects, *Clin. Sci. 69*, 207 (1985).
467. V. J. Stella and K. J. Himmelstein, Prodrug and site-specific drug delivery, *J. Med. Chem. 23*, 1275 (1984).
468. J. W. Simpkins, N. Bodor, and A. Enz, Direct evidence for brain-specific release of dopamine from a redox delivery system, *J. Pharm. Sci. 74*, 1033 (1985).
469. A. W. Segeal, E. J. Willis, G. Slvain, C. D. V. Black, and G. Gregoriadis, Morphological observations on the cellular and subcellular destination of intravascularly administered liposomes, *Br. Exp. Pathol. 55*, 320 (1974).
470. L. R. McDougall, J. K. Dunick, M. S. McNamee, and J. P. Kriss, Distribution and fate of synthetic lipid vesicles in the mouse: a combined radiounclide and spin label study, *Proc. Natl. Acad. Sci. USA 71*, 3487 (1974).
471. G. Gregoriadis and E. D. Neerunjun, Control of the rate hepatic uptake and catabolism of liposome-entrapped proteins injected into the rats. Possible therapeutic applications, *Eur. J. Biochem. 47*, 179 (1974).
472. G. Gregoriadis and E. D. Neerunjun, Homing of liposomes to target cells, *Biochem. Biophys. Res. Comm. 65*, 537 (1975).
473. V. T. Marchesi, T. W. Tillack, R. L. Jackson, J. P. Segrest, and R. E. Scott, Chemical characterization and surface orientation of the major glycoprotein of the human erythrocyte membrane, *Proc. Natl. Acad. Sci. USA 69*, 1445 (1972).

474. R. L. Juliano and D. J. Stamp, Lectin-mediated attachment of glycoprotein-bearing liposomes to cells, *Nature 261*, 235 (1976).
475. G. Weissman, D. Bloomgarden, R. Kaplan, C. Cohen, S. Hoffsteine, T. Collins, A. Gotlier and D. Nagle, A general method for the introduction of enzymes by means of immunoglobulin-coated liposomes of deficient cells, *Proc. Natl. Acad. Sci. USA 72*, 88 (1975).
476. G. Gregoriadis, A. Meehan and M. M. Mah, Interactions of antibody-bearing small unilamellar liposomes with target free antigen *in vitro* and *in vivo*, *Biochem. J. 200*, 203 (1981).
477. G. Poste, R. Kirsch, and T. Koestler, The challenge of liposome targeting in vivo. In, *Liposome Technology*, Vol. III. *Targeted Drug Delivery and Biological Interaction* (G. Gregoriadis, ed.), CRC Press, Boca Raton, 1984, pp. 1–28.
478. M. J. Poznansky and R. L. Juliano, Biological approaches to the controlled drug delivery of drugs: A critical review, *Pharmacol. Rev. 36*, 277 (1985).
479. R. L. Magin and M. R. Niesman, Temperature-dependent drug release from large unilammellar liposomes, *Cancer Drug Delivery 1*, 109 (1984).
480. J. N. Weinstein, R. D. Klausner, T. Innerarity, E. Ralston, and R. Blumental, Phase transition release, a new approach to the interaction of proteins with lipid vesicles: Application to lipoproteins, *Biochim. Biophys. Acta 647*, 270 (1981).
481. V. P. Torchilin, M. I. Tatisov, and V. N. Smirnov, Magnetic Sephadex as a carrier for enzyme immobilization and drug targeting, *J. Biomed. Mater. Res. 19*, 461 (1985).
482. M. Kanke, G. H. Simmons, D. L. Weiss, B. A. Bivins, and P. P. Deluca, Clearance of ^{141}Cr-labeled microspheres from blood and distribution in specific organs following intravenuous and intraarterial administration in beagle dogs, *J. Pharm. Sci. 69*. 755 (1980).
483. J. J. Burger, E. Tomlinson, E. M. A. Mulder and J. G. McVie, Albumin microspheres for intraarterial tumor targeting. I. Pharmaceutical aspects, *Int. J. Pharm. 23*, 333 (1985).
484. R. J. W. Blanchard, I. Grotenhuis, J. W. LaFare, and J. F. Perry, Blood supply to hepatic V2 carcinoma implants as measured by radioactive microspheres, *Proc. Soc. Exp. Biol. Med. 118*, 465 (1965).
485. B. Lindell, K. F. Aronseh, U. Rothman, and H. O. Sjogren, The circulation in liver tissue and experimental liver metastases before and after embolization of the liver artery, *Res. Exp. Med. 171*, 63–70 (1977).
486. S. Dakhil, W. Ensminger, K. Cho, Niederhuber, K. Doan, and R. Wheller, Improved regional selectivity of hepatic arterial BCNU with degradable microsphers, *Cancer 50*, 631 (1982).

487. R. F. Tuma, J. O. Forsberg, and B. Agerup, Enhanced uptake of actinomycin D in the dog kidney by simultaneous injection of degradable starch microspheres into the renal artery, *Cancer 50*, 1 (1982).
488. T. Kato, R. Nemoto, H. Mori, M. Takahashi, Y. Tamakawa, and M. Harada, Arterial chemoembolization with microencapsulated anti-cancer drug, *JAMA 245*, 1123 (1981).
489. S. Benita, Microcapsules: New applications and characterization, *Labo-Pharma. Probl. Tech. 32*, 694 (1984).
490. J. T. Doluisio and L. W. Dittert, Influence of repetitive dosing of tetracyclines on biological half-life in serum, *Clin. Pharmacol. Ther. 8*, 222 (1974).

2

Theory of Mass Transfer

RONALD R. BURNETTE / University of Wisconsin, Madison, Wisconsin

I. INTRODUCTION

Mass transport can be due to either random motion of molecules (diffusion) or bulk fluid motion (convection). The emphasis in this chapter will be on diffusional transport, since in the systems to be described bulk flow effects can generally be neglected. The approach to be taken is to place diffusional processes on a firm thermodynamic foundation, with a discussion of all assumptions employed. Numerical examples will be provided to further illustrate the points being made. Some excellent texts describing the necessary thermodynamic background [1,2] and those dealing with the general subject of mass transport and diffusional processes [3–6] are available. There are also some excellent summaries and reviews [7–10] dealing specifically with mass transport and how it pertains to pharmaceutical systems and biological membranes. It is hoped that this introductory chapter on mass transport will provide an appreciation for the wide applicability of mass transport analysis and will develop an intuitive feel for diffusional processes. In addition, the references cited should provide a good starting point for further study.

II. RANDOM WALK INTERPRETATION OF DIFFUSION

When a drop of dye is placed in a beaker of water at constant temperature one notices that the dye tends to diffuse throughout the water, eventually giving the solution a uniform color. At the molecular level, the dye molecules can be viewed as being in a state of continual random motion. As such, each dye molecule can move in any direction with equal probability. The reason that molecules diffuse away from their source is that there are more dye molecules at the source than in the bulk solution (initially). Therefore more molecules can move away from the source than toward the source. At equilibrium, when a uniform color exists throughout the beaker of water, the dye molecules are uniformly distributed and no further net movement is detectable. For two dimensions, this is illustrated

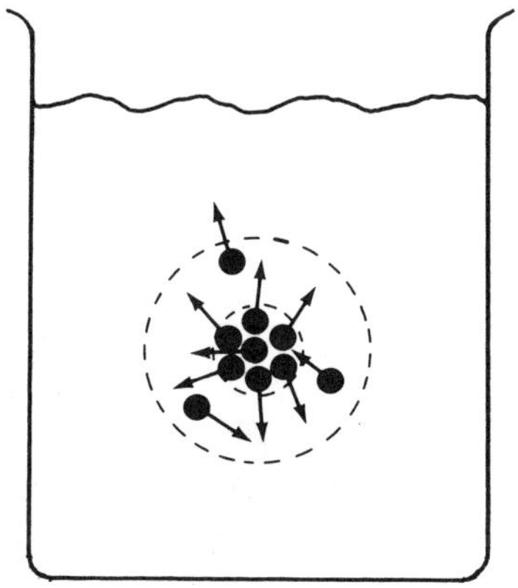

Fig. 1 Diffusion of a drop of dye, which was placed into a beaker of solvent. The two dotted rings represent imaginary boundaries and help to visualize that the net flux is away from the drop of dye into the bulk solution.

in Figure 1. This type of analysis has been employed by Burnette [11] to describe the movement of a solute molecule traversing the skin.

III. FICK'S FIRST AND SECOND LAW [12,13]

A. Free Energy Interpretation of Diffusion

In general, the partial molar free energy of a solute in solution is given by

$$\mu = \mu^0 + RT \ln a \tag{1}$$

where μ is the partial molar free energy, μ^0 is the partial molar free energy in the standard state, R is the universal gas constant, T is the absolute temperature, and a is the activity of the solute. If the solution is dilute, it can be treated as ideal and Eq. (1) may then be written as

$$\mu = \mu^0 + RT \ln C \tag{2}$$

where C is the molar concentration of the solute. Throughout this chapter, we will assume that the solute molecule is uncharged. The change in molar free energy $d\mu$ due to a concentration gradient dC is then

$$\frac{d\mu}{dC} = \frac{d}{dC}(\mu^0 + RT \ln C) \tag{3}$$

or

$$d\mu = RT \left(\frac{dC}{C}\right)$$

This molar free energy difference ($d\mu$) is just the work done on the system in transferring a mole of solute from C + dC to C. The work is the force times the distance, or $d\mu = -Fdx$, so

$$F = \frac{-d\mu}{dx} = \frac{-RT}{C}\left(\frac{dC}{dx}\right) \tag{4}$$

where the negative sign arises because C and x increase in opposite directions.

Since μ refers to one mole so does F. When a driving force is applied to a molecule (or particle), the speed of the molecule increases until the frictional force on the molecule equals the driving force on the molecule. This frictional force (F_f) is proportional to the velocity of the molecule, with the proportionality constant (f) being designated as the frictional coefficient, that is,

$$F_f = Nvf \tag{5}$$

where v = velocity in the x direction and N equals the number of molecules per mole (Avogadro's number). Therefore,

$$Nvf = \frac{-RT}{C}\left(\frac{dC}{dx}\right) \tag{6}$$

or

$$Cv = \frac{-RT}{Nf}\left(\frac{dC}{dx}\right) = \frac{-kT}{f}\left(\frac{dC}{dx}\right)$$

where k is Boltzmann's constant and Cv is the flux (J).

$$\therefore J = -\left(\frac{kT}{f}\right)\frac{dC}{dx} \tag{7}$$

Notice that the flux is just the amount of solute crossing a plane of unit surface area, which is normal to the direction of transport, per unit time.

At this point, the flux has been related to a concentration gradient (dC/dx), and, if temperature is held constant, to a proportionality constant (kT/f) which depends on the molecular quantity f. Einstein showed that this proportionality constant is equal to the diffusion coefficient (D), which is a macroscopic experimentally measurable quantity.

$$\therefore J = -D \left(\frac{dC}{dx}\right) \tag{8}$$

This is the one-dimensional form of Fick's first law. Note the negative sign in Eq. (8), which means that when the concentration gradient is positive, the flux will be in the direction of decreasing concentration, exactly what we observed in our earlier dye diffusion experiment.

As long as we are at steady state (i.e., no time variations in D or C), solutions to Fick's first law provide a completely adequate description of the diffusional process. However, when concentrations are changing with time, as would be the case for a finite amount of dye diffusing from a source, we may know dC/dx at the beginning of the experiment, but the mass flow will continually be changing the concentration gradient. Therefore it is necessary to introduce time as a variable. Eq. (8) then becomes

$$J = -D(x) \left(\frac{\partial C}{\partial x}\right)_t \tag{9}$$

where the partial derivative indicates that the derivative with respect to x is taken at a certain time t. Here the diffusion coefficient has been assumed to be independent of time but can depend on position, hence it is written D(x). Figure 2 depicts the flow of molecules through a rectangular box of length δx and surface area A. From the figure we write

$$J_{in} = J(x) = -D(x) \left[\frac{\partial C(x,t)}{\partial x}\right]_t \tag{10}$$

$$J_{out} = J(x + \delta x) \tag{11}$$

or

$$J_{out} = -D(x) \left[\frac{\partial C(x,t)}{\partial x}\right]_t - \delta \left[D(x) \frac{\partial C(x,t)}{\partial x}\right]_t$$

The change in the amount of solute per unit time inside the rectangular box is the amount of solute which flows into the box

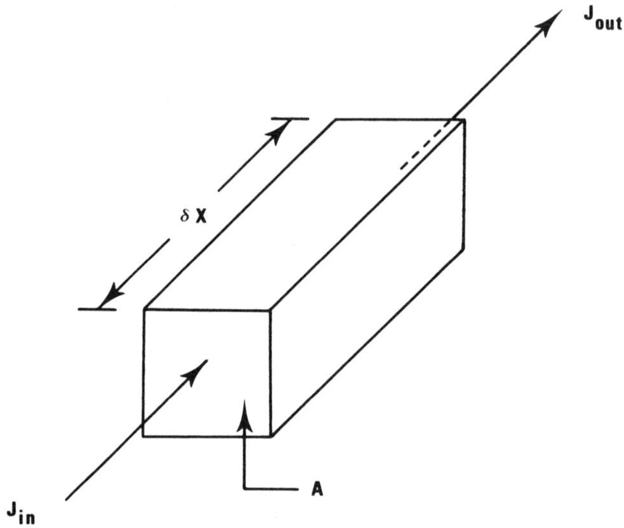

Fig. 2 Mass flow through a rectangular box which has a length equal to δx and a cross sectional area equal to A. J_{in} is the flux into the box and J_{out} is the flux out of the box.

minus the amount of solute which flows out of the box per unit time. This flow equals $J_{in}\, A - J_{out}\, A$, and it must also be equal to

$$\left(\frac{\delta C}{\delta t}\right) V \tag{12}$$

where V is the volume of the rectangular box, so that $V = A\,\delta x$. Therefore,

$$\frac{\delta C}{\delta t} = \frac{(J_{in}\, A - J_{out}\, A)}{A\ \delta x}$$

$$= \frac{-D\left(\frac{\partial C}{\partial x}\right)_t A + \left\{D\left(\frac{\partial C}{\partial x}\right)_t + \delta\left[D\left(\frac{\partial C}{\partial x}\right)_t\right]\right\} A}{A\ \delta x} \tag{13}$$

or

$$\frac{\delta C}{\delta t} = \delta\ \frac{\left[D\left(\frac{\partial C}{\partial x}\right)_t\right]}{\delta x}$$

Taking limits

$$\lim_{\delta t \to o} \frac{\delta C}{\delta t} = \lim_{\delta x \to o} \frac{\delta \left[D \left(\frac{\delta C}{\delta x} \right) \right]_t}{\delta x}$$

gives

$$\frac{\partial C}{\partial t} = \frac{\partial}{\partial x} D \left(\frac{\partial C}{\partial x} \right)_t \tag{14}$$

which is Fick's second law.

If D is independent of position, then Eq. 14 simplifies to

$$\frac{\partial C}{\partial t} = D \left(\frac{\partial^2 C}{\partial x^2} \right) \tag{15}$$

B. Diffusion as an Effective Transport Mechanism over Small Distances

In order to assess whether or not diffusion is an effective mechanism over small distances, we need to have some way of calculating the distance a molecule (or particle) moves in a given length of time. At first glance, trying to find the mean distance moved by the particle might seem like a good idea. However, in a diffusional process, molecules move randomly so the mean distance moved would be zero. This difficulty can be circumvented by calculating the mean squared distance moved in a given time interval and then taking the positive square root of this value. A relationship between the mean squared distance and time can be found by using the general solution to Fick's second law and solving it specifically for an instantaneous plane source placed in liquid perpendicular to the direction of mass transport, as shown in Figure 3.

The general solution to Fick's second law for this case has the following form

$$C(x,t) = k_o \, t^{-1/2} \, e^{-x^2/4Dt} \tag{16}$$

where k_o and D are constants.

The validity of this solution can be checked by substituting it into Fick's second law. Letting the total number of solute molecules be n_o, k_o can be evaluated as follows

$$dn = C(x,t) \, dV = A \, C(x,t) \, dx \tag{17}$$

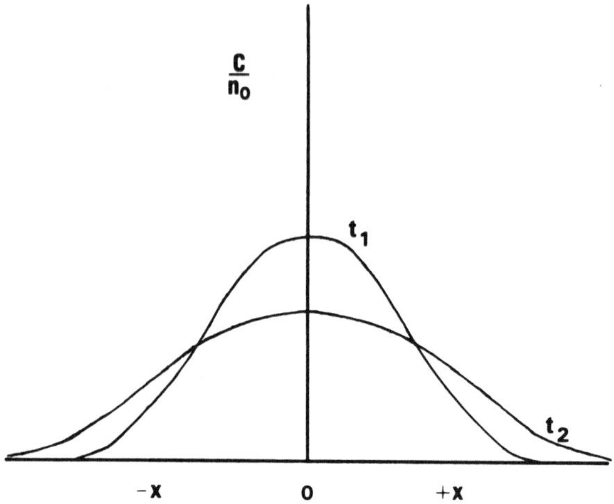

Fig. 3 A plot of normalized concentration (C/n_o) versus position (x). Diffusion is from a plane source perpendicular to the plane of the paper. The curves for time t_1 and t_2 represent snap shots of the distribution of diffusing molecules at times t_1 and t_2. At t = 0, all the diffusing molecules (n_o) are present at x = 0. This represents a volume equal to zero so that the concentration at t = 0 is infinity.

or

$$\int_0^{n_o} dn = A \int_{-\infty}^{\infty} C(x,t)\,dx = k_o A \int_{-\infty}^{\infty} t^{-1/2} e^{-x^2/4Dt} dx$$

or

$$n_o = 2k_o A\,(\pi D)^{1/2}$$

$$\therefore k_o = \frac{n_o}{2A\,(\pi D)^{1/2}} \tag{18}$$

thus

$$C(x,t) = \left[\frac{n_o}{2A\,(\pi D t)^{1/2}}\right] e^{-x^2/4Dt} \tag{19}$$

Now let P(x,t) dx be the probability that a solute molecule will be found between x and x + dx. Using this definition of probability, P(x,t) dx is equal to the number of solute molecules present in the space between x and x + dx divided by the total number of solute molecules (n_o). Therefore,

$$P(x,t)\ dx = \frac{C(x,t)\ dV}{n_o} = \frac{C(x,t)\ A\ dx}{n_o} \tag{20}$$

$$P(x,t)\ dx = \left[\frac{e^{-x^2/4Dt}}{2\ (\pi Dt)^{1/2}}\right] dx \tag{21}$$

Given that the definition of the mean squared distance $\overline{x^2}$ is just the sum over all x^2 weighted by its probability of occurrence, we have

$$\overline{x^2} = \int_{-\infty}^{\infty} x^2\ P\ (x,t)\ dx \tag{22}$$

Substitution for P(x,t) dx via Eq. (21) gives

$$\overline{x^2} = \int_{-\infty}^{\infty} \left[\frac{x^2}{2\ (\pi Dt)^{1/2}}\right] e^{-x^2/4Dt} dx = 2Dt \tag{23}$$

Thus, we get the very simple relationship

$$\overline{x^2} = 2Dt \tag{24}$$

Eq. (24), which relates the mean squared distance moved in a time t to the diffusion coefficient, D, was first derived by Einstein [14]. Typical diffusion coefficients for molecules in liquids or membranes range from 10^{-5} to 10^{-12} $cm^2\ sec^{-1}$.

Example 1:

What is the time required for a protein molecule of molecular weight 20,000 to cross a red blood cell whose diameter is 7×10^{-4} cm or to traverse the length of a 10-cm long nerve cell? Assume that the protein's diffusion coefficient is 8×10^{-7} $cm^2\ sec^{-1}$.

Solution:

$$t = \frac{\overline{x^2}}{2D} = \frac{(7 \times 10^{-4}\ \text{cm})^2}{2\ (8 \times 10^{-7}\ \text{cm}^2\ \text{sec}^{-1})} = 0.3\ \text{sec (red blood cell)}$$

$$t = \frac{(1 \times 10^{1}\ \text{cm})^2}{2\ (8 \times 10^{-7}\ \text{cm}^2\ \text{sec}^{-1})} = 6.25 \times 10^{7}\ \text{sec} \approx 2\ \text{years (nerve cell)}$$

Thus diffusion is an efficient means of transport but only if the distances to be traversed are small.

C. The Size of a Molecule and Its Ability to Diffuse

As the molecular weight of a solute molecule increases, one might expect that the ability of the molecule to diffuse would decrease. This makes intuitive sense because the larger the molecule, the more frictional resistance to its motion will be experienced. This concept was placed on firm theoretical ground by Stokes. His calculations are based on the following assumptions:

1. The diffusing solute molecule can be approximated as a slowly moving solid sphere.
2. The solute molecule is large relative to the solvent molecules. This allows the solvent to be regarded as continuous.
3. Steady-state conditions are assumed.
4. The solvent is isotropic and incompressible.

If these assumptions are made, the following result (Stokes' law) is obtained:

$$F_f = 6\ \pi r \eta v \tag{25}$$

where F_f is the frictional force, r the solute molecule's radius, v the solute molecule's velocity, and η is the viscosity of the diffusing medium. For a more complete derivation, see Tanford [15] or Page [16]. The frictional force can also be expressed as

$$F_f = fv \tag{26}$$

where f is the frictional coefficient. Thus $f = 6\ \pi r \eta$, or, since $D = kT/f$, we have

$$D = \frac{kT}{6\pi r \eta} \tag{27}$$

which is the Stokes-Einstein equation.

Example 2:

A spherical colloidal particle has a diameter of 1×10^{-7} cm. Estimate how long it will take this particle to diffuse through a distance of 1 cm in water at 20.0°C. The viscosity of water equals 1.002×10^{-3} kg m^{-1} sec^{-1} and Boltzmann's constant equals 1.38×10^{-23} J K^{-1}. Note that 1 J = kg m^2 sec^{-2}.

Solution:

$$D = \frac{kT}{6\pi r \eta} = \frac{(1.38 \times 10^{-23}\ \text{J K}^{-1})\ (293\ \text{K})}{(6\ \pi)\ (5 \times 10^{-8}\ \text{m})\ (1.002 \times 10^{-3}\ \text{kg m}^{-1}\ \text{sec}^{-1})}$$

or

$$D = 4.28 \times 10^{-12}\ \frac{\text{J}}{\text{kg sec}^{-1}} = 4.28 \times 10^{-12}\ \text{m}^2\ \text{sec}^{-1}$$

$$t = \frac{\overline{x^2}}{2D} = \frac{(1 \times 10^{-2}\ \text{m})^2}{2(4.28 \times 10^{-12}\ \text{m}^2\ \text{sec}^{-1})} = 1.17 \times 10^7\ \text{sec} = 135\ \text{days}$$

Note once again that diffusion can indeed be a slow process.

If a molecule can be considered to be a sphere, then the molecular weight of the molecule (MW) is

$$MW = N\rho V = N\rho \left(\frac{4\ \pi r^3}{3}\right) \tag{28}$$

where r is the van der Waal's radius of the molecule and ρ is the molecule's density. Therefore, r is proportional to $(MW)^{1/3}$ or

$$D\ \alpha\ \frac{1}{(MW)^{1/3}} \tag{29}$$

From this proportionality, we can see that D is fairly insensitive to changes in MW. This is particularly true when one considers that most drug molecules have molecular weights in the narrow range of 100–500. Table 1 is a list of several molecules with their diffusion coefficients both experimentally determined and calculated from the proportionality given in Eq. (29). Clearly, in some cases, the

Table 1 Observed and Calculated Diffusion Coefficients of Some Molecules

Molecule	MW	$\left(\frac{MW_1}{MW_2}\right)^{1/3}$	D_{obs} $cm^2\ sec^{-1}$	D_{cal} $cm^2\ sec^{-1}$	% error
H_2O[a]	18	–	2.54×10^{-5}	–	–
CH_3OH[a]	32	0.824[d]	1.37×10^{-5}	2.10×10^{-5}	53
Myoglobin[b]	16,000	–	1.13×10^{-6}	–	–
Insulin[a]	41,000	0.731[e]	8.2×10^{-7}	8.3×10^{-7}	1.2
Hemoglobin[a]	68,000	0.617[e]	6.9×10^{-7}	7.0×10^{-7}	1.4
DNA[c]	135,000	0.491[e]	2.5×10^{-8}	5.6×10^{-7}	124
Urease[a]	470,000	0.324[e]	5.3×10^{-8}	3.7×10^{-7}	5.7

[a]Diffusion coefficients from Ref. 13, p. 824.
[b]Diffusion coefficient from Ref. 33, p. 87.
[c]Diffusion coefficient calculated from f value obtained from Ref. 12, p. 721, assuming the diffusing medium to be H_2O at 20°C.
[d]MW_1 = MW of H_2O and MW_2 = MW of CH_3OH.
[e]MW_1 = MW of myoglobin and MW_2 = MW of insulin, hemoglobin, DNA and urease. Note: Myoglobin was chosen as the reference molecule in this series because it is much larger than the imcompresible solvent (H_2O) and is approximately solid and spherical in shape. Thus, Stokes law should approximately hold for myoglobin.

The diffusion medium in all cases is H_2O at 20°C.

Sample calculation for columns 5 and 6 using myoglobin (Myo) and hemoglobin (Hb).

$$D_{Hb\ cal} = D_{Myo\ obs} \left(\frac{MW_{Myo}}{MW_{Hb}} \right)^{1/3}$$

$$\therefore D_{Hb\ cal} = (1.13 \times 10^{-6}\ cm^2\ sec^{-1})\ (0.617) = 7.0 \times 10^{-7}\ cm^2\ sec^{-1}$$

$$\%\ Error = \left(\frac{D_{Hb\ cal} - D_{Hb\ obs}}{D_{Hb\ obs}} \right) (100\%) = 1.4\%$$

calculated diffusion coefficients differ markedly from their experimentally determined diffusion coefficients. This is because, in these cases, the assumptions on which Stoke's law was derived were not valid. For example, the DNA molecule is rod shaped rather than spherical in shape, and the size of CH_3OH is similar to that of the solvent (H_2O). For a more detailed discussion of Stoke's law and some of its extensions, see Tanford [15].

D. Solute Binding and Its Effect on Diffusion

When a molecule diffuses through a membrane lattice, there may be the possibility of binding. Fick's first law as previously written, however, refers only to the freely diffusible solute molecule. The effect of binding can be introduced as follows:

Let

$$C = C_f + C_b \tag{30}$$

where C_f equals the concentration of the freely diffusible solute and C_b is the concentration of the bound solute. If we can assume that the concentration of the bound solute is directly proportional to the free solute concentration, then

$$C_b = K' C_f \tag{31}$$

where K' is the proportionality constant. Now in one dimension

$$J = -D \frac{dC_f}{dx} \tag{32}$$

or since

$$C = C_f + C_b = (1 + K') C_f$$

we have

$$J = - \left(\frac{D}{1 + K'}\right) \frac{dC}{dx} \tag{33}$$

Thus, reversible adsorption occurring within the membrane can decrease the flux by a factor of 1(1 + K'). Flynn et al. [9] suggested that solute binding may well be the reason why water and other polar molecules have such small diffusion coefficients for the skin.

E. The Variable Diffusion Coefficient and the Concept of a Mean Diffusion Coefficient

There are times when the diffusion coefficient cannot be considered a constant. For example, when a polymer swells due to hydration or the skin becomes hydrated after the application of an occlusive bandage, then the diffusion coefficient can become a function of time and/or position. In such cases, it is simpler to replace the diffusion coefficient (which may be a function of position, time, or solute concentration) with its mean value. Let the diffusion coefficient be a function of an arbitrary variable x; position, time, or concentration. Then the mean value of the diffusion coefficient can be written as

$$\overline{D(x)} = \frac{\int_{x_1}^{x_2} D(x)\,dx}{\int_{x_1}^{x_2} dx} \tag{34}$$

or

$$\overline{D(x)} = \frac{\int_{x_1}^{x_2} D(x)\,dx}{x_2 - x_1} \tag{35}$$

The physical meaning of $\overline{D(x)}$ is depicted in Figure 4. From this figure, we can see that $\overline{D(x)}\ (x_2 - x_1)$ represents the area under a rectangle of height $\overline{D(x)}$ and width $x_2 - x_1$. This area also equals the area under the D(x) versus x curve from to $x = x_1$ to $x = x_2$. As such, $\overline{D(x)}$ represents the average value which D(x) takes on over the interval x_1 to x_2. This technique has been applied by Wu [17] in studies relating to transport across the skin.

Example 3:

Show that the mean squared distance defined in Eq. (22) is consistent with the definition of a mean value as given in Eq. (34).

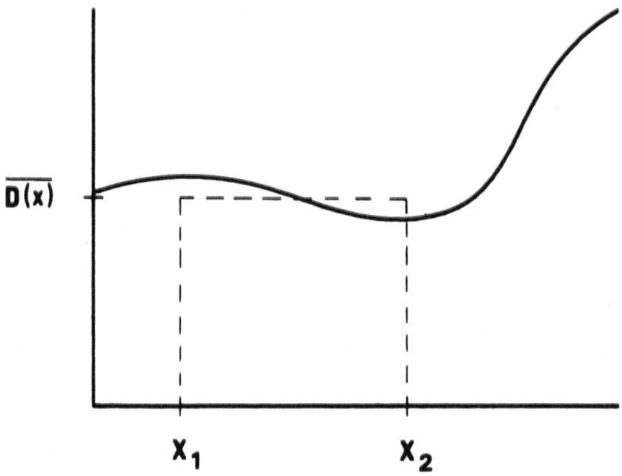

Fig. 4 A plot of D(x) versus x. D(x) is the diffusion coefficient; x is position, time, or concentration; and $\overline{D(x)}$ is the mean diffusion coefficient over the interval from x_1 to x_2.

Solution:

By analogy to Eq. (34) we have

$$\overline{x^2} = \frac{\int_{x_1}^{x_2} x^2 P(x)\, dx}{\int_{x_1}^{x_2} P(x)\, dx}$$

But the range of x covers all possible values of x. Therefore,

$$x_1 = -\infty \text{ and } x_2 = \infty$$

Now the integral of a probability density [P(x)] over all possible values must be equal to unity. Therefore,

$$\int_{-\infty}^{\infty} P(x)\, dx = 1$$

and

$$\overline{x^2} = \int_{-\infty}^{\infty} x^2 \, P(x) \, dx$$

which is Eq. (22).

F. Fick's Second Law in Three Dimensions and Its Coordinate Transformation

Following a derivation identical to that used in the derivation of the one-dimensional form of Fick's second law [Eq. (14)], but extending it to the y and z directions, one obtains the three-dimensional form

$$\frac{\partial C}{\partial t} = \frac{\partial}{\partial x}\left(D\,\frac{\partial C}{\partial x}\right) \frac{\partial}{\partial y}\left(D\,\frac{\partial C}{\partial y}\right) + \frac{\partial}{\partial z}\left(D\,\frac{\partial C}{\partial z}\right) \tag{36}$$

If the diffusion coefficient is constant, we have

$$\frac{\partial C}{\partial t} = D\left(\frac{\partial^2 C}{\partial x^2} + \frac{\partial^2 C}{\partial y^2} + \frac{\partial^2 C}{\partial z^2}\right) \tag{37}$$

At times, the three-dimensional rectangular form of Fick's second law is awkward to use because this form of the equation does not take advantage of the inherent symmetry that may be present in the system under study. For example, cylinders are more easily treated by transforming the rectangular form of Fick's second law into cylindrical coordinates, and spheres are more easily handled by transforming into spherical coordinates. Not only are boundary conditions much easier to deal with, but often times the diffusional process will be independent along one or more of its transformed coordinate axes. The net result is a diffusion equation that is much simpler to solve and one whose solution will be in terms of coordinates more natural for describing the system.

The cylindrical coordinate system is defined by the coordinates r, θ, and z (see Fig. 5), where $x = r\cos\theta$, $y = r\sin\theta$, and $z = z$. By using these relationships for x, y, and z, Fick's second law can be transformed into the following equation

$$\frac{\partial C}{\partial t} = \frac{1}{r}\left[\frac{\partial}{\partial r}\left(r\,D\,\frac{\partial C}{\partial r}\right) + \frac{\partial}{\partial \theta}\left(\frac{D}{r}\,\frac{\partial C}{\partial \theta}\right) + \frac{\partial}{\partial z}\left(r\,D\,\frac{\partial C}{\partial z}\right)\right] \tag{38}$$

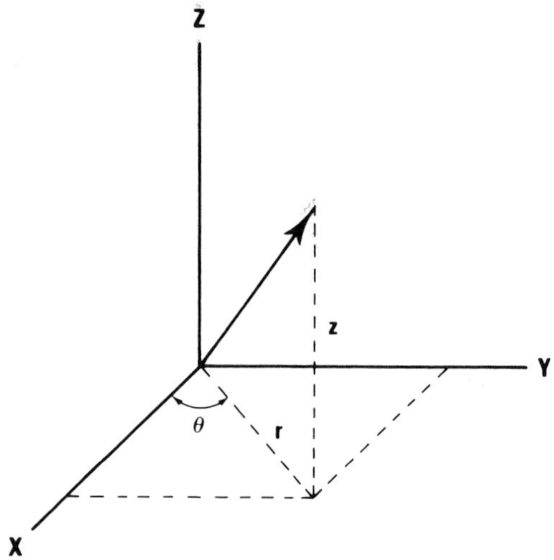

Fig. 5 Cylindrical coordinates (r, θ, and z) and their relationship to rectangular coordinates.

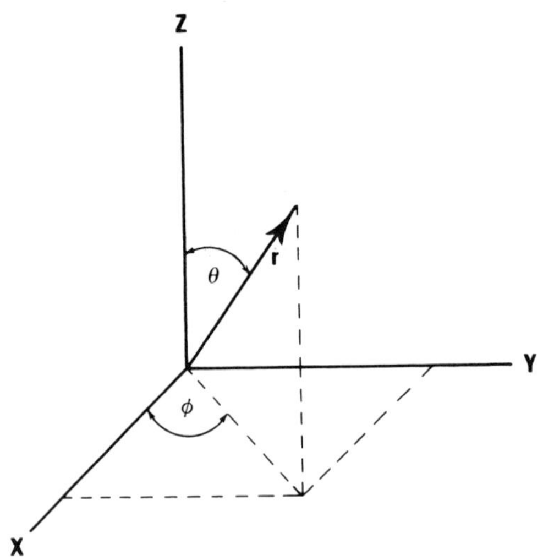

Fig. 6 Spherical coordinates (r, θ, and φ) and their relationship to rectangular coordinates.

Similarly for spherical coordinates (see Fig. 6) we have $x = r \sin\theta \cos\phi$, $y = r \sin\theta \sin\phi$, and $z = r \cos\theta$ which transforms the rectangular form of Fick's second law into

$$\frac{\partial C}{\partial t} = \frac{1}{r^2}\left[\frac{\partial}{\partial r}\left(D\, r^2 \frac{\partial C}{\partial r}\right) + \frac{1}{\sin\theta}\frac{\partial}{\partial \theta}\left(D \sin\theta \frac{\partial C}{\partial \theta}\right) + \frac{D}{\sin^2\theta}\frac{\partial^2 C}{\partial \phi^2}\right] \qquad (39)$$

Example 4:

What form of Fick's second law should be used in studying drug release rates from spherical particles? Assume that the drug is homogenously dispersed throughout the particle and that the particle is uniform in its physical characteristics. Also assume that the diffusion coefficient is constant.

Solution:

Spherical coordinates should be used. Therefore, Eq. (39) is the proper form of Fick's second law to use. Since the particle is uniform and the drug is homogenously dispersed, drug release should not depend on the θ or ϕ coordinates. Fick's second law then becomes

$$\frac{\partial C}{\partial t} = \frac{1}{r^2}\left[\frac{\partial}{\partial r}\left(D\, r^2 \frac{\partial C}{\partial r}\right)\right]$$

Since the diffusion coefficient is a constant

$$\frac{\partial C}{\partial t} = \frac{D}{r^2}\left(r^2 \frac{\partial^2 C}{\partial r^2} + 2r \frac{\partial C}{\partial r}\right)$$

or

$$\frac{\partial C}{\partial t} = D\left(\frac{\partial^2 C}{\partial r^2} + \frac{2}{r}\frac{\partial C}{\partial r}\right)$$

This particular problem has been solved in detail by Guy et al. [18].

IV. PASSIVE DIFFUSION THROUGH A MEMBRANE— THE PARTITION COEFFICIENT

Figure 7 represents a membrane separating two different solutions. Assuming steady state conditions, we have from Fick's first law that

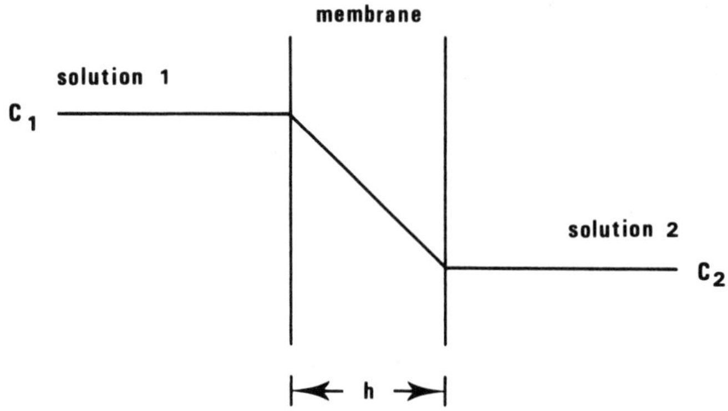

Fig. 7 A membrane of thickness h separating two solutions at concentrations C_1 and C_2. Note that the concentration gradient inside the membrane is linear because steady state conditions were assumed.

$$J = -D \frac{dC}{dx} = -D \left[\frac{C_2 - C_1}{h}\right] = \left(\frac{D}{h}\right) (C_1 - C_2) \tag{40}$$

where C_1 and C_2 are measurable bulk solute concentrations and h is the membrane thickness. The steady state assumption leads to a linear concentration profile within the membrane. This can be seen by application of Fick's second law. At steady state

$$\frac{\partial C}{\partial t} = D \frac{\partial^2 C}{\partial x^2} = 0 \quad \text{thus} \quad \frac{\partial^2 C}{\partial x^2} = 0 \quad \text{and} \quad \frac{\partial C}{\partial x} = C_o \tag{41}$$

where C_o is a constant. Upon integrating Eq. (41), we obtain

$$C = C_o x + C'_o \tag{42}$$

where C'_o is also a constant. From Eq. (42), the linear dependence of C on x can be seen. It is for this reason that the situation depicted in Figure 7 gives

$$\frac{dC}{dx} = \frac{D(C_2 - C_1)}{h} \tag{43}$$

The term h/D is often referred to as a diffusional resistance (R'), thus

$$J = \frac{(C_1 - C_2)}{R'} \tag{44}$$

As R' increases, the flux decreases. This could be due either to a decrease in the diffusion coefficient or to an increase in membrane thickness. Note that Eq. (44) is analogous to Ohm's law from electromagnetic theory:

$$I = \frac{V}{R}$$

Here I is the current, V the voltage, and R is the electrical resistance.

Example 5:

What is the amount of solute which passes through a membrane in 1 hour. Assume $D = 1 \times 10^{-10}\ cm^2\ sec^{-1}$, $h = 2 \times 10^{-3}$ cm, $C_1 = 0.5$ mole l^{-1}, $C_2 \approx 0$, a membrane surface area of 10 cm^2, and a density of unity.

Solution:

$$J = \frac{D}{h}(C_2 - C_1) = \frac{(1 \times 10^{-10}\ cm^2\ sec^{-1})\ (0.5\ mole/1000\ cm^3)}{2 \times 10^{-3}\ cm}$$

or

$$J = 2.5 \times 10^{-11}\ mole\ sec^{-1}\ cm^{-2}$$

$$\text{amount transported} = Amt = JtA$$

or

$$Amt = (2.5 \times 10^{-11}\ mole\ sec^{-1}\ cm^{-2})\ (3600\ sec\ hr^{-1})\ (10\ cm^2)$$

or

$$Amt = 9 \times 10^{-7}\ mole\ hr^{-1}$$

We have assumed, in Figure 7, that the solute molecule is equally soluble in solvents 1 and 2 and the membrane. This is seldom the case because the membrane and solvents generally have different physical chemical characteristics. This results in the solute molecule preferentially partitioning into either the membrane or the solvent. This preferential partitioning may be analyzed by applying Fick's first law to the steady state membrane system shown in Figure 8, which gives

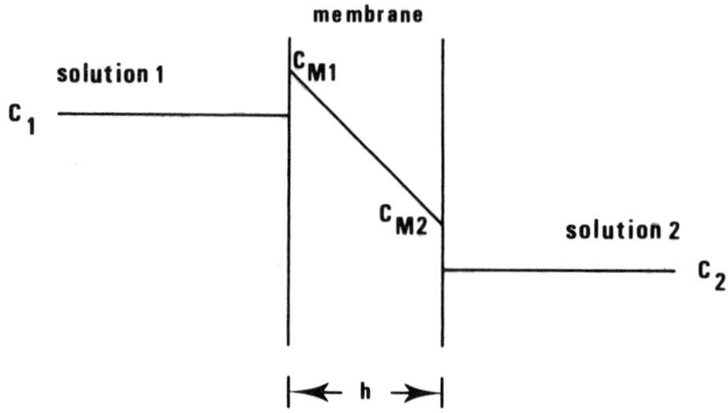

Fig. 8 A membrane of thickness h separated by bulk solutions of concentration C_1 and C_2. Steady-state conditions have been assumed, resulting in a linear concentration gradient inside the membrane. The concentrations of solute immediately inside and outside the membrane are not equal. This is because of the preferential partitioning of the solute into the membrane. C_{M1} and C_{M2} are the membrane solute concentrations at the membrane-bulk solution interface.

$$J = -D\left(\frac{C_{M2} - C_{M1}}{h}\right) \tag{45}$$

where C_{M2} and C_{M1} are the unknown membrane concentrations at the interfaces. In order to express J in terms of the bulk concentrations C_1 and C_2, we assume that equilibrium has been reached at the interfaces, that the temperature is constant, and that the solution are dilute. Then,

$$\mu_1 = \mu_1^o + RT \ln C_1 = \mu_{M1}^o + RT \ln C_{M1} \tag{46}$$

or

$$\ln\left(\frac{C_{M1}}{C_1}\right) = \frac{\mu_1^o - \mu_{M1}^o}{RT}$$

Thus

$$\frac{C_{M1}}{C_1} = e^{(\mu_1^o - \mu_{M1}^o)/RT} = \text{constant} = K_{M1} \tag{47}$$

or

$$\frac{C_{M1}}{C_1} = K_{M1}$$

The constant K_{M1} is a partition coefficient; it is a measure of the relative concentrations of a solute in the membrane and bulk solution at equilibrium.

Similarly

$$K_{M2} = \frac{C_{M2}}{C_2} \tag{48}$$

Therefore

$$J = -D\left[\frac{C_{M2} - C_{M1}}{h}\right] = -D\left[\frac{K_{M2}C_2 - K_{M1}C_1}{h}\right]$$

Often solutions 1 and 2 are similar and the membrane is homogenous, so that

$$K_{M1} \approx K_{M2} \approx K_P \tag{49}$$

where K_P is a general partition coefficient. Then Eq. (48) simplifies to

$$J = -\left(\frac{DK_P}{h}\right)(C_2 - C_1) \tag{50}$$

The set of coefficients DK_P/h is called the permeability coefficient (P). From Eq. (50), it can be observed that as the permeability coefficient increases the flux increases. Experimentally P is obtained by rearranging Eq. (50) and solving for P as in Eq. (51).

$$P = \frac{J}{C_1 - C_2} \tag{51}$$

Notice that the permeability coefficient is a relatively easy parameter to measure, whereas determining the diffusion coefficient, partition coefficient, and membrane thickness separately can be a difficult task. If the objective is only to predict overall fluxes, then permeability coefficients can be very useful. It is necessary to be aware that alterations in the permeability coefficient can be caused by variations in D, K_P, or h.

Solute concentrations on one side of a membrane are often much smaller than on the other side. For example, in a situation where a solute molecule is topically applied to the skin, the concentration on the skin's surface is much greater than in the underlying epidermal layer. This is primarily due to the solute molecule's ability to rapidly diffuse from the epidermis into the systemic circulation, which acts as a sink for solute molecules. When conditions such as this exist, $C_2 \approx 0$ and Eq. (50) becomes

$$J = \frac{DK_P}{h} C = PC \tag{52}$$

where $C = C_1$ in this case.*

Example 6:

What is the maximum flux obtained from topical administration of digitoxin? How much drug can be delivered into the systemic circulation per day, assuming that all the drug that is transported through the skin reaches the systemic circulation? Assume that the principal barrier to diffusion is the uppermost skin layer (the stratum corneum). The following data are given: $K_{M1} = 0.014$, $D = 5.2 \times 10^{-10}$ cm^2 sec^{-1}, stratum corneum thickness = 2×10^{-3} cm, the surface area of the skin covered by a vehicle phase containing digitoxin is 10 cm^2, and the saturation concentration of digitoxin in the vehicle is 0.01 mg/ml.

Solution:

Assume density of the vehicle phase is unity. We use

$$J_{max} \approx \frac{K_{M1}\,D}{h}\,C_s$$

where C_s is the saturation concentration of digitoxin in the vehicle phase. Note that flux is maximized by using a saturated solution of digitoxin. Thus,

$$J_{max} = \frac{(0.014)\ (5.2 \times 10^{-10}\ \text{cm}^2\ \text{sec}^{-1})\ (0.01\ \text{mg/cm}^3)}{2 \times 10^{-3}\ \text{cm}}$$

$$J_{max} = 3.64 \times 10^{-11}\ \text{mg sec}^{-1}\ \text{cm}^{-2}$$

*The author would like to thank P. Mukerjee for helpful discussions concerning this section.

The amount of digitoxin delivered to the systemic circulation per day is

$$\text{Amt} = (J_{max})\ (A)\ (t)$$

$$\text{Amt} = (3.64 \times 10^{-11}\ \text{mg sec}^{-1}\ \text{cm}^{-2})\ (10\ \text{cm}^2)\ (8.64 \times 10^4 \text{sec})$$

$$\text{Amt} = 3.15 \times 10^{-5}\ \text{mg} = 31.5\ \text{ng}$$

This illustrates that, for most drugs, the amount delivered per day is quite small. It is for this reason that only drugs which are highly permeable to the skin and are quite potent can act as effective agents for topical drug delivery. This is the main reason why much current research is being devoted to finding new ways to enhance a drug's permeability through the skin. The reader is referred to Chapter 12 for an evaluation of transdermal drug delivery systems.

V. PASSIVE DIFFUSION THROUGH A MEMBRANE— THE STAGNANT DIFFUSION LAYER

So far in our development, we have assumed that the only barrier to transport has been the membrane itself. However, in any system, the fluid surrounding the membrane becomes less and less well stirred as one approaches the membrane's surface. This effect can be approximated by assuming that there is an unstirred layer of thickness q surrounding the membrane. In this unstirred layer, transport only takes place by diffusion, and the unstirred layer represents an additional diffusional barrier. Figure 9 depicts a membrane with a stagnant diffusion layer on either side of the membrane, and Figure 10 shows an experimental setup for studying this situation. In Figure 9, C_{B1} and C_{B2} are the bulk concentrations on either side of the membrane; C_{I1} and C_{I2} are the concentrations immediately at the surface of the membrane; C_{M1} and C_{M2} are the concentrations actually inside the membrane; q_1 and q_2 are the thicknesses of the stagnant diffusion layers; C_1 and C_2 are the concentrations within the stagnant diffusion layers; and h is the thickness of the membrane, and C_M is the concentration within the membrane. Assuming steady state conditions and equilibrium at the interfaces, we can obtain expressions for C_1, C_2, C_M, and J for the system illustrated in Figure 9. (The derivation which follows is similar to that given in ref. [19].) In general, at steady state,

$$J = -D\,\frac{dC}{dx} = \text{constant} \tag{53}$$

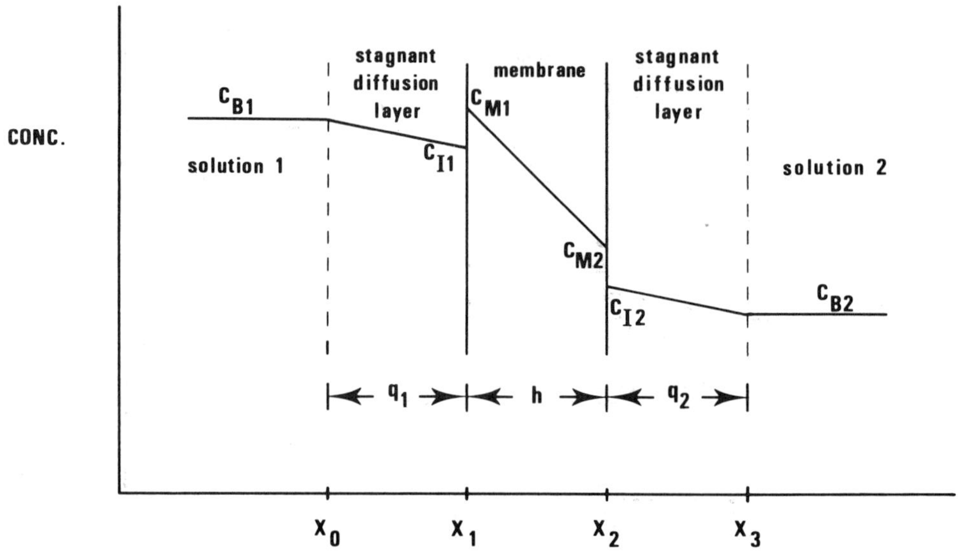

Fig. 9 Concentration profile versus position for a membrane and its associated stagnant diffusion layers. C_{B1} is the concentration in bulk solution 1, C_{B2} is the concentration in bulk solution 2, q_1 and q_2 are stagnant diffusion layer thicknesses, and h is the membrane thickness. C_{I1}, C_{I2}, C_{M1}, and C_{M2} are concentrations at the stagnant diffusion layer-membrane interfaces.

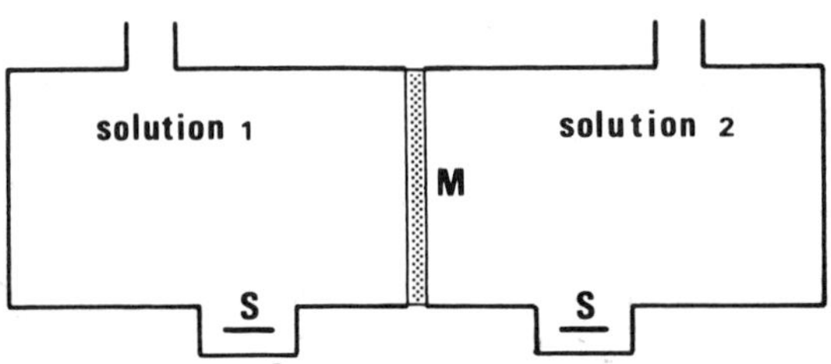

Fig. 10 A diffusion cell. M represents the membrane and S refers to the stirring bars. In a typical experiment, drug is placed into compartment 1 at t = 0 and then compartment 2 is sampled at various time intervals after the initiation of the experiment. The samples obtained from compartment 2 are then analyzed for drug content.

Integrating Eq. (53) gives

$$\int_{x_i}^{x} J\ dx = -\int_{C_i}^{C} D\ dC \tag{54}$$

or

$$J\ (x - x_i) = -D\ (C - C_i)$$

if D is assumed to be independent of position and concentration. Therefore

$$C = C_i - \frac{J}{D}\ (x - x_i) \tag{55}$$

Applying Eq. (55) to the two stagnant diffusion layers and the membrane we obtain

$$C_1 = C_{B1} - \frac{J_1}{D_1}\ (x - x_o) \qquad x_o \leqslant x \leqslant x_o + q_1 = x_1 \tag{56a}$$

$$C_M = C_{M1} - \frac{J_M}{D_M}\ (x - x_1) \qquad x_1 \leqslant x \leqslant x_1 + h = x_2 \tag{56b}$$

$$C_2 = C_{I2} - \frac{J_2}{D_2}\ (x - x_2) \qquad x_2 \leqslant x \leqslant x_2 + q_2 = x_3 \tag{56c}$$

where J_1, J_2, and J_M are the fluxes across the two stagnant diffusion layers and the membrane; and D_1, D_2, and D_M are their associated diffusion coefficients. Now C_{M1} and C_{M2} are experimentally inaccessible concentrations, but they can be related to the experimentally measurable concentrations C_{B1} and C_{B2} via partition coefficients as follows:

$$C_{M1} = K_{M1}\ C_{I1} \tag{57}$$

$$C_{M2} = K_{M2}\ C_{I2} \tag{58}$$

then

$$C_M = K_{M1}\ C_{I1} - \frac{J_M}{D_M}\ (x - x_1) \tag{59}$$

But

$$C_{I1} = C_1 \Big|_{x = x_1} = C_{B1} - \frac{J_1}{D_1}(x_1 - x_o) = C_{B1} - \frac{J_1}{D_1} q_1 \tag{60}$$

$$\therefore C_M = K_{M1}\left(C_{B1} - \frac{J_1}{D_1} q_1\right) - \frac{J_M}{D_M}(x - x_1) \tag{61}$$

Similarly for

$$C_2 = C_{I2} - \frac{J_2}{D_2}(x - x_2)$$

we have,

$$C_2 = \frac{C_{M2}}{K_{M2}} - \frac{J_2}{D_2}(x - x_2) \tag{62}$$

but

$$C_{M2} = C_M \Big|_{x = x_2} = C_{M1} - \frac{J_M}{D_M}(x_2 - x_1) = C_{M1} - \frac{J_M}{D_M} h \tag{63}$$

thus

$$C_2 = \frac{1}{K_{M2}}\left(C_{M1} - \frac{J_M}{D_M} h\right) - \frac{J_2}{D_2}(x - x_2) \tag{64}$$

Again using

$$C_{M1} = K_{M1} C_{I1}$$

$$C_2 = \frac{K_{M1}}{K_{M2}} C_{I1} - \left(\frac{J_M}{K_{M2}}\right)\left(\frac{h}{D_M}\right) - \frac{J_2}{D_2}(x - x_2) \tag{65}$$

but

$$C_{I1} = C_1 \Big|_{x = x_1} = C_{B1} - \frac{J_1}{D_1} q_1$$

thus

$$C_2 = \left(\frac{K_{M1}}{K_{M2}}\right)\left(C_{B1} - J_1\frac{q_1}{D_1}\right) - \left(\frac{J_M}{K_{M2}}\right)\left(\frac{h}{D_M}\right) - \left(\frac{J_2}{D_2}\right)(x - x_2) \tag{66}$$

Alternatively, Eq. (66) can be written in terms of diffusional resistances as follows:

$$C_2 = \left(\frac{K_{M1}}{K_{M2}}\right)(C_{B1} - J_1R'_1) - \left(\frac{J_M}{K_{M2}}\right)R'_M - \frac{J_2}{D_2}(x - x_2) \tag{67}$$

where

$$R'_1 = \frac{q_1}{D_1} \text{ and } R'_M = \frac{h}{D_M}$$

It is illustrative to see how Eq. (67) can be simplified and used to obtain the commonly used expression given in Eq. (52). Assume that the solute concentration in solution 2 is a constant; then

$$C_2\Big|_{x = x_2 + q_2} = C_{B2} = \left(\frac{K_{M1}}{K_{M2}}\right)(C_{B1} - J_1\,R'_1) - \left(\frac{J_M}{K_{M2}}\right)R'_M - J_2\,R'_2 \tag{68}$$

Now assume that we are at steady-state conditions

$$\therefore\ J_1 = J_M = J_2 = J \tag{69}$$

and

$$C_{B2} = \left(\frac{K_{M1}}{K_{M2}}\right)(C_{B1} - JR'_1) - \left(\frac{J}{K_{M2}}\right)R'_M - JR'_2 \tag{70}$$

or

$$J = \frac{K_{M1} C_{B1} - K_{M2} C_{B2}}{(K_{M1} R'_1 + K_{M2} R'_2) + R'_M} \tag{71}$$

The term $K_{M1} R'_1 + K_{M2} R'_2$ is the effective diffusional resistance contributed by the stagnant diffusion layers, whereas R'_M is the diffusional resistance solely from the membrane. The membrane's diffusional resistance can be much greater than the diffusional resistance from the stagnant diffusion layers in the following cases:

1. The membrane itself is very impermeable, i.e. R'_M is large. This could occur if the membrane's thickness is large or if the solute molecule's diffusion coefficient in the membrane is small.
2. R'_1 and R'_2 might be small. This can happen if phases 1 and 2 are well stirred, which is often the case in diffusion cell experiments. The stirring causes a decrease in the stagnant diffusion layer thickness, which results in a corresponding decrease in diffusional resistance.
3. K_{M1} and K_{M2} are small. This would occur if the solute molecule perferentially stays in solutions 1 and 2, rather than partitioning into the membrane. In diffusion cell experiments, solutions 1 and 2 are often aqueous. Therefore, a solute molecule that is hydrophilic in character would stay in solutions 1 and 2, since membranes are generally hydrophobic relative to an aqueous medium. This would result in K_{M1} and K_{M2} being small.

If any of the conditions given in (1), (2), and (3) are met such that

$$R'_M >> K_{M1} R'_1 + K_{M2} R'_2$$

then Eq. (71) simplifies to

$$J = \frac{K_{M1} C_{B1} - K_{M2} C_{B2}}{R'_M} \tag{72}$$

Often solutions 1 and 2 are similar e.g. they might both be aqueous media, as is common in diffusion cell experiments. If the membrane can also be assumed to be homogenous and the solute concentration on one side of the membrane can be assumed to be much less than that on the other side ($C_{B2} < C_{B1}$), then

$$J \approx \frac{K_P C}{R'_M} = \frac{K_P D}{h} C \tag{73}$$

where $K_{M1} = K_{M2} = K_p$ and $C_{B1} = C$, and we have obtained Eq. (52).

The effect of the hydrophobic nature of the solute molecule on the relative importance of the stagnant diffusion layer versus the membrane in controlling transport has been beautifully illustrated by Flynn and Yalkowsky [20]. Some of their results are summarized in an idealized fashion in Figure 11. From Figure 11, notice that as the number of carbons in the alkyl chain of the solute molecule increases the steady state flux eventually reaches a constant value. To understand this, realize that as the alkyl chain length increases the molecule becomes more hydrophobic. Therefore, K_{M1} and K_{M2} increase and eventually cause $K_{M1} R'_1 + K_{M2} R'_2$ to be much larger than R'_M. Thus Eq. (71) becomes

$$J \approx \frac{K_{M1} C_{B1} - K_{M2} C_{B2}}{K_{M1} R'_1 + K_{M2} R'_2} \tag{74}$$

Since the data in Figure 11 were obtained for a homogenous membrane which had aqueous solutions on either side of it, we can assume that

$$K_{M1} = K_{M2} = K_p \tag{75}$$

Therefore

$$J \approx \frac{C_{B1} - C_{B2}}{R'_1 + R'_2} \tag{76}$$

Thus, the flux depends only on the stagnant diffusion layer resistance and is independent of any further changes in the partition coefficient. This case is referred to as diffusion layer controlled transport. Conversely for short alkyl chain lengths, the membrane and partition coefficients will determine the flux and we have instead

$$J \approx \frac{K_{M1} C_{B1} - K_{M2} C_{B2}}{R'_M} \tag{77}$$

which is referred to as membrane controlled transport. This dependence on partition coefficient explains why the flux depends on alkyl

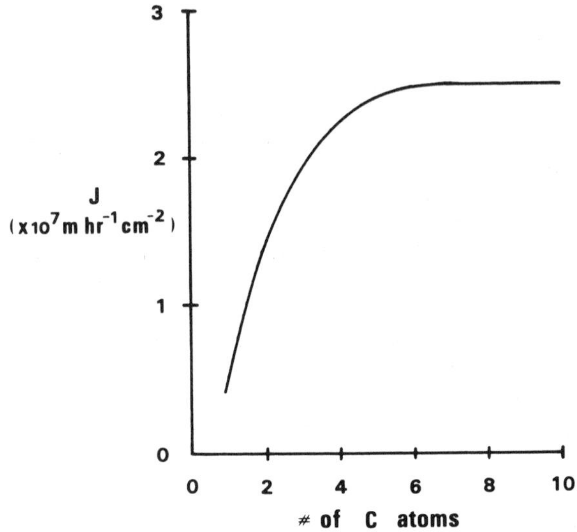

Fig. 11 A plot of the steady-state flux (J) as a function of the number of carbon atoms in the alkyl chain of a homologous series of solute molecules. These data could be obtained by using a diffusion cell such as shown in Figure 10. The data and figure are modeled after information given in Ref. 18.

chain length in the membrane controlled region. If again we assume that $K_{M1} = K_{M2} = K_p$, we see that J is proportional to K_p which is related to the alkyl chain length.

Example 7:

What is the stagnant diffusion layer thickness of a membrane in a diffusion cell whose characteristics are like those shown in Figure 10? Assume that the solute's aqueous diffusion coefficient (D_{aq}) is equal to 5×10^{-6} cm^2 sec^{-1}, $C_{B1} = 1 \times 10^{-3}$ mole l^{-1}, $C_{B2} \approx 0$, and that the density of the aqueous solutions 1 and 2 is unity. Also, assume that the solute has an alkyl chain length of n = 8 and that its flux can be obtained from Figure 11.

Solution:

From Figure 11, diffusion controlled transport occurs when $n \approx 7$ to 10. Therefore, the flux obtained under diffusion control is approximately 2.5×10^{-7} moles hr^{-1} cm^{-2}. Then

$$R_1' + R_2' = \frac{C_{B1}}{J} = \frac{1 \times 10^{-6} \text{ moles cm}^{-3}}{2.5 \times 10^{-7} \text{ moles hr}^{-1} \text{ cm}^{-2}} = 4 \text{ hr cm}^{-1}$$

or

$$R_1' + R_2' = 1.44 \times 10^4 \text{ sec cm}^{-1}$$

Now

$$R_1' + R_2' = \frac{q_1}{D_1} + \frac{q_2}{D_2}$$

Assuming a uniform homogenous membrane and similarity in solutions 1 and 2 we have

$$q_1 = q_2 = q \text{ and } D_1 = D_2 = D_{aq}$$

$$R_1' + R_2' = \frac{2q}{D_{aq}}$$

$$\therefore q = \frac{D_{aq}(R_1' + R_2')}{2} = \frac{(5 \times 10^{-6} \text{ cm}^2 \text{ sec}^{-1})\ (1.44 \times 10^4 \text{ sec cm}^{-1})}{2}$$

or

$$q = 3.6 \times 10^{-2} \text{ cm}$$

Measurement of unstirred diffusion layers shows them to vary from 1×10^{-4} cm to 5×10^{-2} cm, depending on the membrane system studied [10].

VI. APPLICATION OF FICK'S SECOND LAW TO THE DETERMINATION OF THE NON-STEADY-STATE OUTPUT FLUX THROUGH THE SKIN

Referring back to the diffusion cell shown in Figure 10, we will assume that the membrane is excised skin and that solutions 1 and 2 are aqueous and well stirred. One phase (the receptor phase) will not contain any drug at t = 0 and the other phase (the sample phase) will have a known amount of drug added at t = 0. The appearance of drug in the receptor phase will be followed as a function of time. Such experiments are often done for the initial testing of the permeability characteristics of therapeutic or toxic agents. In excised skin, the stratum corneum represents the primary barrier to diffusion with diffusional resistances from other tissue layers and the stagnant diffusion layers generally of minor importance. If it can also be assumed that the aqueous medium and the solute added to the sample phase will not affect the tissue, then our problem simplifies to the transport of solute across a single inert membrane having no associated stagnant diffusion layers. The solution of Fick's second law, Eq. (15), for this single inert membrane is given by Scheuplein [19] and the method of solution may be found in Crank [3]. The solution is

$$\mathrm{Amt}(t)_{out} = (A\ K_p\ h\ C_1)\left[\frac{Dt}{h^2} - \frac{1}{6} - \frac{2}{\pi^2}\sum_{n=1}^{\infty}\frac{(-1)^n}{n^2}\ \exp\left[(-D\ n^2\ \pi^2 t)/h^2\right]\right] \tag{78}$$

A plot of $\mathrm{Amt}(t)_{out}$ versus t obtained by using Eq. (78) is given in Figure 12. As time increases, the series term in the solution goes to zero, resulting in the following steady state expression

$$\mathrm{Amt}(t)^{s.s.}_{out} = A\ K_p\ h\ C_1\left(\frac{Dt}{h^2} - \frac{1}{6}\right) \tag{79}$$

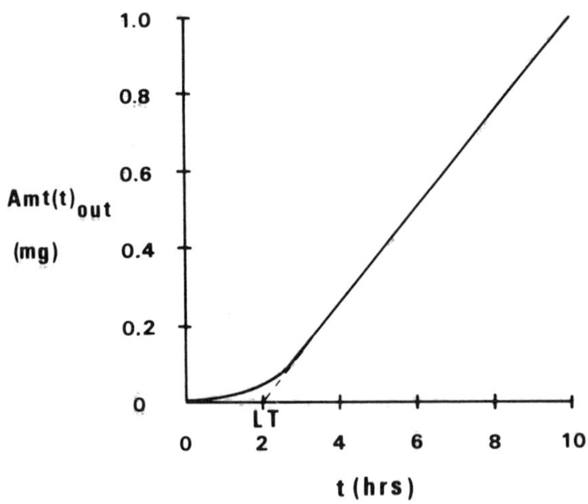

Fig. 12 A plot of the amount of drug passing through a single inert membrane as a function of time. LT is the lag time.

If Eq. (79) is differentiated with respect to time we obtain

$$\frac{1}{A}\frac{d(Amt)}{dt} = \frac{K_p D C_1}{h} = J$$

which is the earlier result we obtained for steady-state conditions by using Fick's first law, Eq. 52.

The time for which $Amt(t)_{out}$ equals zero in Eq. (79) is referred to as the lag time, this is, approximately the time required before solute will appear in the receptor phase. Graphically the lag time may be obtained by extrapolating the steady-state portion of the $Amt(t)_{out}$ versus time curve to $Amt(t)_{out} = 0$ (see Fig. 12). From Eq. (79), we may derive an expression for the lag time as follows

$$0 = A\ K_p\ h\ C_1 \left(\frac{Dt}{h^2} - \frac{1}{6}\right) \tag{80}$$

$$\frac{Dt}{h^2} = \frac{1}{6} \tag{81}$$

or

$$t = \frac{h^2}{6\ D}$$

We therefore have another means of obtaining the diffusion coefficient of a solute in a membrane by use of Eq. (81). However, often times the assumptions underlying the above solution to Fick's second law are not completely valid, resulting in the determination of erroneous diffusion coefficients when Eq. (81) is employed. This is particularly true for skin transport studies, where prolonged hydration will indeed alter the membrane's permeability. For this reason, the diffusion coefficient is often found by using Fick's first law [Eq. (52)].

Example 8:

Using the data given in Figure 12, find the diffusion coefficient for a solute molecule in the stratum corneum. Assume that the thickness of the stratum corneum is 2×10^{-3} cm.

Solution:

From Figure 12, the lag time is approximately 2 hr

$$\therefore D = \frac{h^2}{6t} = \frac{(2 \times 10^{-3}\ \text{cm})^2}{6\ (7.2 \times 10^3\ \text{sec})}$$

$$D = 9.3 \times 10^{-11}\ \text{cm}^2\ \text{sec}^{-1}$$

VII. APPLICATION OF FICK'S FIRST LAW TO THE DETERMINATION OF DRUG RELEASE FROM A POLYMERIC MATRIX OR OINTMENT

As a first step toward characterizing the drug release from a polymeric matrix or ointment (the derivations are identical), consider Figure 13.

Represented here under steady state conditions is an infinite reservior of drug at its saturation concentration C_s. For simplicity, the geometry has been chosen to be that of a semi-infinite slab with only one face exposed to an aqueous medium. Perfect sink conditions are assumed for the surrounding aqueous phase, the partition

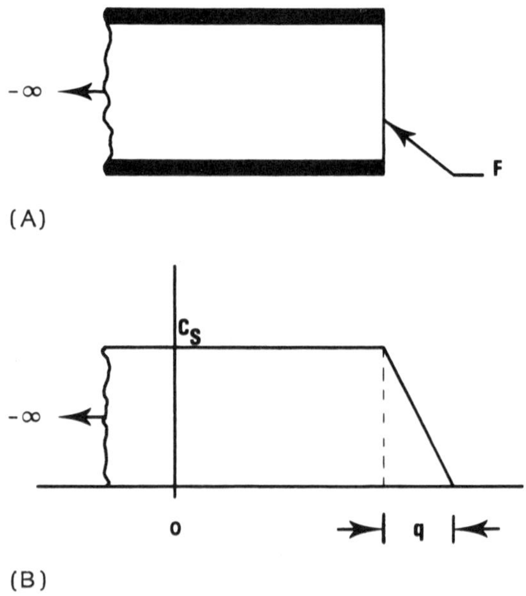

Fig. 13 (A) A semi-infinite slab containing drug at its aqueous saturation concentration C_s. The slab is exposed to an aqueous medium only at one face (F). (B) A concentration profile of the drug in the slab and in the aqueous media. Sink conditions exist in the bulk aqueous phase. There is a stagnant diffusion layer of thckness q, and since steady state conditions exist, the concentration gradient in this stagnant diffusion layer is linear.

coefficient between the slab and aqueous phase is unity, and the stagnant diffusion layer thickness is q. For this system, application of Fick's first law gives

$$J = \frac{DC_s}{q} = \frac{1}{A}\frac{d\,(\text{Amt})}{dt} = \text{constant} \tag{82}$$

where A is the cross sectional surface area. Now consider the polymeric matrix shown in Figure 14. Here the matrix is filled with a homogenously dispersed drug of concentration C_L such that $C_L > C_S$. Once again the flux from the matrix is governed by Eq. 82. However, now the polymeric matrix is allowed to hydrate through a differential distance dq in a differential time dt. This hydration layer makes available for transport an additional amount of drug per unit cross sectional area equal to the shaded area shown in Figure 14. From Figure 15, we can see that

$$\frac{d\,(\text{Amt})}{A} = \text{AREA}_A + \text{AREA}_B \tag{83}$$

where

$$\text{AREA}_A = (C_L - C_s)\,dq$$

and

$$\text{AREA}_B = C_s dq + 1/2\ C_s\ q - 1/2\ C_s\ (q + dq) = 1/2\ C_s\ dq$$

$$\therefore\ \frac{d\,(\text{Amt})}{A} = C_L\ dq - 1/2\ C_s\ dq \tag{84}$$

now this amount of solute (drug) is made available for transport in time dt. Therefore,

$$J = \frac{1}{A}\frac{d\,(\text{Amt})}{dt} = (C_L - 1/2\ C_s)\frac{dq}{dt} \tag{85}$$

Since the flux obtained must also equal that predicted by Fick's first law [Eq. (82)].

$$(C_L - 1/2\ C_s)\frac{dq}{dt} = \frac{D\ C_s}{q} \tag{86}$$

or

$$\frac{2\ C_L - C_s}{2\ D\ C_s}\int q\ dq = \int dt$$

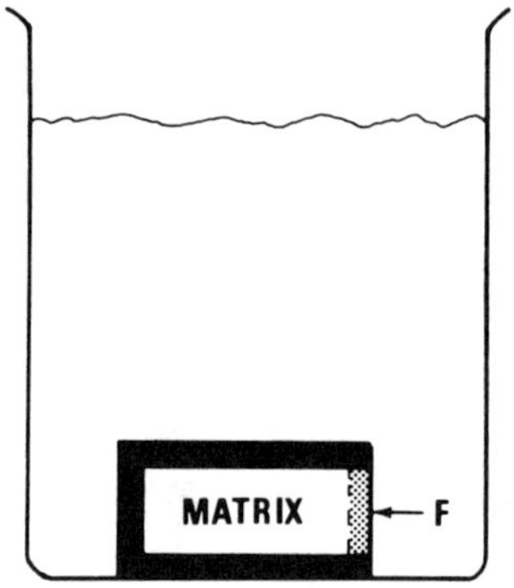

(A)

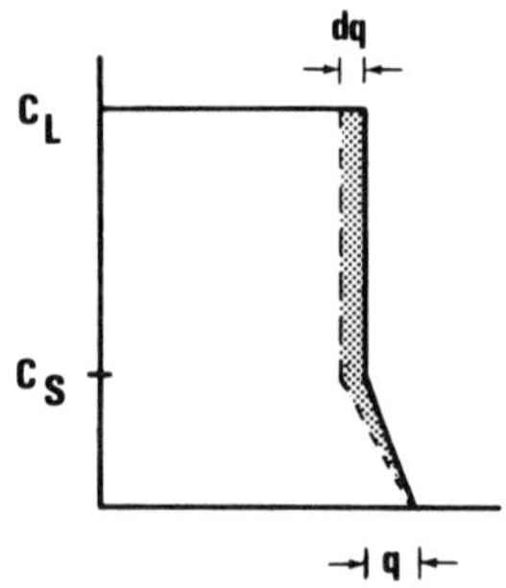

(B)

Fig. 14 (A) A coated polymeric matrix placed in an aqueous medium. Although the polymer matrix is shown to be finite in size, with respect to the change in hydration layer (dq) it can be viewed as semi-infinite. Only one face (F) of the matrix is exposed to the aqueous medium. (B) A concentration profile versus position of the system shown in A. C_L is the loading concentration of drug in the matrix, C_S is the drug's saturation concentration in the aqueous medium, q is the stagnant diffusion layer thickness, and dq is the hydration layer thickness produced in a time dt. The shaded area in part (B) represents the additional amount of drug per unit cross sectional area available for transport due to the hydration occurring in time dt. Note the cross-sectional area is perpendicular to the plane of the paper. The figure in B is adapted from a figure in Ref. 19.

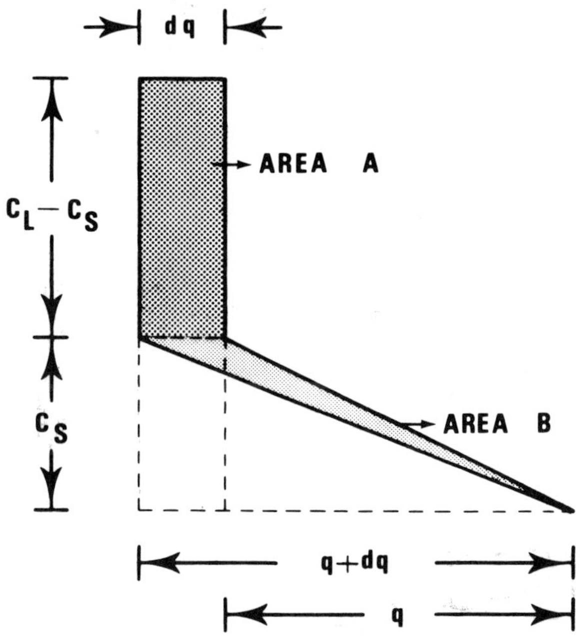

Fig. 15 A detailed diagram of the shaded region given in Figure 10B where C_L = loading concentration of drug in the matrix, C_S = saturation concentration of drug in the aqueous media, q = stagnant diffusion layer thickness, and dq is the thickness of the hydration layer formed in time dt.

$$\left(\frac{2\,C_L - C_s}{4\,D\,C_s}\right) q^2 = t + k_o \tag{87}$$

where k_o is the integration constant, which can be evaluated by using the initial condition that q = 0 at t = 0. Applying this condition shows that k_o = 0, so

$$q = \left(\frac{4\,D\,C_s\,t}{2\,C_L - C_s}\right)^{1/2} \tag{88}$$

Now the amount eliminated per unit cross-sectional area can be obtained by integrating Eq. (84).

$$\frac{1}{A}\int_{o}^{Amt} d\ Amt = (C_L - 1/2\ C_s)\int_{o}^{q} dq \tag{89}$$

$$\frac{Amt}{A} = (C_L - 1/2\ C_s)\ q \tag{90}$$

Substituting for q from Eq. (88) gives

$$Amt = A\ (C_L - 1/2\ C_s)\left(\frac{4\ D\ C_s\ t}{2\ C_L - C_s}\right)^{1/2} \tag{91}$$

$$Amt = A\ [(2\ C_L - C_s)\ (D\ C_s\ t)]^{1/2}$$

which is the Higuchi equation [21]. The above derivation closely follows that originally given by Higuchi. This equation predicts the familiar square root of time dependence on the amount of drug released from a polymeric matrix. If $C_L >> C_s$, then

$$Amt \approx A\ (2\ D\ C_L\ C_s\ t)^{1/2} \tag{92}$$

Example 9:

How much time must pass before a polymeric matrix (protected from hydration except for one face whose surface area is 2 cm^2) will release 1 mg of drug? The loading concentration of drug is 0.1 g cm^{-3}, the drug's saturation concentration is 5×10^{-4} g cm^{-3}, and the diffusion coefficient of drug in the polymeric matrix when hydrated is 1×10^{-7} cm^{-2} sec^{-1}.

Solution:

Since $C_L >> C_s$ we will use Eq. (92).
Rearrangement gives

$$t = \left(\frac{Amt}{A}\right)^2 \left(\frac{1}{2D\ C_L\ C_s}\right)$$

$$\therefore t = \left(\frac{1 \times 10^{-3} g}{2\ cm^2}\right)^2$$

$$\left[\frac{1}{(2)\ (1 \times 10^{-7}\ cm^2 sec^{-1})(0.1\ g\ cm^{-3})(5 \times 10^{-4} g\ cm^{-3})}\right]$$

or

$$t = 2.5 \times 10^4 \text{ sec} \approx 7 \text{ hr}$$

Note that more detailed treatments of this problem may be found [22–24].

VIII. DIFFUSION WITH SIMULTANEOUS REACTION

When a solute molecule diffuses, there is a possibility that it may also undergo a simultaneous chemical reaction. For example, when a drug molecule diffuses through the skin, it may undergo simultaneous enzymatic degradation. Assuming that the diffusion coefficient is constant and that the rectangular one-dimensional form of Fick's second law is an adequate description of our transport system we have

$$\frac{\partial C}{\partial t} = D \frac{\partial^2 C}{\partial x^2} - R \tag{93}$$

Where R is the reactive degradative term and typically has values such as $K''C$ for an irreversible first-order reaction or $V_{max}C(K_M + C)$ for an enzymatic reaction. Here K'' is the first order rate constant, V_{max} is the maximum rate obtainable, and K_M is the Michaelis constant. If steady-state conditions exist, Eq. (93) simplifies to

$$\frac{d^2C}{dx^2} = \frac{R}{D} \tag{94}$$

Several authors who have studied skin drug transport, namely Ando et al. [25], Fox et al. [26], Hadgraft [27], and Guy et al. [28], have solved Eqs. (93) and (94) for the cases where degradation occurs either by an irreversible first-order process or by an enzymatic process. In their treatments they used either analytical or numerical methods to obtain their solutions.

IX. ADDITIONAL CONCERNS IN DIFFUSIONAL MASS TRANSPORT

Not covered in this chapter because of their complexity, but of interest, are diffusion problems associated with heterogeneous structures, non-Fickian diffusion, moving boundary conditions, diffusion of ionic species, an irreversible thermodynamic approach to diffusion, and methods of solution. Most of these additional topics are treated in an excellent fashion by Crank [3]. In addition, articles and texts by Kedem [29], Katchalsky [30], and Hoppe [31,32] provide coverage of irreversible thermodynamics and the diffusion of ionic species as well as their relation to membrane transport problems.

Heterogeneous structures occur when dealing with layered structures (laminates); here each layer can be composed of a different material. Alternatively, heterogeneous structures occur when considering systems in which particulates of one phase are dispersed throughout another continuous phase. Examples of both of these heterogeneous structures can be found in some polymer systems. One result of this heterogeneity is that the diffusion coefficient can no longer be assumed constant throughout the system.

Polymers can also exhibit movable boundary conditions and non-Fickian diffusion. This occurs when the boundries of a polymer change with time upon exposure to an aqueous solution. In this case, as the polymer becomes hydrated it can swell. Fick's first and second laws are often inappropriate to employ in this case because swelling can induce internal stresses which are slow to decay with time. These internal stresses, in turn, alter the solute's ability to diffuse which results in non-Fickian diffusion.

Diffusion of ions, in general, cannot be treated by the simple passive diffusion relationships given by Fick's first and second laws. This is because ions can interact electrostatically with themselves, the solvent, membranes, or with any polymers that they might be associated with. In order to treat ion transport effectively, the techniques of irreversible thermodynamics must usually be used. Basically irreversible thermodynamics provides a theoretical framework for handling coupling between different transport phenomena, such as simultaneous osmotic gradients, pressure differences, and electrical potential differences.

REFERENCES

1. D. Eisenberg and D. Crothers, *Physical Chemistry with Applications to the Life Sciences*, Benjamin/Cummings, Menlo Park, CA, 1979, Chaps. 4 and 7.
2. K. J. Laidler and J. H. Meiser, *Physical Chemistry*, Benjamin/Cumming, Menlo Park, CA, 1982, Chap. 5.
3. J. Crank, *The Mathematics of Diffusion*, 2nd ed., Clarendon Press, Oxford, 1975.
4. R. B. Bird, W. E. Stewart, and E. N. Lightfoot, *Transport Phenomena*, John Wiley & Sons, New York, 1960.
5. D. Hershey, *Transport Analysis*, Plenum/Rosetta, New York, 1973.

6. R. W. Fahien, *Fundamentals of Transport Phenomena*, McGraw-Hill, New York, 1983.
7. Y. W. Chien, *Novel Drug Delivery Systems*, Marcel Dekker, New York, 1982.
8. A. Martin, J. Swarbrick, and A. Cammarata, *Physical Pharmacy*, Lea & Febiger, Philadelphia, 1983, Chap. 15.
9. G. L. Flynn, S. H. Yalkowsky, and T. J. Roseman, Mass transport phenomena and models: Theoretical concepts, *J. Pharm. Sci. 63*, 479 (1974).
10. R. I. Macey, *Physiology of Membrane Disorders* (T. E. Andreoli, J. E. Hoffman, and D. D. Fanestil, Eds.), Plenum Medical Book, New York, 1978, Chap. 7.
11. R. R. Burnette, A Mone-Carlo model for the passive diffusion of drugs through the stratum corneum, *Int. J. Pharm. 22*:89 (1984).
12. D. Eisenberg and D. Crothers, *Physical Chemistry with Applications to the Life Sciences*, Benjamin/Cummings, Menlo Park, CA, 1979, Chap. 15.
13. K. J. Laidler and J. H. Meiser, *Physical Chemistry*, Benjamin/Cummings, Menlo Park, CA, 1982, Chap. 18.
14. A. Einstein, *Investigations on the Theory of Brownian Movement*, Methuen, London, 1926.
15. C. Tanford, *Physical Chemistry of Macromolecules*, John Wiley & Sons, New York, 1961, Chap. 6.
16. L. Page, *Introduction to Theoretical Physics*, D. Van Nostrand, New York, 1928, Chap. 6.
17. M. Wu, Determination of concentration-dependent water diffusivity in a keratinous membrane, *J. Pharm. Sci. 72*, 1421 (1983).
18. R. H. Guy, J. Hadgraft, I. W. Kellway, and M. J. Taylor, Calculations of drug release rates from spherical particles, *Int. J. Pharm. 11*:199 (1982).
19. R. J. Scheuplein and R. L. Bronaugh, *Biochemistry and Physiology of the Skin*, Vol. 2 (L. A. Goldsmith, Ed.), Oxford University Press, New York, 1983, Chap. 58.
20. G. L. Flynn and S. H. Yalkowsky, Correlation and prediction of mass transport across membranes I: Influence of alkyl chain length on flux-determining properties of barrier and diffusant, *J. Pharm. Sci. 61*, 838 (1972).
21. T. Higuchi, Rate of release of medicaments from ointment bases containing drugs in suspension, *J. Pharm. Sci. 50* (10), 874 (1961).
22. S. J. Desai, P. Singh, A. P. Simonelli, and W. I. Higuchi, Investigation of factors influencing release of solid drug dispersed in inert matrices. II Quanitation of procedures, *J. Pharm. Sci. 55*, 1224 (1966).

23. D. R. Paul and S. K. McSpadden, Diffusional release of a solute from a polymer matrix, *J. Memb. Sci. 1*:33 (1976).
24. F. Bottari, G. Di Colo, E. Nannipieri, M. F. Saettone, and M. F. Serafini, Release of drugs from ointment bases II: *in vitro* release of benzocaine from suspension-type aqueous gels, *J. Pharm. Sci. 66*, 926 (1977).
25. H. Y. Ando, N. F. H. Ho, and W. I. Higuchi, Skin as an active metabolizing barrier I: Theoretical analysis of topical bioavailability, *J. Pharm. Sci. 66*, 1525 (1977).
26. J. L. Fox, C. Yu, W. I. Higuchi, and N. F. H. Ho, General physical model for simultaneous diffusion and metabolism in biological membranes. The computational approach for the steady-state case, *Int. J. Pharm. 2*:41 (1979).
27. J. Hadgraft, Theoretical aspects of metabolism in the epidermis, *Int. J. Pharm. 4*:229, (1980).
28. R. H. Guy and J. Hadgraft, Percutaneous metabolism with saturable enzyme kinetics, *Int. J. Pharm. 11*:187, (1982).
29. O. Kedem and A. Katchalsky, A physical interpretation of the phenomenological coefficients of membrane permeability, *J. Gen. Physiol. 45*, 153 (1961–62).
30. A. Katchalsky and P. F. Carran, *Nonequilibrium Thermodynamics in Biophysics*, Harvard University Press, Cambridge, MA, 1965.
31. P. Schuster, *Biophysics* (W. Hoppe, W. Lohmann, H. Markl, and H. Ziegler Eds.), Springer-Verlag, Berlin, 1983, Chap. 8.
32. K. A. Fischer and W. Stoeckenius, *Biophysics* (W. Hoppe, W. Lohmann, H. Markl, and H. Ziegler Eds.), Springer-Verlag, Berlin, 1983, Chap. 12.
33. R. Chang, *Physical Chemistry with Applications to Biological Systems*, 2nd ed., Macmillan, New York, 1981.

3 Fundamentals of Polymer Science

JORGE HELLER / SRI International, Menlo Park, California

I. INTRODUCTION

Polymers, also known as macromolecules, are very large molecules consisting of many repeating units and are formed by a process called polymerization, which links together small molecules known as monomers. The monomers can be linked together in various ways to give rise to linear polymers (Fig. 1a), branched polymers (Fig. 1b), or crosslinked polymers (Fig. 1c). In these representations A is a

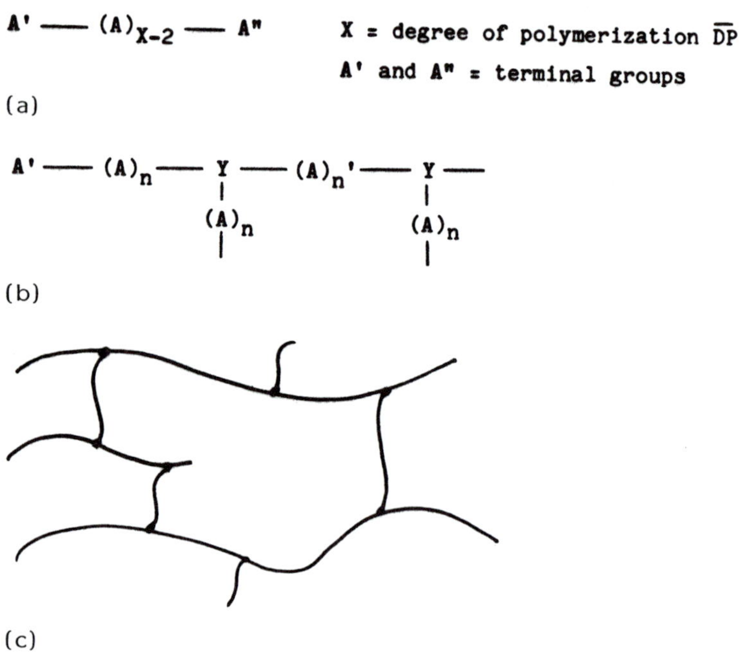

Fig. 1 Various polymer types: (a) linear polymer, (b) branched polymer, and (c) crosslinked polymer.

monomer and A' and A" are the terminal groups. The quantity x is known as the degree of polymerization, usually denoted as $\overline{DP}$, and the molecular weight of the polymer is the product of the degree of polymerization and the molecular weight of the repeat unit. Linear and branched polymers are known as thermoplastic materials because they flow when heated and can thus be fabricated by application of heat and pressure. They are also soluble in certain solvents.

Crosslinked polymers are known as thermosetting materials, and unlike thermoplastic materials they do not flow when heated and thus cannot be fabricated by application of heat and pressure. Because all polymer chains are interconnected by covalent crosslinks, they cannot dissolve and can only swell to the extent allowed by the crosslink density. When these materials are produced in useful form, they are either polymerized directly in a suitable mold or a linear prepolymer is first fabricated by conventional thermoplastic techniques and the fabricated material is then crosslinked by radiation or chemical means.

II. POLYMER CLASSIFICATION AND POLYMERIZATION MECHANISMS

Polymers are usually classified according to the method of polymerization into addition polymers or condensation polymers. In addition polymers, the molecular formula of the monomer is the same as the repeating unit of the polymer, and such polymers are prepared by the polymerization of monomers that contain one or more double or triple bonds or by the ring-opening of cyclic structures. Thus,

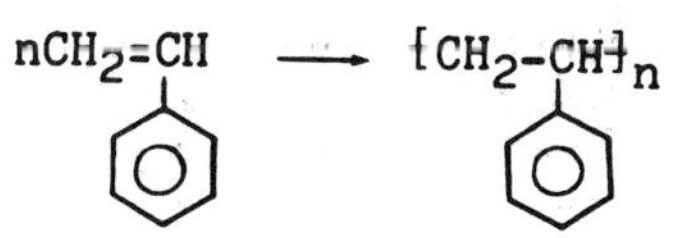

or

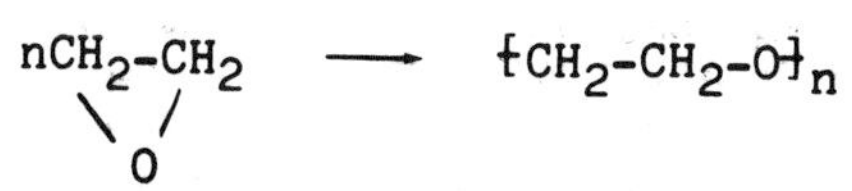

Condensation polymers are formed by successive reactions of functional groups, and because a small molecule by-product forms, the repeating unit of the polymer has fewer atoms than the monomers. Thus,

$$nH_2N(CH_2)_6NH_2 + nHOOC(CH_2)_4COOH \longrightarrow$$

$$\left[NH(CH_2)_6NH-\overset{\overset{\displaystyle O}{\|}}{C}(CH_2)_4-\overset{\overset{\displaystyle O}{\|}}{C}\right]_n + nH_2O$$

However, this common classification does not accommodate condensation reactions where no small molecule is split out, such as in formation of polyurethanes (isocyanate plus diol), polyureas (isocyanate plus diamine), polyacetals (vinyl ethers plus diols), or poly(orthoesters) (ketene acetals plus diols). Thus, for polyurethanes,

$$nO{=}C{=}N-(CH_2)_6N{=}C{=}O + nHO(CH_2)_4OH \longrightarrow$$

$$\left[NH-\overset{\overset{\displaystyle O}{\|}}{C}-O(CH_2)_4O-\overset{\overset{\displaystyle O}{\|}}{C}-NH(CH_2)_6\right]_n$$

Therefore, a more useful classification scheme is one that considers polymerization mechanisms. According to that scheme, polymers can be broadly divided into those that are formed by chain polymerization and those that are formed by a step-growth polymerization. In this scheme addition polymerizations are included in chain polymerization, and condensation polymerizations are included in step-growth polymerizations.

All chain polymerizations are characterized by the following features:

1. Discrete initiation, propagation, and termination steps
2. Rapid preferential growth of each polymer chain once started
3. Monomer concentration that decreases steadily as polymerization proceeds

Mechanistically, all chain polymerizations proceed by three distinct and separate chemical reactions. In one reaction, monomer initiation takes place, in another reaction chain growth takes place, and in the final reaction chain growth terminates. A further feature of chain polymerization is that once initiated, a polymer chain rapidly grows to high molecular weight, so if a chain growth polymerization is stopped at low conversion, the reaction mixture will contain a small amount of high molecular weight polymer and a large amount of unreacted monomer. As a consequence of this process, the concentration of monomer in the reaction mixture steadily decreases as it is converted to high molecular weight polymer.

All step-growth polymerizations are characterized by the following features:

1. No discrete initiation, propagation and termination steps and any two molecular species can react.
2. Polymer molecular weight rises steadily throughout the reaction.
3. Monomer disappears early in the reaction.

Mechanistically, all step-growth polymerizations proceed by specific reactions between functional groups, and any two molecular species bearing appropriate groups can react. As a consequence of this step-growth process, molecular weight of the polymer gradually increases so if a step-growh polymerization is stopped at low conversion, the reaction mixture will contain mainly low molecular weight polymer and only a very small amount of monomer. Thus, in this type of polymerization monomer disappears early in the reaction, and at a degree of polymerization of about 10, less than 1% of the monomer remains in the reaction mixture.

A. Chain Polymerizations

These polymerizations are also known as vinyl polymerizations because most of the monomers of interest are compounds that contain a vinyl group.

Chain polymerizations can, in general, be divided into the following four types according to the nature of the active center:

1. Free radical
2. Anionic
3. Cationic
4. Ziegler-Natta

Not all monomers are capable of undergoing all these polymerizations, and the particular mechanism by which a monomer can be polymerized depends on the chemical structure and, most important, on the nature of the substituent on the vinyl group.

1. Free Radical Polymerizations

A free radical is a species bearing an odd number of electrons and hence has an unpaired electron. Because unstabilized free radicals are extremely reactive molecules, initiation in free radical polymerization involves first the generation of free radicals, which then react with the vinyl monomer in an initiation reaction.

Free radicals can be generated in many ways, but the most common involves homolytic decomposition of covalent bonds having bond energies of about 30–40 kcal/mole, for example

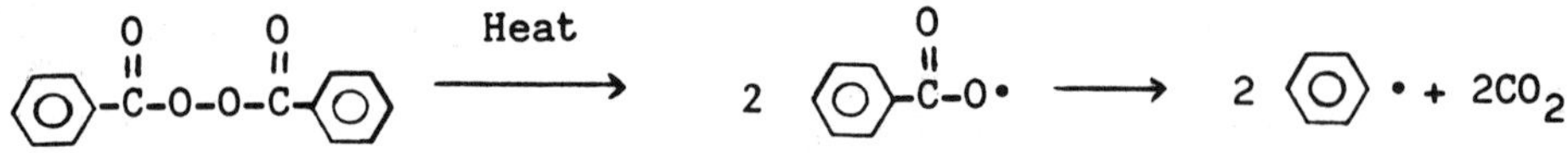

A free radical polymerization process can be schematically represented as follows:

Initiation

$$I{-}I \longrightarrow 2I\cdot$$

$$I\cdot + CH_2{=}CHR \longrightarrow I{-}CH_2{-}CHR\cdot$$

Propagation

$$I{-}CH_2{-}CHR\cdot + CH_2{=}CHR \longrightarrow I{-}CH_2CHRCH_2CHR\cdot \longrightarrow$$

to high polymer

Termination

Free radical polymerizations terminate by two facile reactions: coupling and disproportionation. In addition to termination reactions chain transfer reactions can also take place.

Coupling

$$P{-}CH_2CHR\cdot + \cdot RCHCH_2{-}P \longrightarrow P{-}CH_2CHR{-}CHR{-}CH_2{-}P$$

Disproportionation

$$P{-}CH_2CHR\cdot + \cdot RCH{-}CH_2{-}P \longrightarrow P{-}CH_2{-}CH_2R + CR{=}CH{-}P$$

Chain Transfer

Chain transfer involves abstraction of a hydrogen from another molecule by the growing polymer chain. When the hydrogen is abstracted from another polymer chain, branches are created when that radical initiates monomer molecules.

Abstraction

$$P{-}CH_2CHR\cdot + P{-}CH_2CHR{-}P \longrightarrow P{-}CH_2CH_2R$$

$$+ P{-}CH_2{-}\dot{C}R{-}P$$

Branching

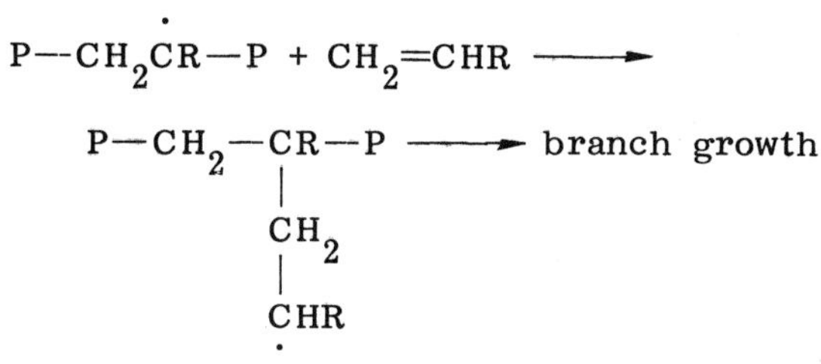

Hydrogen abstraction from a small molecule can also take place.

$$P{-}CH_2CHR\cdot + MH \longrightarrow P{-}CH_2CH_2R + M\cdot$$

When the radical M· is capable of initiating monomer, MH is known as a chain transfer agent, and addition of controlled amounts of MH to the polymerization reactions can be used to control molecular weight of the polymers. When the radical M· is not able to initiate monomer, MH is known as an inhibitor and is used to protect monomers from undesired polymerizations or to protect polymers from free radical oxidative degradation (antioxidant).

2. *Anionic Polymerizations*

Unlike free radical polymerizations, where the growing chain end is neutral, in anionic polymerizations the growing chain end is an anion and is thus associated with a positive counterion. The nature of the counterion and the nature of the solvent determine the degree of association between the anionic chain end and the counterion and thus have important effects on the rate and stereospecificity of the polymerization reaction.

Only monomers that contain an electron-withdrawing substituent on the double bond and can stabilize an anion will undergo anionic polymerizations. The ease of polymerizability is directly related to the stabilizing effect of the substituent(s). An example of a highly activated monomer is methyl cyanoacrylate, which contains two

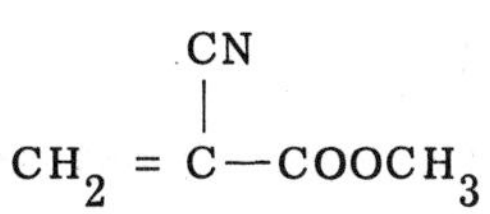

electron-withdrawing groups on one carbon, and even water is sufficiently basic to initiate polymerization.

Anionic polymerizations are commonly initiated with organic bases, such as organometallic compounds, or with electron-transfer agents. Using base initiation as an example, initiation and propagation occur as follows:

Initiation

$$BM \rightleftharpoons B^- + M^+$$

$$B^- M^+ + CH_2{=}CHR \longrightarrow B{-}CH_2CHR^- M^+$$

Propagation

$$B{-}CH_2{-}CHR^- M^+ + CH_2{=}CHR \longrightarrow$$

$$B{-}CH_2CHRCH_2CHR^- M^+ \longrightarrow \text{to high polymer}$$

Because there are no chain transfer reactions, high molecular weight, unbranched polymers are formed.

Unlike free radical polymerizations, anionic polymerization do not have a built-in termination process. Although this is not strictly true for all monomer systems, many monomers can be polymerized in inert solvents and in the rigorous absence of reactive impurities without a termination step, and polymer chains thus formed have active end-groups with long lifetimes.

Such polymers are known as living polymers, and the technique has several important practical applications, including the following:

1. Ability to accurately control molecular weight by controlling ratio of initiator to monomer. Thus,

   $$\overline{DP} = C\,\frac{[\text{Monomer}]}{[\text{Initiator}]} \quad \text{or} \quad \overline{M}_n = C\,\frac{\text{grams monomer}}{\text{moles initiator}}$$

   where

   $C = 1$ for initiation by bases

   $C = 1/2$ for initiation by electron transfer

2. Ability to prepare polymers having an extremely narrow molecular weight distribution
3. Ability to prepare polymers with specific end-groups
4. Ability to prepare block copolymers

Applications (1) and (2) are a consequence of a propagation reaction that occurs without termination so that all chains, once initiated, have an equal probability of growth until the monomer has been depleted. Therefore, no molecular weight broadening due to a random termination process takes place. Applications (3) and (4) are possible because chain-ends remain active and are capable of reacting with small molecules to form specific end-groups or with a second monomer to produce block copolymers.

3. *Cationic Polymerizations*

These are also ionic polymerizations but differ from anionic polymerizations in that the active chain-end is a cation and the associated counterion is a negative species. As in anionic polymerizations, the nature of the counterion and solvent have an important effect on polymerization rate and stereospecificity of the polymerization reaction.

Only monomers that contain an electron-donating substituent on the double bond that is capable of stabilizing a cation will undergo cationic polymerizations. The ease of polymerizability is directly related to the stabilizing effect of the substituent(s). Examples of a highly activated monomer are ketene acetals, which contain two electron donors on a double bond.

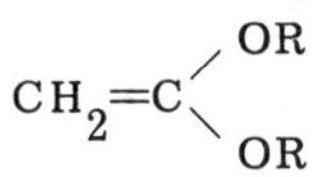

Cationic polymerizations are commonly initiated with acids, either protonic or Lewis. In either case the actual initiating species is a proton. Using a protonic acid as an example, initiation and propagation occur as follows:

Initiation

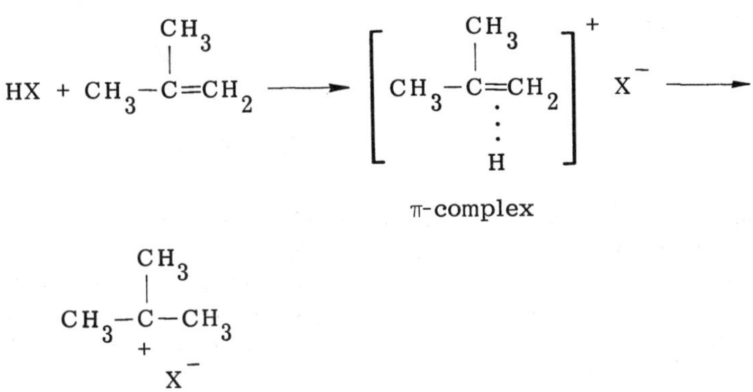

π-complex

Rearrangement of the π-complex always produces the most stable carbonium ion (stability order is III°, II°, I°).

Propagation

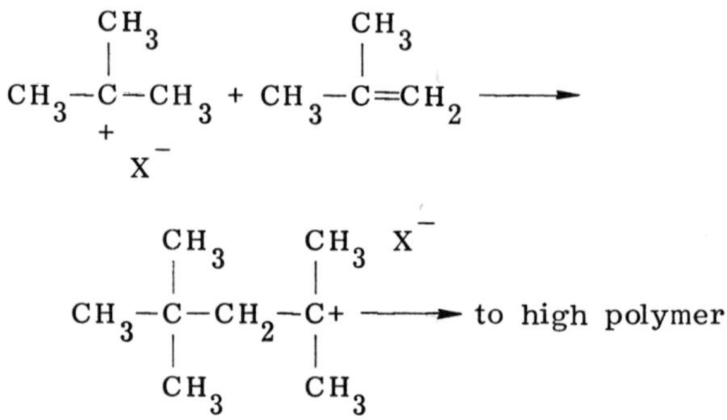

Because there is a strong driving force to form the most stable carbonium ion, rearrangement reactions can take place during propagation.

Unlike anionic polymerizations that have no chain transfer reactions, cationic polymerizations often involve chain transfer, either to monomer or to polymer. The former leads to molecular weight broadening and the latter to branching.

The following two chain transfers to monomer are common:

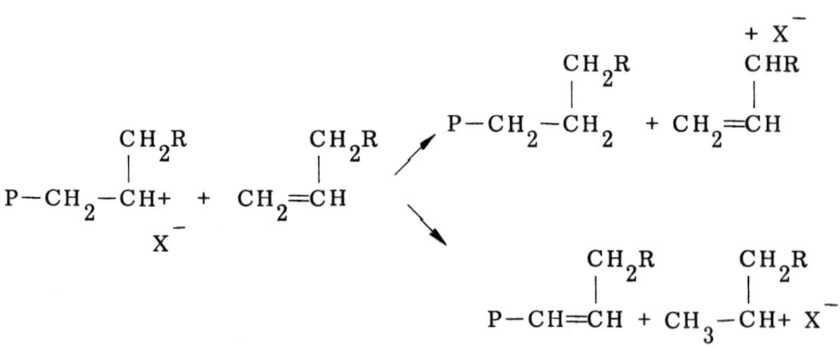

Because the reactivity of the carbonium ions generated by these reactions is sufficient to react with additional monomers, this process leads to considerable broadening of molecular weight distribution.

Chain transfer to polymer also occurs readily, particularly when in the chain-transfer process a secondary carbonium ion is converted to a tertiary carbonium ion.

$$\mathrm{P{-}CH_2\overset{+}{C}HR\ X^- + P{-}CH_2CHR{-}CH_2P \longrightarrow}$$

$$\mathrm{PCH_2CH_2R + P{-}CH_2\overset{+}{C}RCH_2P\ X^-}$$

Although in certain cases cationic polymerizations can be carried out without termination, the majority of cationic polymerizations have a termination reaction so rapid that polymerizations can only be carried out to high conversion by repeated additions of initiator.

One facile termination reaction is deprotonation:

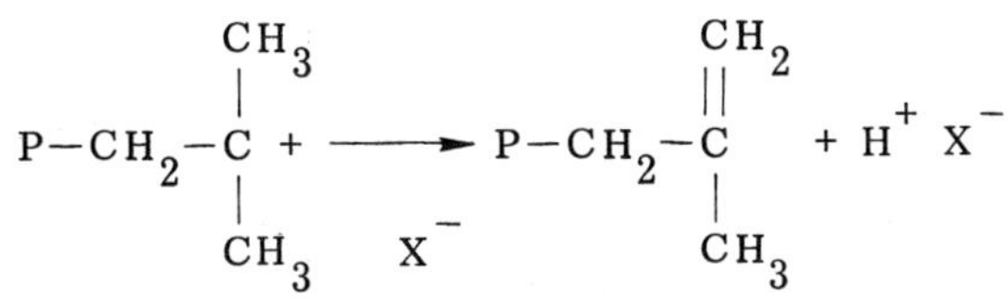

Even though the proton can initiate another monomer so that deprotonation is also a chain-transfer reaction, addition of a proton to a monomer is slow, and the number of chains initiated relative to those that have terminated is low.

4. *Ziegler-Natta Polymerizations*

The combination of metal alkyls and transition metal compounds are known as Ziegler-Natta catalyst systems. Of particular importance are aluminum alkyls, such as aluminum triisobutyl and titanium, or vanadium halides, such as $TiCl_4$, VCl_4, $TiCl_3$, or VCl_3.

These catalyst systems are not only capable of polymerizing olefins, such as ethylene or propylene, at essentially atmospheric pressure to very high molecular weight polymers, but are also capable of producing stereoregular polymers. For these reasons, these catalysts are of enormous industrial importance.

The exact nature of the catalyst system as well as mechanistic details of the polymerization process is complex and not well understood.

5. *Copolymerization*

A copolymer is a polymer chain that contains two or more constituent monomers. Depending on the arrangement of the monomers in the copolymer, various types of copolymers can be identified. Using A and B to denote two different monomers, these can be depicted as follows:

—A—B—B—A—A—B—A—A—A—B—B—A—B—B—

random copolymer

—A—B—A—B—A—B—A—B—A—B—

alternating copolymer

—A—A—A—A—A—A—A—A—A—B—B—B—B—B—B—B—B—

block copolymer

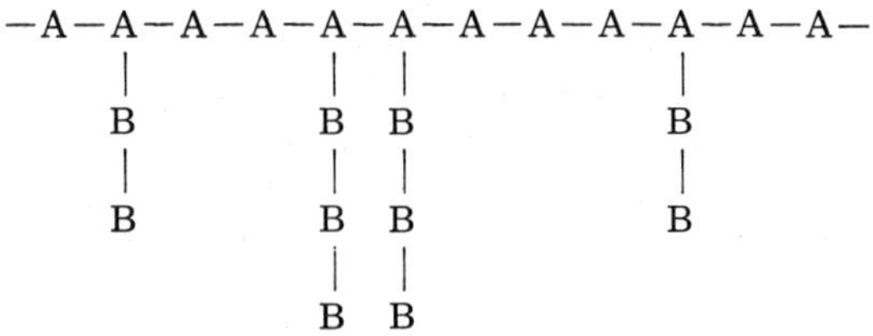

graft copolymer

Graft and block copolymers are prepared by specialized methods, while random copolymers, alternating copolymers or copolymer structures that have elements of random, alternating or block copolymers are prepared by the simultaneous polymerization of two monomers. Copolymers based on three different monomers are known at terpolymers.

Like homopolymerization, copolymerization involves initiation, propagation, and termination steps. Because in polymerizations leading to high molecular weight polymers initiation and terminations are rare events when compared to propagation, only the propagation step will be considered.

In the copolymerization of two monomers, the following propagation steps must be considered:

$$P{-}M_1\cdot + M_1 \xrightarrow{k_{11}} P{-}M_1M_1\cdot$$

$$P{-}M_1\cdot + M_2 \xrightarrow{k_{12}} P{-}M_1M_2\cdot$$

$$P{-}M_2\cdot + M_1 \xrightarrow{k_{21}} P{-}M_2M_1\cdot$$

$$P{-}M_2\cdot + M_2 \xrightarrow{k_{22}} P{-}M_2M_2\cdot$$

where M_1 and M_2 are the two monomers and k_{11}, k_{21}, k_{12}, and k_{22} are the four rate constants. These rate constants define r_1 and r_2, known as reactivity ratios:

$$r_1 = \frac{k_{11}}{k_{12}}$$

and

$$r_2 = \frac{k_{22}}{k_{21}}$$

Reactivity ratio r_1 is a measure of the rate with which radical M_1 reacts with monomer M_1 and M_2, and reactivity ratio r_2 is a measure of the rate with which radical M_2 reacts with monomers M_2 and M_1. When the two radicals display the same preference for either monomer, then

$$k_{11}/k_{12} = k_{21}/k_{22}$$

or

$$r_1 = 1/r_2$$

Because of this lack of preference, a completely random copolymer is obtained. Clearly, when $r_1 r_2 \neq 1$, the composition of the copolymer is not random, and a knowledge of the actual values of r_1 and r_2 allow a prediction of the nature of the copolymer.

B. Step-Growth Polymerizations

Unlike chain polymerizations, step-growth polymerizations do not have discrete initiation, propagation, and termination steps and any two species in the reaction mixture can react by a specific reaction between two appropriate functional groups.

To be useful in the synthesis of high molecular weight polymers, the condensation reaction must proceed in extremely high yields, as illustrated by the Carothers equation:

$$\overline{DP} = \frac{1}{1 - p} \qquad (1)$$

where $\overline{DP}$ is the degree of polymerization and p is the percent conversion of functional groups (yield).

According to this equation a $\overline{DP}$ of 20 requires that 95% of the functional groups react and a $\overline{DP}$ of 50 requires a 98% conversion. Because most condensation polymers are not useful unless the $\overline{DP}$ is at least 50, it is clear that only reactions that proceed in extremely high conversions can be used.

Condensation polymerizations can be carried out by a condensation of two monomers, each monomer bearing two identical functional groups on the same molecule or by the self-condensation of one monomer bearing two appropriate functional groups. In either case, an exact equivalence of functional groups is essential to achieve high molecular weight and the Carothers equation can be modified to show the effect of unbalanced stoichiometry on the degree of conversion.

Thus, when two bifunctional monomers is used,

$$\overline{DP} = \frac{1 + r}{2r(1 - p) + 1 - r} \tag{2}$$

where r is the ratio of the two monomers in the reaction mixture. For an exact equivalence of the two monomers $r = 1$, and the equation reduces to the unmodified Carothers equation.

The Carothers equation can also be modified to take into account a small amount of monofunctional reagents in condensation reactions that use monomers having both functional groups on one molecule. Thus,

$$\overline{DP} = \frac{1 + N_1/N_o}{1 - p + N_1/N_o} \tag{3}$$

where N_o is the number of bifunctional molecules and N_1 the number of monofunctional molecules.

III. POLYMERIZATION METHODS

Polymerization methods can be broadly classified into bulk polymerizations, solution polymerizations, suspension polymerizations, emulsion polymerizations, and interfacial polymerizations. Because the applicability and characteristics of these methods are different in chain and step-growth polymerizations, they are discussed separately.

A. Polymerization Methods for Chain Polymerizations

1. *Bulk Polymerization*

This procedure involves the polymerization of neat monomers and two situations can arise. In one the polymer is not soluble in the monomer, so solid polymer precipitates as the polymerization process takes place. In the other the polymer is soluble in the monomer, so the viscosity of the polymer mass increases with time until it is completely converted to solid polymer. An example of the former situation is the polymerization of acrylonitrile; an example of the latter situation is the polymerization of styrene or methyl methacrylate.

A significant advantage of this method is that very pure polymers can be prepared. However, because chain polymerizations are highly exothermic and because polymers are good insulators, heat dissipation from the bulk of the polymer mass is difficult, and the method is limited to small-scale polymerizations or to industrial situations using specialized equipment.

2. *Solution Polymerization*

In this procedure the monomer or monomers are dissolved in a suitable solvent and then polymerized. The chosen solvent should be a solvent for both monomer and polymer. Because the end-product is a solution of the polymer in the solvent, stirring throughout the polymerization process is possible; thus, heat evolution can be controlled by means of external cooling. The concentration of the monomer in the solvent should be adjusted to avoid an excessively viscous final solution.

The polymer is isolated by either solvent evaporation or precipitation of the polymer solution into a large excess of nonsolvent. Residual solvent is removed from the polymer by heating in a vacuum oven. Because it is difficult to remove solvents from polymers, long heating under vacuum may be necessary.

3. *Suspension Polymerization*

In this procedure the monomer is dispersed in a dispersing medium, and polymerization occurs in the monomer droplets suspended in the dispersing medium. Although nonaqueous media can be used, water is used almost exclusively as the dispersing medium. Clearly, when water is used as the dispersing medium, water-soluble monomers cannot be used unless a salting out procedure is used.

Suspension polymerizations are used with free radical polymerizations where the initiator is dissolved in the monomer, which is then dispersed in water using an emulsifying agent. Polymerization is initiated in the monomer droplets dispersed in the aqueous medium.

In this method, each monomer droplet polymerizes by a bulk polymerization process, but because each droplet is surrounded by water, heat dissipation is not a problem. Furthermore, because the polymer is never dissolved in the suspension medium, excessive viscosity buildup is not a problem and very high monomer concentrations can be used. Polymers obtained by this polymerization method are spheres, typically between 0.01–0.5 cm in diameter.

4. *Emulsion Polymerization*

Experimentally, this polymerization procedure is identical to suspension polymerizations, but differs in that the initiator is insoluble in the monomer and soluble in water. Because of this difference, the kinetics of the polymerization process is distinctly different. Polymer particles produced by this method are typically 0.1 μm in diameter.

When a water-insoluble monomer is dispersed in water that also contains a water-soluble initiator and an emulsifying agent, the various species shown in Figure 2 are present in the polymerization system. A small portion of the emulsifier molecules are dissolved in water, but the bulk aggregate to form colloidal clusters also known as micelles, where the emulsifier molecules arrange their hydrocarbon portions towards the interior and the hydrophilic ends towards the outside.

A small portion of the monomer molecules dissolve in water and a somewhat larger, but still very small portion of the monomer molecules dissolves in the hydrocarbon portion of the micelles. However, the bulk of the monomer is present as dispersed monomer droplets, stabilized by the emulsifier. Typically, the size of these monomer droplets is about 10,000 Å at a concentration of about 10^{10} monomer droplets/cc. This concentration is significantly smaller than that of the micelles which are present at a concentration of about 10^{18}/cc.

Because the concentration of the monomer dissolved in the aqueous phase is extremely low and because the initiator is not soluble in the monomer droplets, polymerization takes place almost exclusively in

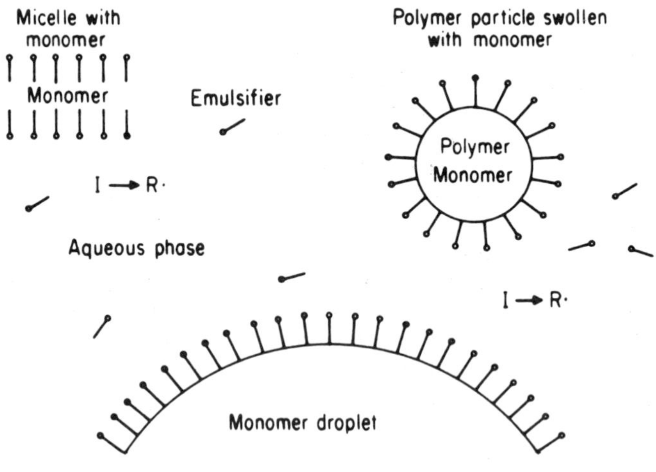

Fig. 2 Simplified representation of an emulsion polymerization system. (Reproduced from G. Odian, *Principles of Polymerizations*, McGraw-Hill Book Co., New York, 1970, p. 283.)

the micelles which serve as the meeting place for the water soluble initiator and water insoluble monomer. As polymerization proceeds, the size of the micelles increases by addition of monomer from the monomer droplets and as the active micelles grow in size, they absorb emulsifier molecules from the solution. When the emulsifier concentration in solution falls below the critical micelle concentration the inactive micelles become unstable and dissolve. At this point, the active micelles are no longer considered micelles, but are in reality monomer swollen polymer particles and all of the emulsifier molecules have adsorbed on the polymer particles.

As polymerization continues in the polymer particles, monomer from the monomer droplets diffuse into the polymer particles and the size of the monomer droplets decreases while the size of the polymer particles increases. At about 50–80% conversion, monomer droplets disappear completely and all the unreacted monomer is contained in the polymer particles.

In this method, polymerization starts when a free radical diffuses into a micelle and initiates the polymerization process. Because termination in free radical polymerizations is a bimolecular process, polymerization in the micelle will continue until a second radical diffuses into the micelle and initiates growth of another chain. Termination can then proceed by coupling or disproportionation, as already discussed. When a third radical diffuses into the micelle, polymerization will again resume and will terminate when a fourth radical diffuses in. Thus, on the average, the micelles are only active one-half of the time.

There are two very important consequences of this unique polymerization process. First, due to the lower frequency of termination, chain growth can continue for longer periods of time and hence polymers prepared by emulsion polymerizations can have very high molecular weights. Second, in conventional free radical polymerization the propagation rate is described by

$$r_p = k_p \, [M][M\cdot] \tag{4}$$

whereas in emulsion polymerization the rate is described by

$$r_p = k_p \, [M][N/2] \tag{5}$$

In these expressions [M] is the concentration of monomer, [M·] is the concentration of radical chain ends, and N is the number of micelles.

Due to bimolecular termination reactions, the concentration of free radical chain-ends [M·] is very much lower than [N/2], so rates of emulsion polymerization are significantly higher than rates of conventional free radical polymerizations.

B. Polymerization Methods for Step-Growth Polymerization

1. *Bulk Polymerizations*

Because step-growth polymerizations are not exothermic, heat dissipation is not a problem, and bulk polymerization is an excellent method for producing polymers by a step-growth polymerization.

2. *Solution Polymerization*

This is also an excellent polymerization method. Because of the critical importance of exact stoichiometry for achievement of high molecular weight, the solvent must be purified to remove impurities that might react with monomer functional groups.

3. *Interfacial Polycondensation*

This is a specialized method using two mutually immiscible solvents, each containing one monomer and where the polycondensation reaction occurs at the interface between the two solvents. The method can only be applied to very rapid reactions such as the reaction between an acid chloride and an amine. Thus, polyamides can be readily formed by this process by placing the amine in water and the diacid chloride in carbon tetrachloride.

IV. POLYMER FABRICATION

Polymer fabrication involves the conversion of monomers or bulk polymer into the desired useful form. Of primary concern in selecting a fabrication method is whether the material is a thermoplastic or a thermoset. Other considerations are polymer softening temperature, thermal stability, and production volume.

Polymer fabrication methods can be generally divided into those used with plastics, fibers, or rubbers. In this brief survey, only methods used with plastics and then only those useful in controlled release applications are described.

A. Molding

In this procedure the polymer is forced to flow into a closed container having the desired shape by the application of heat and pressure. The closed container is known as the mold. Various molding procedures are in use.

1. *Compression Molding*

In this procedure the polymer is placed in the lower half of a heated mold, the mold is closed, air and excess polymer are forced out, and

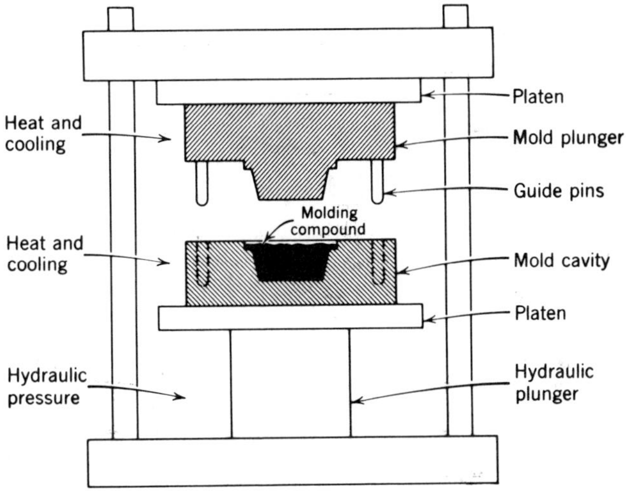

Fig. 3 Diagram of a compression-molding press and mold. (Reproduced from F. W. Billmeyer, Jr., *Textbook of Polymer Science*, 2nd ed., Wiley Interscience, New York, 1962, p. 492.)

final pressure is applied for the selected time period. With thermoplastic materials the mold is then cooled and the object removed. With thermoset materials cooling is not necessary because cured thermoset polymers cannot flow. A schematic of a typical compression-molding apparatus is shown in Figure 3.

2. *Injection Molding*

In this procedure the polymer is first preheated and then forced into a cold mold cavity by means of a hydraulic plunger at pressures ranging between 10,000 and 30,000 psi. Because the mold is cold, this is a high speed method, which, unlike compression molding, does not require a time-consuming cooling step. This methodology has reached an extremely high degree of sophistication. A schematic of an injection molding apparatus is shown in Figure 4.

3. *Transfer Molding*

Because polymers are good insulators, uniform heat transfer throughout the bulk of a sizable molded object is difficult. This may result in uneven cure of thermosetting materials or uneven densities of thermoplastic materials. For this reason, transfer moldings, a combination of compression molding and injection molding was developed.

A schematic diagram of a transfer mold is shown in Figure 5. The molding process consists of heating the polymer in a preheat

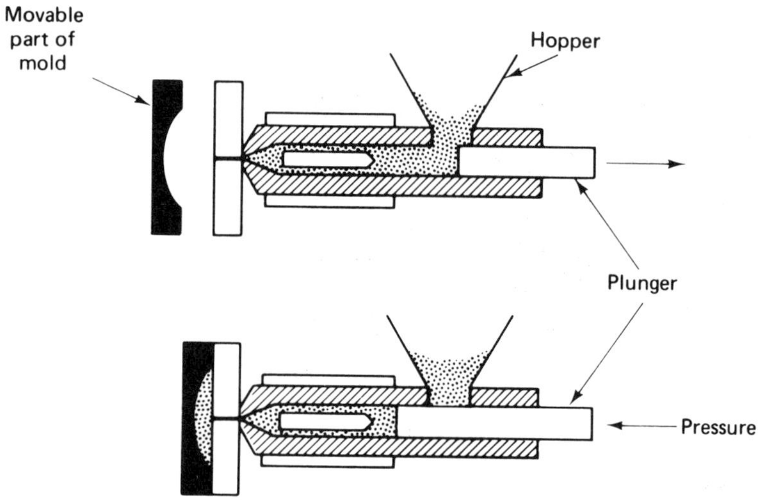

Fig. 4 Injection-molding cycle. (Reproduced from H. R. Allcock and F. W. Lampe, *Contemporary Polymer Chemistry*, Prentice-Hall Inc., Englewood Cliffs, NJ, 1981, p. 524.)

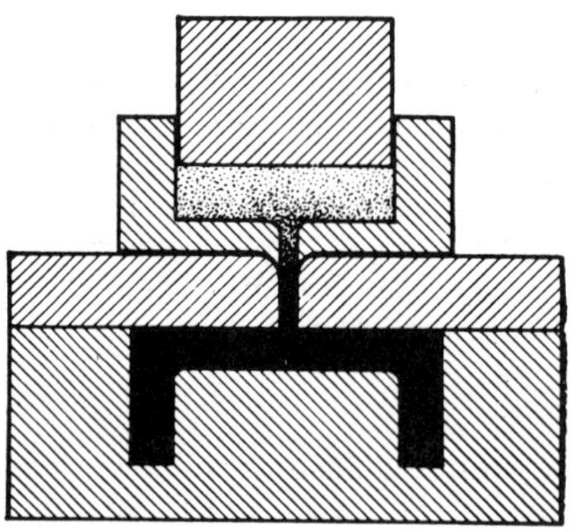

Fig. 5 Schematic of a transfer mold. (Reproduced form B. Golding, *Polymers and Resins*, D. Van Nostrand Co., Inc., Princeton, NJ, 1959, p. 587.)

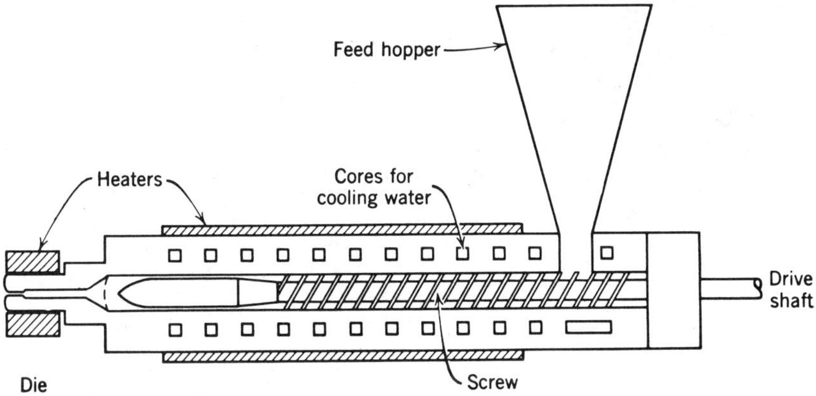

Fig. 6 Diagram of a plastics extruder. (Reproduced from F. W. Billmeyer, Jr., *Textbook of Polymer Science*, 2nd ed., Wiley Interscience, New York, 1962, p. 497.)

cavity until it becomes semifluid and then forcing it by means of a ram through an orifice into the mold cavity. Because the entire mold is heated, thermoplastic materials cannot be removed until the mold has cooled.

B. Extrusion

In this process, polymer is propelled continuously along a screw through regions of high temperature and pressure where it is melted and compacted and finally forced through a die to give the final object. The procedure is useful for preparing rods, tubes, channels and sheets. A schematic diagram of an extruder is shown in Figure 6.

C. Preparation of Films

Polymer films can be made either by a melt-fabrication technique, solution-casting, or polymerization *in situ*.

1. Melt Fabrication

Films can be produced by extrusion through a suitably shaped die or by first extruding a tube and then expanding the hot tube by compressed gas into a tube of thin film. This latter process is shown in Figure 7.

Another process known as calendering is shown in Figure 8. In this procedure the polymer is squeezed into a thin film between heated rollers.

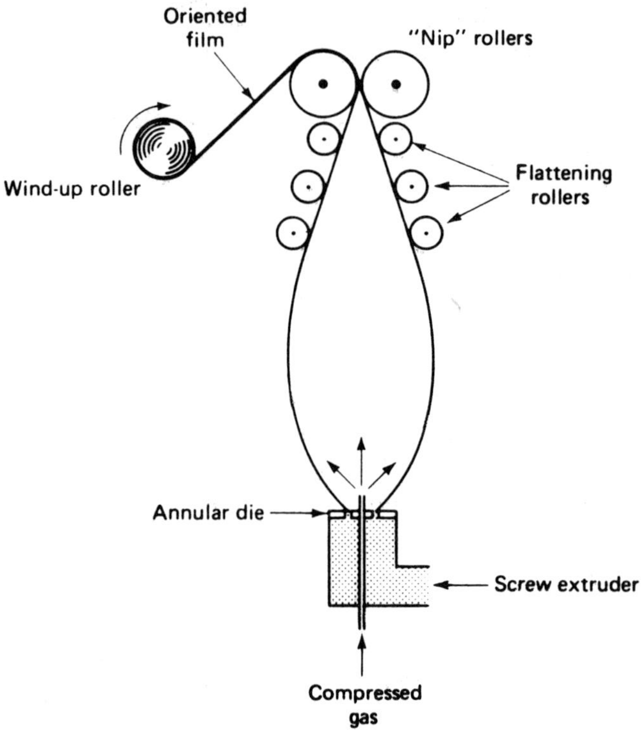

Fig. 7 "Bubble" blowing of films. (Reproduced from H. R. Allcock and F. W. Lampe, *Contemporary Polymer Chemistry*, Prentice-Hall, Inc., Englewood Cliffs, NJ, 1981, p. 513.)

Films can also be produced by melt-pressing where the polymer is placed between two metal plates and the plates then placed between two heated platens in a press, as shown in Figure 9.

2. *Solution-Casting*

In this procedure the polymer is dissolved in a suitable solvent to form a viscous solution that is then spread on a flat, nonadhesive surface; then the solvent slowly evaporates. The resultant polymer film is then peeled from the surface.

On a laboratory scale, the thickness of the polymer solution is usually controlled with a "Gardener knife," a device that allows micrometer adjustments of a blade height above the casting surface. Industrially, rotating metal drums or moving belt systems shown in Figure 10, are used.

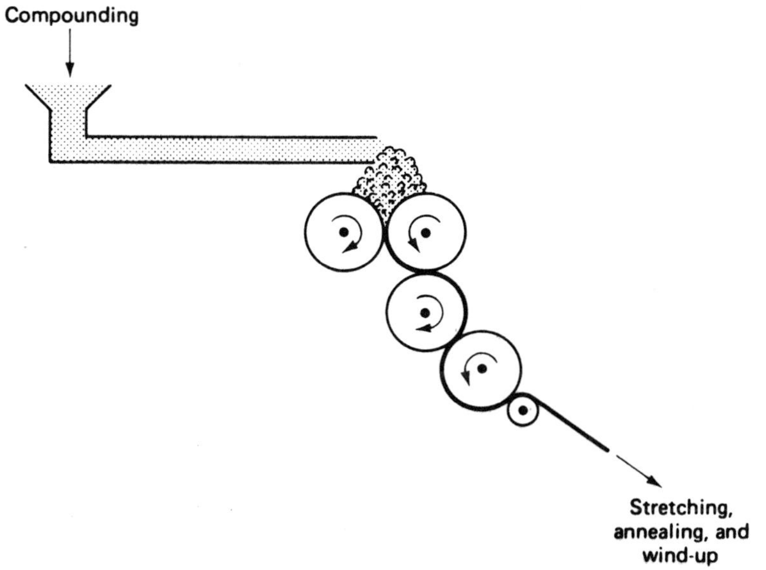

Fig. 8 Film manufacture by calendering. (Reproduced from H. R. Allcock and F. W. Lampe, *Contemporary Polymer Chemistry*, Prentice-Hall Inc., Englewood Cliffs, NJ, 1981, p. 513.)

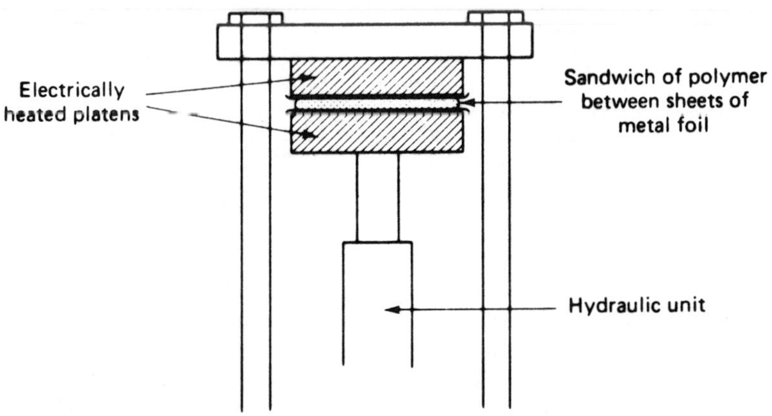

Fig. 9 Hydraulic press for the melt pressing of polymer films. (Reproduced from H. R. Allcock and F. W. Lampe, *Contemporary Polymer Chemistry*, Prentice-Hall Inc., Englewood Cliffs, NJ, 1981, p. 511.)

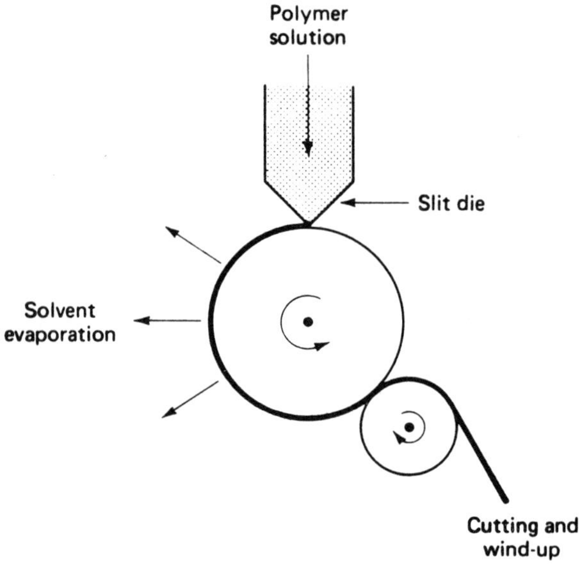

(a)

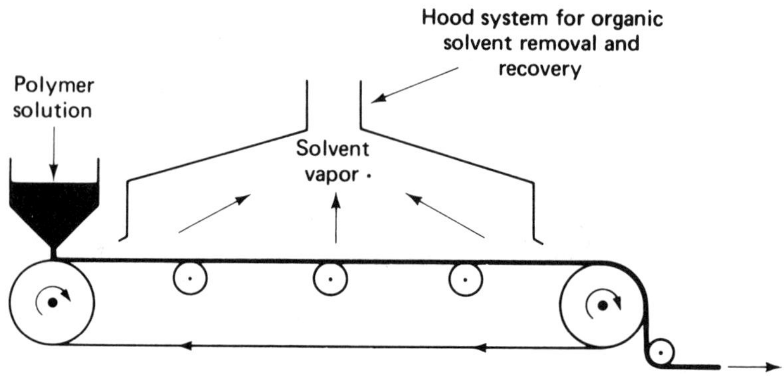

(b)

Fig. 10 (a) Solution casting of films on an industrial scale, with the use of rotating metal drums. (b) Use of a moving-belt system for the continuous solution casting of polymer films. (Reproduced from H. R. Allcock and F. W. Lampe, *Contemporary Polymer Chemistry*, Prentice-Hall Inc., Englewood Cliffs, NJ, 1981, p. 510.)

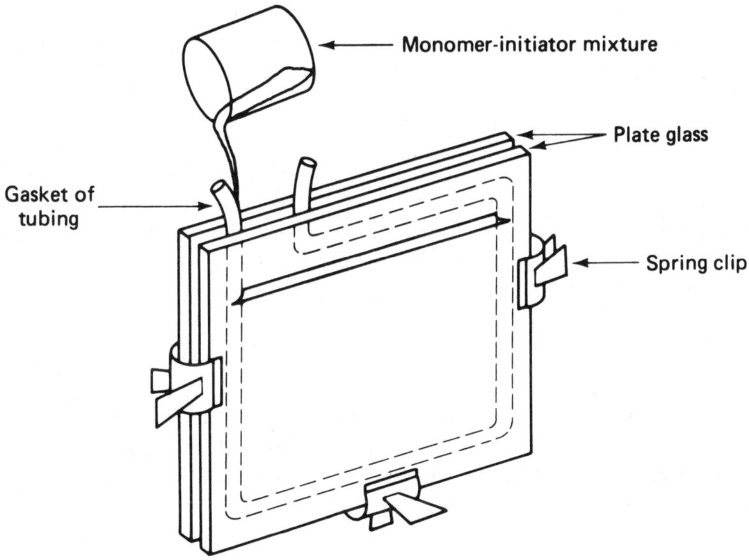

Fig. 11 Procedure for casting sheets of polymer. (Reproduced from H. R. Allcock and F. W. Lampe, *Contemporary Polymer Chemistry*, Prentice-Hall Inc., Englewood Cliffs, NJ, 1981, p. 522.)

3. *Polymerization* In Situ

In this procedure, a liquid polymer or prepolymer is polymerized inside a suitable mold. This procedure is useful for preparing sheets of rigid polymers and is particularly useful for preparing sheets of crosslinked polymer. A typical apparatus for this procedure is shown in Figure 11.

D. Use of Additives

Many polymers in their pure form have properties that make them unsuitable for certain specific applications. However, by use of fillers, plasticizers, and stabilizers, these properties can be substantially improved.

1. *Fillers*

These can be subdivided into particulate and fibrous. In general, fillers substantially improve dimensional stability, impact resistance, tensile and compressive strength, abrasion resistance, and thermal stability. Typical particulate fillers are carbon black, short glass fibers, carbon fibers, asbestos, mica, wood, and flour. Typical fibrous fillers are cellulosic fibers, synthetic fibers (such as nylon or polyesters), carbon fibers, and boron filaments.

2. *Plasticizers*

These additives lower the glass transition temperature of a polymer and hence improve flow and decrease brittleness. To be useful, a plasticizer must be miscible with the polymer and have a low diffusion rate within the polymer to ensure permanence. Typical plasticizers are phthalate esters, adipates and similar compounds, fatty acid esters, and glycol derivatives.

3. *Stabilizers*

These are used to stabilize a polymer against degradation. An important class of stabilizers are antioxidants which are compounds that can be readily oxidized to form unreactive radicals. Common antioxidants are phenols and aromatic amines.

V. POLYMER PROPERTIES

A. Molecular Weight and Molecular Weight Distribution

Because polymerization is a random process, molecules within a given polymer mass will have different molecular weights, and for this reason molecular weights of polymers are described in terms of average molecular weights.

Polymer molecular weights can be defined in different ways, and the most common molecular weights are the number average molecular weight, $\overline{M}_n$, the weight average molecular weight, $\overline{M}_w$, and the viscosity average molecular weight, $\overline{M}_v$. These averages are defined as follows:

$$\overline{M}_n = \frac{w}{\Sigma N_i} = \frac{\Sigma N_i M_i}{\Sigma N_i} \qquad (6)$$

where

$$w = \Sigma N_i M_i$$

$$\overline{M}_w = \frac{\Sigma w_i M_i}{w} = \frac{\Sigma N_i M_i^2}{\Sigma N_i M_i} \qquad (7)$$

$$\bar{M}_v = \left[\frac{\Sigma N_i M_i^{1+a}}{\Sigma N_i M_i}\right]^{1/a} \tag{8}$$

for

$$a = 1,\ \bar{M}_v = \bar{M}_w$$

The ratio of $\bar{M}_w/\bar{M}_n$, also known as the polydispersity index, indicates broadness of molecular weight distribution, and for $\bar{M}_w/\bar{M}_n = 1$ the polymer is monodispersed; that is, all polymer molecules within a polymer mass have the same molecular weight.

The broadness of molecular weight distribution or polydispersity depends on the preparative method used to synthesize the polymer. Anionic living polymer techniques can produce polymers with a polydispersity index close to one, whereas other chain polymerizations can have a polydispersity index as high as 20. Step-growth polymerizations have a polydispersity index of about two, known as the "most probable" molecular weight distribution.

A knowledge of molecular weight and molecular weight distribution of polymers is important because there is a definite relationship between polymer molecular weight and polymer properties. Thus, at very low molecular weights the polymer has essentially no useful mechanical properties, but as the molecular weight rises, the magnitude of the mechanical property of interest also rises.

This effect is illustrated in Figure 12 which shows the increase of tensile strength of polystyrene with increasing number average molecular weight. Thus, a polymer with $\bar{M}_n = 40{,}000$ has essentially no tensile strength but as the molecular weight increases the tensile strength rapidly increases and ultimately levels off at $\bar{M}_n = 150{,}000$. The particular shape of the curve and the $\bar{M}_n$ at which tensile strength levels off depend on the method of polymer synthesis and method used to fabricate tensile specimens.

The relationship between property and $\bar{M}_n$ can in general be represented as

$$\text{Property} = a + b/\bar{M}_n \tag{9}$$

where a and b are constants. This relationship is analogous to one that relates molecular weight and glass transition temperature and, indeed, the relationship between property and molecular weight can be partially attributed to changes in the free volume of the polymer with changing molecular weight. However, molecular entanglement is also important and appreciable tensile strengths cannot be achieved

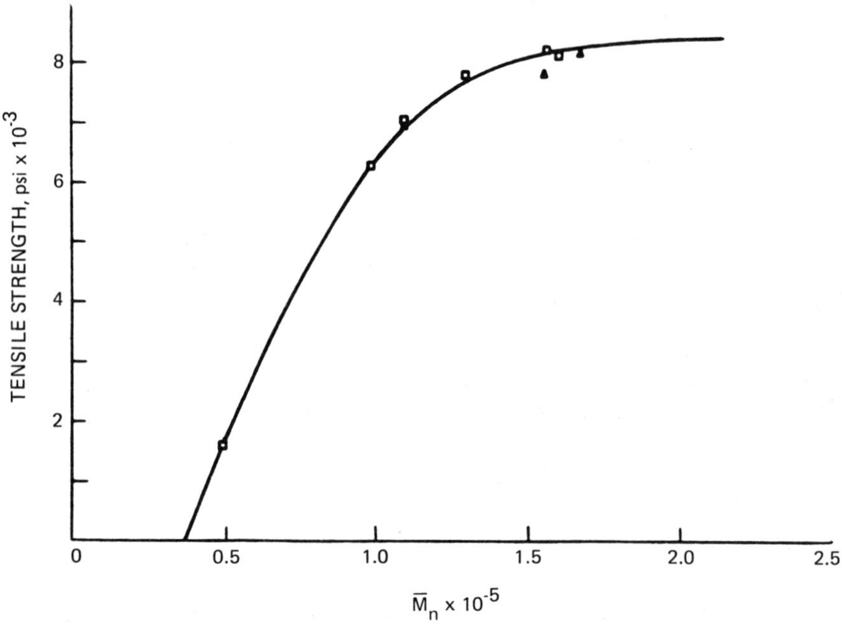

Fig. 12 Plot of tensile strength against number average molecular weight for polystyrene. [Adapted from H. W. McCormick, F. M. Brower, and L. Kin, *J. Polymer Sci. 39*, 87–100 (1959).]

until the molecular weight is high enough for a significant entanglement network to form.

B. Polymer Hydrophobicity

When a polymer is placed in an aqueous environment, it will gradually absorb water, and the amount of absorbed water is determined by the polymer structure. Because use of a polymeric controlled-release device exposes the polymer to an aqueous environment, its interaction with water is of considerable importance.

According to the nature of polymer-water interactions, polymers can be broadly classified into hydrophobic polymers, hydrophilic polymers, water-soluble polymers, and hydrogels.

1. *Hydrophobic Polymers*

These polymers are essentially water impermeable and, when placed in an aqueous environment, will absorb very little water. Clearly, there is no fixed value for the amount of absorbed water below which a polymer is hydrophobic and above which it is hydrophilic, but for purposes of this classification the amount of absorbed water should be less than 5 wt%.

Structural parameters that contribute to polymer hydrophobicity are chain stiffness, high degree of crystallinity, and presence of highly hydrophobic groups where C–H bonds have been replaced by C–F bonds.

2. *Hydrophilic Polymers*

These are polymers that absorb more than 5 wt% water. Clearly, there can be a considerable variation between polymers in their ability to absorb water, and structural parameters that contribute to polymer hydrophilicity are chain flexibility, absence of crystallinity, and presence of certain group such as amino, carboxyl, and hydroxyl, etc.

A useful method for varying the hydrophilicity of a polymer involves the copolymerization of two monomers, one leading to a highly hydrophilic or even water-soluble polymer and the other leading to a hydrophobic polymer. An example of such an approach is the copolymerization of hydroxyethyl methacrylate and methyl methacrylate.

3. *Water-Soluble Polymers*

Some polymers are freely soluble in water, even though they are of very high molecular weight. Examples of such polymers include poly(vinyl alcohol), poly(acrylic acid), poly(N-vinyl pyrrolidone), polyacrylamide, and poly(ethylene oxide).

4. *Hydrogels*

These are highly hydrophilic or water soluble polymers that have been crosslinked by means of covalent bonds. Because the polymer cannot dissolve due to the covalent crosslinks, water uptakes far in excess of those achievable with hydrophilic linear polymers can be obtained.

C. Glass Transition Temperature

At low enough temperatures, all amorphous polymers exist in a glassy state where no large-scale molecular motion can take place, and while in the glassy state, polymers are characterized by their hardness, stiffness, and brittleness. As the temperature is raised, polymers undergo a transition, known as the glass transition temperature, T_g, where they change from a glass to a rubbery elastomer or flexible plastic. This transition takes place over a narrow temperature range and corresponds to the onset of segmental motion of long segments of the polymer chain, which is brought about by the availability of sufficient thermal energy to overcome intermolecular interactions.

As a consequence of this transition, the polymer undergoes an abrupt change in properties. Among these are coefficient of expansion, permeability, heat content, refractive index, and hardness. Thus, in designing a controlled-release device, it must be known whether at use, the polymer will be above or below its glass transition temperature.

The glass transition temperature, also known as the second-order transition, is a characteristic of a particular polymer structure, and its value is closely related to intermolecular forces and chain stiffness. Thus, because above the T_g segmental motions of polymer chains take place, it follows that very flexible polymers, where free rotation about bonds along the polymer chains is possible, will in general have low T_g values. For this reason, poly(dimethyl siloxane), in which virtually unrestricted rotation takes place between the silicon-oxygen bond, has one of the lowest T_g values known (−123°C).

Clearly, the onset of segmental motion of polymer chains will also depend on the magnitude of intermolecular forces because no motion of polymer chains can take place until enough thermal energy is available to overcome those forces. Consequently, polymers with strong intermolecular interactions will tend to have high T_g values.

The glass transition temperature of a random copolymer will usually fall between those of the homopolymers and can be estimated by the following relationship:

$$\frac{1}{T_g} = \frac{w_1}{T_{g1}} + \frac{w_2}{T_{g2}} \tag{10}$$

where w_1 and w_2 are the weight fractions of homopolymers 1 and 2 having glass transitions T_{g1} and T_{g2}.

D. Crystallinity

Polymers that have a regular structure are able to achieve a regular packing of polymer chains and crystallize. The driving force for crystallization is a closer packing of polymer chains with consequent enhancement of intermolecular attractions. However, unlike small molecules, where crystallization results in the regular packing of molecules or ions into a three-dimensional lattice, polymers only exhibit crystallinity in domains that occur within the amorphous polymer. However, a few polymers, among these polyethylene, can be prepared as single crystals.

The presence of crystallinity has a significant effect on polymer properties because crystalline regions act as crosslinks for the regions and for this reason stiffen and toughen the polymer and reduce swelling in solvents. Furthermore, because crystalline regions are impermeable to diffusing molecules, an enhancement of crystallinity results in a decrease in polymer permeability. Crystalline regions are also essentially impermeable to water, so the rate of polymer hydrolysis in crystalline regions is significantly reduced.

IV. POLYMER CHARACTERIZATION

A. Molecular Weight

A comprehensive discussion of the various methods for determining molecular weights is well beyond the scope of this brief outline, and many excellent texts are available. Therefore, this section is limited to a presentation of basic principles only.

1. Osmometry

This method is used to determine the number average molecular weight, $\bar{M}_n$. Although in principle the measurement of any colligative property of a solution (such as freezing point depression, elevation of boiling point, or osmotic pressure) can be used to determine the molecular weight of a dissolved solute, only osmotic pressure is sensitive enough to measure the high molecular weights characteristic of polymeric substances.

Osmotic measurements use a semipermeable membrane through which the solvent can freely pass but which excludes polymer molecules. If this membrane separates two compartments, one filled with pure solvent and the other with a polymer solution, the activity of the solvent in the two compartments is different because polymer molecules cannot pass through the membrane; as a result, an osmotic pressure driving solvent into the polymer solution compartment will develop.

This osmotic pressure π is given, for ideal solutions only, by

$$\frac{\pi}{C} \simeq \frac{RT}{M_n} \qquad (11)$$

For nonideal solutions, ideality can be approached at the limit of infinite dilution, and

$$\lim_{c \to o} \left(\frac{\pi}{c}\right) = \frac{RT}{M_n} \qquad (12)$$

Thus, to obtain M_n, π/c is plotted as a function of c and extrapolated to c = o.

2. *Light Scattering*

Scattering of light by liquids can be related to local fluctuations in density due to thermal motions of molecules. With solutions, additional scattering arises from local fluctuations in the concentration of the solute. From measurements of light scattering of dilute polymer solutions it is possible to derive the weight average molecular weight, $\overline{M}_w$.

Unfortunately, even a simple description of light scattering is fairly complex, and the reader is referred to the excellent treatments available in contemporary textbooks on polymer science.

3. *Viscometry*

Unlike osmometry and light scattering, which are absolute methods in that they allow molecular weight determinations of unknown polymers, viscometry is a relative method and requires calibration with samples of polymer of known molecular weights.

Determination of polymer molecular weight by measurement of the viscosity of polymer solutions is based on the fact that, as polymer molecular weight increases, so does the viscosity of its solutions. The viscosity is measured by timing flow of the solution between two marks in various viscometers, shown in Figure 13. Several viscosity terms can be defined. The simplest of these is the relative viscosity, η_r

$$\eta_r = \frac{t}{t_o} \tag{13}$$

where t_o is the flow time of pure solvent and t is the flow time of the polymer solution.

Another viscosity term is the specific viscosity, η_{sp},

$$\eta_{sp} = \eta_r - 1 \tag{14}$$

Because neither of these viscosities contain a concentration term, no molecular weight information can be derived from these expressions, but they are useful to at least qualitatively estimate whether a particular polymer is of "reasonable" molecular weight.

A viscosity average molecular weight, $\overline{M}_v$, can be obtained by measuring the reduced viscosity, η_{red},

$$\eta_{red} = \frac{\eta_{sp}}{c} \tag{15}$$

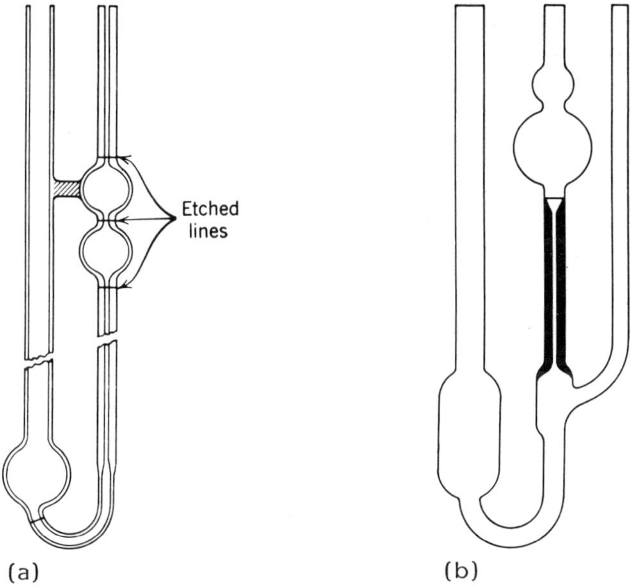

Fig. 13 Capillary viscometers (a) Ostwald-Fenske, (b) Ubbelohde. (Reproduced from F. W. Billmeyer, Jr., *Textbook of Polymer Science*, 2nd ed., Wiley Interscience, New York, 1962, p. 85.)

at a series of decreasing concentrations and extrapolating to c = o. The value at c = o defines the intrinsic viscosity [η] as

$$[\eta] = \lim_{c \to o} \frac{\eta_{sp}}{c} \tag{16}$$

Actual molecular weights can be obtained from measurements of [η] only if the method has previously been calibrated with polymer samples of known molecular weight. To do so, the intrinsic viscosity is measured for a series of narrow-distribution, known molecular weight samples of the same polymer, and a plot is constructed of log M versus log [η]. The resulting straight line is given by

$$\log [\eta] = \log K + a \log M \tag{17}$$

or

$$[\eta] = KM^a \tag{18}$$

The last equation is known as the Mark-Houwink equation and the constants K and a as the Mark-Houwink parameters.

The usefulness of this expression is derived from the fact that Mark-Houwink parameters for a wide range of polymers are available in the literature, so a simple measurement of intrinsic viscosity permits a determination of molecular weights if the Mark-Houwink parameters are available. Clearly, the intrinsic viscosity must be measured under the same set of experimental conditions as those used to determine the Mark-Houwink parameters.

4. *Gel Permeation Chromatography*

Gel permeation chromatography is a procedure whereby polymer molecules are separated according to their size. This method, also a relative method, is capable of measuring not only molecular weight, but also molecular weight distribution.

In this procedure a dilute polymer solution is pumped through a series of columns containing porous beads with different pore sizes but about of the same dimension as the polymer molecules. Then, the smallest polymer molecules will be able to penetrate all pores, the largest polymer molecules will not be able to penetrate any pores, and intermediate size polymer molecules will penetrate some pores but not penetrate others. Therefore, on the average, the smallest molecules will take the longest path through the columns, and the largest molecules will take the shortest paths through the columns flowing only through the interstitial volumes. Therefore, the highest molecular weight species will emerge first and the lowest molecular weight species will emerge last.

A schematic diagram of a typical apparatus is shown in Figure 14. Typical detectors are a differential refractometers, U.V. or IR detectors. Molecular weights can be determined only if the method is first calibrated with polymer samples having known molecular weights and a plot of molecular weight versus retention times constructed.

A useful variation of the method uses a low angle laser light scattering apparatus with a flow-through cell as detector. With this arrangement absolute molecular weights and molecular weight distributions can be determined.

B. Thermal Analysis

The most commonly used method for the thermal analysis of polymers is thermogravimetric analysis (TGA), differential scanning calorimetry (DSC), and thermomechanical analysis (TMA).

1. *Thermogravimetric Analysis*

This method uses a thermobalance that is capable of continuously and very accurately measuring the weight of a sample contained in

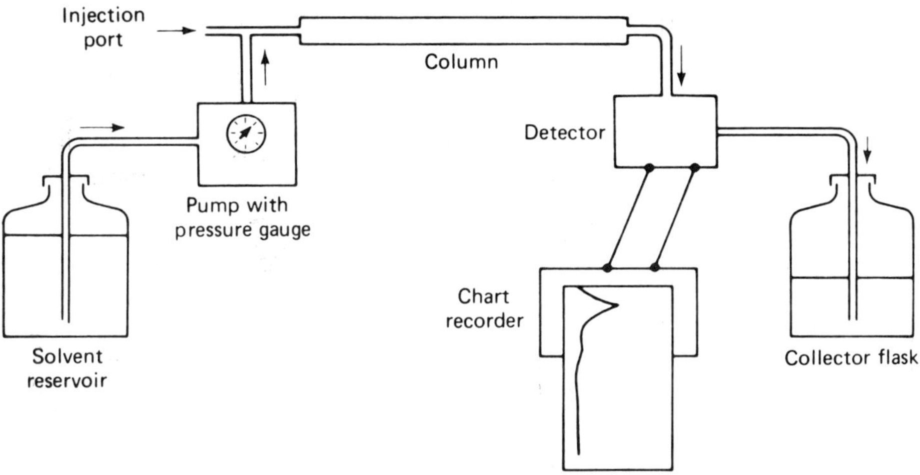

Fig. 14 Schematic diagram of a gel permeation chromatography apparatus. (Reproduced from H. R. Allcock and F. W. Lampe, *Contemporary Polymer Chemistry*, Prentice-Hall Inc., Englewood Cliffs, NJ, 1981, p. 396.)

a pan. The pan is placed in a furnace and the temperature of the furnace slowly raised, usually at 5° to 10°C/min.

The technique is used to determine thermal stability of polymers and the upper limit of thermal stability is usually taken as the temperature at which weight loss of the sample begins. However, the method only measures loss of volatile degradation products from the polymer and is unable to detect chain cleavages that produce degradation fragments that are too large for volatilization.

2. Differential Scanning Calorimetry (DSC)

This is an extremely useful technique for measuring glass transition temperature, crystalline melting points, heats of fusion, and heats of crystallization. The principle on which DSC operates is shown in Figure 15a. The sample and a reference substance, which does not undergo a thermal transition in the temperature range of interest, are placed in two small metal containers and heated by individual electric heaters. The temperature of both samples, monitored by thermocouples, is then gradually raised in such a manner that the temperature of sample and reference remain the same. Then, if the sample suddenly absorbs heat, its heater will supply additional heating to maintain its temperature equal to the reference and if the sample suddenly evolves heat the heater will supply less heat. In

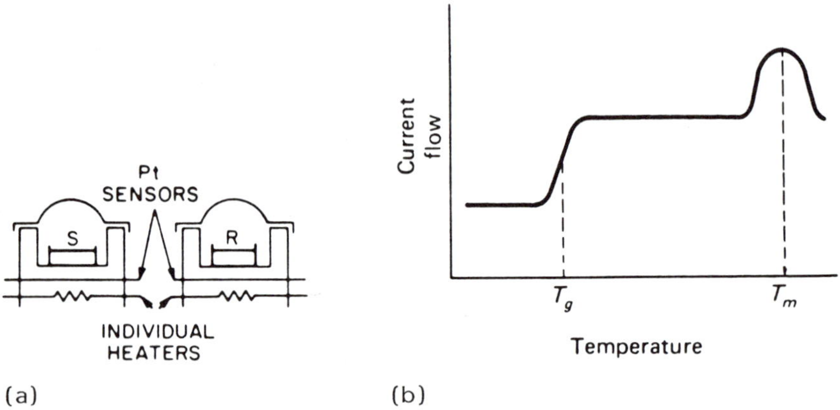

Fig. 15 (a) Schematic of differential calorimetry sample holder. (Reproduced from E. A. Turi, *Thermal Characterization of Polymeric Materials*, Academic Press, New York, 1981, p. 58); (b) Differential scanning calorimetry scan. (Reproduced from F. W. Billmeyer, Jr., *Textbook of Polymer Science*, 2nd ed., Wiley Interscience, New York, 1962, p. 436.)

this way, transition temperatures can be very accurately measured by monitoring the electric current going to the heaters.

Figure 15b shows typical traces for the glass transition temperature and crystalline melting point.

3. *Thermomechanical Analysis* (TMA)

This technique measures deformation of a substance under a nonoscillatory load as a function of the temperature of the sample, which is placed on a platform and contacted with a probe. The probe assembly includes a weight tray that permits a choice of loading on the sample. The probe is connected to the armature of a linear differential transformer that can accurately measure the movement of the probe. A schematic of a typical TMA apparatus is shown in Figure 16.

TMA can conveniently measure transitions from a glassy to a rubbery polymer and can also measure softening temperatures.

C. Mechanical Properties

Mechanical properties of a polymer are most conveniently determined by measuring their stress-strain relationship. Stress is the stretching force applied to the sample, and strain is the elongation of the

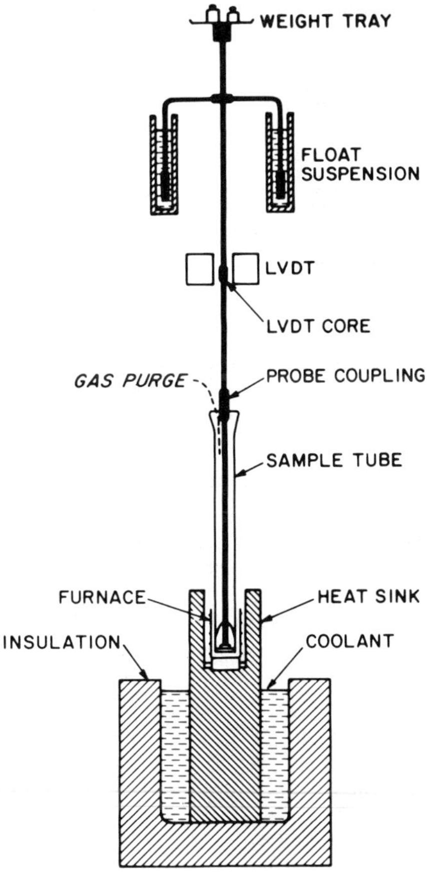

Fig. 16 Typical thermomechanical analyzer apparatus. (Reproduced from E. H. Turi, *Thermal Characterization of Polymeric Materials*, Academic Press, New York, 1981, p. 69.)

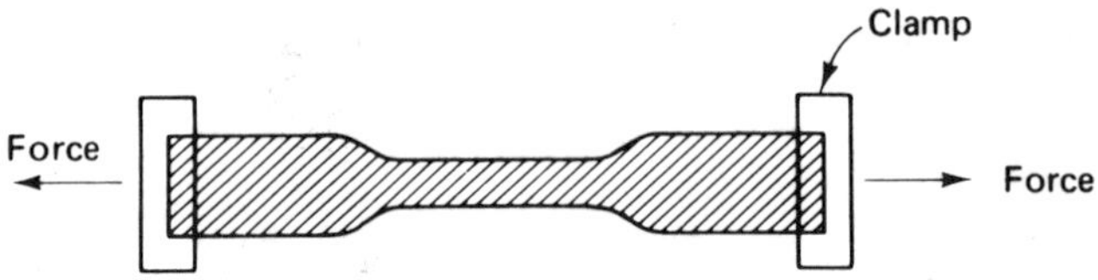

Fig. 17 Typical shape of a flat polymer sample used for stress-strain tests. (Reproduced from H. R. Allcock and F. W. Lampe, *Contemporary Polymer Chemistry*, Prentice-Hall Inc., Englewood Cliffs, NJ, 1981, p. 524.)

sample under a given stress. Because stress-strain relationship in polymers are time-dependent, the speed at which stress is applied is an important experimental parameter.

Stress-strain measurements in polymers are usually performed on dumbell-shaped specimens as shown in Figure 17. The specimen is clamped in a tester, such as an Instron tester, that is capable of extending the specimen at a chosen constant rate and measuring the force that the specimen exerts on a load cell. A typical stress-strain curve for a thermoplastic material, such as polyethylene, is shown in Figure 18. In the initial phase, application of stress causes a

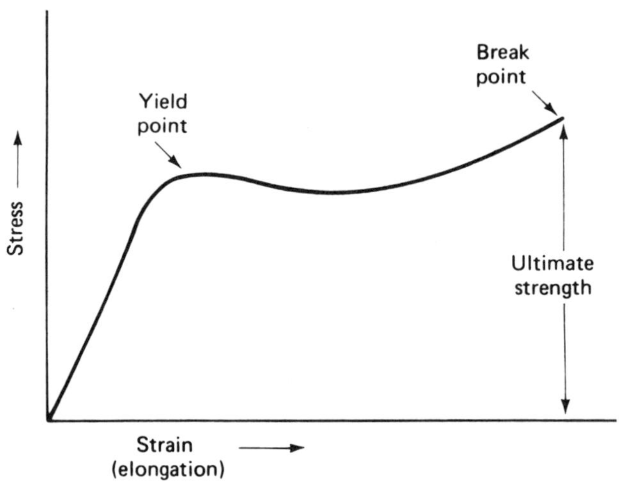

Fig. 18 Stress-strain curve for a thermoplastic material such as polyethylene. (Reproduced from H. R. Allcock and F. W. Lampe, *Contemporary Polymer Chemistry*, Prentice-Hall Inc., Englewood Cliffs, NJ, 1981, p. 536.)

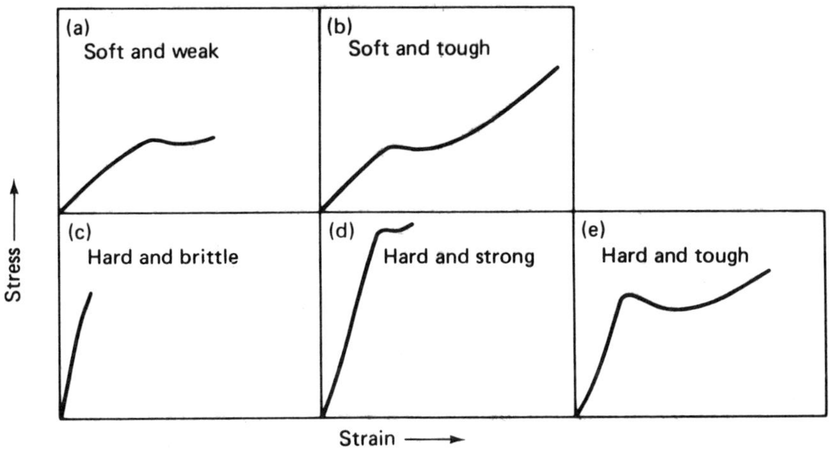

Fig. 19 Characteristic stress-strain curves for five different types of polymeric materials. (Reproduced from H. R. Allcock and F. W. Lampe, *Contemporary Polymer Chemistry*, Prentice-Hall Inc., Englewood Cliffs, NJ, 1981, p. 536.)

moderate elongation to the yield point, after which significant elongation takes place without greatly increased stress. Elongation then continues until the specimen breaks.

Figure 19 illustrates the stress-strain behavior of five typical materials.

4

Use of Polymers in Controlled Release of Active Agents

JORGE HELLER / SRI International, Menlo Park, California

Other than mechanicial pumps, all controlled release devices use polymers in the rate control mechanism. Discussion of the various devices for the release of active agents can be conveniently classified into (a) diffusion-controlled devices, (b) solvent-controlled devices, and (c) chemically controlled devices.

I. DIFFUSION-CONTROLLED DEVICES

With diffusion-controlled devices, two fundamentally different methodologies can be used: release of active agent from monolithic devices and release of active agent from reservoir devices.

A. Monolithic Devices

In a monolithic device the therapeutic agent is intimately mixed in a rate-controlling polymer, and release occurs by diffusion of the agent from the device. It is necessary to consider two types of devices. In one, the active agent is dissolved in the polymer, whereas in the other, the active agent is dispersed in the polymer.

For an active agent dissolved in the matrix, release kinetics can be calculated by two equations [1]. Equation (1), known as the early time approximation, holds true for the first 60% of the release rate, after which it is calculated from Eq. (2), which is known as the late time approximation.

$$\frac{dM_t}{dt} = 2M_x \left(\frac{D}{\pi \ell^2 t}\right)^{1/2} \tag{1}$$

$$\frac{dM_t}{dt} = \frac{8DM_x}{\ell^2} \exp \frac{\pi^2 Dt}{\ell^2} \tag{2}$$

These equations predict active agent release rate from a slab of thickness ℓ where D is the diffusion coefficient, M_x is the total amount of active agent dissolved in the polymer and M_t is the amount released at time t. As Eq. (1) shows, release rate decreases as $t^{-1/2}$ over the first 60% of the release; over the remainder of the release the rate decays exponentially according to Eq. (2). Plots of these two approximations are shown in Figure 1.

When the active agent is dispersed in the polymer, release kinetics have been derived by Higuchi

$$\frac{dM_t}{dt} = \frac{A}{2}\left(\frac{2DC_s C_o}{t}\right)^{1/2} \tag{3}$$

where A is the area, C_s is the solubility of the active agent in the matrix and C_o is total concentration in the matrix (dissolved plus dispersed) [2].

Unlike the slab with dissolved active agent in which the rate is proportional to $t^{-1/2}$ only during the early portion of the release

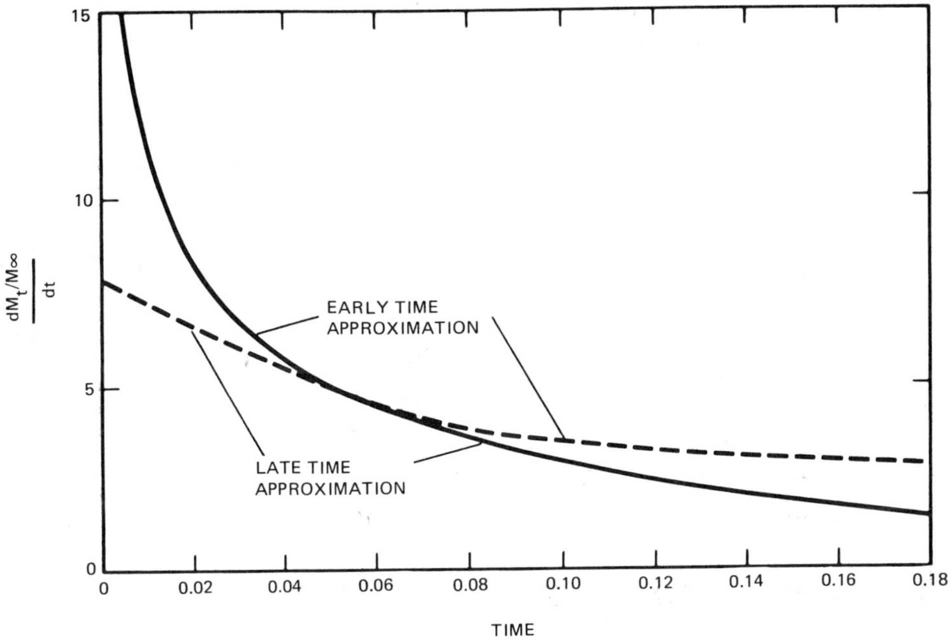

Fig. 1 Release rate of drug initially dissolved in a slab as a function of time. (Reprinted with permission from Ref. 1, p. 43.)

curve, slabs with dispersed active agent maintain a $t^{-1/2}$ dependence over the major portion of the release curve and deviate from this dependence only when the concentration of the active agent remaining in the matrix falls below the saturation value. Because of the $t^{-1/2}$ dependence, a plot of cumulative active agent release versus $t^{1/2}$ will yield a straight line.

Although active agent release from monolithic systems does not proceed by zero-order kinetics, it is the simplest and most convenient way to achieve prolonged release of an active agent. Such devices can be conveniently prepared by using simple polymer fabrication techniques involving a physical blending of the active agent with a polymer matrix, followed by compression molding, injection molding, extrusion, calendering, or solvent casting (see Chapter 3).

B. Reservoir Devices

In a reservoir device the active agent is contained in a core that is surrounded by a rate-controlling membrane. Transport of the material in the core through the surrounding nonporous, homogeneous polymer film occurs by dissolution at one interface of the membrane and then diffusion down a gradient in thermodynamic activity [1]. It can be described by Fick's first law

$$J = -D\frac{dC_m}{dx} \tag{4}$$

where J is the flux in g/cm^2-sec, C_m is the concentration of the permeant in the membrane in g/cm^3, dC_m/dx is the concentration gradient, and D is the diffusion coefficient of the permeant in the membrane in cm^2/sec.

Because the concentration of the permeant just inside the membrane is not known, it is related to the concentration in the medium surrounding the membrane by

$$\begin{aligned} C_{m(o)} &= KC_o \text{ at the upstream side } (x = 0) \\ C_{m(\ell)} &= KC \text{ at the downstream side } (x = \ell) \end{aligned} \tag{5}$$

where K is the distribution coefficient analogous to a liquid-liquid partition coefficient.

The diffusion process is schematically represented in Figure 2. At a steady state, Eq. (4) can be integrated to give

$$J = D\frac{C_{m(o)} - C_{m(\ell)}}{\ell} = D\frac{\Delta C_m}{\ell} \tag{6}$$

Using Eq. (5), Eq. (6) can be rewritten as

$$J = \frac{DK\Delta C}{\ell} \tag{7}$$

where ΔC is the difference in concentration between the solutions on either side of the membrane.

If the thermodynamic activity of the active agent in the reservoir remains constant, if there is no change in the rate-limiting membrane characteristics, and if infinite sink conditions are maintained at the downstream side of the membrane, rate of active agent release will be constant and can be predicted from a knowledge of membrane permeability and device configuration.

Thus, for a slab having a total surface area A, Fick's law can be restated as follows:

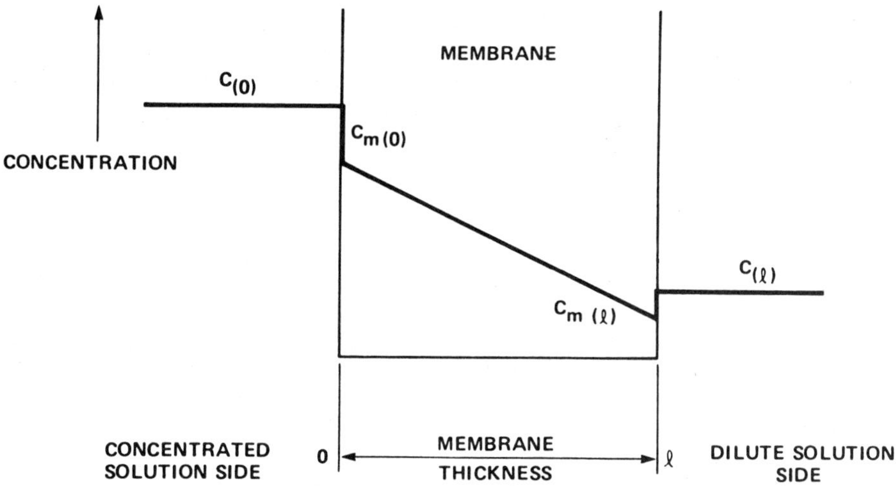

Fig. 2 Schematic representation of the concentration gradient across a membrane. (Reprinted with permission from Ref. 1, p. 19.)

$$\frac{dM_t}{dt} = \frac{ADK\Delta C}{\ell} \tag{8}$$

where M_t is the amount of active agent released and dM_t/dt is the release rate at time t.

Similarly, for a cylinder of inside and outside radii r_o and r_1 and height h, Fick's law is rewritten as

$$\frac{dM_t}{dt} = \frac{2\pi hDK\Delta C}{\ln(r_o - r_1)} \tag{9}$$

Finally, for a sphere of inside and outside radii r_o and r_1, the coresponding expression is

$$\frac{dM_t}{dt} = 4\ DK\ C\ \frac{r_o r_1}{r_o - r_1} \tag{10}$$

In certain applications it may be desirable to replace the dense membrane structure with a microporous, hydrophobic structure. Such membranes have well-defined pores connecting the two sides of the membrane; these pores can be used to immobilize a liquid that is different from the external environment. Diffusion of a permeant then occurs principally by diffusion through the liquid-filled pores.

The flux through such a membrane can be expressed as

$$J = \frac{EDK\Delta C}{\tau \ell} \tag{11}$$

where E is the porosity of the membrane and τ the tortuosity [3].

Even though devices consisting of a reservoir surrounded by a barrier membrane should theoretically be capable of delivering active agents at a constant rate, also referred to as zero-order kinetics, in practice several factors contribute to deviations from zero-order kinetics. The two most important factors are boundary layer effects and the burst effect.

Boundary layer problems arise in applications in which the rate of removal of the active agent from the membrane is slow so that the concentration of the drug at the membrane surface increases with time. Then, as predicted by Eq. (7), the term ΔC decreases and consequently the flux J also decreases. In the extreme case of active agents having very low water solubility, the concentration at the membrane surface can reach saturation value, at which point diffusion will stop and the rate of active agent delivery is completely governed by the rate at which the active agent is removed from the medium surrounding the device.

Burst effects occur when during storage the active agent contained in the core saturates the membrane surrounding the core; then, when the device is placed in desorbing medium, the active agent will rapidly desorb from the membrane. The magnitude of the burst effect is determined by the diffusion coefficient of the active agent in the membrane, the membrane thickness, and the length of storage time.

Although reservoir devices may require more complex fabrication procedures than monolithic devices, they are capable of very long-term, nearly zero-order kinetics and for this reason are of considerable commercial importance.

C. Examples of Diffusion Devices

Because release rate of active agents from monolithic devices is not constant, major commercial utilization has been limited to prolonged release of pesticides, to fertilizers, and to similar applications where manufacturing cost must be low and where constant release is not necessary.

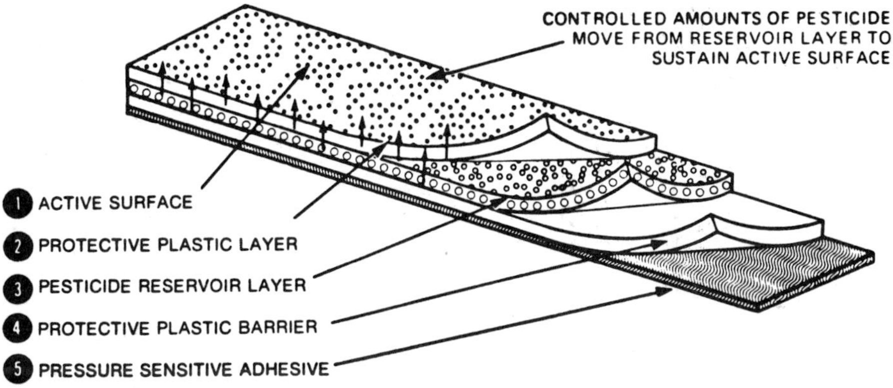

Fig. 3 Schematic of Hercon®, a laminated controlled release structure. [Reprinted with permission from A. F. Kydonieus, in *Controlled Release Pesticides* (H. B. Scher, Ed.), ACS Sypmposium Series, 53, American Chemical Society, Washington, DC, 1977, p. 154.]

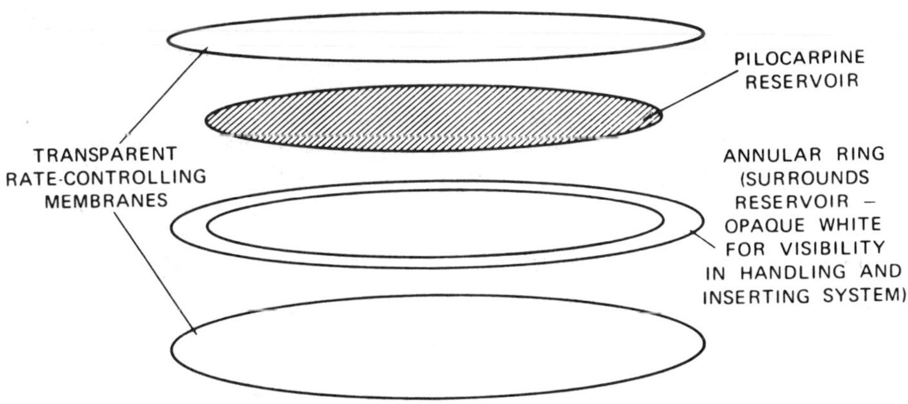

Fig. 4 Schematic diagram of ocular therapeutic system. [Reprinted with permission from S. K. Chandrasekaran, H. Benson, and J. Urquhart, in *Sustained and Controlled Release Drug Delivery Systems* (J. R. Robinson, Ed.), Marcel Dekker, New York, 1978, p. 571.]

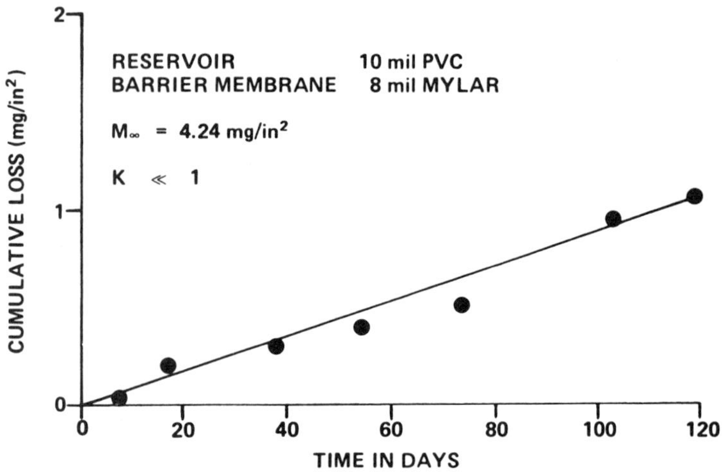

Fig. 5 Release of MGK R-874 fly repellent from a Hercon® multilayered dispenser. [Reprinted with permission from A. F. Kydonieus, in *Controlled Release Pesticides* (H. B. Scher, Ed.), ACS Symposium Series 53, American Chemical Society, Washington, DC, 1977, p. 156.]

One of the first commercial controlled release products was the Shell No-Pest® strip, which contains about 20% dichlorvos dispersed in poly(vinyl chloride) plasticized with 30% dioctylphthalate. Many other devices that contain an active agent dispersed or dissolved in a suitable matrix are also in commercial production.

A number of reservoir devices are also in commercial production. Some are manufactured by relatively simple procedures, such as the Hercon® laminated device for cockroach control shown in Figure 3. Others are manufactured by a significantly more complex procedure, such as the Alza Ocusert® shown schematically in Figure 4.

Release rate from reservoir devices can be constant for long periods of time, as illustrated in Figure 5, which shows release of a fly-repellent from a Hercon® multilayered dispenser. In this particular device the core consists of a 10-mil poly(vinyl chloride) film saturated with the fly repellent, which diffuses through a 8-mil Mylar film. Other devices, such as the Alza Progestasert®, which contains the steroid progesterone in a core surrounded by an ethylene-vinyl acetate copolymer, are capable of maintaining relatively constant release rates for years.

II. SOLVENT-CONTROLLED DEVICES

Solvent-controlled devices release active agents as a consequence of controlled penetration of a solvent into the device. Although non-aqueous solvents can be used, clearly only water is of importance in controlled release applications for human or veterinary applications.

Two general mechanisms have been identified for solvent-controlled devices. These are osmosis and swelling.

A. Osmotically Controlled Devices

The operation of an osmotic pump can be described by referring to Figure 6 [4]. In this device an osmotic agent is contained within a rigid housing and is separated from an active agent compartment by a movable partition. One wall of the rigid housing is a semipermeable membrane so that when the pump is exposed to an aqueous environment, water will be driven osmotically across the membrane; the increased volume within the osmotic compartment will force the active agent out of the device through the delivery orifice.

The volume flux of water across the semipermeable membrane is given by

$$\frac{dV}{dt} = \frac{A}{\ell} L_p \, (\sigma \Delta \pi - \Delta P) \tag{12}$$

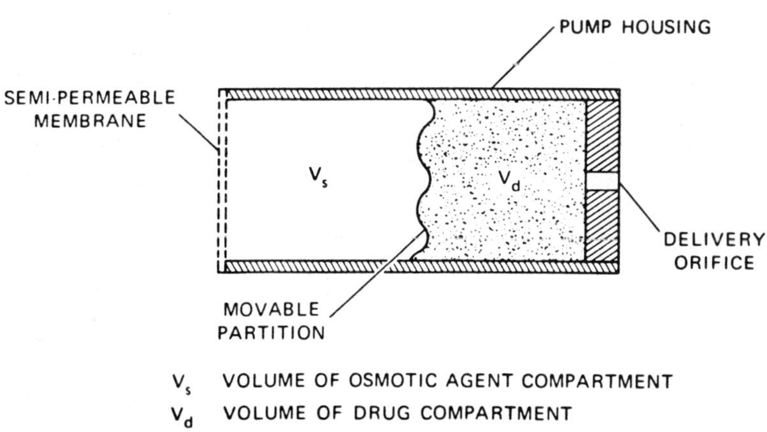

Fig. 6 Schematic representation of an osmotic pump. (Reprinted with permission from Ref. 4.)

where dV/dt is the volume flux; $\Delta\pi$ and ΔP are, respectively, the osmotic and hydrostatic pressure difference across the membrane; L_p is membrane mechanical permeability coefficient; σ is the reflection coefficient; and A and ℓ are membrane area and thickness, respectively.

The active agent delivery rate dM/dt is then given by

$$\frac{dM}{dt} = \frac{dV}{dt} C \tag{13}$$

where C is the concentration of the active agent in the solution pumped out of the orifice.

Devices using osmotic energy to control delivery of active agents have important benefits, including:

1. The devices are generic in that they operate independent of active agent properties.
2. The devices are able to deliver macromolecules.
3. Constant delivery rates much higher than those available from diffusional devices can be realized.

B. Examples of Osmotic Devices

Two osmotic devices, both manufactured by the Alza Corporation, have reached commercial production. One device, shown in Figure 7, is a capsule approximately 2.5 cm long and 0.6 cm in diameter. The active agent is contained in an innermost impermeable flexible reservoir surrounded with an osmotic agent, which in turn is surrounded and sealed within a rigid cellulose acetate semipermeable membrane [4].

When the device is placed in an aqueous environment, water is osmotically imbibed across the semipermeable membrane, and the active agent contained within the flexible reservoir is pumped out of the device. Because the driving force is the osmotic transport of water across the membrane, performance of the device is essentially independent of the environment within which the pump operates. Thus, as shown in Figure 8, about the same drug release rate is observed in isotonic saline at 37°C and from subcutaneous implants in rats or mice [5].

Another device is shown in Figure 9 [6]. This device differs from the one previously described in that the active agent serves as the osmotic agent, which is surrounded by the rigid semipermeable membrane containing a delivery orifice. Major application is for gastrointestinal drug deliveries because delivery rate is pH-independent, as shown in Figure 10 [6].

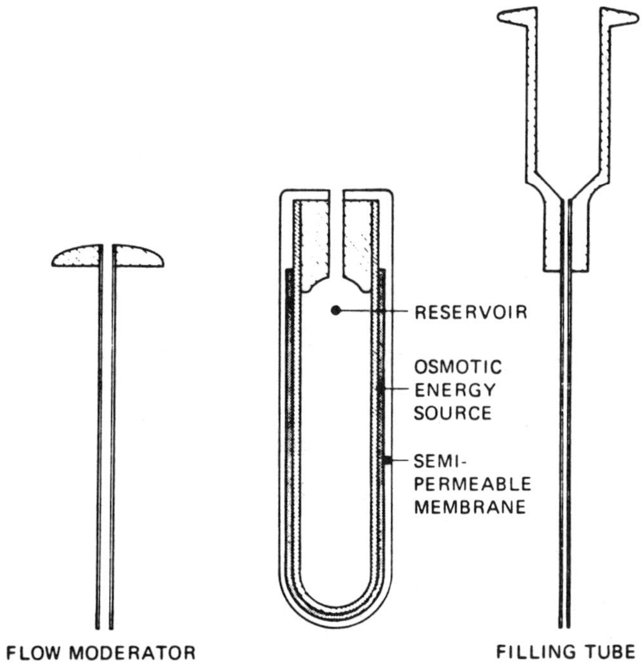

Fig. 7 Osmotic pump and components. (Reprinted with permission from Ref. 4.)

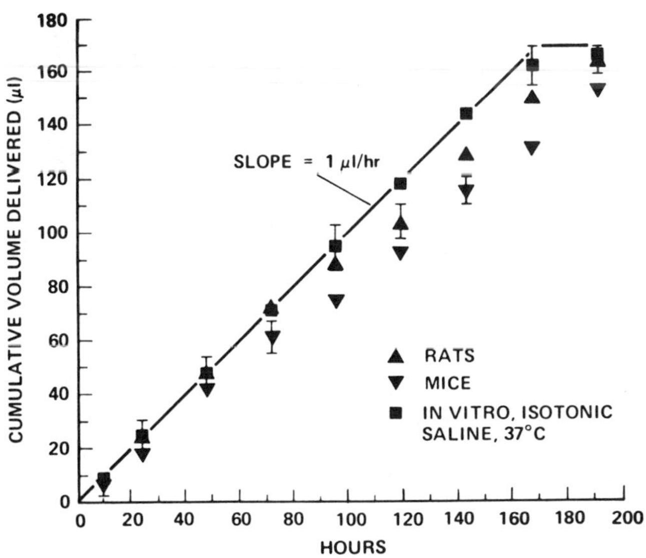

Fig. 8 Cumulative volume delivered from miniaturized osmotic pump. (Reprinted with permission from Ref. 5, p. 201.)

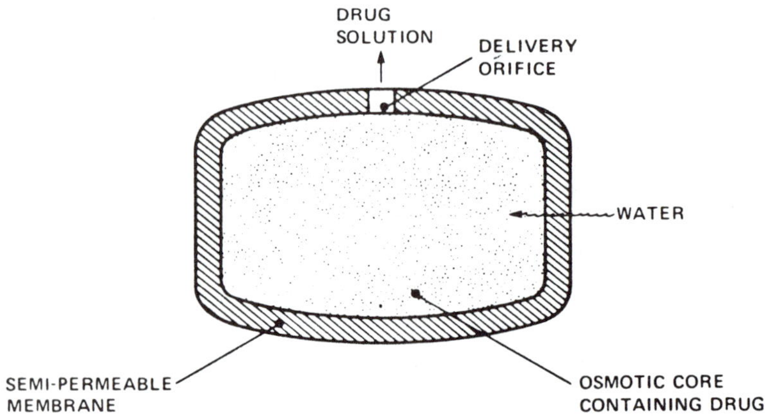

Fig. 9 Elementary osmotic pump cross section. (Reprinted with permission from Ref. 6.)

C. Swelling-Controlled Devices

In swelling-controlled release systems an active agent is homogeneously dispersed in a glassy polymer. Because glassy polymers are essentially impermeable, the active agent is immobilized in the matrix, and no diffusion through the solid polymer phase takes place.

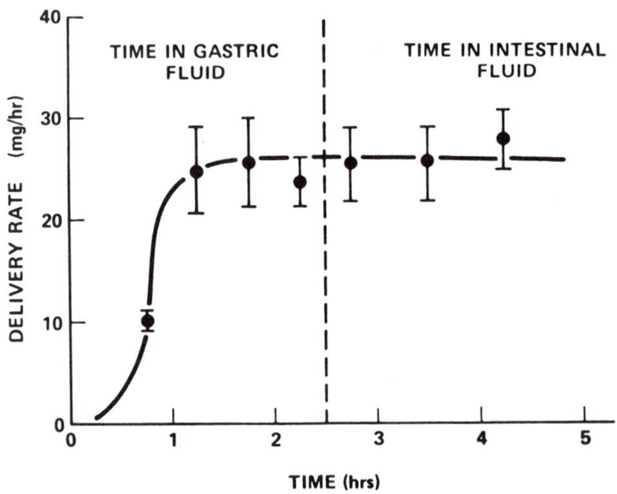

Fig. 10 *In vitro* release rate of sodium phenobarbital from elementary osmotic pump systems. (Reprinted with permission from Ref. 6.)

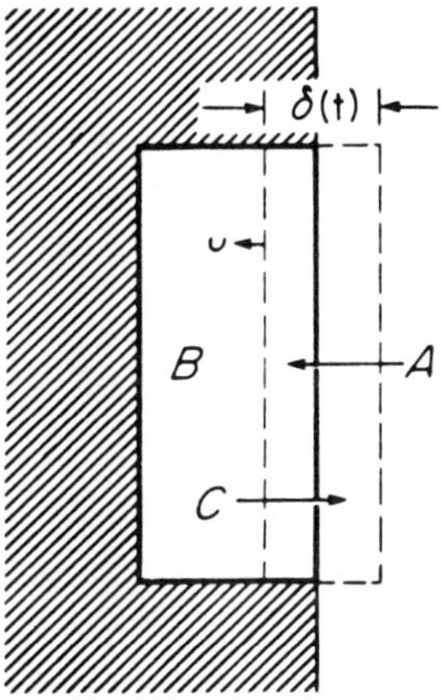

Fig. 11 Schematic representation of swelling-controlled release system. As the penetrant A enters the glassy polymer B, bioactive agent C is released through the gel phase of thickness δ(+). (Reprinted with permission from Ref. 7.)

When such a monolithic device is placed in an aqueous environment, water begins to penetrate the matrix and swelling takes place. As a consequence of the swelling process, chain relaxation takes place, and the incorporated active agent begins to diffuse from the swollen layer.

This process is represented schematically in Figure 11 [7]. One front separating the glassy from the rubbery state moves inward while a second front separating the swollen rubbery polymer from the surrounding aqueous environment moves outward.

In linear amorphous polymers, dissolution follows the swelling process, but crosslinked polymers or those containing significant chain entanglements or partial crystallinity will remain insoluble but will be mechanically weak.

III. CHEMICALLY CONTROLLED DEVICES

In a chemically controlled device, rate of active agent release from the polymer is controlled by a chemical reaction that can be hydrolytic or enzymatic cleavage of a labile bond, ionization or protonation.

The principal rationale for the construction of bioerodible devices is that expended devices need not be removed from their site of application, a feature particularly important with implanted devices.

A. Polymer Erosion Mechanisms

Polymer erosion can be defined as the conversion of an initially water-insoluble material to a water-soluble material and does not necessarily signify a major chemical degradation. The various bioerosion mechanisms can be systematized into the three distinct types shown in Figure 12 [8,9].

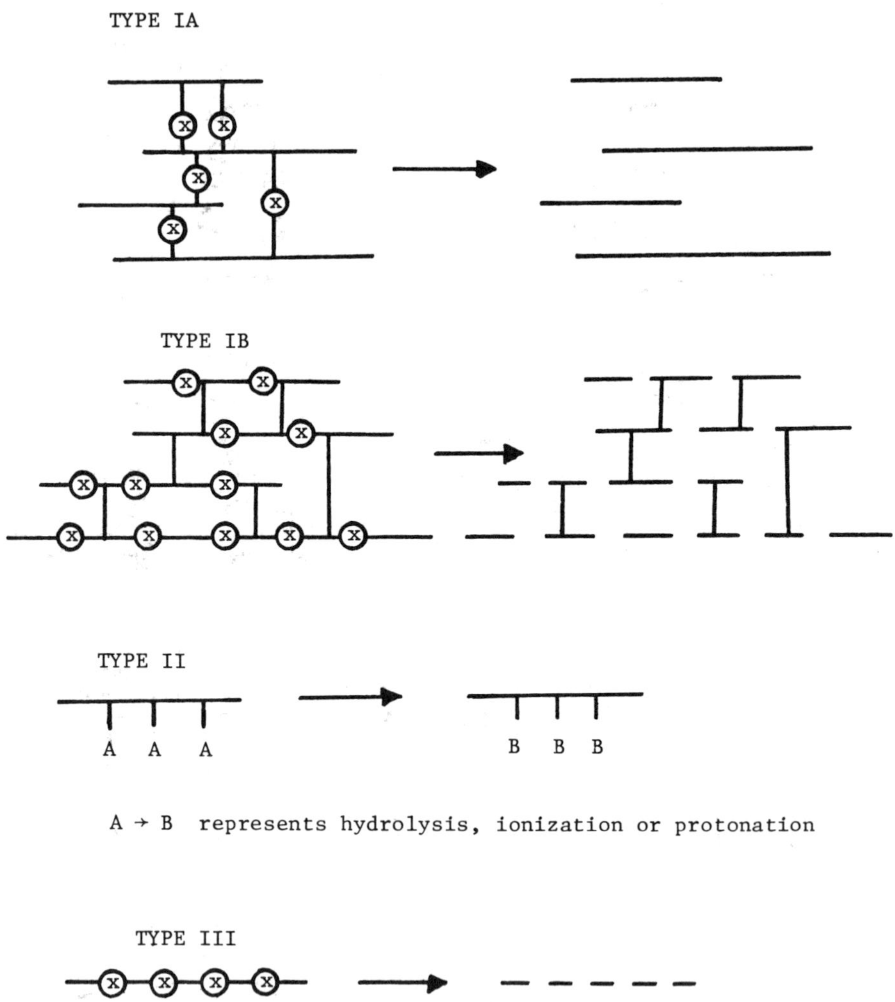

Fig. 12 Schematic representation of bioerosion mechanisms.

1. *Type I Erosion*

In systems based on type I erosion, water-soluble macromolecules are crosslinked to form a three-dimensional network. As long as the crosslinks remain intact, the network is insoluble, and, when placed in an aqueous environment, it can swell only to the extent allowed by the crosslink density. Erosion of these systems can occur by cleavage of cross-links (type IA erosion) or cleavage of the water-soluble polymer backbone (type IB erosion). As bond cleavage takes place, the matrix will begin to swell and eventually it will dissolve.

Such a system has two inherent limitations. First, the progressive swelling of the matrix before dissolution will limit its use to applications where dimensional stability is of little importance. Second, because a system consisting of crosslinked water-soluble polymers is a hydrogel, it is completely permeated by water; therefore, the water solubility of the incorporated therapeutic agent becomes a very important consideration. Clearly, low molecular weight compounds with appreciable water solubility will be rapidly leached, independent of the matrix erosion rate.

2. *Type II Erosion*

In systems based on type II erosion, water-insoluble macromolecules are converted to water-soluble maromolecules by hydrolysis, ionization, or protonation of a pendant group. Because no backbone cleavage takes place, the solubilization does not result in any significant change in molecular weight. However, unless the backbone is also degradable, polymers in this category are only useful in topical applications in which elimination of high molecular weight, water-soluble macromolecules proceeds with no difficulty.

3. *Type III Erosion*

In systems based on type III erosion, high molecular weight, water-insoluble macromolecules are converted to small, water-soluble molecules by a hydrolytic cleavage of labile bonds in the polymer backbone. Because these polymers are converted to small, water-soluble molecules, the principal application of these systems is for the systemic administration of therapeutic agents from subcutaneous, intramuscular, or intraperitoneal implantation sites. Clearly, the development of a useful system mandates that all degradation products be completely nontoxic.

B. Drug Release Mechanisms

Drug release from bioerodible polymers can occur by any one of three basic mechanisms, shown schematically in Figures 13(a), (b), and (c).

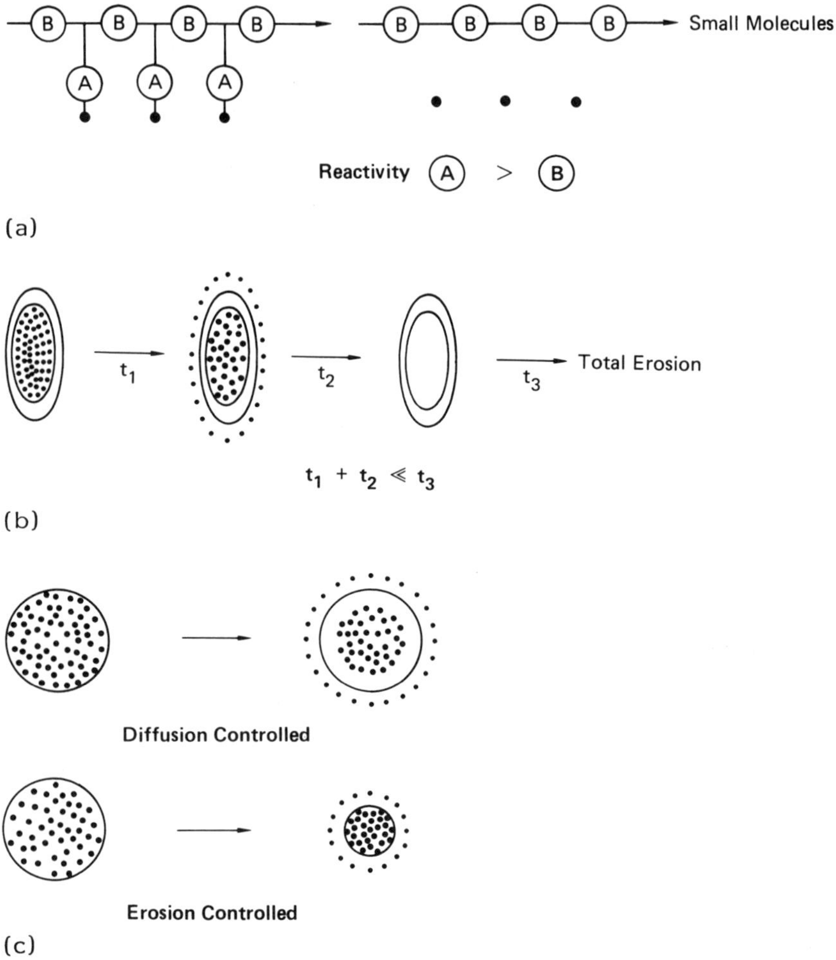

Fig. 13 Schematic representation of drug release mechanisms.

In the mechanism shown in Figure 13(a), the active agent is covalently attached to the polymer backbone and is released as its attachment to the backbone cleaves by hydrolysis of bond A. Because it is not desirable to release active agent molecules with polymer fragments still attached, reactivity of bond A should be significantly higher than reactivity of bond B.

In the mechanism shown in Figure 13(b), the active agent is contained in a core surrounded by a bioerodible rate-controlling membrane. Such a system combines the attributes of a rate-controlling polymer membrane, which provides a constant rate of drug release from a reservoir-type device, with erodibility, which results in bioerosion and makes surgical removal of the drug-depleted device unnecessary. Because constancy of drug release demands that the bioerodible polymer membrane remain essentially unchanged during the delivery regime, significant bioerosion must not occur until after drug delivery has been completed. Thus, polymer capsules will remain in the tissue for varying lengths of time after completion of therapy.

In the mechanism shown in Figure 13(c), the active agent is homogeneously dispersed in a polymer and drug release from this monolith is controlled by diffusion, by a combination of diffusion and erosion, or by erosion.

1. *Drugs Covalently Attached to Polymer Backbone*

This methodology allows the preparation of systems in which the polymer containing the bound therapeutic agent can act either as a depot or as a carrier. In the depot mode the polymer is localized at a certain body site, and the drug is released by gradual cleavage of its attachment to the polymeric backbone. Clearly, the backbone polymer must also undergo a cleavage reaction so that no high molecular weight residues remain in the tissue after all the drug has been released.

One example of a depot system is norethindrone coupled to the water-soluble poly(N^5-hydroxypropyl-L-glutamine) by reaction with phosgene [10]. Reaction of the polypeptide hydroxyl group with the hydrophobic steroid produces a water-insoluble material that gradually solubilizes as hydrolysis of the carbonate linkage removes the steroid. *In vivo* release of tritiated norethindrone, shown in Figure 14, reveals that the drug is released at a fairly constant rate for 144 days [10].

However, it is in the carrier mode that this methodology offers the unique possibility of carrying the drug to specific body sites. To achieve this specificity, the water-soluble polymer carries, in addition to the bound therapeutic agent, a homing group. For example, one such polymer contains as the bioactive agent a *p*-phenylenediamine mustard and as the homing group immunoglobulin from rabbit antisera against mouse lymphoma cells. *In vivo* tests with this material showed

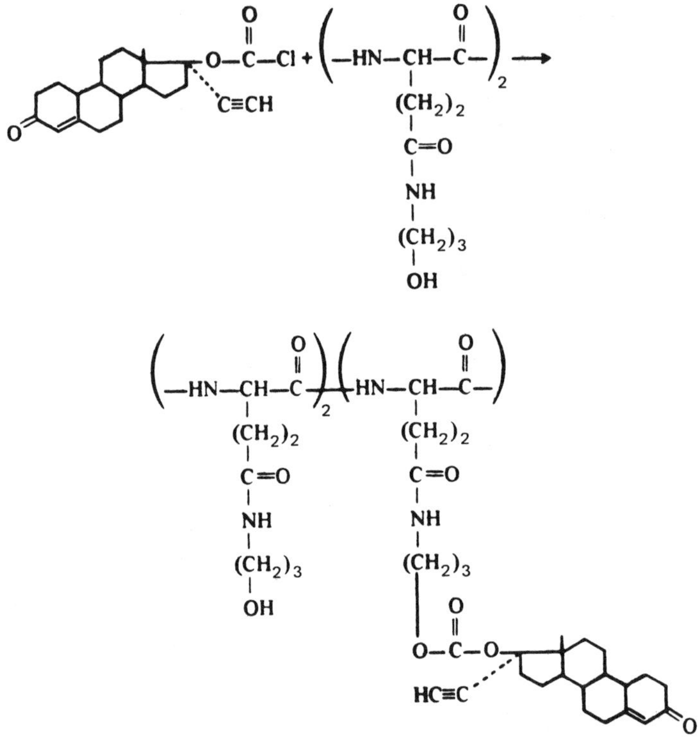

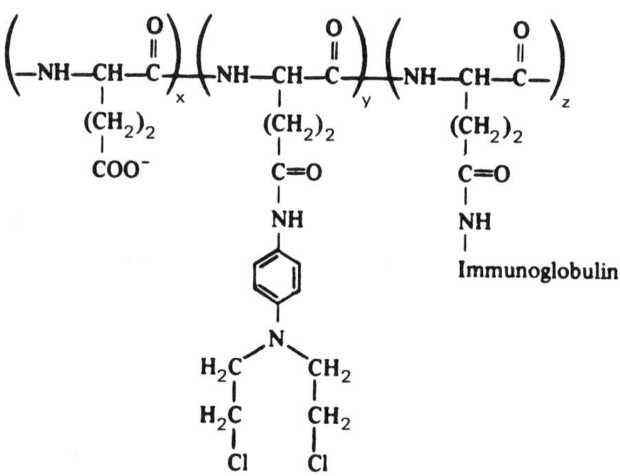

that the polymer is much more effective than the polymer components or a mixture of the components [11].

This methodology has also been used in controlled release pesticide applications in which a pesticide is first made part of an acrylic or methacrylic ester that is then polymerized or copolymerized [12]:

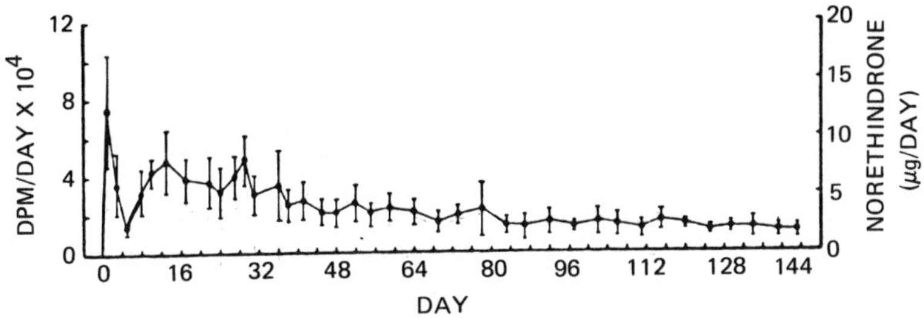

Fig. 14 *In vivo* release of norethindrone from Polymer I. 10 mg Polymer (4.9 mg norethindrone/2.92 × 10^7 dpm), 5 rats average ± S. D. (Reprinted with permission from Ref. 10, p. 57.)

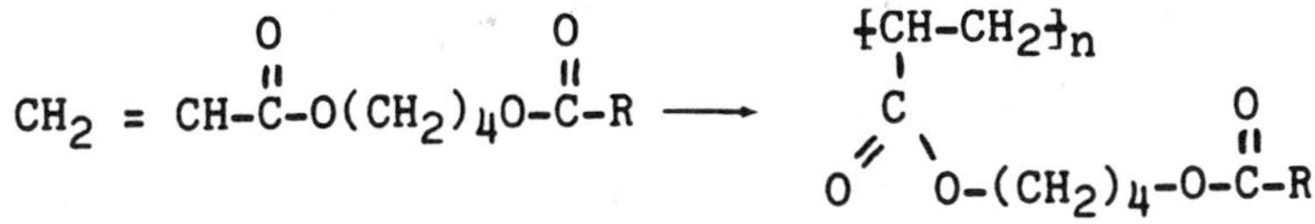

where R is

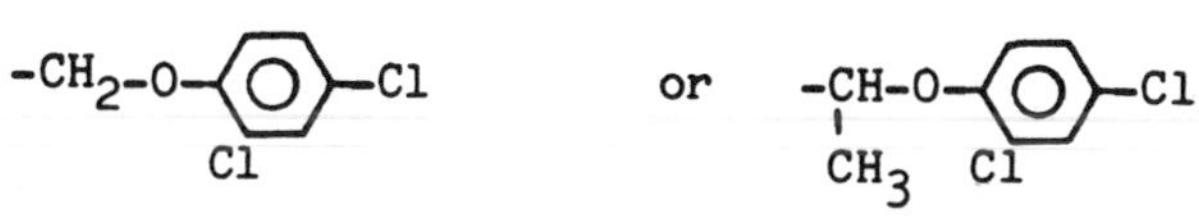

Pesticide release rates are shown in Figure 15. No hydrolysis occurs at pH 8 and 30°C when the hydrophobic polymer shown above is used. However, when a hydrophilic comonomer such as trimethylamine methacrylimide is used, slow hydrolysis of the ester groups takes place.

2. *Drug Contained in a Core Surrounded by Bioerodible Rate-Controlling Membrane*

Major emphasis has been on developing aliphatic polyesters for subdermal delivery of contraceptive steroids and the narcotic antagonist, naltrexone [13–16]. The polyesters investigated were poly(ε-caprolactone), poly(ε-caprolactone-CO-δ-valerolactone), poly(*DL*-lactic acid), poly(ε-caprolactone-DO-*DL*-lactic acid-CO-glycolic acid). The *in vivo* degradation data for various polyesters shown in Figure 16 are consistent with bulk degradation, and because the same rate was observed *in vitro* (water at 40°C) for cylinders and films that had large surface-to-volume differences, cleavage is due to simple hydrolysis with no enzymatic contributions [15].

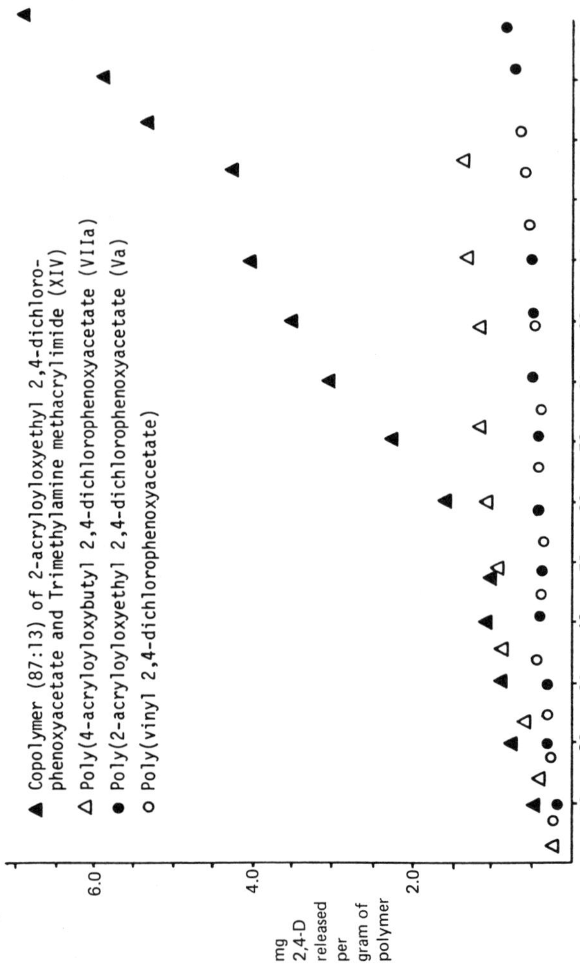

Fig. 15 Hydrolysis data for pendant herbicides. (Reprinted with permission from Ref. 12, p. 226.)

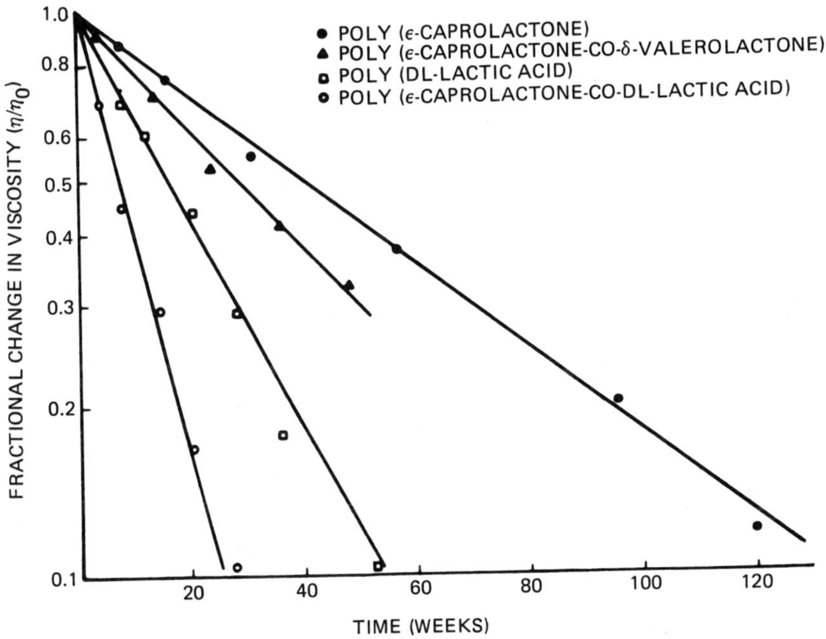

Fig. 16 Fractional change in the intrinsic viscosity of different polyesters implanted in rabbits as a function of time. (Reprinted with permission from Ref. 15, p. 33.)

Because hydrolytic degradation of aliphatic polyesters proceeds for long periods of time before weight loss takes place, diffusional devices that erode only after the drug reservoir has been depleted can be prepared. Furthermore, as shown in Figure 16, rate of polymer degradation can be regulated by varying the nature of the copolymer, so that devices having a range of useful liftimes can be prepared.

Daily rate of release of levonorgestrel from poly (ε-caprolactone) is shown in Figure 17. The capsules were implanted after first measuring release rate *in vitro* for 33 days. The difference in release rate between *in vitro* and *in vivo* experiments is the result of metabolic loss of radioactive label by routes other than urine and feces [15]. Poly (ε-caprolactone) devices (Capronor®) which contain the contraceptive steroid levonorgestrel suspended in tocopherol are now undergoing Phase II clinical trials [17].

3. *Drug Homogeneously Dispersed in Polymer Matrix*

A discussion of these monolithic systems is conveniently divided into hydrophilic polymers and hydrophobic polymers.

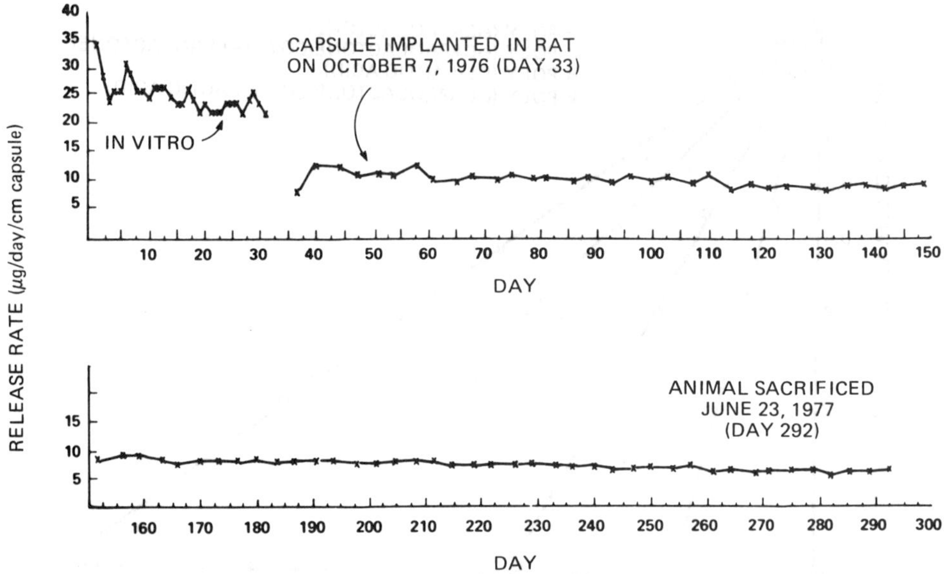

Fig. 17 Daily rate of release of norgestrel from poly(ε-caprolactone) capsule implanted in rat after 32 days *in vitro*. (Reprinted with permission from Ref. 15, p. 36.)

Hydrophilic Bioerodible Polymers

These materials undergo a type I erosion, and because they are completely permeated by water, they undergo a bulk erosion process. Furthermore, they are clearly unable to immobilize small molecules having appreciable water solubility. Consequently, usefulness of these materials is limited to molecules having extremely low water solubility or to macromolecules that can be physically entangled in the hydrogel so that they can not diffuse out of the matrix even though they are freely soluble in water. Escape can only take place after enough polymer chains have cleaved and the degree of entanglement has decreased.

Type I erosion can be subdivided into two subtypes, IA and IB [9]. In subtype IA erosion the hydrogel dissolves when crosslinks that connect the water-soluble polymer chains cleave. The degradation products are high molecular weight, water-soluble polymers. Consequently, if such polymers are to be used as implants, these polymers must degrade further so that the ultimate degradation products are small, water-soluble molecules that can be readily eliminated from the implantation site. However, if the polymers are to be used in topical applications, such as ocular, rectal, or in-utero applications, then degradation to small molecules is not necessary, and, in fact, the formation of nondegradable, water-soluble polymers is a definite toxicological asset.

The most widely investigated type IA erosion system is a hydrogel system prepared by copolymerizing vinyl pyrrolidone or acrylamide with *N,N'*-methylenebisacrylamide [9]. Although such hydrogels are generally not regarded as bioerodible, the crosslinks can nevertheless cleave as follows:

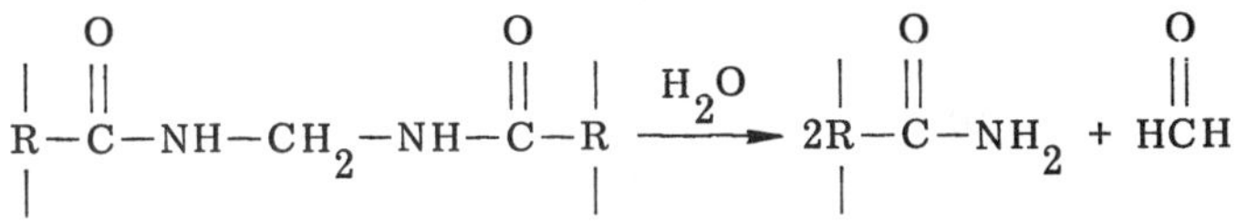

where R represents a polymer chain. However, the rate of the cleavage reaction is extremely slow: a hydrogel prepared with a N,N'-methylene-bisacrylamide crosslinker completely solubilizes within a useful time span only at crosslinker concentrations of less than 1% [18].

The distribution and elimination of acrylamide microspheres crosslinked with *N,N'*-methylenebisacrylamide in rats and mice has been studied. The data indicate that the microspheres are broken down by hydrolysis of crosslinks and subsequent elimination of the water soluble polymer fragments [19].

In subtype IB erosion the hydrogel solubilizes by cleavage of the water-soluble polymer chains, so the degradation products are relatively low molecular weight molecules. Thus, provided all degradation products are toxicologically innocuous, such systems can be considered for implantation applications.

One example of such a system is a material prepared by copolymerizing dextran that has been reacted with acrylic acid glycidyl ester and *N,N'*-methylenebisacrylamide [20]. Microparticles have been shown to be stable at pH 2 through 7 and to hydrolyze at increasingly rapid rates as the pH is increased. Macromolecules, such as carbonic anhydrase, human serum albumin, immunoglobulin, and catalase, have been immobilized in the microspheres with no loss of activity. *In vivo* degradation of these microspheres depends on enzymatic activity. Release of various proteins by diffusion from the microspheres is shown in Figure 18. No *in vivo* release studies have been described.

Another system that bioerodes by cleavage of water-soluble chains insolubilized by covalent crosslinks is schematically represented as follows [21]:

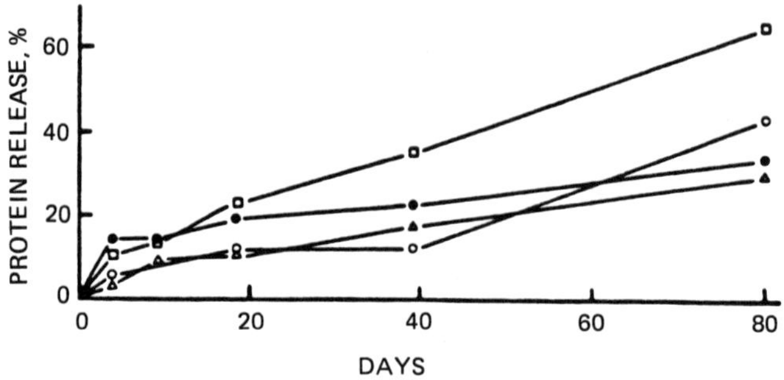

Fig. 18 Leakage of proteins from microspheres during storage at room temperature at pH 7.4. The immobilized proteins were carbonic anhydrase (□), human serum albumin (•), immunoglobulin (○), and catalase (△). (Reprinted with permission from Ref. 20.)

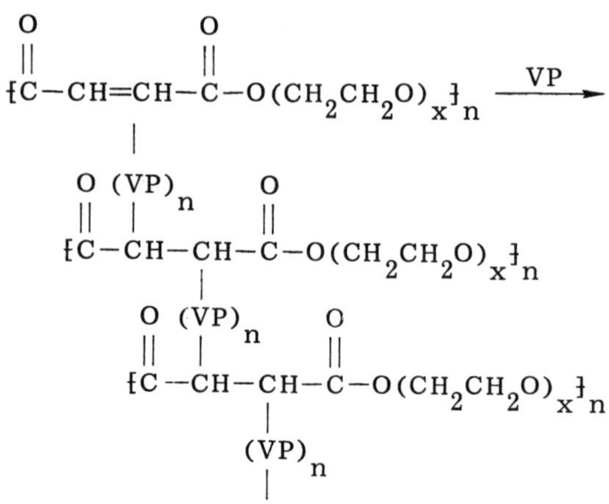

where VP is vinyl pyrrolidone, but could be other water-soluble vinyl monomers. Water-soluble macromolecules, such as bovine serum albumin (BSA), are entangled in the hydrogel by performing the cross-linking reaction in an aqueous solution that contains dissolved macromolecule. Chain cleavage takes place by a hydrolysis of ester links with consequent generation of poly(ethylene glycol) and a poly(*N*-vinyl pyrrolidone) modified by vicinal carboxylic acid functions.

However, hydrolysis rate of aliphatic polyesters at pH 7.4 and 37°C is too slow for useful rates of release, but hydrolysis rates of the polyester backbone can be accelerated by using diacids with electron-withdrawing groups, denoted as R in the structure shown below:

$$\left[O-\overset{\overset{O}{\|}}{C}-CH{=}CH-\overset{\overset{O}{\|}}{C}-O(CH_2CH_2O)_x\overset{\overset{O}{\|}}{C}-R-\overset{\overset{O}{\|}}{C} \right]_n$$

where R is $-CH_2-O-CH_2-$ for diglycolic acid, $-\overset{\overset{O}{\|}}{C}-$ is for ketomalonic acid, and $-CH_2-CH_2-\overset{\overset{O}{\|}}{C}-$ is for ketoglutaric acid [22].

Release of BSA from the activated unsaturated polyesters crosslinked with 60 wt% *N*-vinyl pyrrolidone is shown in Figure 19, which for comparison also includes a hydrogel containing no activating diester. Clearly, enhancing the hydrolytic instability of the polyester hydrogels increases the rate of BSA release, thus confirming that

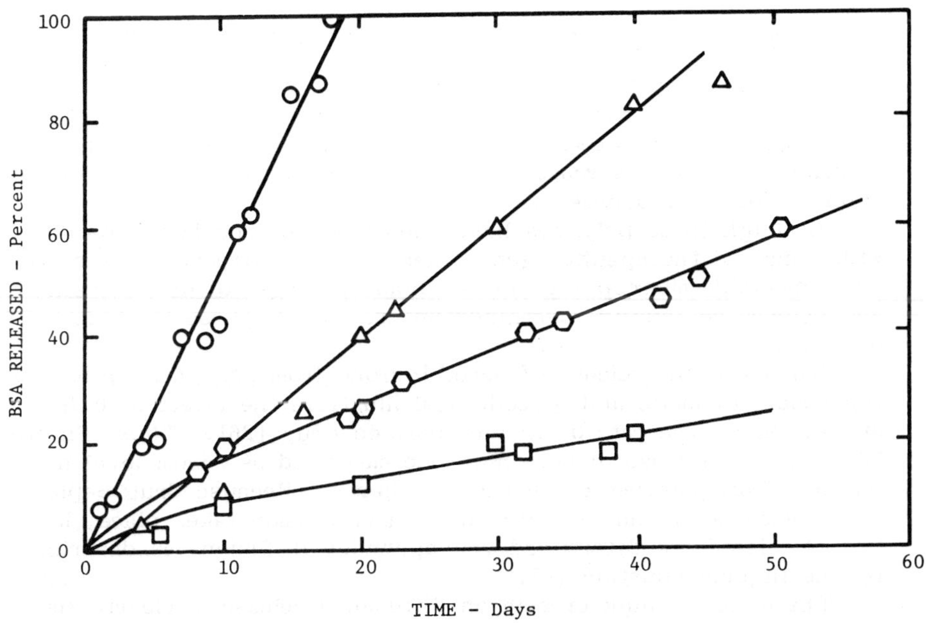

Fig. 19 Release of BSA at pH 7.4 and 37°C from microparticles prepared from various water-soluble unsaturated polyesters crosslinked with 60 wt% *N*-vinyl pyrrolidone.

○ 4:1 ketomalonic/fumaric △ 1:1 ketoglutaric/fumaric
⬡ 1:1 diglycolic/fumaric □ fumaric

(Reprinted with permission from Ref. 21.)

release occurs principally by matrix erosion and not simply by diffusion.

Hydrophobic Bioerodible Polymers

Erosion of hydrophobic polymers can proceed by two distinct mechanisms: bulk erosion and surface erosion. Because kinetics of drug release and behavior of the devices are significantly different in bulk erosion and surface erosion, they are discussed separately.

Bulk Erosion: In a bulk erosion process hydrolysis occurs throughout the bulk of the polymer, and in general, an analysis of kinetics of drug release is complex because it combines diffusion and erosion [23]. Thus, because the bulk erosion process changes the matrix, permeability of the polymer to the drug will increase with time, but this increase is not predictable, so the increase in drug release rate is also not predictable. Furthermore, the matrix can disintegrate before drug depletion, and a large burst in rate of drug delivery can take place. Such bursts have been observed [24].

The most extensively investigated hydrophobic bulk eroding polymers are poly(lactic acid) and copolymers of glycolic and lactic acids [9]. These polymers were originally developed as bioerodible sutures and degrade to the natural metabolites glycolic or lactic acid. Thus, they satisfy the requirement of degrading to toxicologically innocuous products and for this reason to this day occupy a preeminent place among bioerodible polymers.

Although these polymers have been used for the delivery of a wide range of therapeutic agents, delivery of contraceptive steroids from injectable microspheres is in advanced stages of development, and devices containing norethindrone are now in phase II clinical tests [25].

Studies of the release of norethindrone from poly(lactic acid) and copolymers of lactic and glycolic acid illustrate the effect of bulk erosion on release rate of an incorporated drug [26]. Thus, Figure 20 shows the release of norethindrone measured as serum level in baboons from poly(lactic acid) microspheres. Because drug depletion takes place before any significant polymer erosion takes place, kinetics of release are determined principally by diffusion, as described by the Higuchi equation [2].

The effect of bulk erosion on diffusional release is clearly shown in Figure 21. In this study, the more rapidly eroding copolymer of lactic and glycolic acid was used, and in Figure 21 the biodegradation of the polymer is shown along with baboon plasma levels of norethindrone [26].

During the early stages where little polymer erosion occurred, rate of drug release is typically first order and is determined by simple diffusion. However, as the polymer begins to bioerode,

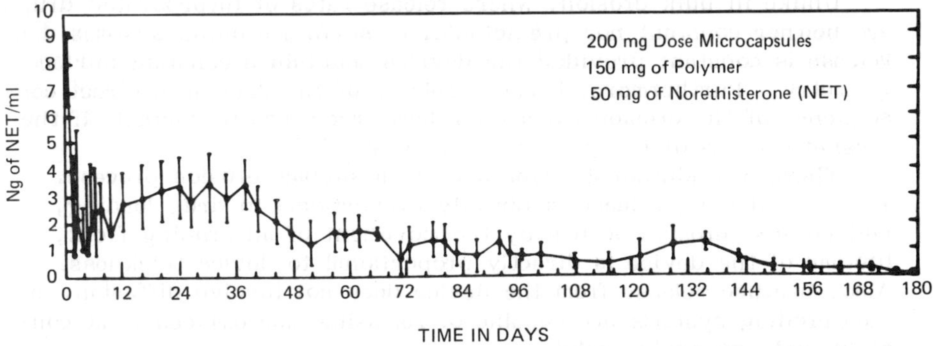

Fig. 20 Mean serum levels of NET ± SD (vertical bars) in baboons treated with 200 mg of the prototype system. [Reprinted with permission from L. R. Beck, D. R. Cowsar, D. H. Lewis, J. W. Gibson, and C. E. Flowers, *Am. J. Obstet. Gynecol.*, *135*, 491–426 (1979).]

release rate accelerates because it is determined by a combination of diffusion and polymer erosion.

Surface Erosion: In a surface erosion process hydrolysis of the polymer is confined to the outer surface, and the interior of the matrix remains essentially unchanged.

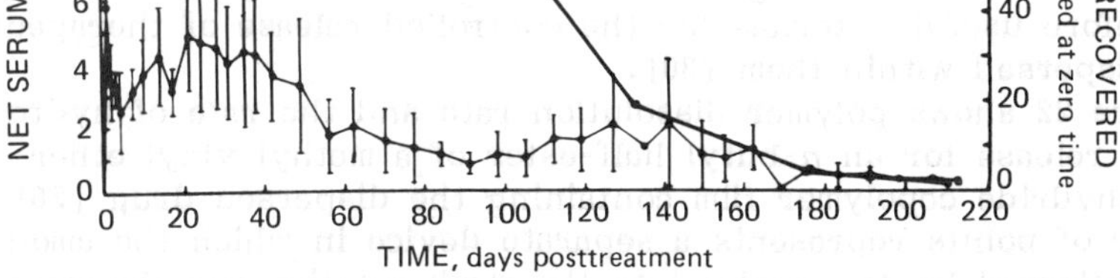

Fig. 21 Biodegradation curve of copolymer superimposed on mean serum levels of NET ± SD (vertical bars) in baboons treated with the copolymer formulation (88:12). [Reprinted with permission from L. R. Beck, V. Z. Pope, C. E. Flowers, Jr., D. R. Cowsar, T. R. Tice, D. H. Lewis, R. L. Dunn, A. B. Moore and R. M. Giley, *Biol. Reprod.*, *28*, 186–195 (1983).]

Unlike in bulk erosion, where release rates of incorporated drugs are neither constant nor predictable, in surface eroding systems drug release is constant provided the devices maintain a constant surface geometry. Furthermore, because release of the drug is a direct consequence of the erosion process, release rates are predictable if the erosion process of the polymer is understood.

There are additional advantages to a surface erosion process. The rate of drug release is directly proportional to drug loading, and because erosion occurs by the movement of an eroding front, lifetime of the device is directly proportional to device thickness. Also, because release from the device does not involve diffusion, surface eroding systems are capable of releasing macromolecules at constant and predictable rates.

At present, there are three polymer systems with demonstrated surface erosion characteristics. These are partially esterified copolymers of methyl vinyl ether and maleic anhydride, poly(ortho esters), and polyanhydrides.

Partially esterified copolymers of methyl vinyl ether and maleic anhydride solubilized by ionization of carboxylic acid groups and are insoluble when the carboxyl group is un-ionized [27–29].

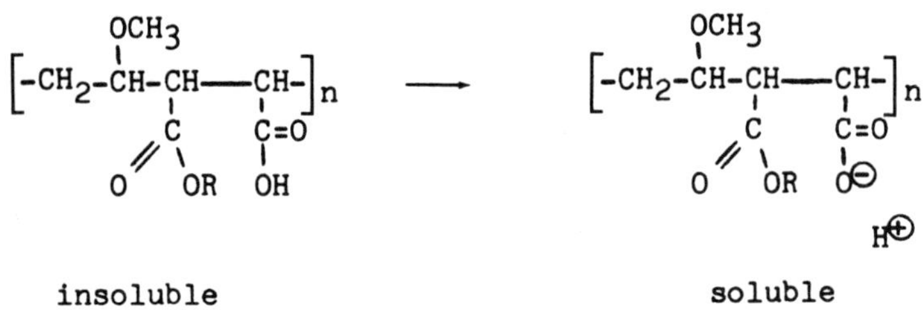

Although these polymers were originally designed to dissolve abruptly with a significant increase in external pH, in a constant pH environment they undergo a controlled dissolution process and are therefore useful materials for the controlled release of therapeutic agents dispersed within them [30].

Figure 22 shows polymer dissolution rate and the rate of hydrocortisone release for an *n*-butyl half-ester of a methyl vinyl ether-maleic anhydride copolymer film containing the dispersed drug [26]. Each pair of points represents a separate device in which the amount of drug released by the device into the wash solution was determined by uv measurements and the amount of polymer dissolved was calculated from the total weight loss of the device. The excellent linearity of both polymer erosion and drug release over the lifetime of the device provides strong evidence for a surface-erosion mechanism and for negligible diffusional release of the drug. The latter result was independently verified by placing a drug-containing film in water at a

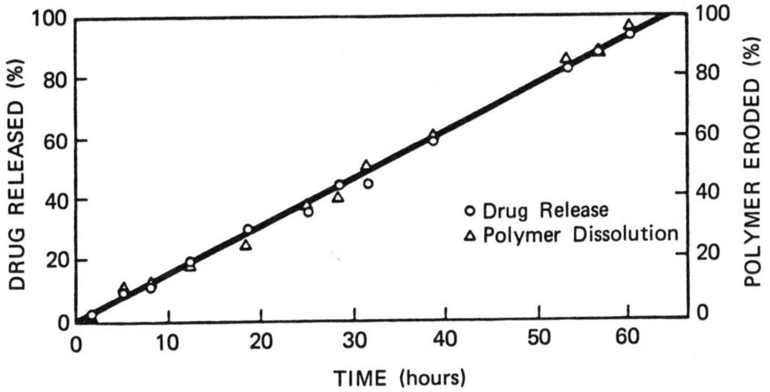

Fig. 22 Rate of polymer dissolution and hydrocortisone release from *n*-butyl half-ester of methyl vinyl ether-maleic anhydride copolymer containing 10 wt% drug. (Reprinted with permission from Ref. 30.)

pH low enough that no dissolution of the matrix took place and periodically analyzing the aqueous solution for hydrocortisone. None was found over several days. However, this polymer degrades by a Type II erosion, and the degradation product is a high molecular weight water-soluble polymer that has a hydrocarbon backbone and will not undergo further degradation. Consequently, the usefulness of this system is limited to topical applications.

Poly(ortho esters) have been prepared by adding alcohols to diketene acetals shown schematically as follows [31]:

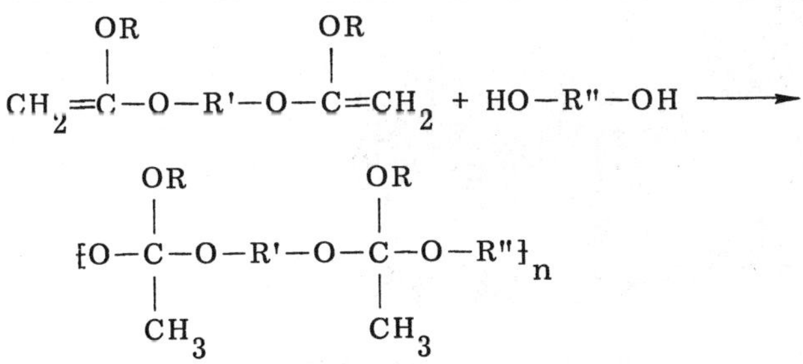

The reaction proceeds either spontaneously or can be catalyzed by traces of acid, is exothermic, and proceeds to completion virtually instantaneously. Because no small molecule by-products are produced, dense, crosslinked matrices can be produced by using varying proportions of monomers having a functionality greater than two.

Principally because of ease of monomer synthesis, polymers were prepared by adding various diols to 3,9-*bis*(methylene 2, 4, 8,

10-tetraoxaspiro[5,5]undecane) as shown below, where R = H or for 3,9-bis(ethylidene-2,4,8,10-tetraoxaspiro[5,5]undecane), R = CH_3:

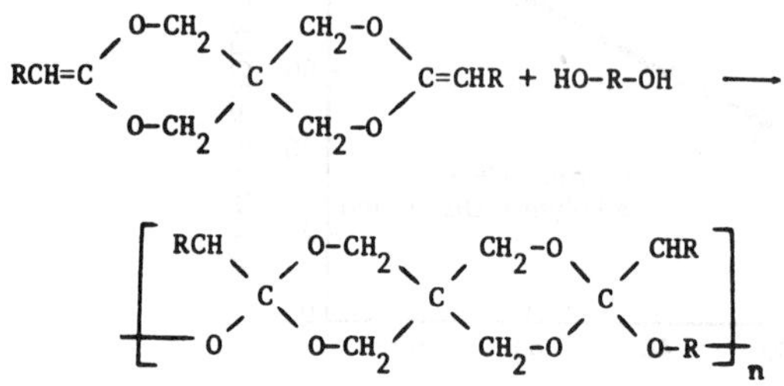

The ultimate degradation products are diol, pentaerithrytol and either acetic acid or propionic acid.

Poly(ortho esters) are stable in base, hydrolyze at slow rates at the physiological pH of 7.4, and become progressively more labile as the pH to which they are exposed is lowered.

As a result of this pH dependence, rate of polymer erosion can be manipulated within a very wide range by means of excipients physically incorporated into the matrix. Devices that release contraceptive steroids for very long times have been prepared by using highly hydrophobic polymers and catalyzing surface erosion by incorporating the slightly acidic salt calcium lactate or by using a more hydrophilic

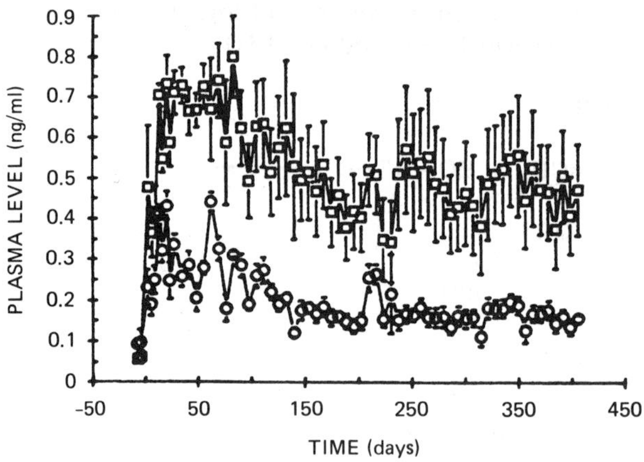

Fig. 23 Daily rabbit bollod plasma levels of levonorgestrel from poly(ortho ester) rods, 2.4 × 20 mm, containing 30 wt% levonorgestrel and 2 wt% calcium lactate. Total drug content 32.0 mg. Devices implanted subcutaneously.

○ 1 device per rabbit. □ 3 devices per rabbit.

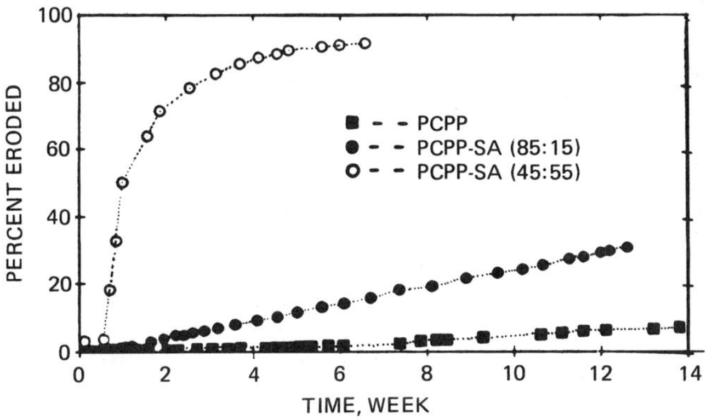

Fig. 24 Erosion profiles of poly bis(p-carobxyphenoxy) propane (PCPP) and its copolymers with sebacic acid (SA) at 37°C and pH 7.4. (Reprinted with permission from Ref. 38.)

polymer and stabilizing the interior of the matrix with $Mg(OH)_2$ so that only the surface layers can erode where the $Mg(OH)_2$ has been neutralized by the external medium [32,33]. Figure 23 shows levonorgestrel blood plasma levels in rabbits with implanted devices using the excipient calcium lactate.

Devices with shorter delivery times have been developed using acid anhydride excipients whose catalytic action depends on reaction with water to yield a diacid, which then catalyzes erosion of the matrix. Devices using anhydrides have been prepared that have lifetimes ranging from a few hours to weeks [34,35].

Poly(ortho esters) containing incorporated model drugs have been shown to exhibit all the properties expected of a surface eroding system, and proportionality of erosion rate and loading and that of device thickness and lifetime have been demonstrated [35].

The deterioration of mechanical properties of fibers prepared from aliphatic polyanhdrides was recognized many years ago as being due to their hydrolytic instability. However, aromatic polyanhydrides are quite stable, and their stability has been attributed to the crystalline nature of the polymer [36].

Polyanhydrides formed from aliphatic and aromatic diacids are being investigated as a surface eroding system for the delivery of incorporated therapeutic agents, and results of *in vitro* erosion studies are shown in Figure 24 [37,38]. Clearly, incorporation of an aliphatic segment into the polymer has a significant effect on rate of erosion, and variations in the amount of aliphatic segments relative to the aromatic segments provide a means of varying erosion times within a very wide range.

REFERENCES

1. R. W. Baker and H. K. Lonsdale, Controlled release: Mechanism and rates. In, *Controlled Release of Biologically Active Agents*, (A. C. Tanquary and R. E. Lacey, Eds.) Plenum Press, New York, 1974, pp. 15–71.
2. T. Higuchi, Rates of release of medicaments from ointment-bases containing drugs in suspension, *J. Pharm. Sci. 50*, 874–875 (1961).
3. W. P. O'Neill, Membrane systems. In, *Controlled Release Technologies: Methods, Theory and Applications*, Vol. I (A. G. Kydonieus, Ed.), CRC Press, Boca Raton, FL, 1980, pp. 129–182.
4. F. Theeuwes and S. I. Yum, Principles of the design and operation of generic osmotic pumps for the delivery of semi-solid or liquid drug formulations, *Ann. Biomed. Eng. 4*, 343–353 (1976).
5. F. Theeuwes, Delivery of active agents by osmosis. In, *Controlled Release Technologies: Methods, Theory and Applications*, Vol. II (A. G. Kydonieus, Ed.) CRC Press, Boca Raton, FL, 1980, pp. 195–205.
6. F. Theeuwes, Elementary osmotic pump, *J. Pharm. Sci. 64*, 1987–1991 (1975).
7. R. Langer and N. Peppas, Chemical and physical structure of polymers as carriers for controlled release of biactive agents: A review, *Rev. Macromol. Chem. Phys. C23*, 61–126 (1983).
8. J. Heller, Controlled release of biologically active compounds from bioerodible polymers, *Biomaterials 1*, 51–57 (1980).
9. J. Heller, Biodegradable polymers in controlled drug delivery. *CRC Crit. Rev. Ther. Drug Carrier Systems 1*, 39–90 (1984).
10. R. V. Petersen, C. G. Anderson, S. M. Fang, D. E. Gregonis, S. W. Kim, J. Feijen, J. M. Anderson and S. Mitra, Controlled release of progestins from poly(α-amino acid) carriers. In, *Controlled Release of Bioactive Materials*, (R. W. Baker, Ed.), Academic Press, New York, 1980, pp. 45–60.
11. G. R. Rowland, G. J. O'Neill, and D. A. L. Davies, Suppression of tumour growth in mice by a drug-antibody conjugate using a novel approach to linkage, *Nature (London) 255*, 487–488 (1975).
12. F. W. Harris, A. E. Aulabaugh, R. D. Case, M. K. Dykes, and W. A. Feld, Polymers containing pendent herbicide substituents: Preliminary hydrolysis studies, In, *Controlled Release Polymeric Formulations* (D. R. Paul and F. W. Harris, Eds.), American Chemical Society, ACS Symposium Series 33, Washington, DC, 1976, pp. 222–230.
13. C. G. Pitt, A. R. Jeffcoat, R. A. Zweidinger, and A. Schindler, Sustained drug delivery systems. I. The permeability of poly

(ε-caprolactone), poly(*DL*-lactic acid) and their copolymers, *J. Biomed. Mat. Res. 13*, 497–507 (1979).
14. C. G. Pitt, M. M. Gratzl, A. R. Jeffcoat, R. Zweidinger, and A. Schindler, Sustained drug delivery systems II: Factors affecting release rates from poly(ε-caprolactone) and related biodegradable polyesters, *J. Pharm. Sci. 68*, 1534–1538 (1979).
15. C. G. Pitt, T. A. Marks, and A. Schindler, Biodegradable drug delivery systems based on aliphatic polyesters: Application to contraceptives and narcotic antagonists. In, *Controlled Release of Bioactive Materials*, (R. W. Baker, Ed.), Academic Press, New York, 1980, pp. 19–43.
16. C. G. Pitt and A. Schindler, The design of controlled drug delivery systems based on biodegradable polymers. In, *Biodegradables and Delivery Systems for Contraception*, (E. S. E. Hafez, and W. A. A. van Os, Eds.), G. K. Hall Medical Publishers, Boston, 1980, pp. 17–46.
17. S. J. Ory, C. B. Hammond, S. G. Yancy, W. R. Hendren, and C. G. Pitt, The effect of biodegradable contraceptive capsule (Capronor) containing levonorgestrel on gonadotropin, estrogen and progesterone levels, *Am. J. Obstet. Gynecol. 145*, 600–605 (1983).
18. V. P. Torchilin, E. G. Tishenko, V. N. Smirnov, and E. I. Chazov, Immobilization of enzymes in slowly soluble carriers, *J. Biomed Mat. Res. 11*, 223–235 (1977).
19. I. Sjoholm, and P. Edman, Acrylic microspheres *in vivo*. I. Distribution and elimination of polyacrylamide microparticles after intravenous and intraperitoneal injection in mouse and rat, *J. Pharmacol. Exp. Ther. 211*, 656–662 (1979).
20. P. Edman, B. Ekman, and I. Sjoholm, Immobilization of proteins in microspheres of biodegradable polyacryldextran, *J. Pharm. Sci. 69*, 838–842 (1982).
21. J. Heller, R. W. Baker, R. F. Helwing, and M. E. Tuttle, Controlled release of water-soluble macromolecules from bioerodible hydrogels, *Biomaterials 4*, 262–266 (1983).
22. P. Y. Wang, and B. P. Arlitt, Structural requirements for the degradation of condensation polymers *in vivo*. In, *Biomedical Applications of Polymers*, (H. P. Gregor, Ed.), Plenum Press, New York, 1975, pp. 173–182.
23. J. Heller and R. W. Baker, Theory and practice of controlled drug delivery from bioerodible polymers. In, *Controlled Release of Bioactive Materials* (R. W. Baker, Ed.), Academic Press, New York, 1980, pp. 1–17.
24. D. L. Wise, J. B. Gregory, D. M. Newberne, L. C. Bartholow, and J. B. Stanbury, Results on biodegradable cylindrical subdermal implants for fertility control. In, *Polymeric Delivery*

Systems (R. J. Kostelnik, Ed.) Gordon and Breach Science Publishers, New York, 1978, pp. 121–138.

25. L. R. Beck, C. E. Flowers, V. Z. Pope, W. H. Wilborn, and T. R. Tice, Clinical evaluation of an improved injectable microcapsule contraceptive system, *Am. J. Obstet. Gynecol. 147*, 815–821 (1983).
26. L. R. Beck and T. R. Tice, Poly(lactic acid) and poly(lactic acid-co-glycolic acid) contraceptive delivery systems. In, *Long-Acting Steroid Contraception* (D. R. Mishell, Jr., Ed.), Raven Press, New York, 1983, pp. 175–199.
27. L. C. Lappas and W. McKeehan, Synthetic polymers as potential enteric and sustained-release coatings, *J. Pharm. Sci. 51*, 808 (1962).
28. L. C. Lappas and W. McKeehan, Polymeric pharmaceutical coatings materials, I. Preparation and properties, *J. Pharm. Sci. 54*, 176–181 (1965).
29. L. C. Lappas and W. McKeehan, Polymeric pharmaceutical coatings materials II. *In vivo* evaluation as enteric coatings, *J. Pharm. Sci. 56*, 1257–1261 (1967).
30. J. Heller, R. W. Baker, R. M. Gale, and J. O. Rodin, Controlled drug release by polymer dissolution, I. Partial esters of maleic anhydride copolymers—properties and theory, *J. Appl. Polymer Sci. 22*, 1991–2009 (1978).
31. J. Heller, D. W. H. Penhale, and R. F. Helwing, Preparation of poly(ortho esters) by the reaction of ketene acetals and polyols, *J. Polymer Sci., Polym. Lett. 18*, 619–624 (1980).
32. J. Heller, B. K. Fritzinger, S. Y. Ng, and D. W. H. Penhale, *In vitro* and *in vivo* release of levonorgrestrel from poly(orthoesters). I. Linear polymers, *J. Controlled Release 1*, 225–232 (1985).
33. J. Heller, B. K. Fritzinger, S. Y. Ng, and D. W. H. Penhale, *In vitro* and *in vivo* release of levonorgestrel from poly(ortho esters). II. Crosslinked polymers, *J. Controlled Release 1*, 233–238 (1985).
34. C. Shih, T. Higuchi, and K. J. Himmelstein, Drug delivery from catalyzed erodible polymeric matrices of poly(ortho ester)s, *Biomaterials 5*, 237–240 (1984).
35. R. V. Sparer, C. Shih, C. D. Ringeisen, and K. J. Himmelstein, Controlled Release from erodible poly(ortho ester) drug delivery systems, *J. Controlled Release 1*, 23–32 (1984).
36. A. Conix, Aromatic polyanhydrides, a new class of high melting fiber-forming polymers, *J. Polymer Sci. 29*, 343–353 (1958).
37. H. B. Rosen, J. Chang, G. E. Wnek, R. J. Linhardt, and R. Langer, Bioerodible polyanhydrides for controlled drug delivery, *Biomaterials 4*, 131–133 (1983).
38. K. W. Leong, B. C. Brott, and R. Langer, Bioerodible polyanhydrides as a drug carrier matrix, *Polymer Reprints 25*(1), 201–202 (1984).

5

Pharmacokinetic/Pharmacodynamic Basis of Controlled Drug Delivery

B. MICHAEL SILBER, MEIR BIALER,* and AVRAHAM YACOBI
American Cyanamid Company, Pearl River, New York

I. INTRODUCTION

The pharmacological action of a drug correlates better with the concentration-time course of the drug (or its active metabolite) in the blood or some other biophase than with the absolute dose administered. This proposition is based on empirical evidence demonstrating variability

*On sabbatical leave from the Department of Pharmacy, School of Pharmacy, Hebrew University, Jerusalem, Israel.

in drug disposition both between and within individuals, particularly in the rates of drug absorption, distribution, and elimination. The goal of drug therapy is to produce therapeutic drug concentrations that elicit desired pharmacological action(s) and to minimize the incidence and severity of unwanted adverse effects. To achieve this goal it would be advantageous and more convenient to maintain a dosing frequency to once, or at most, a twice daily regimen [1–3].

Conventional dosage forms are rapidly absorbed, with the ascending and descending portions of the concentration versus time curve reflecting primarily the rate of absorption and elimination, respectively. Because of the rapid rate of drug absorption from conventional dosage forms, drugs are usually administered more than once daily, with the frequency being dependent on biological half-life ($t_{1/2}$) and duration of pharmacological effect. The rate of dosing may also be affected by the therapeutic index (TI) of a drug.

The TI is commonly defined as the ratio of the concentration eliciting an unwanted effect to that eliciting a desired therapeutic effect. This parameter is important in determining the relative safety of a drug. For drugs with small TI values (i.e., 2 to 4), the monitoring of drug concentrations in blood (or plasma) may be particularly useful in designing drug dosage regimens, maintaining effective concentrations, and, at the same time, reducing the likelihood of exposing the patient to either potentially toxic peak concentrations, or subtherapeutic concentrations. The attainment of this objective is not a trivial one, particularly since TI values may be small and since many effective drugs have relatively short elimination half-lives. Therefore, the results for a drug with a small TI and short elimination half-life are situations in which:

1. Drug is given at a dose low enough to assure attainment of effective and nontoxic concentrations, but at frequent intervals.
2. Drug is dosed such that peak concentrations (C_{max}) are high enough to elicit the desired pharmacological effect, but dosed at a frequency less than that of its elimination half-life, resulting in long periods of subtherapeutic concentrations over the dosing interval.
3. Drug is administered in large doses infrequently, resulting in a high C_{max}, with therapeutic concentrations maintained over a prolonged period of time. The high initial concentration, however, may result in adverse reactions.

To avoid many potential problems associated with the use of conventional dosage forms, sustained release concepts have been applied to the development of new dosage formulations.

There are various factors that can influence the performance of a sustained release product; these are indicated in Table 1. The physiological, biochemical, and pharmacological factors listed in Table 1 can complicate the evaluation of the suitability of a sustained release dosage formulation. Even if a specific formulation exhibits minimal variability in release characteristics *in vitro*, *in vivo* factors can be important enough to result in a vastly different drug disposition profile between indivudals and even within the same individual given the formulation on different occasions. These concerns are expected to be heightened when single dose studies are performed. In order to minimize the impact of these factors on the evaluation of the concentration versus time course of a drug given as a sustained release dosage form, it may be prudent to conduct studies under steady-state conditions, over the entire therapeutic plasma concentration range.

From a pharmacokinetic standpoint, there are two fundamental approaches to the design of formulations that allow for the attainment of desired therapeutic concentrations which are maintained throughout a dosing interval. The first approach is to select drugs (such as warfarin and phenobarbital) that have elimination half-lives long

Table 1 Factors Influencing the *In Vivo* Performance of Sustained Release Dosage Formulations

Physiological
Prolonged drug absorption
Variability in GI emptying and motility
Gastrointestinal blood flow
Influence of feeding on drug absorption
Pharmacokinetic/biochemical
Dose dumping
First-pass metabolism
Variability in urinary pH; effect on drug elimination
Enzyme induction/inhibition upon multiple dosing
Pharmacological
Changes in drug effect upon multiple dosing
Sensitization/tolerance

enough to be administered infrequently. This approach can be successful sometimes if an analog from a class of biologically active drugs can be found that demonstrates a long elimination half-life. Although this approach could be adopted at the early stages of developing a new drug candidate, it would likely be time consuming and costly since it would require an extensive research and development program in animals and possibly in humans.

The second major approach involves the modification of the drug formulation in such a way that the fluctuation in drug concentrations during a dosing interval is reduced. This latter approach has the inherent advantage of potentially not restricting the drug selection process to drugs having long elimination half-lives. Theoretically, such an approach would be desirable for potent drugs with short half-lives and low TIs for which maintenance of therapeutic concentrations with minimal fluctuations over an extended period of time are essential (e.g., quinidine and procainamide). For these drugs, development of sustained release dosage forms may result in better patient management and potentially a lower incidence of toxicity.

The ultimate purpose of a sustained action dosage form, therefore, would be to improve therapeutic management through assuring a uniform plasma concentration of drug at steady state, and through reducing the ratio of maximum and minimum plasma levels (C_{max}/C_{min}) following each dose. Ideally, this could be achieved if the release of the active ingredients from a product resulted in slow first-order or slow zero-order absorption of the drug from the gastrointestinal tract. Once steady state was achieved, drug concentration in plasma would remain within the therapeutic range throughout the dosing interval.

Practically, preparing such an ideal sustained release dosage form is difficult since there are a number of physiological and physicochemical variables influencing drug release and absorption of a drug in the gastrointestinal tract. The *in vivo* release and absorption of drugs from most commercially available sustained action oral dosage forms follows an apparent first-order process with considerably slower absorption rates than those observed after conventional oral preparations. Sustained release dosage forms would be most applicable for drugs having low TIs and short elimination half-lives. It should be emphasized that as drug half-life increases, formulation factors become less important in the development of a dosing regimen.

The most serious restriction to the use of oral sustained release dosage forms would be the limited residence time of the dosage form in the small intestine. Literature data suggests that 9–12 hr would be a reasonable estimate of average effective absorption time after oral administration of a well-absorbed drug in a dosage form that remains intact in the gastrointestinal tract. This suggests that the dissolution half-lives of drugs from dosage forms that release the

Table 2 Drugs Available in Controlled Release forms with Literature References of Pharmacokinetic Evaluations of These Drug Products

Drugs	Reference
Minerals	
Fluoride	[90]
Potasium chloride	[91]
Diuretics and cardiovascular drugs	
Chlorthalidone	[112]
Disopyramide	[66]
Furosemide	[77]
Heptaminol	[111]
Isosorbide dinitrate	[74, 75]
Metipranolol	[114]
Metoprolol	[94, 110]
Mexiletine	[82]
Nitroglycerin	[87]
Oxprenolol	[92]
Papaverine	[97]
Prenalterol	[76]
Procainamide	[84, 100]
Propranolol	[59, 70, 121]
Quinidine	[83]
Trimazosin	[78]
Vinacamine	[96]
CNS drugs	
Aminosalicylic acid	[106]
Amitriptyline	[101]
Aspirin	[72]
Butriptyline	[109]
Dihydrocodeine	[105]
Diazepam	[67, 88]
Indomethacin	[79, 85]
Ketoprofen	[65]
Lithium Carbonate	[63, 99]
Morphine	[71]
Naltrexone	[120]
Phenytoin	[107]
Salicylic acid	[72]
Trihexyphenidyl	[62]
Valproic acid	[61]

Table 2 (Continued)

Drugs	Reference
Respiratory agents	
Aminophylline	[81]
Betamethasome	[68]
Brompheniramine	[98]
Chlorpheniramine	[116, 117]
Dyphylline	[102]
Hydroxyethyltheophylline	[95]
Phenylpropanolamine	[108]
Pseudoephedrine	[89, 116]
Proxyphylline	[103]
Terbutaline	[69]
Theophylline	[38, 64, 86]
Triprolidine	[89]
Antimicrobial agents	
Diethylcarbamazine	[118]
Nitrofurantoin	[93]
Sulphamethizole	[104]
Other Drugs	
Bezafibrate	[113]
Coumarin	[115]
7-Hydroxycoumarin	[115]
Glibenclamide	[73]
Metformin	[80]
Metoclopramide	[60]
Urodeoxycholic acid	[119]

active ingredient in a first-order manner should not exceed 3–4 hr. Because there should be a limit to the reduction in the release rate of a drug from a sustained release dosage form without a compromise in the extent of absorption (bioavailability), there also should be a limit to the prolongation of the duration of drug effect by means of altering the dosage form [4]. Since the most important criteria for the evaluation of sustained release dosage forms are bioavailability and fluctuations at steady state, it would certainly be desired that the formulation demonstrate less fluctuations and have a bioavailability of at least 80% relative to that of the conventional dosage form.

The primary purpose of this chapter is to discuss the principles of pharmacokinetics and pharmacodynamics, particularly as they relate to sustained action dosage forms and under realistic conditions. This discussion will focus on drugs given orally as sustained-release formulations, as listed in Table 2.

II. REVIEW OF GENERAL PRINCIPLES

A. Pharmacokinetics

The compartmental analysis approach was initially proposed to describe the multiexponential time course of plasma concentrations of drug in the body following drug administration [5,6]. Physiological models were subsequently derived relating drug transfer on the basis of organ and tissue blood flows and extraction ratios of the active moiety(s) [5–7]. These classical concepts were developed for conventional dosage forms, wherein the rate of drug absorption generally greatly exceeded the rate of elimination. Under such conditions, a distribution phase can be seen following a conventional dosage form. However, a sustained release dosage form for a drug with a relatively short elimination half-life ($t_{1/2} \leqslant 4$ hr) represents a substantially different situation, where the rate of absorption is so slow that it ultimately obscures the distribution phase and if the rate constant of absorption becomes less than that of the rate constant of elimination, a "flip-flop" model results [5,6]. In this case, the terminal phase is actually a reflection of the rate constant for absorption. This is true because most sustained release dosage forms are deliberately designed to release their content over a prolonged period of time; a period usually longer than a typical dosing interval for a conventional formulation. When the absorption and elimination rates of a drug or a drug product are of the same order of magnitude, absorption will proceed throughout the disposition phase of the drug, resulting in a pseudo steady state where there is very little change in drug concentration in blood occurring during each dosing interval. Pharmacokinetic factors, therefore, can have a significant impact on the design of sustained release formulations.

The ideal formulation is one that releases the drug at a constant rate, associated with a constant rate of absorption and producing sustained therapeutic concentrations over a prolonged period of time. The size of the dose should allow adequate drug release in the gastrointestinal tract until the administration of the next scheduled dose. In reality, the performance of a sustained release dosage form in the gastrointestinal tract is governed by many variables, seldom allowing an ideal situation. As previously stated, a good sustained release dosage form has to exhibit a more prolonged and uniform absorption rate, yielding more sustained plasma levels after ingestion and has to be bioequivalent and therapeutically equivalent to a conventional (standard) formulation of the same drug. In order to define the pharmacokinetic parameters which will help in understanding the *in vivo* absorption and elimination of the drug, the following four models were proposed [8]:

1. Models of Drug Input and Elimination

1. Zero-order absorption followed by first-order elimination
2. Slow first-order absorption followed by first-order elimination
3. Rapid first-order absorption of part of the dose, then release and absorption of the remainder over an extended period of time by a zero-order kinetic process followed by a first-order elimination process
4. Rapid first-order absorption of part of the dose, then release and absorption of the remainder over an extended period of time by a slower first-order kinetic process followed by a first-order elimination process

These models will be described very briefly here, as the mathematical considerations are presented in greater detail in another chapter of this book [8]. In this chapter, it is assumed that: (a) the elimination of a drug is by a first-order process; (b) the rate of drug distribution in the body, which is usually rapid, is governed by the rate of drug absorption (and/or drug elimination when $k_a < k_e$); and (c) all kinetic processes, except for drug absorption, are linear.

Zero-Order Absorption Followed by First-Order Elimination

This model presents a situation where the orally administered drug is absorbed by an apparent zero-order process, or at a constant rate, and is being eliminated by a first-order process. In this case, the release of the drug out of the drug product is the rate limiting step. Following a single dose of a drug, the concentration versus time course of the drug is provided by the following relationship [5,6], which is equivalent to that for a drug during and after a constant rate intravenous infusion [5]:

$$C = \frac{Fk_0(e^{k_eT} - 1)\ e^{-k_et}}{k_e V} \tag{1}$$

where k_0 is the apparent zero-order absorption rate, t is the time after drug administration, T is a constant corresponding to the absorption time (when peak drug concentration is attained), V is the volume of distribution, and F is the bioavailability factor indicating the fraction of the dose reaching the systemic circulation. During absorption, T = t. In the postabsorption phase, t = T + t' where t' is the time from the start of the postabsorption phase. Equation (2) is derived from Eq. (1) (since T = t during absorption) and describes drug plasma concentrations during the absorption phase.

$$C = \frac{Fk_0 (1 - e^{-k_e T})}{k_e V} \tag{2}$$

Theoretical plots have been provided that describe the concentration time course of a drug given at various zero-order rates of absorption and first-order rates of elimination [8]. In general, the greater the value of k_e (the shorter the half-life), the greater the amount needed to maintain concentrations close to a desired value. If a drug follows an apparent zero-order absorption process and an apparent first-order elimination process following multiple dosing at steady state, the equation describing the concentration time course will be defined by Eq. (3):

$$C_{ss} = \frac{Fk_0}{k_e V} \tag{3}$$

where C_{ss} is the drug concentration at steady state and the product of $k_e V$ is the total body clearance (CL) of the drug. When F = 1, i.e. complete absorption, the equation can be simplified to one describing an intravenous infusion as shown by Eq. (4):

$$C_{ss} = \frac{k_0}{CL} \tag{4}$$

First-Order Absorption Followed by First-Order Elimination

This is the most frequently selected model describing drug pharmacokinetics following conventional oral dosage formulations. Following a single dose, the concentration versus time curve for a drug at any time can be described by Eq. (5):

$$C = \frac{Fk_a D (e^{-k_e t} - e^{-k_a t})}{V (k_a - k_e)} \tag{5}$$

where D is the dose. For some conventional formulations where $k_a >> k_e$, this relationship can be approximated by Eq. (6):

$$C = \frac{Fk_a D e^{-k_e t}}{V(k_a - k_e)} \tag{6}$$

However, this might not be the case for a sustained release formulation since the absorption process will be slower, k_a will be smaller and its value may approach or become smaller than that of k_e.

Rapid First-Order Absorption of Part of the Dose, Then Release and Absorption of the Remainder over an Extended Period of Time by a Zero-Order Kinetic Process Followed by a First-Order Elimination Process

This model presents a case where the release of the drug from the dosage form occurs in two ways. First, a fraction of the total dose is released for immediate availability (burst effect) to be absorbed by a first-order process and the remaining fraction is absorbed at a constant rate, i.e., a slow zero-order process which results in zero-order absorption over a prolonged time period. Following a single oral dose, the concentration at any time after such a dosage form can be described by Eq. (7) [8]:

$$C = \frac{k_0 (e^{k_e T} - 1) e^{-k_e t}}{k_e V} + \frac{(k_a D - k_0)(e^{-k_e t} - e^{-k_a t})}{V(k_a - k_e)} \tag{7}$$

where k_0 is the "slow," zero-order absorption rate, T is the duration of the zero-order input period, and k_a is the "fast" first-order absorption rate constant.

Rapid First-Order Absorption of Part of the Dose, Then Release and Absorption of the Remainder over an Extended Period of Time by a Slower First-Order Kinetic Process Followed by a First-Order Elimination Process

This model is very similar to model "3" except that a small portion of the administered dose is absorbed by a first-order kinetic process. Plasma drug concentration at any time after oral administration of such a dosage form can be described by Eq. (8):

$$C = A\,(e^{-k_e t} - e^{k_r t}) + B\,(e^{-k_e t} - e^{-k_a t}) \tag{8}$$

where k_r and k_a are the fast and slow first-order absorption rate constants, respectively, and A and B are hybrid rate constants which incorporate the elimination and absorption rate constants, the burst release and slow release doses and the volume of distribution [8].

It may be difficult to unambiguously select one of the four models [Eqs. (1,5,7,8)] for fitting and analyzing experimental data obtained after oral administration of a sustained release dosage form. Although the absorption rate for a sustained release product may be slower than after a conventional dosage form, it may be a mixed or a combined first and zero-order process, and therefore, probably cannot be precisely described by a single model-dependent equation. Additionally, the kinetic order of the absorption process may be time- or site-dependent as the drug traverses through the gastrointestinal tract where absorption takes place. The importance of these considerations will depend on the drug, the formulation and whether the drug can potentially be absorbed from wide or restrictive areas along the gastrointestinal tract. General approaches which can potentially overcome these practical concerns are the Loo-Riegelman [9] and Wagner-Nelson methods [10] and model-independent statistical moment methods [5,11,12].

2. *Loo-Riegelman and Wagner-Nelson Pharmacokinetic Methods*

For many drugs, after intravenous (i.v.) administration, the plasma concentration versus time curve can be described by an apparent biexponential equation. This is not the case after oral administration due to the apparent multiexponential nature of the disposition processes involving absorption, distribution and elimination. Theoretically, after oral administration, the disposition of a drug in the body is not affected by the formulation used but the distribution phase might be obscured by the slower process(es) of drug release in the gastrointestinal fluids and its subsequent absorption. This experimental phenomenon observed after oral administration presents the problem of a vanishing exponential term, usually describing the distribution phase [13].

The pharmacokinetics of a drug after i.v. administration can, in general, be described by a two-compartment model. The Loo-Riegelman method is a very powerful method for assessing drug absorption, in general, and absorption from sustained release formulations, in particular [5,9]. This method states that the amount of drug absorbed at any given time is equal to the sum of the amount of drug present in the central and peripheral compartments and of the amount eliminated by all routes. This method is not predicated on any assumption regarding the kinetic order of the absorption process. The absorption kinetics of the drug can be zero-order, first-order, or a combination of the two. Therefore, the Loo-Riegelman method is particularly useful in the assessment of the drug absorption process and, therefore, the pharmacokinetic evaluation of drugs using sustained release formulations. The only assumption with this approach is that drug pharmacokinetics can be described by at least a two-compartment model. Because most drugs fall into this category after i.v. administration, this is not a restrictive assumption, especially since this method can be applied to any multicompartmental model. However, to use the Loo-Riegelman method, a drug must be given by the i.v. route as a reference. This method can be used not only to measure the rate and extent of drug absorption but also to determine the pharmacokinetic order of the absorption process by the following [9]:

$$\frac{(X_A)_T}{(X_A)_\infty} = \frac{C_T + k_{10} \int_0^T Cdt + (X_p)_T / V_c}{k_{10} \int_0^\infty Cdt} \qquad (9)$$

where $(X_A)_T$ and $(X_A)_\infty$ are the amount of drug absorbed in the body at time T and time infinity, respectively, and the ratio between $(X_A)_T$ and $(X_A)_\infty$ is the fraction absorbed at any time t. C_T and $(X_p)_T$ are drug plasma concentration and amount of drug in the peripheral compartment at time t, respectively. The rate constant k_{10} is the apparent first-order elimination rate constant of the drug from the central compartment, and V_c is the volume of distribution of the central compartment.

If a plot of percent unabsorbed (i.e., $100\{1-[(X_A)_T/(X_A)_\infty]\}$) versus time on semilogarithmic coordinates approximates a straight line, suggesting an apparent first-order absorption, the absorption rate constant (k_a) can be estimated from the slope of this plot. A linear relationship between percent unabsorbed and time on rectilinear coordinates suggests apparent zero-order absorption with a zero input rate k_0 [5,9].

The classical method which preceded the Loo-Riegleman method was the Wagner-Nelson approach [5,10]. This method has the advantage of not needing results from an i.v. reference standard, but is restricted to drugs displaying one-compartment open-body-model characteristics, which adequately describe the actual disposition of some drugs after i.v. administration. The Wagner-Nelson model is given as follows [10]:

$$\frac{(X_A)_T}{(X_A)_\infty} = \frac{C_T + k_e \int_0^T Cdt}{k_e \int_0^\infty Cdt} \qquad (10)$$

where k_e is the overall elimination rate constant. The kinetic order of the absorption process and the values of k_a or k_0 can be determined by using the Wagner-Nelson method.

The Wagner-Nelson method and its subsequent modification [14] are not recommended for the analysis of data obtained after oral administration displaying multicompartmental disposition characteristics. Therefore, use of the Wagner-Nelson method for assessing drug absorption kinetics after oral administration will be more suitable for drugs known to demonstrate, or to be approximated by, one-compartment model characteristics after rapid i.v. injection. In the absence of this information, or with knowledge to the contrary, the Loo-Riegelman method might be a better method for assessing absorption kinetics after oral administration [15]. However, for many drugs which are given as sustained release formulations and have a rapid distribution phase relative to drug absorption, the Wagner-Nelson model can provide a reasonable basis for the estimation of absorption parameters.

3. *Model Independent Pharmacokinetic Analysis*

The use of moments in pharmacokinetics was first described by Yamaoka et al. (11) and allows one to state that for any theoretical relationship between plasma concentration and time, nonnormalized moments about the origin can be calculated. The zero and first nonnormalized moments allow for the calculation of area under the curve (AUC) and area under the moment curve (AUMC), respectively.

By using statistical moment theory, one also can calculate the mean residence time (MRT) of a drug after administration of standard and sustained release dosage formulations. The MRT is defined as the mean time for the intact drug molecule to transit through the body and involves a composite of all kinetic processes including release from the dosage form, drug absorption into the body and drug disposition and can be calculated after any single oral administration using Eq. (11) [11,12,16–19]:

$$\mathrm{MRT} = \frac{\int_0^\infty tC\,dt}{\int_0^\infty C\,dt} = \frac{\mathrm{AUMC}_{0\to\infty}}{\mathrm{AUC}_{0\to\infty}} \tag{11}$$

where AUC is the area under the concentration versus time curve (the zero moment) and AUMC is the area under the curve of the product of concentration and time (the first moment) versus time. The MRT can be used in a comparative way to evaluate the *in vivo* performance of a sustained release dosage form. The longer the MRT the more sustained or prolonged is the absorption of the drug assuming a constant elimination rate constant. If an intravenous reference dosage form is available, a more rigorous assessment of the drug absorption process can be performed. Subtraction of the MRT obtained after i.v. administration ($MRT_{i.v.}$) from the MRT obtained after oral (or any noninstantaneous manner) administration (MRT_{oral}) will give the mean absorption time (MAT) [Eq. (12)] [11, 12].

$$MAT = MRT_{oral} - MRT_{i.v.} \tag{12}$$

MAT is more closely related to the absorption process than is the MRT_{oral}. The longer the MAT, the more sustained or prolonged is the absorption of the drug. If additional information about the absorption kinetics of a drug is available, one can estimate the apparent absorption rate constant, which is k_a in the case of a first-order absorption process, and absorption time (T) in the case of a zero-order absorption process [Eqs. (13) and (14), respectively and Eq. (12)].

$$MAT = \frac{1}{k_a} \tag{13}$$

$$MAT = \frac{T}{2} \tag{14}$$

Equations 13 and 14 are not compartmental-model-dependent but depend on the absorption kinetic order which ought to be defined and must be homogeneous throughout the period of absorption. If the kinetic order for absorption is complex, or time dependent, the MRT or MAT can be used as an estimate to perform a model-independent pharmacokinetic evaluation of a sustained release dosage form.

When drug is absorbed by first- or zero-order kinetic input processes, the MRT_{ni} can be described by Eqs. (15) and (16), respectively [5]:

$$MRT_{ni} = MRT_{i.v.} + \frac{1}{k_a} \tag{15}$$

$$MRT_{ni} = MRT_{i.v.} + \frac{T}{2} \tag{16}$$

When a drug is absorbed by a zero-order process, T is equal to the quotient of the dose absorbed (D) divided by k_0. Therefore, Eq. (16) can be rewritten as follows:

$$MRT_{ni} = MRT_{i.v.} + \frac{D}{2k_0} \tag{17}$$

The MRT, after any mode of administration, can also be described by Eq. (11) [5,11,12,16–19].

Because k_a or k_0 appears in the expanded equation defining the AUMC [10], but not in the final equation describing AUC, the input rate constant k_a or the zero-order input rate k_0 will not affect the AUC but will affect the AUMC. Therefore, changes in these parameters should result in changes in MRT.

According to Eqs. (15) and (17), there is a linear relationship between MRT_{ni} and $1/k_a$ when a drug is absorbed by a first-order kinetic process and between MRT_{ni} and $1/k_0$ when a drug is absorbed (or administered) by a zero-order process. These models were explored by a series of computer simulations which were run for a hypothetical drug with the following pharmacokinetic parameters: The oral dose (D) was equal to 500 mg; the volume of distribution (V) was set at 35 liters and various elimination rate constants (k_e) equal to: 0.0575, 0.077, 0.12, 0.23, and 0.46 hr^{-1}. In all cases, complete bioavailability (F) was assumed. This assumption is not absolutely required since the F term is present in both the AUMC and AUC terms and cancel each other out when the MRT is calculated. The MRT was calculated by using Eq. (11).

The relationship between MRT and $1/k_a$ at each value of k_e is provided in Fig. 1 and shows that Eq. (15) holds over a given range of $1/k_a$ depending on the k_e value. Beyond this point, the line begins to bend in an apparent convex fashion and eventually reaches a plateau. When k_a is equal to k_e, the MRT is equal to $2/k_a$ as shown in Eq. (18).

$$MRT = \frac{1}{k_a} + \frac{1}{k_e} = \frac{1}{k_a} + MRT_{i.v.} = \frac{2}{k_a} \tag{18}$$

A plot of MRT versus $1/k_a$ for this special case will give a straight line which will pass through the origin with a slope of 2 (Fig. 1). Assuming the same k_e, the linear line obtained by Eq. (18) will intersect with the curve of MRT versus $1/k_a$ [Eq. (15)] at the point where linearity ends and curvature begins. The reason for this deviation from theory was examined. It was noted that the method of extrapolation for AUC and AUMC from time t* (the time of the last observed plasma concentration) to infinity can result in an underestimation of the contribution to MRT_{ni}. Under normal circumstances, the extrapolations for AUC and AUMC are done according to Eqs. (19) and (20), respectively [5]:

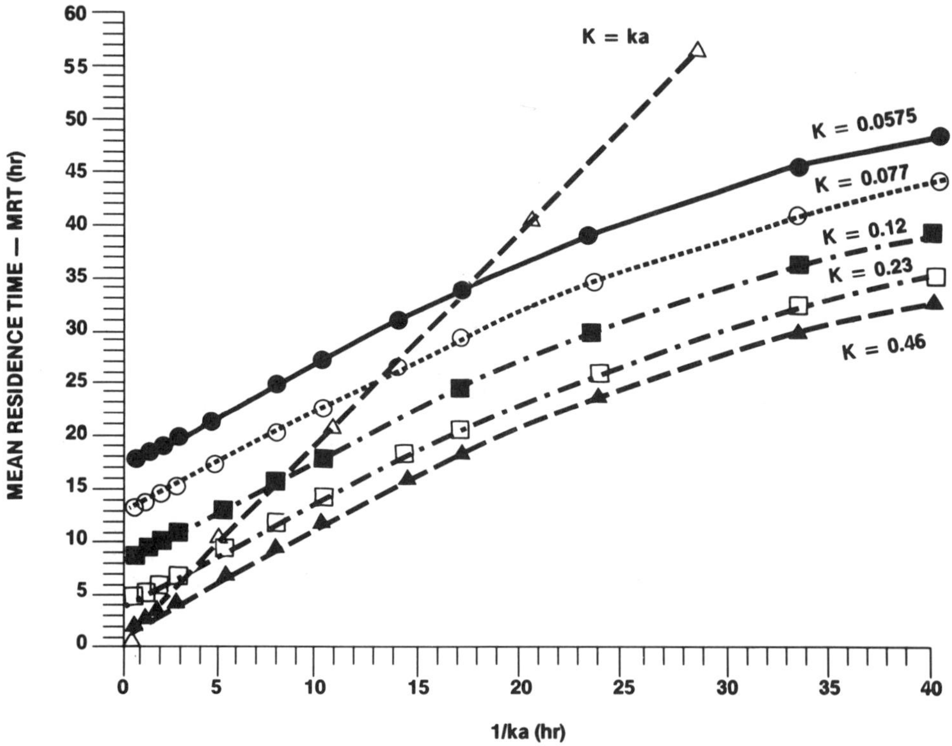

Fig. 1 The relationship between the mean residence time $(MRT)_{ni}$ and $1/k_a$ for the following K values (● – 0.0575 hr^{-1}; ○ – K = 0.077 hr^{-1}; ■ – K = 0.12 hr^{-1}; □ – K = 0.23 hr^{-1}; ▲ – K = 0.46; △ – K = k_a hr^{-1}) (inappropriately calculated).

$$AUC \Big|_{t^*}^{\infty} = \frac{C^*}{k_e} \tag{19}$$

$$AUMC \Big|_{t^*}^{\infty} = \frac{t^* \, C^*}{k_e} + \frac{C^*}{k_e^{\,2}} \tag{20}$$

This is true when $k_a > k_e$. In the "flip-flop" case (where $k_e > k_a$), however, the correct approach to extrapolate for AUC and AUMC from t* to infinity is to use k_a instead of k_e in Eqs. (19) and (20). These latter calculations resulted in a correction of the deviation from theory shown previously in Fig. 1. The linear relationship between MRT_{ni} and k_a with a slope of unity and an intercept of

$1/k_a$, as predicted by Eq. (15), was fully restored as shown in Fig. 2.

The relationship between MRT and $1/k_0$ at each value of k_e given in Fig. 3 shows that there is a linear relationship between the MRT and $1/k_0$ along the entire range of k_0 (with the same dose given over T hours; varying from 1 to 24 hr). In Figs. 1-3, the intercepts of all plots of MRT_{ni} versus $1/k_a$ or versus $1/k_0$ are equal for the reciprocal of each respective k_e value and represent the value of $MRT_{i.v.}$. The mean slope for the linear portions of each of the five curves presented in Figs. 1 and 2 was 253 mg [which is essentially equal to D/2, as predicted from Eq. (17)]. It can, therefore, be concluded that the MRT_{ni} is always a linear function of either $1/k_a$ or $1/k_0$. Deviations from this relationship may occur in special cases, such as the "flip-flop" situation where correct

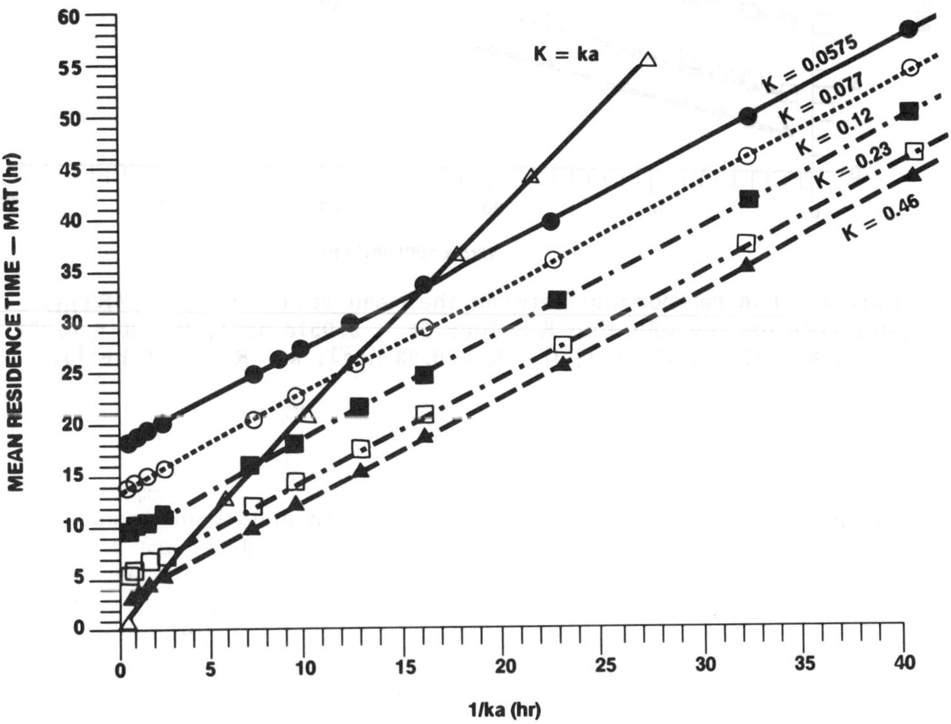

Fig. 2 The relationship between the mean residence time $(MRT)_{ni}$ and $1/k_a$ for the following K values (● – 0.0575 hr^{-1}; ○ – K = 0.077 hr^{-1}; ■ – K = 0.12 hr^{-1}; □ – K = 0.23 hr^{-1}; ▲ – K = 0.46; △ – K = k_a hr^{-1}) (appropriately calculated).

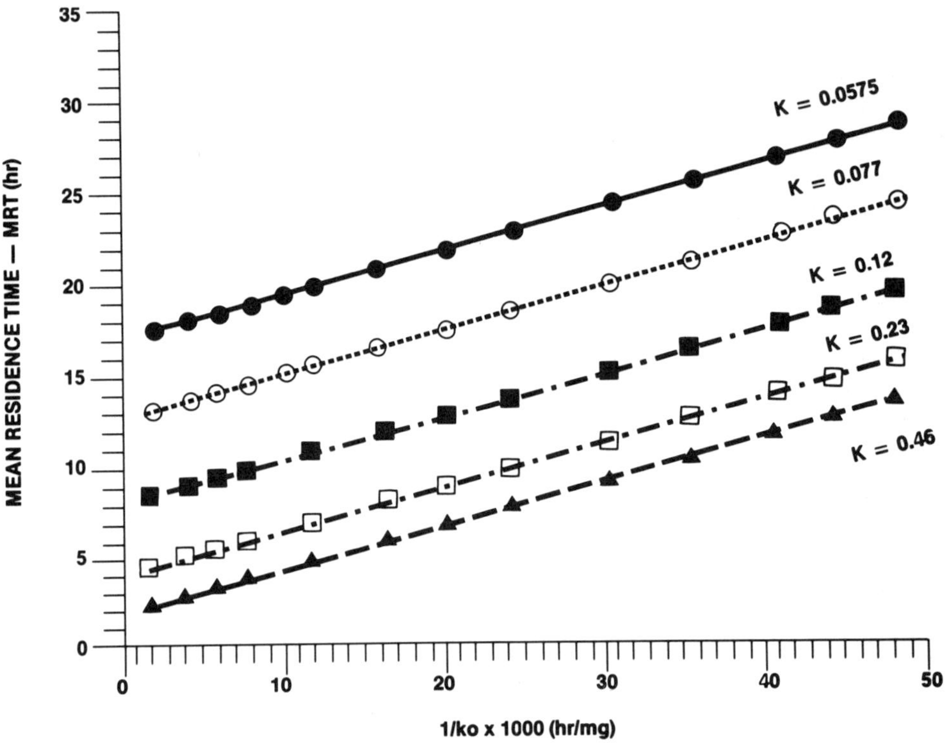

Fig. 3 The relationship between the mean residence time (MRT_{ni}) and $1/k_0$ for the following K values (● – 0.0575 hr^{-1}; ○ – K = 0.077 hr^{-1}; ■ – K = 0.12 hr^{-1}; □ – K = 0.23 hr^{-1}; ▲ – K = 0.46 hr^{-1}).

calculations of AUC and AUMC are essential to yield valid results.

Although the relationship based on Eq. (1) and (5) are derived from a one-compartment body model, the relationships between MRT_{ni} and $1/k_a$ or $1/k_0$ [Eqs. (15–17)] are model independent [5,11,12]. Therefore, the results illustrated in Figs. 1–3 (by determining AUC and AUMC) are independent of the model describing the disposition of the drug as long as the drug is eliminated by linear pharmacokinetics [20].

4. *Pharmacokinetics on Multiple Dosing*

Sustained release dosage forms offer the potential of extending drug effect well beyond what is usually observed after a single dose given as a conventional dosage form and of minimizing fluctuations in plasma drug concentrations over a dosing interval. As previously stated, by minimizing fluctuations in drug plasma concentrations, it may be possible to reduce the total dosage required, improve the effectiveness and decrease the incidence and severity of adverse effects related to drug therapy. The most important criteria for evaluating the performance of sustained release dosage forms are: (a) the amount of drug intended to be absorbed is actually absorbed in a reproducible manner; and (b) the ratio of steady-state maximum to minimum drug concentrations (obtained after multiple or chronic administration) are not greater than, or ideally, less than that produced by the more frequently administered conventional oral dosage form [21].

The fluctuations (or oscillations) in drug plasma concentrations at steady state after consecutive doses of a drug are usually evaluated by directly determining the peak to trough plasma concentration as shown in Eq. (21) [21].

$$\% \text{ Fluctuation} = 100 \cdot \frac{(\text{Peak plasma concentration} - \text{trough plasma concentration})}{(\text{Trough plasma concentration})} \tag{21}$$

The merits of estimating fluctuations in drug plasma concentrations according to Eq. (21) are called into question when trough plasma concentrations are low. In this case, the percentage of fluctuation may vary considerably between subjects. An alternative approach was proposed by Caldwell et al. [22], who used the fluctuations index [FI; Eq. (22)] for evaluating the performance of sustained release tablets of lithium at steady state,

$$\text{FI} = \frac{(\text{Peak plasma concentration} - \text{trough plasma concentration})}{(\text{Average drug plasma concentration})} \tag{22}$$

The average drug plasma concentration is calculated from the quotient of the area under the drug plasma concentration versus time curve (AUC) during a steady-state dosing interval and the dosage interval (AUC_{ss}/τ).

Ideally, the ratio of maximum to minimum drug concentrations in plasma at steady state should be less than the therapeutic index (TI) of the drug. Theeuwes and Bayne [23] derived an equation [Eq. (23)] relating the required dosing interval to drug elimination half-life and the TI of the drug,

$$\tau \leqslant t_{1/2} \cdot \frac{\ln \text{TI}}{\ln 2} \tag{23}$$

A drug with a therapeutic index of 2 and an elimination half-life of 6 hr must be given no less frequently than every 6 hr to avoid excessive (toxic) or subtherapeutic concentrations. A drug with a similar half-life but a therapeutic index of 4 may be given every 12 hr. The derivation of Eq. (23) assumes that the drug has very rapid and complete absorption. A similar expression [Eq. (24)] can be written in terms of mean residence time (MRT) [24]:

$$\tau \leqslant 0.693\ \text{MRT} \cdot \frac{\ln \text{TI}}{\ln 2} \qquad (24)$$

Fluctuations in drug plasma concentrations are related not only to the release rate of the drug from the dosage form and the dosage interval but also to the drug elimination rate. Jackson and Wright [25] recently observed an apparently linear relationship between percent fluctuation of theophylline serum concentrations at steady-state after regular dosing of a prolonged release product and theophylline clearance in individual subjects.

B. Pharmacodynamics

Pharmacokinetic theory is useful not only in facilitating predictions of the time course of drug concentrations in the body, but also in developing a better understanding of the time course of drug action on the body. This may be accomplished by linking the relationship between the dose, the concentration time course and the time course of drug action. While pharmacokinetics can describe what the body does to the drug, pharmacodynamics can relate pharmacokinetics to the drug's effects on the body once it has reached its site of action.

Pharmacodynamics can be defined as a quantitative assessment of the time course of drug effect on the body after administration by any route. Inherent in this definition is that drug effect can be objectively measured. The measured response to a drug may be all or none or it may be graded. In addition, a drug effect may be reversible. This section will be limited to drugs that elicit measurable pharmacodynamic effects that are reversible, graded, and objectively quantifiable.

There are two fundamental ways that pharmacodynamic principles can be applied to the drug development process. These will be applicable whether classical or sustained release dosage forms are under investigation. In the first case, the pharmacokinetics of a drug will be known and a pharmacokinetic model can be established for the drug in humans or in some animal species. This pharmacokinetic model can then be linked to available pharmacodynamic data resulting in a unified concept relating the kinetics of the drug (or an active metabolite) to the time course of drug effect.

In the second case where the pharmacokinetic characteristics of a drug cannot be adequately defined (i.e., AUCs cannot be accurately measured because of assay sensitivity limitations) or where drug effect is apparently unrelated to concentrations, alternative approaches can be utilized. We will describe both cases and illustrate how each approach can be utilized to allow pharmacodynamic considerations to play an important role in the development of dosage forms, particularly sustained release formulations.

Implicit to many pharmacodynamic models is that measured drug and/or active metabolite concentrations in a sampled biophase are in equilibrium with concentrations at the receptor or the site of drug action (i.e., heart, brain, kidney, etc.) [26,27]. Concentration data obtained at steady state may be particularly useful in defining a pharmacodynamic model since single-dose data alone may not be adequate to describe the effect of drug and/or active metabolite accumulation on the drug's pharmacological action upon multiple dosing [28]. Pharmacodynamic data obtained from several steady-state concentrations and appropriate washout periods may also be required to characterize the dynamic effects of a drug since time- and concentration-related effects must also be assessed and evaluated.

Pharmacodynamic models are generally mathematical and can rely heavily on parameters which are believed to be important in defining drug disposition in the body. These models can be particularly useful if they not only help to explain empirical data, but also provide a rationale for elucidating fundamental mechanisms, thereby facilitating a prediction of drug activity in different subjects or under altered physiological/disease-state conditions. The potential usefulness of pharmacokinetic-pharmacodynamic models as predictors of drug action cannot be overstated. Although there is a plethora of data in the literature describing drug pharmacokinetics in the body, there is a paucity of data delineating the time course of drug action *in vivo*.

One of the most significant breakthroughs in allowing scientists to test various hypotheses relating to various proposed pharmacodynamic models is the increasing availability and accessibility of measuring drug and active metabolites with greater specificity and sensitivity. Of equal importance, more sophisticated methods have been successfully applied providing means by which drug action can be objectively and reproducibly measured and quantified. Quantitation of drug effect can be a formidable endeavor if one considers that a drug or active metabolite may, and frequently does, have the potential to elicit a multitude of pharmacodynamic actions, some of which may have antagonistic effects.

The earliest reports describing quantifiable pharmacological activity were documented for *d*-tubocurarine [27–29]. Pharmacodynamic models have since been proposed and tested for: antiarrhythmics [30–35], antiasthmatics [36–38], cardiovascular agents [39–46], and anticoagulants [47–49].

A preprequisite to a rigorous mathematical analysis of pharmacodynamic data is an adequate description of a model describing the pharmacokinetics of the drug *in vivo* [50,51]. Complex pharmacokinetic models are not necessarily required and often can limit the interpretation of pharmacodynamic data because of the assumptions inherent to these models. The absence of pharmacokinetic data does not, however, preclude the analysis of pharmacodynamic data. In a later section, a description of how pharmacodynamic data can be used in the absence of pharmacokinetic data in the development process will be discussed.

Many useful pharmacodynamic models are based on concentration versus time data that are obtained at an "effect" site [26,37]. These models are based on the assumption that the actual blood sampling site is in equilibrium with drug at its effect site. This condition is generally believed to be true only at steady state or at quasi-steady state [28].

1. *Pharmacodynamic Models*

One of the simplest and oldest pharmacodynamic models described is the *fixed-effect model*, where drug concentration can be related to a pharmacological effect which is either observed or not observed. This can also be used to refer to a partial effect (i.e., percentile of baseline). This model requires no particular assumption about the relationship between concentration and the effect measured. One limitation of this model, however, is that at a given drug concentration, the effect may or may not be observed in a given individual. This problem can be overcome by including a probability factor that allows for an assessment of the anticipated percent of the patients or individuals that will respond in a particular way at a given drug concentration. The major drawback of the *fixed-effect model* is its inherent inability to relate a range of drug concentrations to a broad range of pharmacological effects *in vivo* [51].

The most fundamental model directly linking drug concentration and effect is the *linear model*, which can be described mathematically by Eq. (25):

$$E = P \cdot C \tag{25}$$

where E is the quantified effect, C the drug concentration, and P a linear parameter best linking E and C. Depending on the drug and the effect being elicited, a baseline effect may be measured (i.e., intraocular pressure, heart rate, etc.) in the absence of drug (i.e., when C = O at time t = O), and in this case, the relationship can be rewritten as Eq. (26):

$$E = P \cdot C + E_0 \tag{26}$$

where E_0 is the effect at time t = 0 when C = 0. The parameter P will then be estimated from a plot of $E - E_0$ versus C. Estimating E_0 may not be a trivial matter necessarily and a variety of problems and methods for their solution have been proposed [32,39,51–53]. This model has been successfully applied to many drugs including verapamil [30], quinidine [32], disopyramide [35], and digoxin [52]. An improved relationship between drug concentration and effect may be obtained after logarithmic transformation of concentration data as shown in Eq. (27) (*logarithmic model*):

$$E = P \cdot \text{Log } C + E_0 \tag{27}$$

If a dosage form is given chronically, and concentrations at steady state are measured, this equation can be rewritten as Eq. (28):

$$E_{ss} = P \cdot \text{Log } C_{ss} + E_{0_{ss}} \tag{28}$$

where the subscript *ss* indicates the parameter at steady state. This equation, however, may not be directly comparable to Eq. (27) since effect data obtained at steady state may be different from that obtained after single doses [e.g., if there is accumulation of an active metabolite(s)]. Equation (28) may also be used to assess pharmacodynamic data obtained using sustained release formulations. Again, depending on whether metabolites contribute to drug effect, and the importance of metabolite accumulation on multiple dosing, the slope of this line may or may not be equivalent after classical versus sustained release formulations.

A frequently employed method describing the relationship between drug effect and drug concentration is derived from the *sigmoidal model* describing the relationship between drug concentration and effect over the range of 0–100%. However, this approach may only be applicable to isolated tissues or receptors. With this model, E cannot be predicted when C is close to zero, and the maximal effect cannot be predicted. The major problem intrinsic to the application of this model to an *in vivo* case is the unlikely possibility of reaching a maximal effect and, therefore, the general difficulty of anticipating the range of concentrations necessary to result in a linear change in effect.

None of the preceding models can account for a maximal drug effect. The *E_{max} model*, however, incorporates concepts from enzymology and equilibirum theory and allows for a prediction of C_{max}. This is shown in Eq. (29) [51]:

$$E = \frac{E_{max} \cdot C}{E_{50} + C} \tag{29}$$

where E_{max} is the theoretical maximal attainable effect attributable to the drug and E_{50} is the concentration of drug eliciting 50% of this maximal effect. As written, this *E_{max} model* predicts E to equal 0 when C = 0, as with previous models. Where a baseline effect is present in the absence of drug, an E_0 may be incorporated into the equation to account for non-drug-related baseline measurements, as in Eq. (30) [51]:

$$E = E_0 + \frac{E_{max} \cdot C}{E_{50} + C} \tag{30}$$

Where the drug effect is to reduce an effect measurable in the absence of drug, such as a drug given to reduce blood pressure or heart rate, this equation can be transformed to Eq. (31) [51]:

$$E = E_0 - \frac{E_{max} \cdot C}{I_{50} + C} \tag{31}$$

where I_{50} is the drug concentration producing a 50% reduction in the baseline measured biological parameter. Equations describing the *E_{max} model* (also for enzyme kinetics and equilibrium theory) assume a hyperbolic relationship between concentration and effect. Such a relationship may not always be observed. One of the explanations for this finding is that implicit to this model is that each receptor site combines with a single drug molecule. However, where not all of the receptors are occupied or where a receptor interacts with more than one drug molecule, the exponent of C may differ from a value of one to that greater than one, and can even be a non integer value. Therefore, under certain conditions, a modified *E_{max} model* may be useful in describing the drug concentration-effect relationship. In this *sigmoid-E_{max} model*, there is a modified hyperbolic function which can be described mathematically by Eq. (32) [51]:

$$E = \frac{E_{max} \cdot C^n}{E_{50} + C^n} \tag{32}$$

where n is a parameter which affects the hyperbolic nature of the curve. This relationship was originally applied by Hill to describe the interaction between oxygen and hemoglobin [54] and has been extensively discussed by Wagner [50].

If upon inspection of the graphical relationship between drug concentration and effect, a counterclockwise hysteresis loop is observed, this may be suggestive of a delay in drug equilibration between plasma and the effect compartment [55]. This phenomenon can arise, theoretically (although not likely), if an active metabolite is formed at an increasing rate with increasing drug concentration, and its disposition is significantly different from that of the parent drug [51]. This phenomenon can be circumvented by a multiple dosing scheme with dosing and pharmacodynamic measurements made at steady state. Under these conditions, the rate of drug and metabolite elimination are equal to the corresponding rates of drug and metabolite input.

Other more sophisticated approaches involve the use of multicompartment, deconvolution, and mixed-compartment models [28,55]. One common key feature dropping out of some of these complex models is the concept of equilibration time, a concept of particular importance under non-steady-state conditions, which is of lesser importance during chronic dosing or steady-state studies.

There is no *a priori* reason why, nor is it likely, that the active site of a drug corresponds to a pharmacokinetically accessible site (i.e., the plasma or blood). Therefore, the basic premise of the active site being in direct equilibrium with a pharmacokinetically accessible site is possibly invalid. To address this issue, Sheiner and co-workers have proposed that an "effect compartment" should be modeled as a separate compartment linked to the plasma compartment by a first-order process. This compartment receives a negligible amount of drug. This approach has been found to be valuable in describing pharmacokinetic/pharmacodynamic data for *d*-tubocurarine [28].

Complete pharmacokinetic characterization of a drug in humans or in some animal model may not always be possible. For example, it may be impossible to adequately define the area under the concentration time curve after a single dose of a drug or to calculate the elimination half-life or bioavailability because of assay limitations (e.g., inadequate sensitivity). In spite of these limitations, one can study the relationship of drug effect and steady state drug concentration at various drug dosing levels in the same individual (Figs. 4 and 5). By using sustained release dosage forms resulting in varying release rates or rate constants, one can derive valuable information regarding a drug product.

Often, there may be no apparent correlation between drug concentration and effect. One may still employ pharmacodynamic data in the development process. These pharmacodynamic data can often reveal valuable information regarding the efficacy of the dosage form and even shed some light on drug pharmacokinetics not otherwise available. Levy first proposed the concept of relating drug effect with time following administration of a drug [26]. Utilizing this

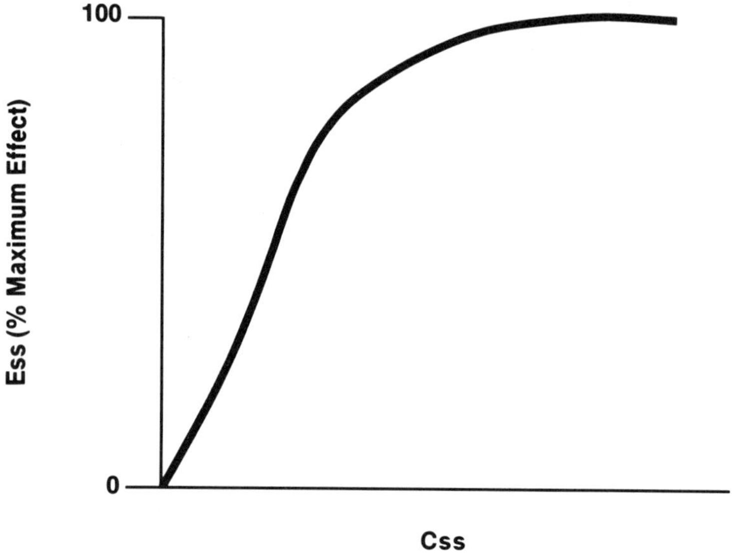

Fig. 4 A linear concentration-response (effect) curve for a theoretical drug.

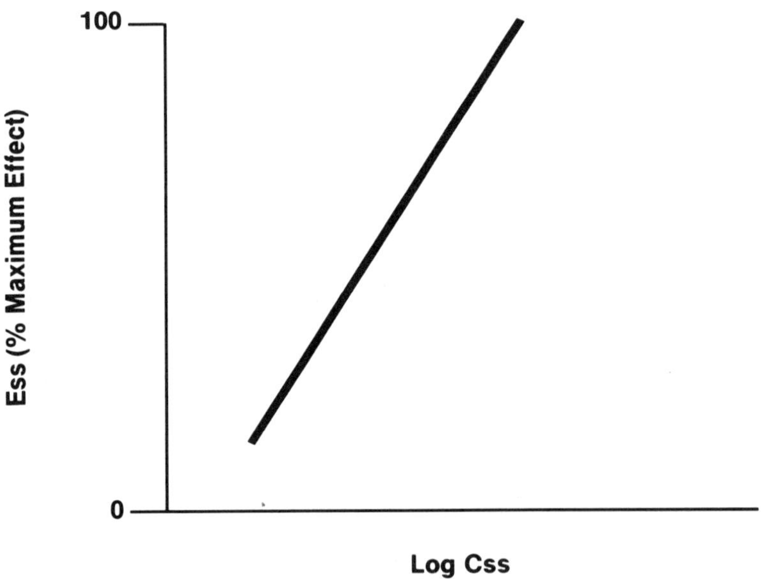

Fig. 5 A semilogarithmic concentration response curve for a drug and emphasizing the apparent linearity between log concentration and response.

approach, it can be shown that there is a maximal effect following varying dosing levels and the duration of effect for each dosing level can be determined. From these results, one can determine what dose or dosage form would be needed to elicit a given effect and how long the effect should last. This information may be valuable in supporting claims of single-daily dosing based on prolonged efficacy throughout a dosing interval. The realtionship between effect and time is given by Eq. (33) [29]:

$$E = E_0 - \frac{mk_e t}{2.3} \tag{33}$$

where m is the slope of the linear phase of the plot of E versus t. Therefore, with a knowledge of drug effect with time, and a prior knowledge of the slope (m) from Eq. (33), one can estimate the drug's apparent elimination half-life, which for various reasons, may not be otherwise easily calculated. With knowledge of a drug's elimination half-life, it would be possible to design a sustained release dosage form with a desired MRT in the body.

Examples of pharmacodynamic evaluations of sustained release dosage forms is shown in the work of Falliers [36], who evaluated the pharmacodynamics, including spirometric measurements, in asthmatic patients receiving a sustained release theophylline capsule formulation. In these patients, after isoproterenol inhalation, an average of 25% improvement in forced expiratory volume in 1 sec (FEV) was observed while after placebo there were very minimal changes. After the administration of a sustained release theophylline capsule formulation to steady state, an average 20% improvement in FEV was observed at the 5-hr time period and sufficient bronchodilation expressed as FEV was observed for a 10–12-hr period.

A comparative pharmacokinetic and pharmacodynamic study of slow release and conventional formulations of oxprenolol showed that a single dose of the conventional dosage form produced a significant reduction in exercise induced tachycardia for 8 hr, whereas the high dose of the slow release preparation produced a similar reduction which lasted for at least 14 hr [57]. In a similar study with propranolol, the percentage reduction in exercise heart rate over the 3–24-hr period after the dose was similar for the slow release formulation and the two standard regimens of the conventional tablets when compared with placebo. In the 2-hr period following the dose, the 80 mg twice-a-day regimen produced a significant reduction in the postexercise systolic blood pressure when compared with the long-acting formulation [58]. In both cases the results deomonstrated that pharmacodynamic measurements might be utilized for the comparison of drug efficacy when given in different formulations.

III. SUMMARY

Pharmacokinetic and pharmacodynamic evaluation of a drug can yield information that can be crucial to the development and design of drug dosage forms in general, and sustained release formulations in particular. The selection of a particular pharmacokinetic model or approach is subject to individual preferences although, in general, model-independent methods are mathematically less complex and require fewer restrictive assumptions.

Pharmacokinetic parameters can be used to compare sustained release with conventional formulations. The mean residence time (MRT) is a term which describes the time a drug molecule takes to traverse through the body and can be used to compare dosage forms, particularly for sustained release formulations.

The most serious restriction to the use of oral sustained release dosage forms is the limited residence time of the dosage form in the small intestine. Literature data suggests that 9–12 hr is a reasonable estimate of average effective absorption time after oral administration of a well-absorbed drug in a dosage form that remains intact in the gastrointestinal tract. This means that ordinarily the dissolution half-lives of drugs from dosage forms that release the active ingredient in a first-order manner should not exceed 3–4 hr. Because there may be a limit to the reduction in the release rate of a drug from a sustained release dosage form without compromising the extent of absorption (bioavailability), there may also be a limit to the prolongation of the duration of drug effect by means of altering dosage forms [4,122]. Since the most important criteria for the evaluation of sustained release dosage forms are bioavailability and fluctuations at steady state, it is of interest that the desired formulation demonstrate less fluctuation and have a bioavailability of at least 80% relative to a conventional dosage form. Table 2 lists drugs available in controlled release forms for which pharmacokinetic evaluation of these drug products has been reported in the literature.

Recent findings [12,20,21,23,24] suggest that concepts derived from statistical moment theory can be helpful in the design of drug products in general, and for sustained release products in particular. In the case of a product having a slow first-order release (and absorption) rate, it is important to use the correct approach to the estimation of area under the curve (AUC), area under the moment curve (AUMC), and oral mean residence time (MRT_{ni}). In the case where the first order absorption rate constant (k_a) is less than the elimination rate constant (k_e), it is important to note that area extrapolation to infinity from the last measured concentration must be made by C^*/k_a rather than by C^*/k_e (Figs. 1 and 2). Where a plot of MRT_{ni} versus $1/k_a$ does not yield a linear relationship, an exploration into the "flip-flop" situation is warranted. These results have important practical implications for drugs with very short elimination half-lives. When a drug is intended to be released (and absorbed) by a first-order rate process, the k_a value should be decreased and MRT_{ni} should be increased sufficiently to achieve and maintain effective plasma concentrations over each dosing interval. Similarly, when a drug is intended to be released and absorbed by an apparent zero-order process, it has been shown that the MRT_{ni} can be appreciably increased simply by reducing k_0 (or increasing $1/k_0$) (Fig. 3). In summary, with a prior knowledge of a drug's elimination and distribution pharmacokinetics and the use of the correct approach to the estimation of MRT, it is possible to design formulations having particular release characteristics with predictive impacts on the mean residence time of a drug in the body.

Pharmacodynamic measurements can have a significant impact on the design and development of sustained release products. Selection of a pharmacodynamic model does not require having a complex pharmacokinetic model in-hand. In fact, in general, the simpler the pharmacokinetic model, the more useful the results may be. The most important approach, however, is the assessment of pharmacokinetic and pharmacodynamic parameters at steady state, rather than after single dose administration. The benefits of steady state studies include:

1. Improved reproducibility of the *in vivo* absorption process is achieved.
2. More consistent and reliable estimates of pharmacokinetic parameters of the drug are attainable.
3. Estimates of steady state concentrations of drug and active metabolites are available.
4. Urinary excretion kinetics of unchanged drug and major metabolites(s) should be more reproducible at steady state.
5. Clinical observations (if any) can be made at steady state.

Evaluation of sustained release formulations is recommended after multiple dosing where steady state prevails. Under these conditions, the physiological variables are minimized and all pharmacokinetic measurements reflect therapeutic conditions.

REFERENCES

1. B. E. Ballard, An overview of prolonged action drug dosage form, In, *Sustained and Controlled Release Drug Delivery Systems* (J. R. Robinson, ed.), Marcel Dekker, Inc., New York, 1978, pp. 1–69.
2. P. G. Welling, Oral controlled drug administration: Pharmacokinetic considerations, *Drug Dev. Ind. Pharm.* 9, 1185–1225 (1983).

3. M. Rowland, Drug administration and regimens, In, *Clinical Pharmacology*, 2nd ed. (K. L. Melmon and H. F. Morrelli, eds.), Macmillan Publishing Co., Inc., New York, 1978, pp. 25–70.
4. H. G. Boxenbaum, Physiological and pharmacokinetic factors affecting performance of sustained release dosage forms, *Drug Dev. Ind. Pharm.* *8*, 1–25 (1982).
5. M. Gibaldi and D. Perrier, *Pharmacokinetics*, 2nd ed., Marcel Dekker, Inc., New York, 1982.
6. J. G. Wagner, *Fundamentals of Clinical Pharmacokinetics*. Drug Intelligence Publication, Hamilton, IL, 1975.
7. K. J. Himmelstein and R. J. Lutz, A review of the applications of physiologically based pharmacokinetic modeling. *J. Pharmacokin. Biopharm.* *7*, 127 (1979).
8. P. G. Welling and M. R. Dobrinska, Dosing considerations and bioavailability assessment of controlled drug delivery systems, In, *Sustained and Controlled Drug Delivery Systems*, 2nd ed. (J. R. Robinson and V. H. L. Lee, eds.), Marcel Dekker, Inc., New York, 1986, pp. 253–290.
9. J. C. K. Loo and S. Riegelman, New method for calculating the intrinsic absorption rate of drugs, *J. Pharm. Sci.* *57*, 918–928 (1968).
10. J. G. Wagner and E. Nelson, Kinetic analysis of blood levels and urinary excretion in absorptive phase after single doses of drug, *J. Pharm. Sci.* *53*, 1392–1403 (1964).
11. K. Yamaoka, T. Nakagawa, and T. Uno, Statistical moments in pharmacokinetics, *J. Pharmacokin. Biopharm.* *6*, 547–558 (1978).
12. S. Riegelman and P. Collier, The application of statistical moment theory to the evaluation of *in vivo* dissolution time and absorption time, *J. Pharmacokin. Biopharm.* *8*, 509–534 (1980).
13. J. G. Wagner, Linear pharmacokinetic models and vanishing exponential terms: Implication in pharmacokinetics, *J. Pharmacokin. Biopharm.* *4*, 395–425 (1976).
14. J. G. Wagner, Application of the Wagner-Nelson absorption method to the two-compartment open model, *J. Pharmacokin. Biopharm.* *2*, 469–486 (1974).
15. K. K. H. Chan and M. Gibaldi, Evaluating drug absorption after oral administration: Some problems and some solutions. *Eur. J. Clin. Pharmacol.* *26*, 255–259 (1984).
16. F. H. Dost, Uber ein einfaches statistisches Dosis-Umsatzgesetz, *Klin. Wochenschr.* *36*, 655–657 (1958).
17. D. J. Cutler, Theory of the mean absorption time, an adjunct to conventional bioavailability studies, *J. Pharm. Pharmacol.*, *30*, 476–478 (1978).
18. L. Z. Benet and R. L. Galeazzi, Noncompartmental determination of steady state volume of distribution, *J. Pharm. Sci.*, *68*, 1071–1074 (1979).

19. A. Rescigno and G. Segre, *Drug and Tracer Kinetics*, Blaisdell, Waltham, MA, 1966, pp. 161–167.
20. M. Bialer, Z. M. Look, B. M. Silber, and A. Yacobi, The relationship between drug input and mean residence time in the body, *Biopharm. Drug Dispos.*, in press.
21. M. Gibaldi, Prolonged-release medication II, *Perspect. Clin. Pharmacol. 2*, 25–27 (1984).
22. H. C. Caldwell, W. J. Westlake, R. C. Shriver, and E. E. Bumbier, Steady state lithium blood level fluctuations in man following administration of lithium carbonate conventional and controlled-release dosage form, *J. Clin. Pharmacol. 21*, 106–109 (1981).
23. F. Theeuwes and W. Bayne, Dosage form index: An objective criterion for evaluation of controlled-release drug delivery systems, *J. Pharm. Sci. 66*, 1388–1392 (1977).
24. M. Gibaldi, Prolonged-release medication I, *Perspect. Clin. Pharmacol. 2*, 17–20 (1984).
25. S. H. D. Jackson and J. M. Wright, Sustained serum theophylline concentrations during chronic twice daily administration of a slow release preparation, *Eur. J. Clin. Pharmacol. 24*, 205–208 (1983).
26. G. Levy, Kinetics of pharmacologic effects, *Clin. Pharmacol. Ther. 7*, 362–372 (1966).
27. G. Levy, Relationship between elimination rate of drugs and rate of decline of their pharmacological effects, *J. Pharm. Sci. 53*, 342–343 (1964).
28. L. B. Sheiner, D. R. Stanski, S. Vozeh, R. D. Miller, and J. Ham, Simultaneous modeling of pharmacokinetics and pharmacodynamics: Application to *d*-tubocurarine, *Clin. Pharmacol. Ther. 25*, 358–371 (1979).
29. G. Levy, Relationship between rate of elimination of tubocurarine and rate of decline of its pharmacological activity, *Br. J. Anaesth. 36*, 694–695 (1964).
30. M. Eichelbaum, P. Birkel, E. Grube, U. Gutgemann, and A. Somogyi, Effects of verapamil on P-R intervals in relation to verapamil plasma levels following single i.v. and oral administration and during chronic treatment, *Klin. Wochenschr. 58*, 919–925 (1980).
31. R. L. Galeazzi, L. Z. Benet, and L. B. Sheiner, Relationship between the pharmacokinetics and pharmacodynamics of procainamide, *Clin. Pharmacol. Ther. 20*, 278–289 (1976).
32. N. H. G. Holford, P. E. Coates, T. W. Guentert, S. Riegelman, and L. B. Sheiner, The effect of quinidine and its metabolites on the electrocardiogram and systolic time intervals: Concentration-effect relationships, *Br. J. Clin. Pharmacol. 11*, 187–195 (1981).

33. P. J. Meffin, R. A. Winkle, T. F. Blaschke, J. Fitzgerald, and D. C. Harrison, Response optimization of drug dosage: Antiarrhythmic studies with tocainide, *Clin. Pharmacol. Ther. 22*, 42–57 (1977).
34. T. Meinertz, W. Kasper, F. Kersting, H. Just, H. Bechtold, and E. Janchen, Lorcainide II. Plasma concentration-effect relationship, *Clin. Pharmacol. Ther. 26*, 187–195 (1979).
35. B. Whiting, N. H. G. Holford, and L. B. Sheiner, Quantitative analysis of the disopyramide concentration-effect relationship, *Br. J. Clin. Pharmacol. 9*, 67–75 (1980).
36. C. J. Falliers, Pharmacodynamic and spirometric responses to sustained-release theophylline capsule, *Int. J. Clin. Pharmacol. Biopharm. 17*, 125–130 (1979).
37. P. A. Mitenko and R. I. Ogilvie, Rational intravenous doses of theophylline, *N. Engl. J. Med. 289*, 600–603 (1973).
38. L. Hendeles, R. P. Iafrate, and M. Weinberger, A clinical and pharmacokinetic basis for the selection and use of slow-release theophylline products, *Clin. Pharmacokin. 9*, 95–135 (1984).
39. M. Esler, A. Zweifer, O. Randall, and V. DeQuattro, Pathophysiologic and pharmacokinetic determinants of the antihypertensive response to propranolol, *Clin. Pharmacol. Ther. 22*, 299–308 (1977).
40. B. N. Singh, F. M. Williams, R. M. Whitlock, J. Collett, and C. Chew, Plasma timolol levels and systolic time intervals, *Clin. Pharmacol. Ther. 27*, 159–166 (1980).
41. W. D. Hager, H. J. Pieniaszek, Jr., D. Perrier, M. Mayersohn, and V. Goldberger, Assessment of beta blockade with propranolol, *Clin. Pharmacol. Ther. 30*, 283–290 (1981).
42. T. Ishizaki, J. Hirayama, K. Tawara, H. Nakaya, M. Sato, and K. Sato, Pharmacokinetics and pharmacodynamics in young normal and elderly hypertensive subjects: A study using sotalol as a model drug, *J. Pharmacol. Exp. Ther. 212*, 173–181 (1980).
43. D. G. McDevitt and D. G. Shand, Plasma concentrations and the time-course of beta blockade due to propranolol, *Clin. Pharmacol. Ther. 18*, 708–713 (1975).
44. R. A. Winkle, P. J. Meffin, J. W. Fitzgerald, and D. C. Harrison, Clinical efficacy and pharmacokinetics of a new orally effective antiarrhythmic tocainide, *Circulation 54*, 884–889 (1976).
45. R. Zacest and J. Koch-Weser, Relation of propranolol plasma level to β-blockade during oral therapy, *Pharmacology 7*, 178–184 (1972).
46. B. Ablad, K. O. Borg, G. Johnsson, C. G. Regardh, and L. Solvell, Combined pharmacokinetic and pharmacodynamic studies on alprenolol and 4-hydroxy alprenolol in man, *Life Sci. 14*, 693–704 (1974).

47. R. Nagashima, R. A. O'Reilly, and G. Levy, Kinetics of pharmacologic effects in man: The anticoagulant action of warfarin, *Clin. Pharmacol. Ther. 10*, 22–35 (1969).
48. P. A. Routledge, P. H. Chapman, D. M. Davies, and M. D. Rawlins, Pharmacokinetics and pharmacodynamics of warfarin at steady-state, *Br. J. Clin. Pharmacol. 8*, 243–247 (1979).
49. L. R. Whitfield and G. Levy, Relationship between concentration and anticoagulant effect of heparin in plasma of normal subjects: Magnitude and predictability of interindividual differences, *Clin. Pharmacol. Ther. 28*, 509–516 (1980).
50. J. G. Wagner, Kinetics of pharmacologic response. I. Proposed relationships between response and drug concentration in the intact animal and man, *J. Theor. Biol. 20*, 171–201 (1968).
51. N. H. G. Holford and L. B. Sheiner, Kinetics of pharmacologic response, *Pharmacol. Ther. 16*, 143–166 (1982).
52. W. G. Kramer, A. J. Kolibash, R. P. Lewis, M. S. Bathala, J. A. Visconti, and R. H. Reuning, Pharmacokinetics of digoxin: Relationship between intensity and predicted compartmental drug levels in man, *J. Pharmacokinet. Biopharm. 1*, 47–61 (1979).
53. A. W. Kelman and B. Whiting, Modeling of drug response in individual subjects, *J. Pharmacokinet. Biopharm. 8*, 115–130 (1980).
54. A. V. Hill, The possible effects of the aggregation of the molecules of haemoglobin on its dissociation curves, *J. Physiol. (London) 40*, iv–vii (1910).
55. N. H. G. Holford and L. B. Sheiner, Pharmacokinetic and pharmacodynamic modelling *in vivo*, *Crit. Rev. Bioeng. 5*, 273–322 (1981).
56. V. F. Smolen, Theoretical and computational basis for drug bioavailability determinations using pharmacologic data, I. General considerations and procedures, *J. Pharmacokinet. Biopharm. 4*, 337–353 (1976).
57. M. J. West, M. J. Kendall, and M. Mitchard, A comparison of slow release with conventional oxprenolol: Plasma concentration and clinical effects, *Br. J. Clin. Pharmacol. 3*, 439–443 (1976).
58. J. McAnish, N. S. Baber, R. Smith, and J. Young, Pharmacokinetic and pharmacodynamic studies with long-acting propranolol, *Br. J. Clin. Pharmacol. 6*, 115–121 (1978).
59. P. B. Bottini, E. M. Caulfield, J. G. Devane, E. J. Geogheran, and D. E. Panoz, Comparative oral bioavailability of conventional propranolol tablets and a new controlled-absorption propranolol capsule, *Drug Dev. Ind. Pharm. 9*, 1475–1493 (1983).
60. G. Berner, F. Leuschner, H. H. Wagener, and A. Becker, Bioavailability of metoclopramide in a sustained release preparation, *Arzneim. Forsch./Drug Res. 34*, 637–639 (1984).

61. M. Bialer, M. Friedman, and J. Dubrovsky, Comparative pharmacokinetic analysis of novel sustained release formulation of valproic acid in dogs, *Drug Dispos.* 5, 1–10, (1984).
62. J. P. Devissaguet, S. Garbarg, M. Prost, and Y. Bogaievsky, Comparative pharmacokinetic study of two dosage forms of 5 mg trihexyphenidyl tablets (Artane) and sustained release capsules (Parkinane retard), *Therapie*, 39, 231–236 (1984).
63. G. A. Hart, Aspects of the pharmacokinetics of slow-release lithium carbonate, *S. Afr. Med. J.* 66, 178–179 (1984).
64. R. A. Upton, J. F. Theircelin, T. W. Guentert, L. Sansom, J. R. Powell, P. E. Coates, and S. Riegelman, Evaluation of the absorption from some commercial sustained release theophylline products, *J. Pharmacokinet. Biopharm.* 8, 149–151 (1980).
65. G. W. Houghton, M. J. Dennis, E. D. Rigler, and R. L. Parsons, Comparative pharmacokinetics of ketoprofen derived from single oral doses of ketoprofen capsules or a novel sustained release pellet formulation, *Biopharm. Drug Dispos.* 5, 203–209 (1984).
66. K. L. Liem and J. M. R. Hollander, Maintenance therapy after i.v. administration of disopyramide with an oral sustained release preparation, a pharmacokinetic study, *Br. J. Clin. Pharmacol.* 18, 226–228 (1984).
67. J. H. Gustafson, L. Weissman, R. E. Weinfeld, A. A. Holazo, K. C. Khoo, and S. A. Kaplan, Clinical biavailability evaluation of a controlled release formulation of diazepam, *J. Pharmacokin. Biopharm.* 9, 679–691 (1981).
68. J. C. V. Loo, N. Jordan, C. Charette, R. Brien, and I. J. McGilvery, Pharmacokinetic evaluation of a conventional and controlled release product of betamethasone, *Biopharm. Drug Dispos.* 5, 97–100 (1984).
69. L. Nyberg and B. M. Kennedy, Pharmacokinetics of terbutaline given in slow-release tablets, *Eur. J. Respir. Dis. C Suppl.* 134, 119–169 (1984).
70. E. Perucca, R. Grimaldi, G. Gatti, M. Caravaggi, F. Crema, S. Lecchini, and G. M. Frigo, Pharmacokinetics and pharmacodynamic studies with a new controlled-release formulation of propranolol in normal volunteers: A comparison with other commercially available formulations, *Br. J. Clin. Pharmacol.* 18, 37–43 (1984).
71. M. Vater, G. Smith, G. W. Aherne, and A. R. Aitkenhead, Pharmacokinetics and analgesic effect of slow-release oral morphine sulfate in volunteers, *Br. J. Anaesth*, 56, 821–827 (1984).
72. C. G. Wilson, G. D. Parr, J. W. Kennerley, M. J. Taylor, S. S. Davis, J. G. Hardy, and J. A. Rees, Pharmacokinetics and *in vivo* scintigraphic monitoring of a sustained release acetylsalicylic acid formulation, *Int. J. Pharm.* 18, 1–8 (1984).

73. G. Ayanoglu, P. U. Witte, and M. Badian, Bioavailability and pharmacodynamics of a sustained release glibenclamide product (Deroctyl) in comparison to a standard tablet formulation (Euglucon, Daonil), *Int. J. Clin. Pharmacol. Ther. Toxicol. 21*, 479–482 (1986).
74. L. F. Chasseaud, E. Doyle, T. Taylor, A. Darragh, and R. F. Lambe, Bioavailability of isosorbide dinitrate and its two mononitrate metabolites from sustained release formulations, *Int. J. Clin. Pharmacol. Ther. Toxicol. 21*, 514–518 (1983).
75. L. F. Chasseaud, T. Taylor, R. M. Major, I. W. Taylor, and V. Luckow, Pharmacokinetics of ^{14}C-isosorbide dinitrate after different sustained release formulations, *Arnzneim. Forsch./Drug Res. 33*, 1298–1301 (1983).
76. U. Dahlstorm, C. Graffner, G. Johnsson, K. J. Hoffman, E. Karlsson, and P. O. Lagerstrom, Pharmacokinetics of prenalterol after single and multiple administration of controlled-release tablets to patients with congestive heart failure, *Eur. J. Clin. Pharmacol. 24*, 495–502 (1983).
77. A. Ebihara, K. Tawara, and T. Oka, Pharmacodynamic and pharmacokinetic study of a slow-release formulation of furosemide in man, *Arzneim. Forsch./Drug Res. 33*, 163–167 (1983).
78. B. Flouvat, F. Fodor, A. Roux, and J. R. Bianchine, Pharmacokinetics of a sustained release trimazosin tablet formulation, *Am. Heart J. 106*, 1228–1234 (1983).
79. W. H. Helfand and B. L. Pejouan, New indomethacin pharmaceuticals. Pharmacokinetic profile of an oral osmotic controlled-release form, *Ann. Pharm. Fr. 41*, 401–408 (1983).
80. P. Karttunen, M. Uusitupa, and U. Lamminsivu, The pharmacokinetics of metformin: a comparison of the properties of a rapid-release and a sustained-release preparation, *Int. J. Clin. Pharmacol. Ther. Toxicol. 21*, 31–36 (1983).
81. V. W. Steinijans, K. Zech, and R. Fischer, Comparison of aminophylline and theophylline sustained release formulations by their bioavailability and steady-state serum levels, *Int. J. Clin. Pharmacol. Ther. Toxicol. 21*, 624–630 (1983).
82. Y. Santoni, R. Bruno, M. Fornaris, A. Egre, T. Danays, and J. P. Cano, Pharmacokinetics and relative bioavailability of a new oral sustained-release form of mexiletine in healthy subjects, *Therapie 38*, 341–344 (1983).
83. W. V. Taggart and W. Holyoak, Steady state bioavailability of two sustained release quinidine preparations: Quinidine gluconate versus quinidine sulfate, *Clin. Ther. 5*, 357–364 (1983).
84. P. H. Vlasses, M. L. Rocci, K. A. Porrini, A. J. Greenspan, and R. K. Ferguson, Immediate release and sustained release procainamide: Bioavailability at steady state in cardiac patients, *Ann. Intern. Med. 98*, 613–614 (1983).

85. K. R. H. Adams, L. D. C. Halliday, R. G. Sibeon, N. Baber, T. Littler, and M. L'E. Orme, Clinical and pharmacokinetic study of indomethacin in standard and slow-release formulations, *Br. J. Clin. Pharmacol. 14*, 286–289 (1982).
86. P. W. Trembath and S. W. Boobis, Pharmacokinetics of a sustained release theophylline formulation, *Br. J. Clin. Pharmacol. 9*, 365–369 (1980).
87. R. J. Erb, Bioavailability of controlled-release buccal and oral nitroglycerin by digital plethysmography, *Adv. Pharmacother. 1*, 35–43 (1982).
88. R. J. Will and W. A. Colburn, Multiple-dose pharmacokinetics of diazepam once-daily administration of a controlled-release capsule, *Ther. Drug Monit.* 5, 423–426 (1983).
89. J. G. Perkins, R. Bressler, D. Heatherington, A. Cato, and J. Dickerson, Bioavailability and safety study comparing actifed-sustained action (SA) capsules to Actifed immediate release (IR) tablets, *Curr. Ther. Res. Clin. Exp. 28*, 650–668 (1980).
90. W. Suess and M. Kuntze, Investigations on release and bioavailability of fluoride tablets with sustained drug release, *Zentralbl. Pharm. Pharmakother. Labor. 119*, 511–514 (1980).
91. W. Suess and B. Haaser, Investigation on release and bioavailability of potassium preparations, *Zentralbl. Pharm. Pharmakother. Labor. 119*, 503–506 (1980).
92. C. P. Charmaine, M. J. Kendall, and P. G. Welling, Bioavailability of conventional slow-release oxprenolol in fasted and non-fasted individuals, *Br. J. Clin. Pharmacol. 7*, 299–302 (1979).
93. R. Groning, Study of the bioavailability of nitrofurantoin. Part 3. Comparative evaluation of commercial sustained release drug forms, *Dtsch. Apoth. Ztg. 119*, 983–985 (1979).
94. C. P. Quaterman, M. J. Kendall, and P. G. Welling, Plasma levels and negative chronotropic effect of metoprolol following single doses of a conventional and sustained release formulation, *Eur. J. Clin. Pharmacol. 15*, 97–103 (1979).
95. P. L. Sharma and R. M. Sharma, Comparative bioavailability of sustained-release and conventional tablets of hydroxyethyltheophylline in man, *Int. J. Clin. Pharmacol. Biopharm. 17*, 394–396 (1979).
96. W. Erking, P. W. Luecker, G. Metz, M. Specker, and K. Wetzelsberger, Relative bioavailability of vincamine slow-release formulation. Pharmacokinetic study in normal subjects, *Arzneim. Forsch./Drug Res. 28*, 2332–2336 (1978).
97. B. Y. Lee, H. Sakamoto, F. Trainor, G. Brody, and Y. W. Cho, Comparison of soft gelatine capsule versus sustained release formulation of papaverine hydrochloride: vasodilation and plasma levels, *Int. J. Clin. Pharmacol. Biopharm. 16*, 32–39 (1978).

98. C. D. Steuart, Brompheniramine bioavailability from two oral sustained-release nasal decongestant formulations with identical active drugs but with different release systems, *Curr. Ther. Res. 24*, 960–966 (1978).
99. D. P. Thornhill, Pharmacokinetics of ordinary and sustained release lithium carbonate in manic patients after acute dosage, *Eur. J. Clin Pharmacol. 14*, 267–271 (1978).
100. W. J. Tilstone, D. H. Lawson, W. Campbell, I. Hutton, and T. D. Lawrie, The pharmacokinetics of slow-release procainamide, *Eur. J. Clin. Pharmacol. 14*, 261–265 (1978).
101. A. Joergensen, Comparative bioavailability of a sustained release preparation of amitriptyline and conventional tablets, *Eur. J. Clin. Pharmacol. 12*, 187–190 (1977).
102. K. J. Simons, E. R. Simons, and E. W. Bierman, Bioavailability of a sustained release dyphylline formulation, *J. Clin. Pharmacol. 17*, 237–242 (1977).
103. C. Graffner, G. Johnsson, and J. Sjogren, Comparative absorption and pharmacokinetic studies on proxyphylline in ordinary and slow-release tablets, *Acta. Pharm. Suec. 11*, 125–132 (1974).
104. K. A. Javaid and C. W. Hartman, Blood levels of sulfamethizole in dogs following administration of time-release tablets employing lipase-lipid-drug systems, *J. Pharm. Sci. 61*, 900–902 (1972).
105. B. Muehlenbruch, H. Strauss, and H. Glaubitz, Studies on the bioavailability of resinates as oral sustained release drug dosage forms. Part I. Pharmaceutical availability of dihydrocodeine resinates, *Pharmazie 37*, 200–203 (1982).
106. S. N. Rasmussen, S. Bondesen, E-F. Hvidberg, S-H. Hassen, V. Binder, S. Halskov, and H. Flachs, 5-aminosalicylic acid in a slow-release preparation: bioavailability, plasma level, and excretion in humans, *Gastroenterology 83*, 1062–1070 (1982).
107. R. J. Sawchuk, S. M. Pepin, I. E. Leppik, and R. J. Gumnit, Rapid and slow-release phenytoin in epileptic patients at steady-state: Assessment of relative bioavailability utilizing Michaelis-Menten parameters, *J. Pharmacokinet. Biopharm. 10*, 383–391 (1982).
108. W. E. Barrett, J. J. Hanigan, and D. L. Snyder, The bioavailability of sustained release tablets which contain phenylpropanolamine and chlorpheniramine, *Curr. Ther. Res. 30*, 640–654 (1981).
109. J. Bourgouin, M. A. Gagnon, R. Elie, D. Dvornik, R. Gonzalez, and M. Kraml, Butriptyline: Human pharmacokinetics and comparative bioavailability of conventional and sustained release formulations, *Biopharm. Drug. Dispos. 2*, 123–130 (1981).

110. R. C. Browning, V. A. John, R. J. L. Till, and W. Theobald, A pharmacokinetic comparison between different slow-release formulations of Metoprolol (Lopresor, SR and Betaloc SA), *Br. J. Clin. Pharmacol. 12*, 600–602 (1981).
111. F. Chanoine, W. Rovei, and M. Strolin Benedetti, Pharmacokinetics of heptaminol in man. Bioavailability of sustained release tablet, *C. R. Cong. Eur. Biopharm. Pharmacokinet. 1*, 125–133 (1981).
112. M. J. Kendall, L. Lambert, C. P. Quarterman, and V. A. John, Pharmacokinetic and pharmacodynamic assessment of a combined slow-release metoprolol-chlorthalidone preparation, *J. Clin. Hosp. Pharm. 6*, 259–265 (1981).
113. H. Ledermann and B. Kaufmann, Comparative pharmacokinetics of 400 mg bezafibrate after a single oral administration of a new slow-release preparation and the currently available commercial form, *J. Int. Med. Res. 9*, 516–520 (1981).
114. J. Marinow, W. Akpan, H. Ledermann, and U. Abshagen, Comparative studies of the pharmacokinetics and pharmacodynamics of metipranalol and slow-release metipranolol in healthy volunteers, *Herz/Kreislauf. 13*, 548–554 (1981).
115. W. A. Ritschel and K. A. Hoffman, Pilot study on bioavailability of coumarin and 7-hydroxycoumarin upon peroral administration of coumarin in a sustained release dosage form, *J. Clin. Pharmacol. 21*, 294–300 (1981).
116. A. Yacobi, R. G. Stoll, G. C. Chao, J. E. Carter, D. M. Baaske, B. L. Kamath, A. N. Amann, and C. M. Lai, Evaluation of sustained-action chloropheniramine-pseudophedrine dosage form in humans, *J. Pharm. Sci. 69*, 1077–1081 (1980).
117. J. J. Vallner, J. A. Kotzan, J. T. Stewart, W. J. Brown, I. L. Honigberg, T. E. Needham, and S. V. Dighe, Blood levels following multiple oral dosing of chlorpheniramine conventional and controlled-release preparations, *Biopharm. Drug Dispos. 3*, 95–104 (1982).
118. S. K. Baveja, K. V. Ranga Rao, and A. Singh, Sustained release tablet formulation of diethylcarbamazine, *Int. J. Pharm. 19*, 229–231 (1984).
119. C. Sama, A. M. Morselli Labate, C. Chiodarelli, A. Roda, M. Briganti, and E. Roda, Bioavailability of a delayed-release preparation of urodeoxycholic acid in man, *Curr. Ther. Res. 33*, 558–564 (1983).
120. R. H. Reuning, S. H. T. Liao, A. E. Staubus, S. B. Aschcraft, D. A. Downs, D. E. Harrigan, J. N. Wiley, and D. L. Wise, Pharmacokinetic quantitation of naltrexone controlled-release from a copolymer delivery system, *J. Pharmacokinet. Biopharm. 11*, 369–387 (1983).

121. A. A. Mishriki and D. J. Weidler, Long acting propranolol (Inderal LA); pharmacokinetic, pharmacodynamics and therapeutic use. *Pharmacotherapy 3*, 334–341 (1983).
122. M. Gibaldi and P. J. McNamara, Steady-state concentrations of drugs with short half-lives when administered in oral-sustained release drug formulations, *Int. J. Pharm. 2*, 167–172 (1979).

6

Dosing Considerations and Bioavailability Assessment of Controlled Drug Delivery Systems

PETER G. WELLING / Warner-Lambert/Parke-Davis Research Division, Ann Arbor, Michigan

MICHAEL R. DOBRINSKA / Merck Sharp & Dohme Research Laboratories, West Point, Pennsylvania

I. INTRODUCTION

The success of sustained or controlled release systems for a number of agents has provided unprecedented impetus for this dosage form. With ever improving techniques and methodologies, and with ever increasing pressure to find novel and clinically viable dosage forms for new and old drugs, it has become almost mandatory to examine this dosage form for practically every drug in pharmaceutical research and development.

Despite the extraordinary proliferation of this dosage form, regulatory authorities have exercised great caution in suggesting guidelines for their standardization and testing. This is understandable when one considers the inherent problems of making a successful controlled release dosage form, and possibly even greater problems of their standardization.

Although great clinical advantages are claimed, and sometimes realized, for controlled release drug products, and great advances have been made in pharmacokinetics during the past two decades, most sustained or controlled release formulations are prepared on an empirical basis. While exceptions to this generalization exist, as exemplified by the work of Theeuwes and associates [1], there are few examples in the literature of controlled release dosage form design based on accepted pharmacokinetic, as well as physical and chemical, principles.

There are a number of possible reasons for this. One may be that of inadequate communication between formulator and pharmacokineticist, especially when their respective development time-frames do not coincide. Another may be the difficulty in establishing a relationship between *in vitro* and *in vivo* data, and this will be discussed in greater length later. The third reason may be the unpredictable performance of oral controlled release systems under different dietary conditions, thereby rendering accurate pharmacokinetic prediction difficult. The fourth reason, again pertinent for oral controlled release systems, is the capricious and often unpredictable absorption characteristics in different regions of the GI tract. Despite these factors, it is unfortunate that more use is not made of a now rather sophisticated science to provide working estimates at least, and to provide precise and predictable characteristics at best, of a controlled release dosage form.

The objectives of this chapter are to discuss in a qualitative sense some of the advantages and disadvantages of controlled release formulations, to consider some of the contentious issues regarding the feasibility for controlled release systems for certain drugs, some *in vitro* and *in vivo* aspects and models, and also to provide some comments on bioavailability testing. Attention will focus primarily on oral dosage forms.

II. ADVANTAGES OF CONTROLLED RELEASE DOSAGE FORMS

The importance of controlled release dosage forms is illustrated by the list of representative compounds, separated into major therapeutic areas, in Table 1. As noted previously [2], it is interesting that so much attention has focused on diuretic, cardiovascular, CNS, and respiratory drugs, and so little attention on antimicrobial agents. To our knowledge tetracycline is the only antibiotic that is currently available in sustained release form, which is marketed in Europe as Tetrabid[R]. The major reason for lack of attention in this area is possibly the size of the conventional dose, making a controlled release dosage prohibitively large. However, this is not the case with all antimicrobials. Many agents are given at conventional doses of 150 mg or less, and are thus potential candidates for controlled release dosing. Provided that it is desirable to obtain antimicrobial levels above a certain minimum concentration for as long a period as possible for optimum therapy, there is no more reason not to produce a controlled release dosage form for this class of drugs than any other.

As controlled release dosages are often more expensive than conventional formulations, they cannot be justified unless they offer some clinical or practical advantages. Some advantages are: (a) reduction in dosing frequency, (b) reduced fluctuation in circulating drug levels, (c) increased patient compliance, (d) avoidance of night time dosing, (e) more uniform effect, and (f) reduction in GI irritation and other dose-related side effects. The ideal controlled release dosage form will offer all of these advantages. Clearly, justification is directly related to the number and extent of the advantages compared to cost. The second and third advantages are concerned with circulating drug levels, which influence many of the other possible advantages and may be predicted from pharmacokinetic principles. The fifth advantage, achieving a more uniform pharmacological response, is one of the major goals of controlled release dosing. However, there is little documentation to support this claim and, for the most part, improved pharmacological profiles of controlled release dosage forms have to be implied from blood concentration data.

Table 1 Some Substances Available in Controlled Release Form

Vitamins, minerals, and hormones
Ascorbic acid
Iron preparations
Methyltestosterone
Nicotinic acid

Table 1 (Continued)

[Vitamins, minerals, and hormones]

- Potassium
- Pyridoxine
- Vitamin combinations

Diuretic and cardiovascular drugs

- Acetazolamide
- Ethaverine HCl
- Isosorbide dinitrate
- Nicotinyl alcohol
- Nitroglycerin
- Papaverine HCl
- Pentaerythritol tetranitrate
- Procainamide
- Quinidine gluconate and sulfate
- Reserpine

CNS drugs

- Amphetamine sulfate
- Aspirin
- Caffeine
- Chlorpromazine
- Dextroamphetamine sulfate
- Diazepam
- Diethylpropion HCl
- Fluphenazine
- Indomethacin
- Lithium
- Meprobamate
- Methamphetamine HCl
- Orphenadrine citrate
- Pentobarbital
- Pentylenetetrazole
- Perphenazine
- Phenmetrazine HCl
- Phenobarbital
- Phentermine HCl
- Prochlorperazine

Respiratory agents

- Aminophylline
- Brompheniramine maleate
- Carbinoxamine maleate

Table 1 (Continued)

[Respiratory agents]
Chlorpheniramine maleate
Combination, antitussive
Combination, expectorant
Combination, upper respiratory
Dexchlorpheniramine maleate
Dimethindene maleate
Dyphenylpraline HC1
Dyphylline
Phenylpropanolamine HC1
Psuedoephedrine HC1 and sulfate
Theophylline
Trimeprazine
Tripelennamine HC1
Xanthine combinations
Antimicrobial
Tetracycline
Gastrointestinal drugs
Belladonna alkaloids
Hexocyclium methylsulfate
Hyoscyamine sulfate
Isopropamide iodide
Prochlorperazine maleate
Tridihexethyl chloride
Other
Pyrodostigmine bromide

Source: Reproduced by permission from Ref. 2.

III. DISADVANTAGES OF CONTROLLED RELEASE DOSAGE FORMS

Controlled release dosage forms have several potential disadvantages. They include cost, unpredictable and often poor *in vitro–in vivo* correlations, dose dumping, reduced potential for dosage adjustment, and increased potential for first-pass clearance and also of poor systemic availability in general. For oral dosage forms there is the additional disadvantage that the effective drug release period is influenced and limited by GI residence time.

The high cost of sustained release dosage forms must again be taken into account when the advantages and disadvantages of a particular drug formulation are being considered. *In vitro–in vivo* correlations for conventional dosage forms are often poor, and this problem has occupied the minds of many for a long time. For controlled release dosages, in which the rate of release is deliberately reduced to achieve drug release over a greater region of the GI tract with potential reduction in systemic availability, there is no reason to suspect that *in vitro–in vivo* correlations would not be worse.

Dose dumping is a phenomenon whereby the relatively large quantity of medication in a controlled release formulation is rapidly released, introducing potentially toxic quantities of drug into the systemic circulation. This has been reported for a bronchodilator [3]. However, dose dumping should not be a problem with good manufacturing practice and the types of rigid controls that have become standard in industry. For the same reason, it is also prudent to indicate in product labeling relevant statements concerning alteration of the dosage form by the patient prior to its ingestion (e.g., chewing or grinding and dispersing in food or liquids).

Reduced potential for dosage adjustment is a major disadvantage of some controlled release products, and this should be considered when preparing controlled release formulations for drugs that are available in a variety of strengths in conventional dosages. The controlled release formulation should also be available in a variety of strengths or in a form that can easily be subdivided without losing controlled release properties.

Hepatic metabolism is a saturable process. Saturable elimination has been reported for only a small number of drugs following intravenous administration, including alcohol, phenytoin, carbamazepine, valproate, theophylline, and probenecid. These observations have been based on drug/concentration dependent elimination rates. The small number of drugs that have exhibited this phenomenon indicates that most drugs do not achieve drug levels that saturate hepatic metabolizing enzymes at therapeutic dose levels. After oral dosing, on the other hand, drug reaches the liver via the portal vein at far greater concentrations than normally observed in the systemic circulation. In fact, the levels may be high enough to exceed the capacity of the hepatic metabolizing enzymes. Thus, the higher the oral dose the greater the possibility of saturating hepatic drug metabolizing enzymes. Conversely, the smaller the dose, or the slower the dose is released from the formulation, the smaller the possibility of saturating first pass metabolism. The potential for reduced drug availability due to first-pass metabolism is therefore greater with controlled or sustained release formulations than with conventional dosages.

Reduced drug absorption is an intrinsic hazard with all controlled release dosage forms. Apart from the obvious limitation of GI residence time, a controlled release formulation is likely to cause a fraction of administered drug to be released in regions of the GI tract that are distal to the optimum absorptive region of the small intestine. The so called "absorption window" becomes important, and may give rise to unsatisfactory drug absorption *in vivo* despite excellent release characteristics *in vitro*. There is generally poor agreement in estimates of effective GI residence time for drug absorption. This may vary for different drugs and formulations depending on (a) absorption efficiency in distal regions of the intestine and (b) susceptibility of the drug or dosage form to intestinal bacterial degradation.

The transit time of a dosage form through the gastrointestinal tract depends not only on the physical characteristics of the formulation but also on physiological factors [4–6]. Stomach emptying is perhaps the single most important factor controlling the overall transit time. Following food intake, the stomach enters the 'fed mode' in which liquids and digested material are readily emptied but solid materials are selectively retained until particle size is reduced to about 2 mm in diameter [7]. When digestion is complete, the stomach enters the 'fasting mode' in which intense contractions (part of the interdigestive myoelectric complex or housekeeper) recur briefly in a 2-hr cycle and result in complete emptying of any residual or indigestible material from the stomach [5]. Hence, gastric residence time of a slowly-eroding or nondisintegrating dosage form may differ substantially between fed and fasting modes. Gastric residence times of such formulations also appear to increase as the caloric content of the ingested meal increases; times reported for an osmotic delivery device, for instance, range from about 10 hr when given after a heavy breakfast to as little as 0.5 hr after a very light meal [8,10]. Notwithstanding direct effects of food on the absorption process, administration of sustained-release dosage forms with food therefore has the potential for increasing the duration and extent of absorption of a drug, particularly if the optimum absorption region is in the small intestine. Hence, bioavailability studies should be conducted under both fasting and nonfasting conditions.

IV. COMPOUNDS THAT ARE UNSUITABLE FOR CONTROLLED RELEASE

Some characteristics that may make a drug a poor candidate for controlled release dosing are given in Table 2. For drugs with an elimination half-life of less than two hours, as well as those that are administered in large doses, a controlled release dosage form may contain a prohibitively large quantity of drug. On the other hand, drugs with elimination half-lives of 8 hr or more are sufficiently sustained in the body from conventional doses, and controlled release is generally not necessary. Dose dumping of a very potent drug or of a compound with a narrow therapeutic index may give rise to very high circulating drug levels, with possibly disastrous consequences.

Absorption of poorly water-soluble drugs is often dissolution rate-limited. Incorporating such compounds into controlled release formulations is therefore unrealistic and may reduce overall absorption efficiency. Administering drugs like warfarin, whose pharmacological effect is delayed relative to its blood profile, offers no clinical advantage. Similarly, incorporating drugs such as fluorouracil, and perhaps some beta lactam antibiotics and thiazide diuretics that appear to exhibit an "absorption window" may reduce absorption efficiency. Problems of first-pass hepatic clearance of sustained-release drugs has been discussed.

While the above comments may provide useful guidelines for decision making regarding the feasibility of controlled release dosage forms, they may not apply in specific situations. For instance, many of the drugs in Table 1 have very short elimination half-lives, while others have half-lives greater than 8 hr.

The best example of the former is nitroglycerin. The present consensus is that nitroglycerin has a short biological half-life of

Table 2 Characteristics That May Make a Drug Unsuitable for Controlled Release Dosing

1. Short elimination half-life
2. Long elimination half-life
3. Narrow therapeutic index
4. Large doses
5. Poor absorption
6. Active absorption
7. Low or slow solubility
8. Time course of circulating drug levels different to that of pharmacological effect
9. Extensive first-pass clearance

Table 3 Some Categories of Oral Controlled Release Dosage Forms

Category	Product	Active Ingredient
Slow erosion with initial fast release dose	Tedral SA	Theophylline, ephedrine HCl, phenobarbital
Erosion core only	Tenuate Dospan	Diethylpropion HCl
Repeat action tablets	Chlor-Trimeton	Pseudoephedrine sulfate, chlorpheniramine maleate
Pellets in capsules	Combid	Isopropamide iodide, prochlorperazine maleate
Pellets in tablets	Theo-dur	Theophylline
Leaching	Desbutal Gradumet	Methamphetamine HCl, pentobarbital sodium
Ion-exchange resins	Biphetamine	Amphetamine, dextroamphetamine
Complexation	Rynatan	Chlorpheniramine, phenylephrine, and pyrilamine tannates
Microencapsulation	Nitrospan	Nitroglycerin
Flotation-diffusion	Valrelease	Diazepam
Osmotic delivery	Acutrim	Phenylpropanolamine HCl

about 10 min and that it undergoes considerable first-pass hepatic metabolism. Nitroglycerin is therefore given by the buccal route for treatment of angina pain. Bucally administered drug avoids first-pass metabolism and ensures rapid availability of active drug to the circulation. There are thus two excellent reasons why nitroglycerin should not be given in a controlled release dosage forms and particularly not by the oral route. However, most of the dosage forms of nitroglycerin are controlled release in nature and both oral and transdermal routes are used. The reason for this apparent anomaly lies in the indication for this drug. Buccal administration is used to provide high circulating levels of nitroglcycerin to relieve acute pain of angina, while controlled release is used as prophylaxis. It is claimed that with oral doses sufficient compound escapes first-pass metabolism to provide adequate circulating drug levels to prevent angina. Transdermal dosing is claimed to provide the additional advantage of not only delivering drug slowly but also avoiding first-pass hepatic metabolism. These various claims are under regulatory review.

Controlled release of drugs that have long biological half-lives is difficult to rationalize. The most plausible reason is that by reducing the absorption rate it is possible to prevent the occurrence of high peak drug levels shortly after dosing. This may be important for drugs that have a narrow therapeutic index, but is less important for drugs that exhibit a relatively flat dose-response profile. The current active interest in controlled drug release, together with improved technology, has given rise to a rush of new formulations. Examples of well established and also more novel oral dosage forms are summarized in Table 3. Undoubtedly, this list will increase further as more novel dosage forms are introduced. Microencapsulation and osmotic pressure systems will likely find more applications. Other products that prolong GI residence time, either by means of adhesion or by the use of low density hydrated gels have been introduced (Susadrin®, Valrelease®). These types of dosage forms may undergo extensive development in the future.

V. *IN VITRO* CONSIDERATIONS

Despite the large variety of formulations devoted to oral controlled drug release, and also the varied physical properties that influence drug release from these formulations, the number of kinetic models necessary to describe overall drug release is relatively small. The four major release patterns are illustrated in Figure 1.

The release patterns can be divided into those that release drug at a slow zero- or first order-rate and those that provide an initial rapid dose, followed by slow zero- or first-order release of sustained component. Formulations that release drug at a slow first-order or zero-order rate are more common than those containing a fast-release component. Arguments presented later in this chapter will show that this is appropriate from a pharmacokinetic viewpoint.

The sustained nature of drug release from these dosage forms presents problems in the development of *in vitro* dissolution standards. Dissolution is now accepted as an *in vitro* standard for drug release from conventional dosage forms. The use of such tests to determine drug product bioavailability or bioequivalence has been advocated by the United States Food and Drug Administration [11]. While dissolution rate has proven to be an excellent criterion for product uniformity, it has been less successful in predicting product bioavailability [12–14].

For conventional oral drug products, *in vitro* dissolution criteria are based on the fastest possible dissolution rate. The situation is

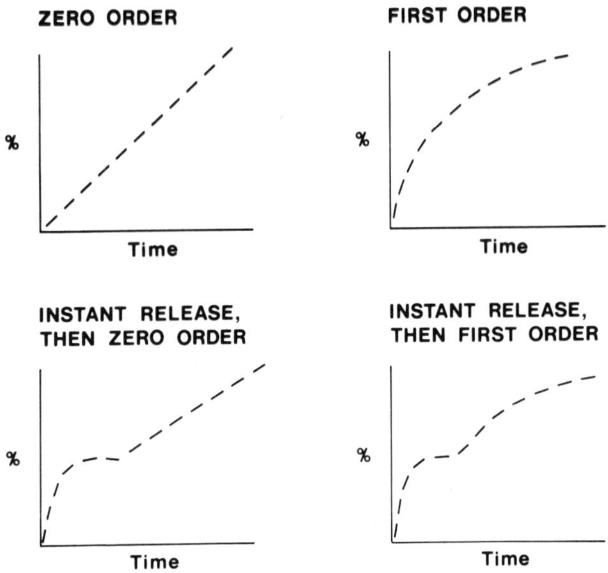

Fig. 1 Drug release characteristics from oral controlled release formulations. (Reproduced by permission from Ref. 2.)

quite different, however, for controlled release products for which the optimum dissolution rate is not the fastest that can be obtained, but rather an intermediate value that will hopefully result in prolonged release of drug *in vivo*. Thus for these products a dissolution windows is required, and deviation from the optimum rate can be in terms of being too fast or too slow.

Given (a) the enormous variety of formulations that are currently available, (b) the different release patterns indicated in Figure 1, and (c) the rapid development of other novel drug release forms such as the osmotic pump, adhesion formulations, and hydrated gels, it is not surprising that there are currently limited compendial (USP XXI, 1985) guidelines for *in vitro* dissolution tests for controlled release products. Also due to the relatively poor correlations that are generally observed between *in vitro* and *in vivo* characteristics, bioavailability and bioequivalence determinations must currently be carried out *in vivo*.

VI. *IN VIVO* CONSIDERATIONS

In this section, attention will focus on the pharmacokinetics associated with the four release patterns shown in Figure 1, the blood-level profiles that may be achieved from these dosage forms, and how these profiles may be influenced by GI transit time.

Drugs may obey single- or multi-compartment pharmacokinetic models depending on their affinity for various body tissues. Multi-compartment characteristics are more readily identified after rapid drug administration compared to slow administration as the distribution phase is not obscured by absorption processes. Slow absorption of drugs from controlled release formulations generally precludes description of resulting drug profiles by kinetic models more complex than the simple one-compartment model. That approach will be used here. For ease of presentation the following simplifying assumptions are made: (a) drug absorption, metabolism, and excretion are first-order processes, (b) drug absorption and elimination are irreversible, (c) drug that is released into the GI tract is completely absorbed in its unchanged form, and (d) drug release from the sustained release formulation is rate-limiting in the absorption process.

The model is shown in Scheme I [15].* In this scheme, D_s denotes slowly released drug, D_i denotes instantaneously released

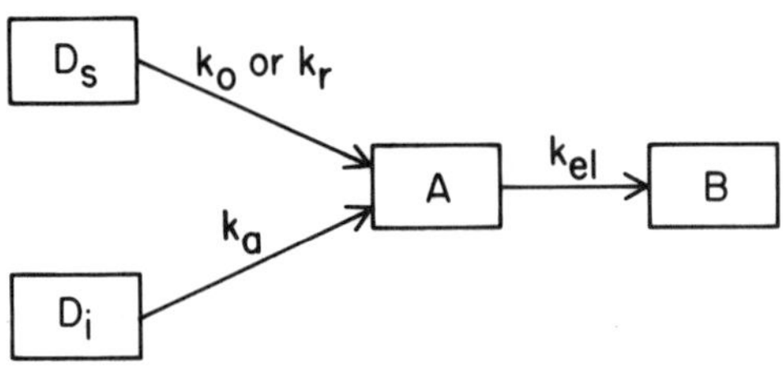

Scheme I

drug, A denotes unchanged drug in the body, B denotes cumulative amount of drug excreted in urine or metabolized, k_a is a first-order rate constant for drug transfer from the absorption site into the systemic circulation, k_o and k_r are zero-order (k_o) or first-order (k_r) rate constants for release of drug from D_s, respectively, and k_{el} is a first-order rate constant for elimination of drug by combined urinary excretion, metabolism, etc.

---

*In the original model an additional absorption step was incorporated for the slowly released component D_s. However, as k_o or k_r are generally significantly smaller than k_a, deletion of that step does not significantly affect resulting drug profiles [15].

A. First-Order Release

1. *Single Dose*

The amount of drug in the body following a single dose is given by Eq. (1), in which k_r is the rate constant governing absorption ($k_r << k_a$).

$$A = \frac{D_s k_r}{k_r - k_{el}} \left[e^{-k_{el}t} - e^{-k_r t} \right] \tag{1}$$

Eq. (1) can be converted to describe drug concentration, C, by adding the distribution volume, V, to the denominator, as in Eq. (2).

$$C = \frac{D_s k_r}{V(k_r - k_{el})} \left[e^{-k_{el}t} - e^{-k_r t} \right] \tag{2}$$

With this model, drug profiles can be influenced by the absorption and elimination rate constants, as shown in Figures 2 and 3, respectively. From Figure 3, the drug profile is markedly influenced by its biological half-life ($t_{1/2} = \ln 2/k_{el}$). The peak level, A_{max}, and time of peak level, T_{max}, both increase as the half-life increases. The curves generated with $k_{el} = 0.3\ hr^{-1}$ and $0.5\ hr^{-1}$ have the same elimination slopes with values of $0.2\ hr^{-1}$. This is an example of the "flip-flop" model, where $k_{el} > k_r$ [16] and where the apparent elimination slope is controlled by the rate at which drug is released from the formulation. This is a common situation with controlled release formulations.

From Figure 2, for a given value of k_{el}, drug profiles are lowered and more prolonged as k_r is reduced. In this case, A_{max} is reduced while T_{max} is prolonged as the drug release rate constant is reduced.

Reduction in the value of A_{max} (or C_{max}) in controlled release products is of concern, particularly for drugs that have a well defined minimum effective concentration in the body. The controlled release dose, D_s, that is necessary in order to achieve the same A_{max} as its fast release counterpart can be calculated by Eq. (3) [15]. For a drug with an elimination $t_{1/2}$ of four hr ($k_{el} = 0.17$

$$\frac{D_s}{D_i} = \left(\frac{k_a}{k_{el}}\right)^{\left(\frac{k_{el}}{k_{el} - k_a}\right)} \cdot \left(\frac{k_r}{k_{el}}\right)^{\left(\frac{k_{el}}{k_r - k_{el}}\right)} \tag{3}$$

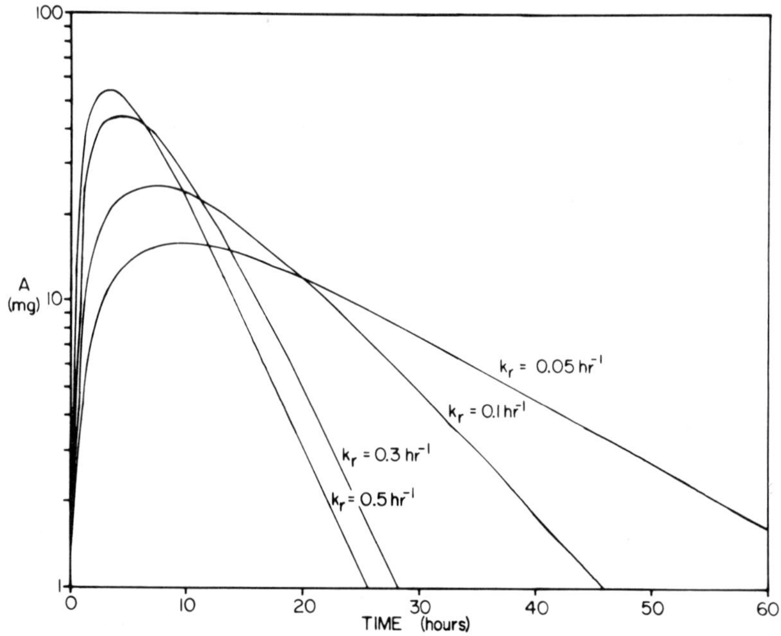

Fig. 2 Drug levels following a single dose. Curves generated from Eq. (1) with D_s = 100 mg, k_{el} = 0.2 hr^{-1}, and k_r = 0.05, 0.1, 0.3, and 0.5 hr^{-1}. (Reproduced by permission from Ref. 15.)

hr^{-1}) and a k_a of 1.0 hr^{-1} and a controlled release rate constant k_r of 0.5 hr^{-1} (release $t_{1/2}$ = 1.4 hr), a controlled release dose would have to be 1.2 times greater than the fast release dose to achieve the same A_{max}. If k_r were reduced further to 0.2 hr^{-1} (release $t_{1/2}$ = 3.5 hr), then the controlled release dose would have to be 1.8 times the fast release dose. A k_r of 0.1 hr^{-1}, which is practical only in cases of prolonged GI residence time, would require a 2.5-fold dose increase.

2. *Repeated Dose*

The same rules govern drug accumulation following repeated doses of both controlled release and conventional dosage forms. Provided the dosage interval τ is less than the time taken for all drug to be cleared from the body, accumulation will occur with each subsequent dose until steady state is reached. The time taken to reach steady state is controlled by the drug elimination rate and is independent of the absorption or drug release rate (k_r, k_a > k_{el}). Thus, prolonging the absorption of a drug by controlled release does not influence its accumulation rate.

As it takes $4.3 \times t_{1/2}$ to reach 95% of steady state the number of doses required to attain this condition depends upon the relationship between the dosage interval and the elimination half-life. For a compound that is dosed once every half-life it will take between four and five doses to reach 95% of steady-state. If drug is administered every second half-life, 95% of steady state will be achieved between two and three doses.

The major difference between controlled and conventional dosage forms is in the maximum A_{max}^{∞} and minimum A_{min}^{∞} values at steady-state. These values are obtained from Eqs. (4) and (5), and the time of peak values, T_{max}^{∞} is given by Eq. (6).

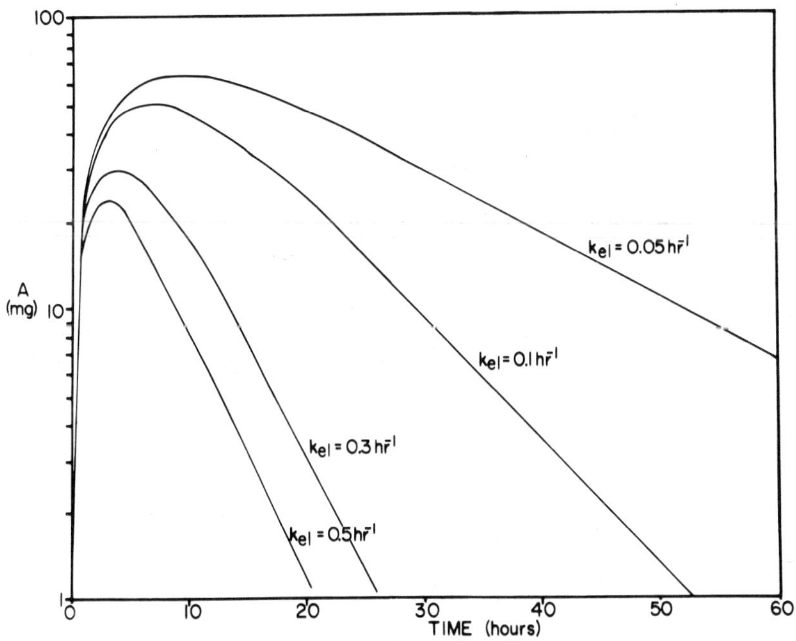

Fig. 3 Drug levels following a single dose. Curves generated from Eq. (1) with $D_s = 100$ mg, $k_r = 0.2$ hr^{-1}, and $k_{el} = 0.05$, 0.1, 0.3, and 0.5 hr^{-1}. (Reproduced by permission from Ref. 15.)

$$A^{\infty}_{max} = D_s \left[\frac{1}{1 - e^{-k_{el}\tau}}\right] \left[\frac{k_r(1 - e^{-k_{el}\tau})}{k_{el}(1 - e^{-k_r\tau})}\right] \left(\frac{k_{el}}{k_{el} - k_r}\right) \tag{4}$$

$$A^{\infty}_{min} = \frac{D_s k_r}{k_r - k_{el}} \left[\frac{e^{-k_{el}\tau}}{1 - e^{-k_{el}\tau}} - \frac{e^{-k_r\tau}}{1 - e^{-k_r\tau}}\right] \tag{5}$$

$$T^{\infty}_{max} = \frac{1}{k_r - k_{el}} \ln\left[\frac{k_r(1 - e^{-k_{el}\tau})}{k_{el}(1 - e^{-k_r\tau})}\right] \tag{6}$$

From Eq. (6), the time of peak level increases as the release rate is decreased. For example, if $k_{el} = 0.17\ hr^{-1}$ and τ is 12 hr, k_r values of 0.5, 0.2, and 0.1 hr^{-1} would yield T^{∞}_{max} values of 2.3, 3.9, and 4.4 hours, respectively, compared to two hours with a conventional formulation with a k_a of 1.0 hr^{-1}. Thus, a ten-fold decrease in the absorption rate constant yields only a 2.2-fold increase in the value of T^{∞}_{max}.

It is generally believed that controlled drug release results in lower C_{max} and higher C_{min} values compared to conventional release. However, this is not always the case. Consider Figure 4. A conventional dosage form of drug ($k_a = 1.0\ h^{-1}$, $k_{el} = 0.1\ hr^{-1}$) administered 100 mg every six hours yields peak and trough amounts of the drug in the body of 105 and 54 mg, respectively. A controlled release dose ($k_r = 0.5\ hr^{-1}$) administered 200 mg every 12 hr results in increased peak and decreased trough levels. The value of k_r would need to be reduced to <u>ca</u> 0.25 hr^{-1} in order to obtain similar peak and trough levels to those from the conventional dosage form.

B. Zero-Order Release

1. *Single Dose*

The amount of drug in the body following a single dose is given by Eq. (7), in which k_o is the rate constant governing absorption ($k_o << k_a$).

$$A = \frac{k_o}{k_{el}}\left[1 - e^{-k_{el}t}\right] \tag{7}$$

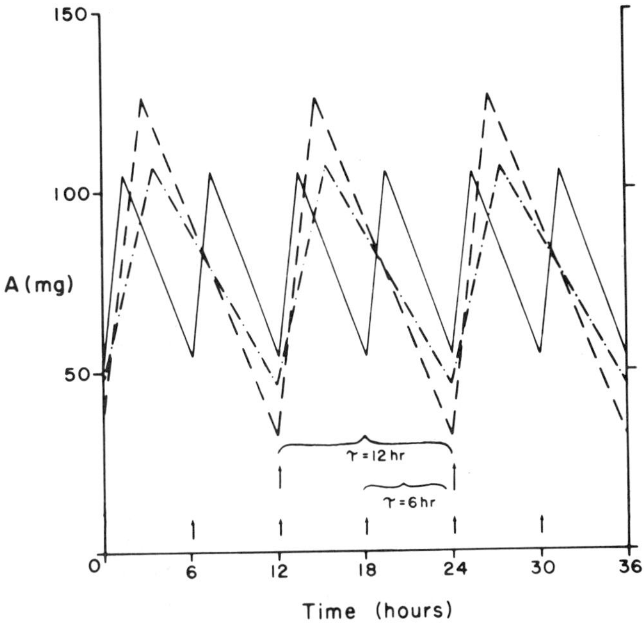

Fig. 4 Drug levels at steady-state during repeated doses, 400 mg per day in divided doses, of a conventional formulation (k_a = 1.0 hr^{-1}) and controlled release formulations (k_r = 0.5 hr^{-1} [---] and 0.25 hr^{-1} [-·-·], τ = 6 hr for the conventional formulation and 12 hr for the others, and k_{el} = 0.2 hr^{-1}). (Reproduced by permission from Ref. 2.)

Eq. (7) can be converted to describe drug concentrations as in Eq. (8).

$$C = \frac{k_o}{Vk_{el}}\left[1 - e^{-k_{el}t}\right] \tag{8}$$

Drug profiles from this type of dosage form are influenced by the rate at which drug is released from the dosage form and also the elimination rate, as shown in Figures 5 and 6. It is clear from Figure 5 that, while drug levels are directly proportional to the controlled release rate, the time course of accumulation following a single dose is independent of release rate and is dependent solely on the elimination rate constant. It is also clear that, even with a short

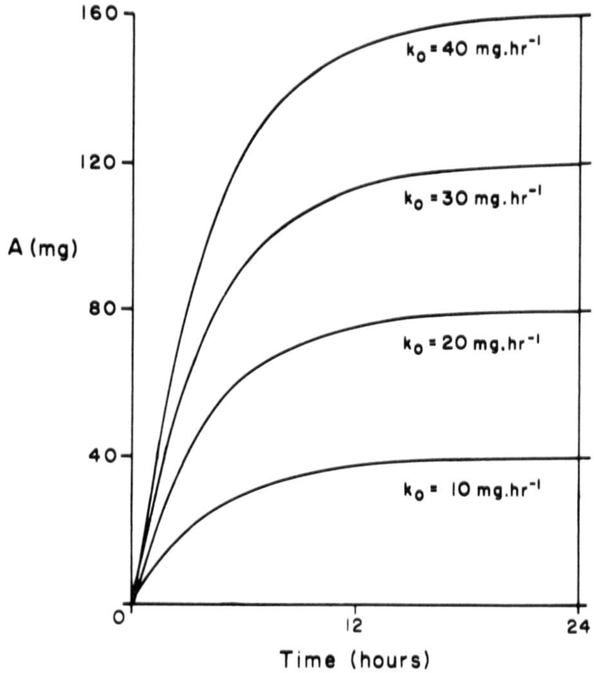

Fig. 5 Accumulation of drug in the body from a single dose of zero-order release formulations (k_o = 10, 20, 30, and 40 mg·hr^{-1} and k_{el} = 0.25 hr^{-1}). (Reproduced by permission from Ref. 2.)

drug elimination half-life of 2.8 hr, plateau drug levels are not achieved with a GI residence time of 12 hr. To achieve a plateau level, the residence time would have to be increased to 20–25 hr. For drugs with longer elimination half-lives, it is unlikely that plateau drug levels are achieved from a single dose. For example a drug with a $t_{1/2}$ of 10 hr would have to be released continuously for 45 hours before steady-state levels were approached.

This argument is illustrated in Figure 6. A drug with an elimination $t_{1/2}$ of 1.7 hr (k_{el} = 0.4 hr^{-1}) will approach steady state at 12 hr. A drug with a $t_{1/2}$ of 7 (k_{el} = 0.1 hr^{-1}) will not achieve steady state at 24 hr. These examples illustrate the misconception that it is possible to achieve plateau or steady-state drug levels with a single dose of a zero-order release formulation.

When a zero-order formulation has released all of its medication, or when the partially spent formulation is voided in the feces, drug levels decline at a first-order rate regardless of whether or not steady-state levels have been reached. Typical profiles for drugs with elimination half-lives of 2 hr (k_{el} = 0.35 hr^{-1}) and 8 hr (k_{el} = 0.087 hr^{-1}) are shown in Figure 7.

2. *Repeated Dose*

Despite the discontinuous nature of drug levels from zero-order release formulations, as shown in Figure 8, the dependency of both the ascending and descending components of the curves on drug elimination half-life lends itself to sustained and controlled levels of medication with repeated dosing.

Consider the two situations in Figure 7. If the drug with the shorter half-life is administered every 12 hr as in Figure 8, then

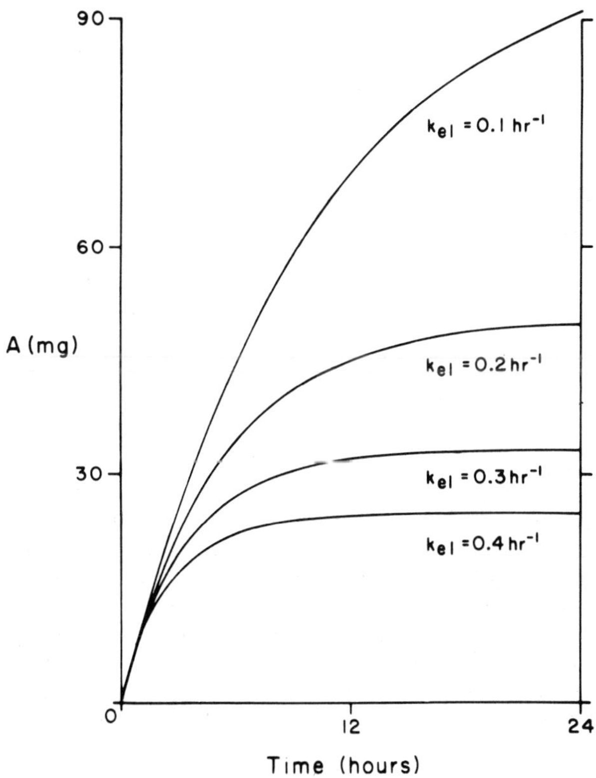

Fig. 6 Accumulation of drug in the body from a single dose of a zero-order release formulation (k_o = 10 mg.hr^{-1} and k_{el} = 0.1−0.4 hr^{-1}). (Reproduced by permission from Ref. 2.)

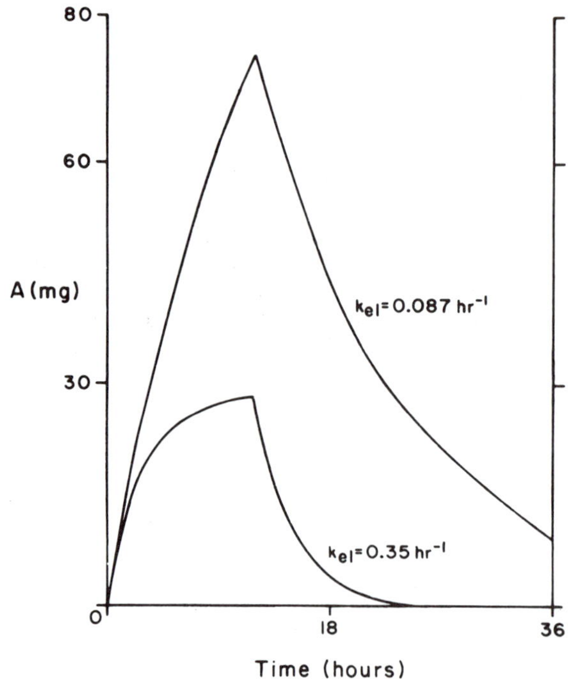

Fig. 7 Drug levels during and after a single dose of a zero-order release dosage form (k_o = 10 mg hr^{-1}, release time T = 12 hr, and k_{el} = 0.087 and 0.35 hr^{-1}). (Reproduced by permission from Ref. 2.)

plateau drug levels are maintained with successive doses. If the drug with the longer half-life is given every 12 hr, then, as shown in Figure 9, accumulation will continue with successive doses until the steady-state level is achieved. Ninety-five percent of steady-state level will be reached at $4.3 \times t_{1/2}$, or between the fourth and fifth doses. Once steady-state is reached, plateau drug levels, with minimal fluctuation, can theoretically be obtained. Zero-order release formulations thus represent an ideal controlled release system and several recently introduced products are based on this principle. Obviously, actual blood levels obtained *in vivo* will depend not only on drug release rate, but also on drug stability, absorption efficiency from various regions of the GI tract, and a host of other factors.

From this discussion on first-order and zero-order release systems, it is clear that, whether considering single dose or multiple dose, the time taken to achieve desired levels in the body depends on the elimination rate constant. The slower the elimination, the more time will be required to reach steady-state. Methods for calculating appropriate loading doses under a variety of situations are well documented [17].

A number of formulations have been designed incorporating a fast release drug component in addition to a controlled release component. While such formuations may be useful when administered either as single doses or as widely spaced intermittent doses, their usefulness for repeated dosages in order to maintain drug levels in the body is less obvious. The next sections will consider some advantages and disadvantages of this type of dosage form.

C. Zero-Order Release with a Fast Release Component

1. *Single Dose*

Incorporation of a fast release component into a controlled release formulation is intended to rapidly obtain a desired drug level in the body and to maintain this level by means of the controlled release component.

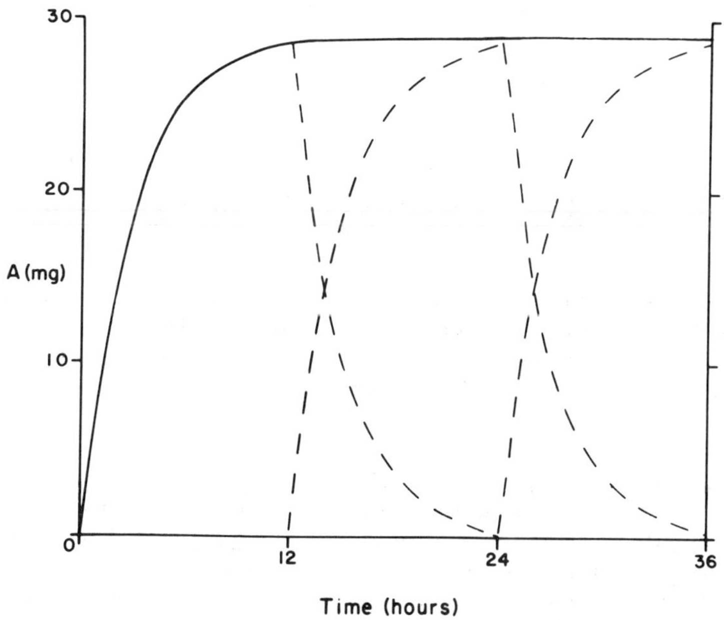

Fig. 8 Drug levels during 12-hourly repeated doses of the rapidly eliminated dosage form from Figure 7. Solid lines indicate total drug levels while dashed lines indicate the individual levels from successive doses. (Reproduced by permission from Ref. 2.)

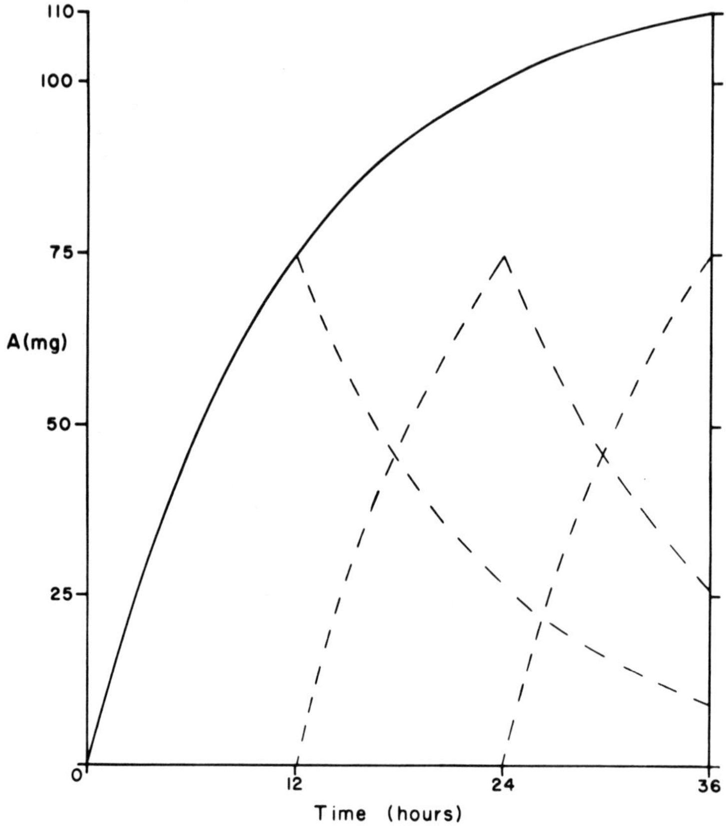

Fig. 9 Drug levels during 12-hourly repeated doses of the slowly eliminated dosage form from Figure 7. Solid lines indicate total drug levels while dashed lines indicate the individual levels from successive doses. (Reproduced by permission from Ref. 2.)

The pharmacokinetics associated with this type of drug release are complex because of contributions from both the fast and slow release components. Although the temporal relationship between initiation of release of the two components may vary, discussions here will assume that release of both components starts simultaneously.

Again assuming $k_o << k_a$, the amount of drug in the body following a single dose is given by Eq. (9).

$$A = \frac{D_i k_a}{k_a - k_{el}} \left[e^{-k_{el}t} - e^{-k_a t} \right] + \frac{k_o}{k_{el}} \left[1 - e^{-k_{el}t} \right] \tag{9}$$

The two parenthetical terms on the right hand side of this equation represent the contributions of the fast and slow release components. The first portion is similar to Eq. (1) (released by first-order process) while the second portion is identical to Eq. (7) (zero-order release). The quantity of drug in the controlled release component, D_s, is given by k_oT, where T is the duration of drug release. The drug profile obtained from a single dose is a composite of a rapidly increasing and then declining component and of a slowly increasing component. This dosage form is ideally suited for all drugs other than those with very short elimination half-lives, that would not achieve steady-state without a fast release component.

With this dosage form, both the rate of deline in drug levels from the fast-release component and the rate of increase in levels from the slow zero-order release component are controlled by the drug elimination rate constant [Eq. (9)]. Several methods have been described to calculate the proportions of D_i and D_s that are required to rapidly achieve and maintain therapeutic drug levels [18–21]. The most recent method is based on the assumption that the fast release component should provide the quantity of drug that would yield the desired therapeutic response at steady-state, A_{ss}, as in Eq. (10) [21].

$$D_i = A_{ss} = k_o/k_{el} \tag{10}$$

This approach ignores the possible additive effect from the fast and slow release components at early times and may yield drug levels higher than the desired steady-state levels shortly after dosing. However, this effect is likely to be slight, and the method is simple and practical.

Application of the method is demonstrated for theophylline. Theophylline has an elimination $t_{1/2}$ of approximately 4 hr ($k_{el} = 0.17\ hr^{-1}$) and a distribution volume of 32 liters [22]. A steady-state level of 5 μg/ml is thus equivalent to $A_{ss} = D_i = 160$ mg, and $k_o = 160 \times 0.17 = 27.2$ mg/hr [Eq. (10)]. Substitution into Eq. (9) and assigning $k_a = 1.3\ hr^{-1}$ [22] and a zero-order release time of 12 hr yields the drug levels in Figure 10. The required level of 5 μg/ml is achieved by 2 hr and maintained through 12 hr, after which time the zero-order component is exhausted of drug. Levels then fall exponentially at a rate determined by k_{el}.

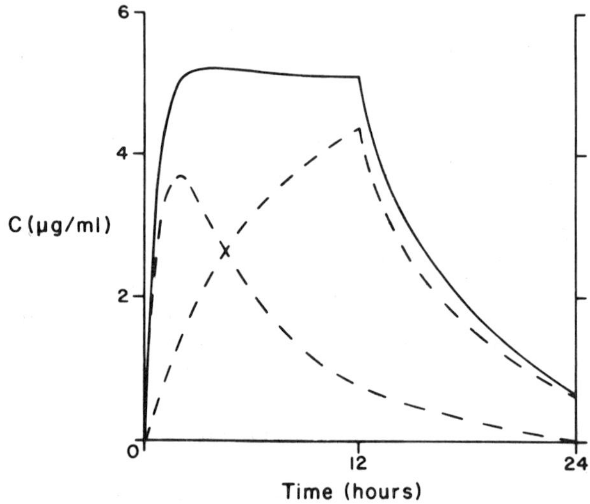

Fig. 10 Plasma theophylline concentration profile from a single dose of an oral formulation containing 160 mg as a fast-release component and a slow component releasing 27.2 mg.hr^{-1} during 12 hr. Solid lines indicate total drug levels while dashed lines indicate the contributions from individual components. (Reproduced by permission from Ref. 2.)

The above method clearly is successful in rapidly achieving a desired drug level, but the level reached is only one half the minimum therapeutic concentration of 10 µg/ml. This is intentional and reflects two problems associated with controlled release drug formulations. The first is dose size. Rapidly obtaining and then maintaining a theophylline level of 5 µg/ml for a 12-hr period requires (160 + 27.2 × 12) mg or ca. 500 mg. This is probably the upper limit for a single oral dosage unit. A theophylline level of 10 µg/ml under the same conditions would require a total dose of 1000 mg (320 mg as D_i and 680 mg as D_s released over 12 hr). This is too large for a single dosage unit, but can be obtained by giving 2 × 500 mg units. Similarly 15 µg/ml and 20 µg/ml levels can be obtained with three and four dosage units, respectively. Thus, whatever the dosage size for a drug, multiples of a minimum drug level are achieved by taking the appropriate number of tablets. While this process is simple, the reverse is not. It is often not possible to subdivide single controlled release formulations to achieve a smaller dose. Thus, it is appropriate for maximum flexibility in dosing to prepare controlled release dosage forms in the smallest practical dosage units.

2. *Repeated Dose*

The objective with repeated doses for this case is not so much to achieve increasing drug levels with each subsequent dose, but to maintain plauteau levels obtained with the initial dose. It is at this point that the argument for a fast release component in an oral controlled release dosage form becomes tenuous.

While formulations that release all of the drug at a slow, zero-order rate yield continuous drug levels with no peaks or troughs with repeated doses at intervals equal to the total release time of each dose (Figs. 8 and 9), this type of drug level pattern cannot be achieved when a fast release component is added.

Consider the theophylline example again. If this formulation were taken every 12 hr, then, unlike the situation in Figure 8, there would be sharp increases in drug levels with successive doses and undue accumulation may occur if drug levels do not return to required C_{ss} levels at the end of each dosing interval. This is demonstrated in Figure 11 using a dosing interval of 12 hr and the same kinetic values as in Figure 10. Although a plateau level of ca. 5 μg/ml is rapidly achieved with the initial dose, levels are transiently increased to 8.7 and 9.2 μg/ml shortly after the second and third doses, respectively. This could clearly give rise to transient yet potentially toxic side effects after each dose with this type of formulation.

Several approaches may be used to prevent transient fluctuations in drug levels with this type of formulation. One can minimize the transient increase by decreasing the loading dose in all doses after the first, or by administering the dosages at time intervals greater than the zero-order release period. Unfortunately, these approaches are either impractical from a formulation viewpoint or cumbersome with respect to drug administration. A more realistic approach is not to include a fast-release component at all, but rather to administer a conventional dosage form initially to establish therapeutic levels, followed by repeated doses of a zero-order controlled release dosage form to maintain constant levels with minimum fluctuation.

For the theophylline example, an initial conventional dose of 300 mg, together with (a) a zero-order release formulation that releases 600–650 mg during 12 hr and (b) subsequent 12-hourly doses of the controlled release formulation, would rapidly achieve and maintain a theophylline plasma level of ca. 10 μg/ml.

D. First-Order Release with a Fast Release Component

1. *Single Dose*

Both the fast and slow components of this dosage form release drug at a first-order rate. If release of both components starts simultaneously, the resulting drug profiles are described by Eq. (11).

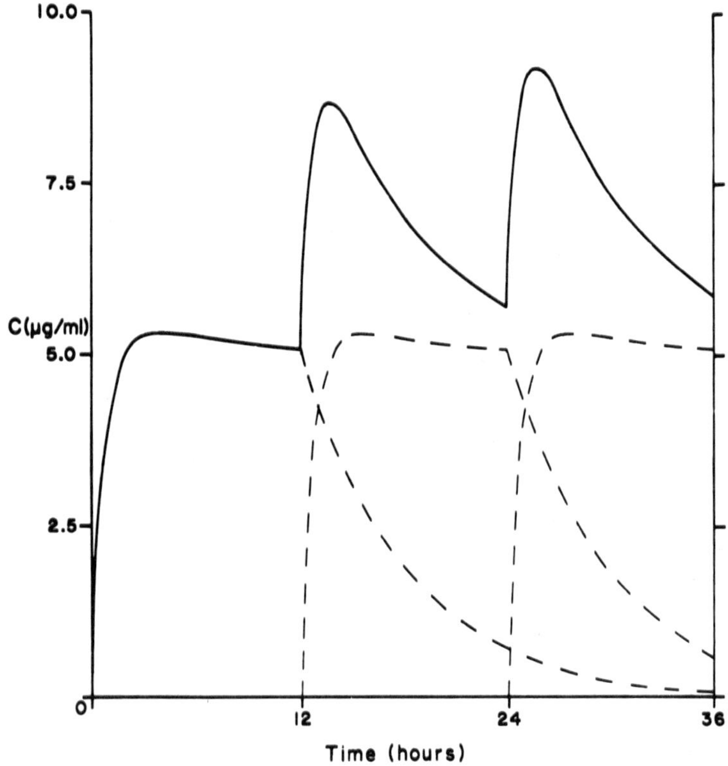

Fig. 11 Plasma theophylline concentration profile from three successive doses of the formulation in Figure 10. Pharmacokinetic parameters are the same as in that figure. Dosage interval is 12 hr. Solid lines indicate total drug levels while dashed lines indicate the individual levels from successive doses. (Reproduced by permission from Ref. 2.).

$$A = \frac{D_i k_a}{k_a - k_{el}} \left[e^{-k_{el} t} - e^{-k_a t} \right] + \frac{D_s k_r}{k_r - k_{el}} \left[e^{-k_{el} t} - e^{-k_r t} \right] \tag{11}$$

This equation is the sum of two separate, simultaneous first-order absorption and elimination profiles, with different apparent absorption rate constants k_a and k_r.

With this pattern of drug release, which is probably more common than the previous model, a strong argument can be made for delaying the release of the slow component until some time later compared to the fast component. Consider the profiles in Figure 12. In this figure the slow component is threefold greater in size than the fast component. The curve generated when all the dose is in the fast-release form is included for comparison. When $k_r = 0.5\ k_a$ there is a negligible sustained effect, and drug profiles are not significantly prolonged until k_r is reduced to $0.1\ k_a$. Unfortunately, between 25 and 50% of the slow release proportion may not be absorbed due to limited GI residence time so that the sustained component during 12–24 hr would be lost.

An alternative method to achieve prolonged circulating drug profiles with this type of formulation is to delay release of the slow component

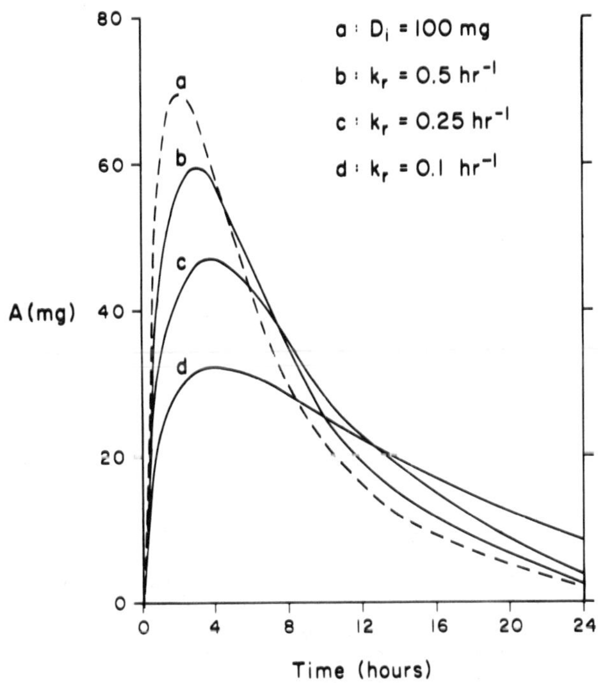

Fig. 12 Drug levels following single oral doses of a dosage form containing fast and slow first-order release components, released simultaneously. The pharmacokinetic values are as follows: D_i = 25 mg, D_s = 75 mg, $k_a = 1.0\ hr^{-1}$, $k_{el} = 0.17\ hr^{-1}$ ($t_{1/2}$ = 4 hr), and k_r = 0.1, 0.25, and 0.5 hr^{-1}. The curve obtained when D_i = 100 mg and D_s = 0 mg is also shown. (Reproduced by permission from Ref. 2.)

to provide a second input at a certain time after the release of the fast component. Arguments can then be made for fast or slow release of the second drug component. The first of these is similar to administering repeated doses of a conventional dosage form except that the second portion will be released lower down the GI tract. The second component therefore will be less susceptible to gastric degradation but more susceptible to poor absorption from distal parts of the intestine, bacterial degradation, and limited GI transit time. Apart from these problems, which may be drug specific, the general pharmacokinetic treatment from two- or three- step fast release formulation does not differ conceptually from repeated doses of conventional dosage forms.

The alternative approach of a delayed, controlled-release component is also a viable method to maintain drug levels. The principal

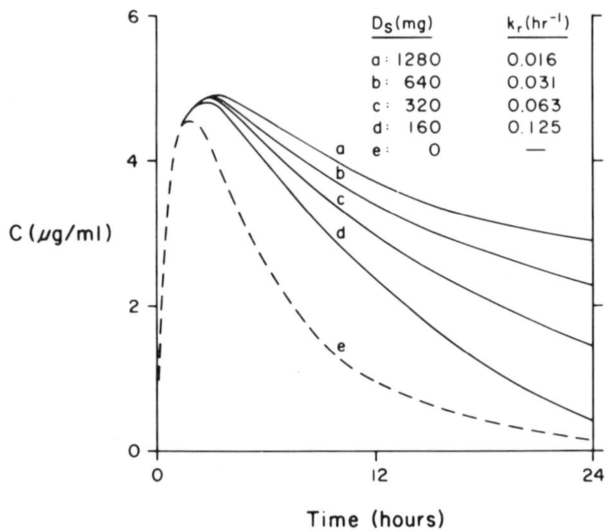

Fig. 13 Plasma theophylline concentration profiles from a single dose of an oral formulation in which first-order release of the slow component is initiated when plasma levels from the fast release component are at a maximum. The curves are calculated from Equation 12 with the value of t for the slow component reduced by T_{max} = 1.8 hr. The pharmacokinetic values are as follows: k_a = 1.3 hr^{-1}, k_{el} = 0.17 hr^{-1}, V = 32L, D_i = 200 mg, and D_s = 160 mg (k_r = 0.125 hr^{-1}), 320 mg (k_r = 0.063 hr^{-1}), 640 mg (k_r = 0.031 hr^{-1}), and 1280 mg (k_r = 0.016 hr^{-1}). (Reproduced by permission from Ref. 2.)

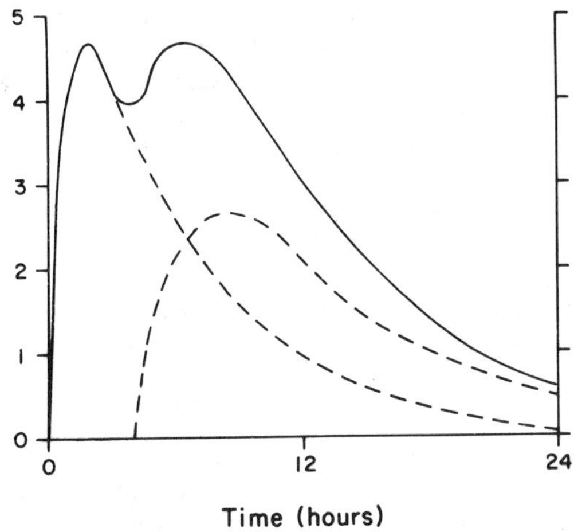

Fig. 14 Predicted plasma theophylline concentration profile from a single dose of an oral formulation in which first-order release of the slow component is initiated when release of the fast component is 99% complete. The pharmacokinetic values are as follows: $D_i = 200$ mg, $D_s = 180$ mg, $k_a = 1.3\ hr^{-1}$, $k_{el} = 0.17\ hr^{-1}$, and $k_r = 0.3\ hr^{-1}$. Delay time for the slow component is four hours. Solid lines indicate total drug levels while dashed lines indicate the individual levels from the two components. (Reproduced by permission from Ref. 2.)

questions in this approach are: (a) when should the slow release component be released and (b) what are the optimal proportions of drug in the fast and slow release components. Regarding the first question, two possible approaches are (a) to release the second component when levels from the first component are at a maximum, or (b) to release the second component when essentially all of the first component has been released [20].

The first approach is based on the argument that if the slow component can approximate zero-order release, then initiating the second component when the drug levels from the fast component are at a peak should yield a plateau effect similar to that achieved with the third case. This approach does not work well in practice. First-order release approximates zero-order only when the amount of drug is large and the first-order release rate constant is small. This is illustrated for the theophylline example in Figure 13. An ideal plateau affect is achieved only when D_s is six-fold greater than D_i and k_r is reduced to $0.016\ hr^{-1}$. This is wasteful as only 20% of the slowly released dose would be absorbed during a 12 hour period, and only 30% during 24 hr.

The second approach of releasing the slow component when most of the fast component has been released is more realistic. If the delay is equal to the time when D_i is essentially completely released, then drug level curves similar to those shown in Figure 14 can be achieved. In this example the slow release component is released four hours, or 7.5 absorption half-lives, after the fast component. Despite the fluctuations in drug levels, reasonably sustained levels are obtained using a relatively small maintenance dose. This type of formulation is also efficient from a drug utilization viewpoint. In this example, approximately 80% of the sustained dose would be absorbed by 12 hr, and absorption would be quantitative in 24 hr.

2. *Repeated Dose*

A dosage form that contains fast and slow first-order release components presents the same problems for multiple dosing regimens as those described for the preceding case (Case C). For that model it was shown that more satisfactory multiple dose drug profiles are

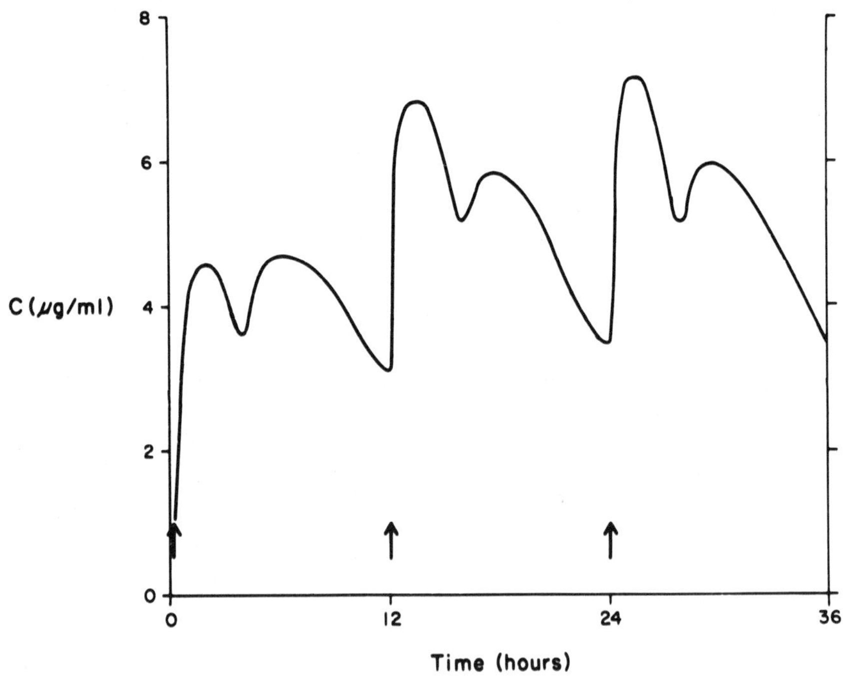

Fig. 15 Predicted plasma theophylline concentration profile during repeated doses of the formulation in Figure 14. (Reproduced by permission from Ref. 2.)

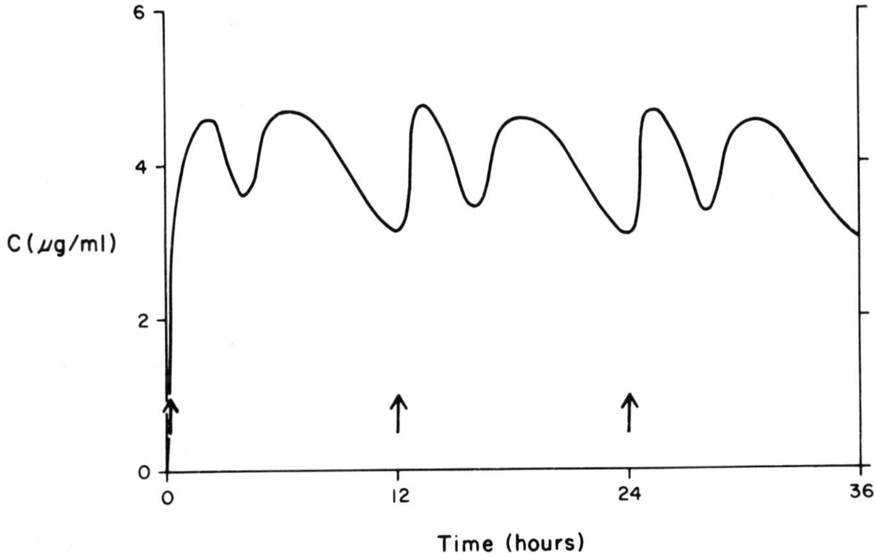

Fig. 16 Predicted plasma theophylline concentration profile during repeated doses of the oral formulation in Figure 14. D_i has been reduced to 100 mg for the second and third doses [τ = 12 hr]. (Reproduced by permission from Ref. 2.)

obtained without a fast release component. In the present case, a variety of multiple dose profiles can be obtained by judicious selection of drug quantities and release rates [15].

Consider the formulation in Figure 14. Multiple doses of this formulation could be given with the sustained and fast drug components unchanged, or with the quantity D_i reduced to compensate for drug remaining in the body from the previous dose. Typical profiles are shown in Figures 15 and 16.

The profile in Figure 15 shows that, once again, repeated dosing of a formulation containing a fast release component that yields the required therapeutic profile after the initial dose will lead to marked oscillation, the possibility of yielding toxic levels shortly after each dose, and also undue accumulation with repeated dosing. If, on the other hand, the amount of drug in the fast component is appropriately reduced [15], then the more acceptable profile in Figure 16 is obtained. Thus, by judicious dose adjustment, drug levels can be generated, at least in theory, to oscillate within a relatively narrow range.

It is impractical to have varying amounts of instantly released drug in different tablets, so that one is presented with a compromise of either achieving required levels rapidly and accepting the wide range of drug levels subsequently, or achieving the ideal drug profile at steady-state and accepting a delay in achieving that level. It is not possible to rapidly achieve required drug levels and then maintain them with minimum oscillation from this type of formulation.

VII. BIOAVAILABILITY TESTING

Bioavailability is generally defined as the rate and extent of absorption of unchanged drug from its site of application to the general circulation. Bioavailability is necessarily defined in terms of a specific drug moiety, usually the active therapeutic entity, which may be the unchanged drug or, as with prodrugs for instance, a metabolite. In contrast, the term "absorption" often refers to net transport of drug-related mass from its site of application into the body. Hence, a compound may be completely absorbed but only partially bioavailable as would occur, for example, with a pharmacologically active agent which is efficiently absorbed from the gut to the portal circulation but undergoes extensive first-pass degradation to inactive metabolites in the liver before it reaches the systemic circulation. When low bioavailability is caused by incomplete absorption, pharmaceutical optimization of the dosage form may be warranted to improve absorption characteristics of the drug and thereby also its bioavailability. Throughout this chapter, it is assumed that the orally administered drug is the pharmacologically active agent which is absorbed in unchanged form so that absorption and bioavailability are synonymous.

The assessment of extent of absorption from a sustained-release formulation does not differ fundamentally from that for standard, immediate-release dosage forms. Mass balance dictates that the amount of drug absorbed must be equivalent to the amount of drug eliminated. In other words, after a single oral dose the bioavailable fraction (F^X) of the administered oral dose (D^X) is equivalent to the product of the plasma clearance (CL) of the drug and the total area under the plasma drug concentration curve (AUC^X):

$$F^X D^X = CL.AUC^X \tag{12}$$

Once the CL of the drug is known, F^X can be determined. CL is estimated in a separate reference treatment following an intravenous dose of the drug (X = i.v.) since $F^{i.v.}$ in Eq. (12) is, by definition, unity. In this case, the "absolute bioavailability" of the oral dose is determined. When intravenous dose administration is not possible an oral solution or other reference standard(s) is used and the "relative bioavailability" determined:

$$F^{X}/F^{s} = (AUC^{X}/AUC^{s}).(D^{s}/D^{X}) \tag{13}$$

Equation (13) is valid as long as $CL^{X} = CL^{s}$; alternatives to the constant clearance assumption have been delineated [23,24].

Equation (13) provides an estimate of the extent of absorption but gives no information on the rate, or time-course, of the absorption (input) process. Equivalence in rate of absorption between immediate-release and reference formulations is often inferred from the observed maximum and time of maximum plasma drug concentration (C_{max}, t_{max}). The two formulations are termed "bioequivalent" if their rate and extent of absorption are similar. Since rate is intentionally modulated in a sustained release formulation, it is, by definition, not bioequivalent to an immediate release dosage form. Rather, an objective of bioavailability testing of sustained-release formulations is to document in a quantitative sense how the input process has been modulated. Again, mass balance considerations provide one means to determine the absorption, or input, profile of the drug. The amount of drug absorbed through time t after dose administration A(t), must be equal to the sum of that which is in the body at time t, B(t), and that which has been eliminated from the body by time t. That is,

$$A(t) = V.C(t) + CL \ . \ AUC^{o \to t} \tag{14}$$

where B(t) is given by the product of the volume of distribution of the drug, V, and its plasma concentration at time t, C(t), and the cumulative amount eliminated is the product of drug clearance and the area under the curve from time 0 to 5, $AUC^{o \to t}$. The absorption profile [A(t) vs t] is obtained by successive application of Eq. (14) to each of the plasma sampling time points. The experimental design should accomodate a plasma sampling scheme sufficient to define the entire time course of the absorption process.

Equation (14) is applicable for drugs which exhibit monoexponential disposition kinetics and is known as the Wagner-Nelson method [25] for estimating the time course of absorption. The method is model-dependent and requires estimates of V and CL obtained following an i.v. dose. If i.v. dose administration is not feasible, the amount of drug absorbed relative to its distribution volume can be obtained as:

$$A(t)/V = C(t) + k_{el} \ AUC^{o \to t} \tag{15}$$

since CL/V is the elimination rate constant of the drug (k_{el}). Application of Eq. (15) requires an estimate of the true value of k_{el}. With conventional, fast release dosage forms, where $k_a > k_{el}$, k_{el} is obtained from the terminal slope of the log-concentration versus time profile ($k_{el} = 0.693/t_{1/2}$). With a sustained release formulation, where a prolonged absorption phase is intended, the observed terminal portion of the profile may not be free from the effects of absorption and, in the extreme, may represent the release rate constant of drug from the formulation (k_r) as shown in Figures 2 and 3, where $k_r < k_{el}$. Notwithstanding intersubject variability in k_{el}, comparison of the plasma profile after the sustained-release formulation with that after an immediate release formulation would provide assurance that the proper k_{el} is used.

When drug disposition kinetics are more complex than a one-compartment model, the amount of drug in the body term in Eq. (14) must account for drug in the peripheral as well as central compartments, as has been described for biexponential [26,27] or more complex [28] disposition models.

Owing to the absence of suitable *in vitro* tests for sustained release drug products, and also the uncertain relationship between *in vitro* release and *in vivo* absorption, bioavailability and bioequivalence testing of sustained and controlled release products must be conducted *in vivo* in man.

The FDA requirements for bioequivalency testing between controlled release and conventional release products, or between two controlled release products, have been set out in the Federal Register [11]. The regulations provide the following guidelines to assist in conducting and presenting bioequivalence studies in support of a New Drug Application for controlled release products.

The purpose of an *in vivo* bioavailability study involving a drug for which a controlled release claim is made is to determine if all of the following conditions are met:

1. The drug product meets the controlled release claims made for it.
2. The bioavailability profile established for the drug product rules out the occurrence of any dose dumping.
3. The drug product's steady-state performance is equivalent to a currently marketed non-controlled release or controlled release drug product that contains the same active drug ingredient or therapeutic moiety and that is subject to an approved full New Drug Application.
4. The drug product's formulation provides consistent pharmacokinetic performance between individual dosage units.

The reference material(s) for such a bioavailability study shall be chosen to permit an appropriate scientific evaluation of the controlled release claims made for the drug product. The reference material shall be one of the following or any combination thereof:

1. A solution or suspension of the active drug ingredient or therapeutic moiety
2. A currently marketed non-controlled release drug product containing the same active drug ingredient or therapeutic moiety and administered according to the dosage recommendations in the labeling of the noncontrolled release drug product
3. A currently markedted controlled release drug product subject to an approved full New Drug Application containing the same active drug ingredient or therapeutic moiety and administered according to the dosage recommendations in the labeling proposed for the controlled release drug product
4. Another reference material that is appropriate for valid scientific reasons

The guidelines have been described recently by Malinowski [29]. It is the position of the FDA that the above requirements apply to essentially all controlled release prescription as well as over-the-counter (OTC) products. It is important to note that, *in vivo* tests must be done at steady-state, as pointed out in item 3. Single dose data are insufficient. However, single dose data have been accepted for some OTC products in the past.

In addition to *in vivo* data, the FDA requires *in vitro* data to ensure lot uniformity and hopefully to provide information that is predictive of *in vivo* bioavailability. The key elements of *in vitro* tests, as outlined by Malinowski, are method reproducibility, correct choice of dissolution medium, maintenance of perfect sink conditions, and control of solution hydrodynamics.

The FDA are concerned with the possibility of dose dumping, and criteria for evaluating this consists essentially of administering the quantity of drug contained in the controlled release product as an immediate release bolus dose. The rate of absorption from the test formulation should be substantially slower compared to the bolus dose.

Whether testing a new controlled release formulation against conventional release or another controlled release product, similar criteria for bioequivalence apply, notwithstanding the different dosage intervals for slow release and fast release products.

One problem that is being addressed by the FDA is that of therapeutic equivalence. The current guidelines indicate that for two products to be therapeutically equivalent thay must by definition be bioequivalent with the same rate and extent of absorption. Thus, for therapeutic equivalence, the reference product needs to be an approved controlled release formulation, and the blood level curves from the test and reference products should be statistically superimposable. Products that do not meet these criteria exactly, as well as situations where a controlled release product is compared to a conventional formulation, need to be considered on a case by case basis.

VIII. CONCLUSIONS

The development of sustained or controlled release products is now one of the most active research areas in the pharmaceutical industry. Controlled release has inherent advantages and disadvantages, and these should be considered together before embarking on a formulation program for a drug candidate. Controlled release formulations have developed principally for cardiovascular, CNS, and respiratory drugs. The antimicrobial drugs have been largely neglected. For drugs such as nitroglycerin, the particular indication has to be considered as well when assessing the merits of controlled release compared to conventional release.

Despite the ever increasing number of controlled release products available in the United States and elsewhere, there have been few attempts to predict *in vivo* drug level data from *in vitro* or theoretical release patterns, or to address the unique problems that accompany single and repeated doses of these dosage forms. There are some notable exceptions. Attempts to develop a truly zero-order release dosage form have found expression in the osmotic pump [30, 31] and also in a matrix system for controlled release [32].

Basic pharmacokinetic principles can be used in the development of controlled release prducts to achieve desirable release properties. Different criteria may apply when one is considering single and repeated doses. The methods described here, while containing some simplifying assumptions, provide a rational basis for controlled release dosage design. The methods represent a compromise between ideality and practical feasibility. They may not always apply to individual cases. Some drugs may exhibit a marked apparent absorption window or may be susceptible to bacterial degradation in the lower GI tract, thus reducing absorption efficiency. The opposite effect occurs with formulations designed to extend GI transit time. First-pass clearance may also be important for drugs that undergo extensive hepatic metabolism or are excreted extensively in the bile.

In the final analysis, controlled release dosage forms are entering an era of unprecedented sophistication, not only in terms of new dosage forms but also in terms of more rigid testing and characterization with respect to *in vitro–in vivo* relationships, predicted and actual release patterns, and pharmacokinetic/pharmacodynamic relationships. Appreciation and application of simple kinetic principles, similar to those described in this chapter, is an essential component of controlled release development and offers a greater opportunity for success compared to the empirical approach.

REFERENCES

1. F. Theeuwes, Drug delivery system, *Pharmac. Ther. 13*, 149–191 (1981).
2. P. G. Welling, Oral controlled drug administration: Pharmacokinetic considerations, *Drug Dev. Ind. Pharm. 9*, 1185–1225 (1983).
3. L. Hendeles, R. P. Iafrate, and M. Weinberger, A clinical and pharmacokinetic basis for the selection and use of slow release theophylline products, *Clin. Pharmacokin. 9*, 95–135 (1984).
4. A. F. Hofmann, J. H. Dressman, C. F. Code, and K. F. Witztum, Controlled entry of oral administered drugs: Physiological considerations, *Drug Dev. Ind. Pharm. 9*, 1077–1109 (1983).
5. K. A. Kelly, Motility of the stomach and gastroduodenal junction. In, *Physiology of the Gastrointestinal Tract* (L. R. Johnson, Ed.), Raven Press, New York, 1981, Chap. 12, pp. 393–410.
6. J. W. Fara, Gastrointestinal transit of solid dosage forms, *Pharm. Tech. 7* (Suppl.), 23–26 (1983).
7. J. H. Meyer, H. Ohashi, D. Jehn, and J. B. Thomson, Size of liver particles emptied from the human stomach, *Gastroenterology, 80*, 1489–1496 (1981).
8. S. S. Davis, J. G. Hardy, M. J. Taylor, D. R. Whalley, and C. G. Wilson, A comparative study of the gastrointestinal transit of a pellet and tablet formulation, *Int. J. Pharm. 21*, 167–177 (1984).
9. S. S. Davis, J. G. Hardy, M. J. Taylor, D. R. Whalley, and C. G. Wilson, The effect of food on the gastrointestinal transit of pellet and an osmotic device (Osmet), *Int. J. Pharm. 21*, 331–340 (1984).
10. S. S. Davis, J. G. Hardy, M. J. Taylor, A. Stockwell, D. R. Whalley, and C. G. Wilson, The *in vivo* evaluation of an osmotic device (Osmet) using gamma scintigraphy, *J. Pharm. Pharmacol. 36*, 740–742 (1984).
11. Drug products, bioequivalence requirements and *in vivo* bioavailability procedures, *Fed. Register 42*, 1624–1653 (1977).
12. C. MacLeod, H. Rabin, J. Ruedy, M. Caron, D. Zarowny, and R. O. Davies, Comparative bioavailability of three brands of ampicillin, *Can. Med. Assoc. J. 107*, 203–209 (1972).
13. P. G. Welling, R. B. Patel, U. R. Patel, W. R. Gillespie, W. A. Craig, and K. S. Albert, Bioavailability of tolazamide from tablets: Comparison of *in vitro* and *in vivo* results, *J. Pharm. Sci. 71*, 1259–1263 (1982).

14. R. B. Patel, M. C. Rogge, A. Selen, T. J. Goehl, V. P. Shah, V. K. Prasad, and P. G. Welling, Bioavailability of hydrocortisone from commercial 20 mg tablets, *J. Pharm. Sci.* (in press).
15. P. G. Welling and M. R. Dobrinska, Multiple dosing of sustained release systems. In, *Sustained and Controlled Release Drug Delivery Systems* (J. R. Robinson, Ed.), Marcel Dekker, Inc., New York, 1978, pp. 631–716.
16. M. Gibaldi and M. A. Schwartz, The pharmacokinetics of penamecillin, *Br. J. Pharmacol. Chemother. 28*, 360–366 (1966).
17. M. Gibaldi and D. Perrier, *Pharmacokinetics*, Marcel Dekker, Inc., New York, 1975, p. 108.
18. E. Nelson, A note on mathematics of oral sustained-release products, *J. Amer. Pharm. Assoc. (Sci. Ed) 46*, 572–573 (1957).
19. M. Rowland and A. H. Beckett, Mathematical treatment of oral sustained-release drug formulations, *J. Pharm. Pharmacol. 16* (*Suppl.*), 156T–162T (1964).
20. J. R. Robinson and S. P. Eriksen, Theoretical formulation of sustained release dosage forms, *J. Pharm. Sci. 55*, 1254–1263 (1966).
21. M. R. Dobrinska and P. G. Welling, Blood levels from a sustained-release dosage form, *J. Pharm. Sci. 64*, 1728–1729 (1975).
22. J. W. Jenne, E. Wyze, F. S. Rood, and F. M. MacDonald, Pharmacokinetics of theophylline: Application to adjustment of the clinical dose of aminophylline, *Clin. Pharacol. Ther. 13*, 349–360 (1972).
23. K. C. Kwan and A. E. Till, Novel method for bioavailability assessment, *J. Pharm. Sci. 62*, 1494–1497 (1973).
24. S. Hwang and K. C. Kwan, Further considerations on model-independent bioavailability estimation, *J. Pharm. Sci. 69*, 77–80 (1980).
25. J. G. Wagner and E. Nelson, Percent absorbed time plots derived from blood level and/or urinary excretion data, *J. Pharm. Sci. 52*, 610–611 (1963).
26. J. C. K. Loo and S. Riegelman, New method for calculating the intrinsic absorption rate of drugs, *J. Pharm. Sci. 57*, 918–928 (1968).
27. H. G. Boxenbaum and S. A. Kaplan, Potential source of error in absorption rate calculations, *J. Pharmacokin. Biopharm. 3*, 257–264 (1975).
28. K. C. Kwan, Pharmacokinetic considerations in the design of controlled and sustained release drug delivery systems. In, *Sustained and Controlled Release Drug Delivery Systems* (J. R. Robinson, Ed.), Marcel Dekker, Inc., New York, 1978, Chap. 8, pp. 605–607.

29. H. J. Malinowski, Biopharmaceutics aspects of the regulatory review of oral controlled-release drug products, *Drug. Dev. Ind. Pharm. 9*, 1255–1279 (1983).
30. W. Bayne, V. Place, F. Theeuwes, J. D. Rogers, R. B. Lee, R. O. Davies, and K. C. Kwan, Kinetics of osmotically controlled indomethacin delivery systems after repeated dosing, *Clin. Pharmacol. Ther. 32*, 270–276 (1982).
31. J. D. Rogers, Biopharmaceutical evaluation of "Osmosin," *Curr. Med. Res. Op. 8(Suppl. 2)*, 38–54 (1983).
32. P. O. Fagerstrom, T. Mellstrand, and N. Svedmyr, Absorption of theophylline from conventional and sustained-release tablets, *Int. J. Clin. Pharmacol. 19*, 128–131 (1981).

7

Regulatory Assessment

JEROME PHILIP SKELLY / Center for Drugs and Biologics, Food and Drug Administration, Rockville, Maryland

WILLIAM H. BARR / Medical College of Virginia, Richmond, Virginia

I. INTRODUCTION

A discussion of regulatory assessment is usually limited to providing an explanation of the governing regulations, how they should be implemented and the type of studies that should be conducted in order to provide the required data. The area of controlled release drug delivery is evolving so rapidly that it is necessary to go beyond definitions, regulations and data requirements. Accordingly, it is our intention to also discuss the rationale and pharmacokinetic basis of controlled release labeling claims, types of problems that can be anticipated with controlled release drug products, and type of studies necessary to establish labeling claims and rule out problems. In addition, the complex relationship of *in vitro* dissolution rate data to *in vivo* blood level data for controlled release products will be explored and compared to the simpler relationships found with conventional release dosage forms.

II. TERMINOLOGY

Controlled release drug delivery systems are rapidly expanding from the originally marketed depot injections to include many types of new oral delivery systems, intra-uterine devices, transdermal drug delivery systems, implantable pumps, etc. Accompanying this rapid development in delivery systems has been an equally rapid expansion in the terminology, due partly to the competitive forces of the marketplace. These include sustained release, controlled release, modified release, delayed release, and numerous others. Some of these terms are intended to be used interchangeably since they mean essentially the same thing, e.g., sustained release or prolonged release. On the other hand, some terms are employed by a particular group, firm or regulatory body to convey one idea of controlled release (e.g.,

Table 1 Terminology

FDA Controlled release dosage forms	U.S.P. Modified release dosage forms
Oral dosage	
1. Prolonged release drug products	1. Extended release
2. Delayed release drug products	2. Delayed release
Intramuscular dosage	
1. Depot injections	
2. Water immiscible injections (i.e., oils)	
Cutaneous/subcutaneous dosage	
1. Implants	
2. Transdermal preparations	
Targeted dosage	
1. Ocusert	
2. Intrauterine devices (IUDs)	

delayed release for prolonged release) but are employed by others to convey a more limited idea (e.g., delayed release for enteric coated tablets). To make matters worse, the two official regulatory bodies, the Food and Drug Administration (FDA) and the United States Pharmacopeial Convention (USP), have developed separate lexicons: one codified in federal regulations; the other officially recognized by the USP Convention.

While meetings between the two regulatory bodies are resulting in a move toward a unified nomenclature, both systems as they exist today are discussed. The USP's "Modified Release Dosage Forms" publication [1] encompasses two of the major entities (extended and delayed release) included in FDA's "Controlled Release Dosage Form Policy" (Table 1) [2]. Both the FDA and USP policies specifically recognize enteric coated tablets as being different from other controlled release products, since they are intended to release drug rapidly once they reach the intestine. Both the FDA and USP employ the term "delayed release" for enteric coated products.

The term, however, has been used by others in the context of extended or controlled release, and some confusion may presently exist. If the USP proposal leads to a standardization of the terminology, the authors feel the final result will be well worth the short term confusion.

Besides delayed release dosage forms, the other category presently recognized by the USP is that of extended release preparations. The FDA terminology, on the other hand, employs the term "prolonged release" for these oral preparations formulated for the purpose of maintaining drug and/or metabolite concentrations at the site of action for longer intervals than is possible with conventional preparations. The FDA has also employed the term "slow release" to include those preparations formulated for the purpose of avoiding the toxicity associated with a peaking effect. The term, "long acting" has been used to encompass those drugs with an inherently long pharmacological effect, because of their pharmacokinetic properties (say a biological half-life greater than 12 hours).

The FDA terminology also recognizes intramuscular injections; implants (dosage forms implanted beneath the skin); and targeted dosage forms (drug delivery systems intended only for local rather than systemic effects, e.g., IUD's, Ocusert, etc.).

III. RATIONALE FOR CONTROLLED RELEASE DOSAGE FORMS

There are some obvious advantages to the use of controlled release products which effectively prolong absorption of a drug:

1. Increase in the time interval required between doses. This provides a reduction in the total number of doses required per day. The decrease in frequency of daily doses is more convenient to the patient and can lead to improved patient compliance. Reduction of dosing from three or four times daily to once or twice daily has been shown to increase patient compliance. While there is little published evidence that going from twice daily to once daily provides greater compliance, this may be due to the fact that once a day prescription delivery systems are only a recent addition to the medical armamentarium. In institutions where drug administration costs are significant there may be a net reduction in medication costs. Evaluation of cost-benefit as opposed to risk-benefit, however, are considerations for the market place rather than regulatory assessment.
2. Reduction in fluctuation of drug blood levels about the mean. In cases where a constant drug level is desirable, a controlled release dosage form may decrease the drug concentration's fluctuation by (a) reducing the peak blood levels (C_{max}), thus potentially reducing dose-related adverse effects, and (b) increasing the minimum plasma concentrations (C_{min}), thereby increasing efficacy if a threshold concentratio

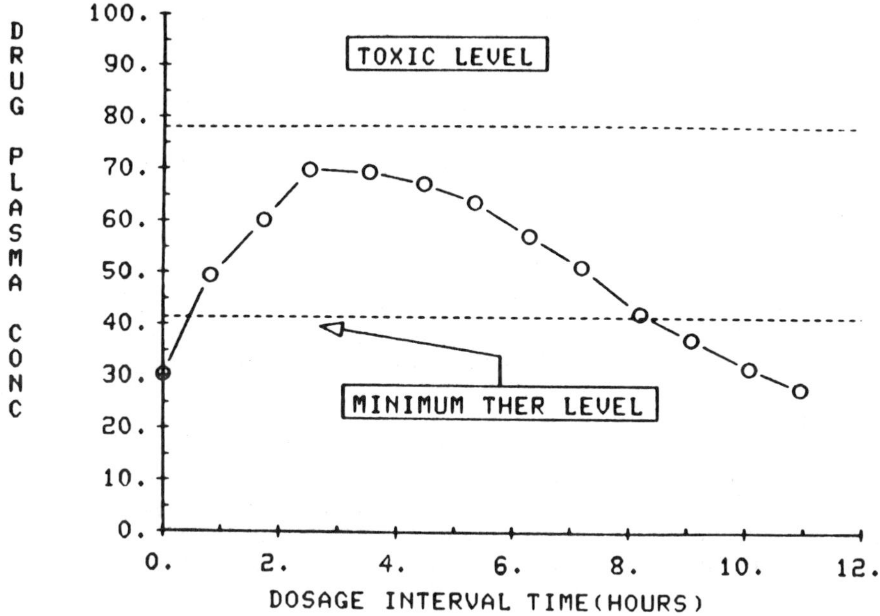

Fig. 1 Therapeutic occupancy time. Therapeutic occupancy time is defined as that fraction of the dosage interval that the dosage form maintains drug and/or metabolite concentrations above the minimum therapeutic level and below the toxic plasma level. In the selected example, therapeutic occupancy time is 8 hr for a b.i.d. dosage form.

is required. The degree of fluctuation about the mean plasma level is therefore an important parameter for regulatory assessment of controlled release forms. A second criterion is the time that the plasma concentration stays within therapeutic range, the so-called "therapeutic occupancy time" (Fig. 1).

The extent to which these potential advantages are realized must be evaluated for each specific drug, particularly with respect to the therapeutic window. There are also some potential disadvantages particular to controlled release drugs which must be assessed in evaluating the therapeutic effectiveness of dosage forms that deliver a constant, rather than an oscillating plasma level. This requires an understanding of the relationship between plasma levels and the pharmacodynamics of a drug, as well as the relationship between the input function and oscillations of plasma levels.

IV. POTENTIAL PHARMACODYNAMIC PROBLEMS WITH CONTINUOUS RELEASE PRODUCTS

Although it is usually assumed that an ideal plasma level is a constant steady-state, the relationship between plasma levels and pharmacologic effect must be established on both an acute and chronic basis. A constant blood level is not necessarily the most advantageous. Corticosteroids given at a constant blood level can cause suppression of endogeneous ACTH and produce adrenocorticoatrophy, whereas blood levels alternating every other day do not. As another example, the bactericidal effects of penicillin are believed more effective given as pulses rather than continuously. Finally, transdermal patches which provide continuous nitroglycerin plasma levels appear to lead to the development of tolerance when used chronically.

Most biological systems show diurnal or cyclical behavior. Many are complex homeostatic systems with a variety of feedback loops. It should not be assumed, a priori, that nonvarying drug blood levels will be universally optimal. In addressing this issue the Workshop cosponsored by the Food and Drug Administration, the Academy of Pharmaceutical Sciences and the American Society for Clinical Pharmacology and Therapeutics [3] proposed the following:

1. Where there is a well-defined relationship between plasma concentration of drug and/or active metabolite(s) and clinical response (therapeutic and adverse), it may be possible to rely on plasma concentration data alone as a basis for the approval of the controlled release product. This is particularly so when the degree of fluctuation (C_{max}/C_{min}) for the immediate release product administered is already small.
2. Where the therapeutic effect is substantially delayed, where there is irreversible toxicity, where there is evidence of functional (pharmacodynamic) tolerance, where peak to trough differences of the immediate release product are very large, or where there is any other reasonable uncertainty concerning the relationship between plasma concentration and therapeutic and adverse effects, it will probably be necessary to carry out clinical studies.
3. Where there is no well defined relationship between the pharmacokinetics and pharmacodynamics of a drug, the premarketing evaluation of the controlled release product should include consideration of the possible development of functional tolerance to the drug.
4. The premarketing evaluation should include consideration of the possible occurrence of sensitivity reactions or local tissue damage due to dosage form dependent persistence or localization of the drug, the clinical implications of dose dumping,

or unexpected decrease of bioavailability (by physiological or physiochemical mechanisms), and quantitative alteration in the metabolic fate of the drug due to nonlinear or site specific disposition.

Elucidation of the relationships between therapeutic effects, adverse effects and blood levels is probably the most critical step in validating a controlled release product. For drugs, such as sedatives and antihistamines, it may be most important to keep C_{max} below a certain level to avoid adverse effects. For others, such as certain bacteriostatic antibiotics, it may be most important for C_{min} to stay above some minimum level to assure continuous therapeutic activity. Finally, for other drugs, such as theophylline, phenytoin, and salicylate, it is important to stay within a narrow range of plasma levels.

V. IDEAL INPUT FUNCTION

It is instructive to first define an "ideal input function" for a given "drug delivery system" and then delineate the extent that deviation from this ideal can be permitted, relative to the pharmacodynamic characteristics and clinical use of the drug. A drug delivery system is defined as the dosage form and dosage regimen (i.e., the dose and time interval between doses) that is recommended for the labeled indications of a given drug.

The input function may be defined as a cumulative amount of drug entering the systemic circulation as a function of time. Alternatively, one may conceptualize the input function as the amount of drug in the body at any given time, if the drug is allowed to enter the body from the dosage form, but not allowed to leave. The input function is a very useful concept for examining different dosage forms and dosage regimens of a given drug, because it allows us to focus on the absorption process without having to worry about the complexities and variabilities of elimination processes.

An ideal input might be one of the following types:

1. Multiple dose regimen of a given dose (D) of a conventional release dosage form given at regular time intervals (τ) that has been shown to be safe and effective in clinical trials.
2. First-order controlled release. The rate constant of absorption (Ka) is sufficiently reduced (or the corresponding absorption half-life ($T_{1/2a}$) is increased) to prolong absorption over the dosage interval.
3. Zero-order controlled release. The input is a continuous constant rate of delivery of all of the drug within the dosage interval.

Table 2 Input Functions

Multiple-Dose, Conventional (Standard or Immediate Release) Dosage form

The first order rate is very rapid (ka – 1.386, $T_{1/2a}$ = 0.5 hr; dosage interval (Tau) – 6 hrs).

Twice daily dosage form—zero order

Zero order infusion for 12 hr. This would be considered an ideal or "perfect" twice daily, zero order.

Twice daily—first order

$T_{1/2a}$ is 3 hr (ka = 0.231). This is an acceptable dosage for twice daily (q12h) dosing because 94% of the drug has been released with in the 12-hr interval (4 half-lives).

Once daily—zero order—24-hr release

This represents the perfect once-daily dosage form.

Once daily—zero order—18-hr release

This represents an acceptable, though not perfect, once-daily dosing form.

Once daily—first order

$T_{1/2a}$ = 6 hr. This represents an acceptable once-daily dosage form since 94% is released within the 24-hr dosage interval (4 half-lives).

In actuality, most input functions are combinations of zero-order and first order—and the ideal is seldom seen. The following specific input functions serve as examples (Table 2).

These input functions listed above are represented in Figure 2 and the simulated corresponding "plasma concentrations" for the hypothetical drug with a half-life of elimination of 6 hr are shown in Table 3. The degree of fluctuation (% Δ C) given in Table 3 for the various input functions can be compared with that produced by the conventional input function of an immediate release product given four times a day (every 6 hr), which serves as a reference standard where,

$$\%\Delta C = \frac{C_{max} - C_{min}}{\bar{C}} \times 100\%, \quad \bar{C} = \frac{AUC}{\tau}$$

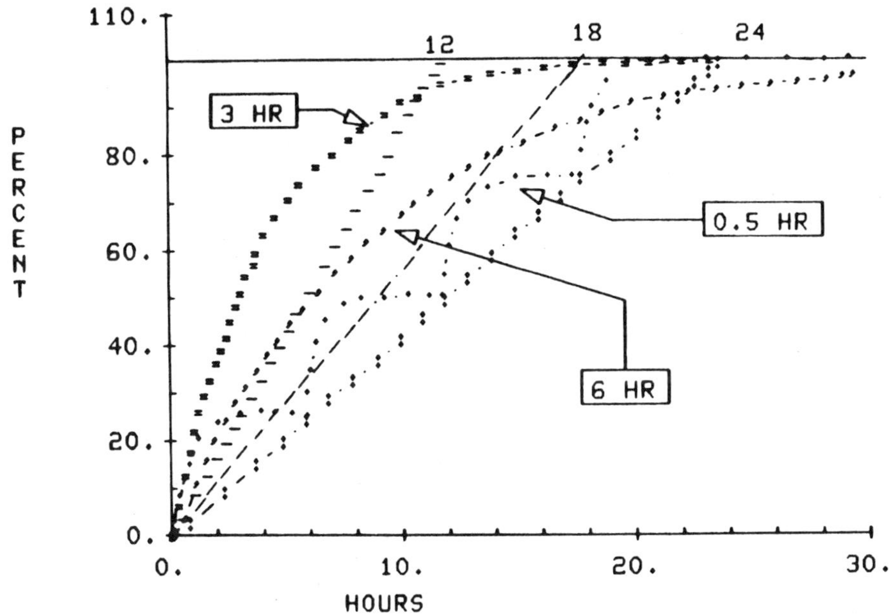

Fig. 2 Dose input functions. (See text.)

or

$$\%\Delta C(\text{appx.}) = \frac{C_{max} - C_{min}}{C_{avg}}, \quad C_{avg} = \frac{C_{max} + C_{min}}{2}$$

The following generalizations regarding the rate and type of input for once daily (every 24 hr) or twice daily (every 12 hr) dosage forms for a drug with a 6-hr elimination half-life appear to be warranted.

1. For those situations where a defined narrow therapeutic window exists and tolerance does not develop with zero order input; the ideal input is zero order because it produces minimal fluctuation.
2. First order input with an absorption half-life of 6 hr is suitable for once daily dosing and is comparable to a zero-order input of 18 hr for a once daily dosage form.
3. First order input with an absorption half-life of 3 hr is suitable for twice daily dosing.
4. First order absorption has the disadvantage that when the dosage interval is less than four times the half-life of the

Table 3 Fluctuation of Input Functions

Form	interval (τ)	Resulting plasma concentrations		ΔC ($C_{max} - C_{min}$)	C_{avg}	Fluctuation (%ΔC)
		C_{max}	C_{min}			
Conventional form						
1. *($T_{1/2a}$ = 0.5 hr)	q6	14	9	5	11.5	43%
Once-daily dosage form						
2. Perfect zero order (24-hr release)	q24	12	12	0	12	0%
3. Minimum zero order (18-hr release)	q24	15	8	7	11.5	61%
4. Minimum first order ($T_{1/2a}$ = 6 hr)	q24	16	7	9	11.5	78%

Twice-daily dosage form						
5. Zero order (12-hr release) used once daily	q24	19	6	13	12.5	104%
6. First order ($T_{1/2a}$ = (3 hr) used once daily	q24	19	5	14	12	117%
7. First order ($T_{1/2a}$ = 3 hr) used once daily	q12	14	9	5	11.5	43%
Once-daily dosage form given in multiple doses						
8. First order ($T_{1/2a}$ = 6 hr) used twice daily	q12	13	11	2	12	17%
9. First order ($T_{1/2a}$ = 6 hr) used four times daily (at 1/2 total dose)	q6	13	12.5	0.5	12.8	4%

drug, there must be a "gut residual," i.e., an amount of drug still remaining in the gut at the time the next dose is given [4]. This can contribute to the variability of the dosage form or decreased bioavailability.

VI. POTENTIAL BIOAVAILABILITY PROBLEMS OF ORAL CONTROLLED RELEASE PRODUCTS

The potential problems inherent in oral controlled release dosage forms generally relate to (1) interactions between the rate, extent, and location that the dosage form releases the drug; and (2) the regional differences in gastrointestinal tract physiology. Some potential problems requiring evaluation are as follows:

A. Gastrointestinal Transit Times and Regional Absorption

Total gastrointestinal transit time in the normal population varies from 5 to 36 hr, with an average total transit time of approximately 24 hr. There is still much to be learned about the physiological processes involved and factors that influence gastric empyting, intestinal transit, and colon residence. A major influence is food administration which delays the "housekeeper wave," causing a significant delay in gastric emptying. A high-fat meal may delay gastric emptying from 3 to 5 hr, and the total gastrointestinal transit delay is largely a function of delay in gastric emptying in this case.

Recent scintographic data [5] show that many prolonged release products, particularly those intended for twice or once daily administration, actually release some of their drug in the colon where it may be absorbed into the systemic circulation. It is anticipated that conditions of dissolution, absorption, and metabolism in the distal portions of the intestine are different than in the proximal regions, due to differences in pH, lumen fluid, mucosal morphology, and motility. The extent and significance of these differences are largely unknown, since these differences have not been systematically studied.

B. Decreased Systemic Availability due to Incomplete Absorption

Many controlled release products are somewhat less bioavailable than their immediate release counterparts. This can be due to incomplete release from the dosage form or release at such a slow rate that the drug has passed the optimal sites of absorption.

C. Decreased Bioavailability due to Increased First Pass Metabolism

The fraction of drug metabolized during first pass by hepatic or intestinal enzymes can be altered by dosage forms which markedly alter the rate at which the drug is presented to the enzyme system(s). If the enzyme systems are saturable, then a slower rate of presentation may result in a greater fraction of drug metabolized. Phenytoin is an example [6]. The steady-state plasma levels of phenytoin observed with equal doses of the prolonged release product are less than for the prompt release product. The difference in plasma levels appears not to be due to decreased absorption, but rather increased metabolism as the amount of total drug in the urine is the same for both formulations. Because of its narrow therapeutic ratio, nonlinear kinetics and different clinical uses, the USP recognizes two dosage forms: prompt (for immediate release) and extended (for controlled release) [7].

It is also possible that intestinal metabolism due to enzymes in the mucosa may be different in the distal portion of the small intestine (ileum) or large intestine (colon) compared to the proximal intestine (duodenum, jejunum). The regional differences in metabolism that may exist would be important only for poorly absorbed drugs or drug products intentionally designed to release drug lower in the gut. Also, bacterial enzymes (largely reductases) in the lower ileum and large intestine are known to extensively metabolize some drugs (e.g., digoxin). This bacterial flora varies greatly in the population.

We know very little about metabolism in the distal portion of the gastrointestinal tract and about the interactions between formulation variables of controlled release drugs and metabolic processes of the intestine. In general, however, it can be expected that differences in systemic availability due to metabolism during the absorptive process will be greater for controlled release drug dosage forms than for immediate release drug products.

D. Dose Dumping

One of the major problems of once or twice daily dosage forms is that they contain from 2 to 4 times the usual dose of the drug. Any event that results in more than the usual fraction being released is termed "dose dumping," and could result in toxicity. The effect of food or other physiological or formulation variables may result in dose dumping.

Dose dumping of a controlled release product, then, can be defined as the product releasing drug at a greater rate than the customary amount of drug per dosing interval, such that potentially adverse plasma levels could be reached.

E. Effect of Food

Although food may not significantly affect drug absorption from some tablet and capsule controlled release and partially enteric coated dosage forms [8–10], it can greatly affect both the rate and extent of absorption of other dosage forms or products of the same drug. Lagas and Jonkman [11] showed that input changed dramatically when Theo-grad® (a controlled release theophylline tablet not available in the United States) was administered in the presence of a high fatty meal, as opposed to drug administered under fasting conditions. They demonstrated that not only did the rate of input increase, the extent of bioavailability was also increased. Pedersen and Moeller-Petersen [12] demonstrated that the rate of drug absorption from Nuelin Retard® was significantly delayed when dosed with food but claimed that the extent of bioavailability did not change. The same authors showed that both the rate and extent of absorption of theophylline from the coated beads of Theodur Sprinkle^R are significantly decreased when the drug was administered with a meal [13]. In contrast, Hendeles et al. [14] have reported a significant increase in the rate and extent of absorption of another coated bead theophylline controlled release formulation (Theo 24®) following administration with food as compared to the same dosage form administered in the fasting state. Additional studies by Karim [15] on this dosage form have been reported indicating that the extent of this food effect depends upon the type of meal. A high carbohydrate/low fat meal produces less effect than a medium or high fat meal.

It should be pointed out that most prescription controlled release dosage forms have not been appropriately tested to determine the effect of food on drug administration, since food effect challenge studies are only recent requirements of the FDA.

F. Effect of Diurnal Variation

There are examples in which the pattern of release of controlled release products varies depending upon the time that the product was administered (morning versus evening). The reasons for these diurnal differences are not clear. In some cases they may be simply related to the fact that the evening doses were given with meals. In other cases, however, the effect of meals can be ruled out and changes in GI motility or drug disposition at night may be the factor producing differences. Because of the potential for differences in AUC at different times of the day, it is necessary to sample the entire dosage period when testing a 24-hr product. Also if the product is to be given at night, it is necessary to test the product at night.

G. Increased Variability

The total variability of C_{max} and C_{min} at steady state are a function of all variables including the variability of gut residual, diurnal variation, food effects, variability related to absorption in the lower gut and colon, and dosage form variability. The net affect of all factors associated with controlled release dosage forms demonstrates increased variability of steady-state plasma levels.

Because first order absorption has the disadvantage that absorption half-lives which exceed four times the dosage interval have a gut "residual" (i.e., drug still remaining in the gut at the time

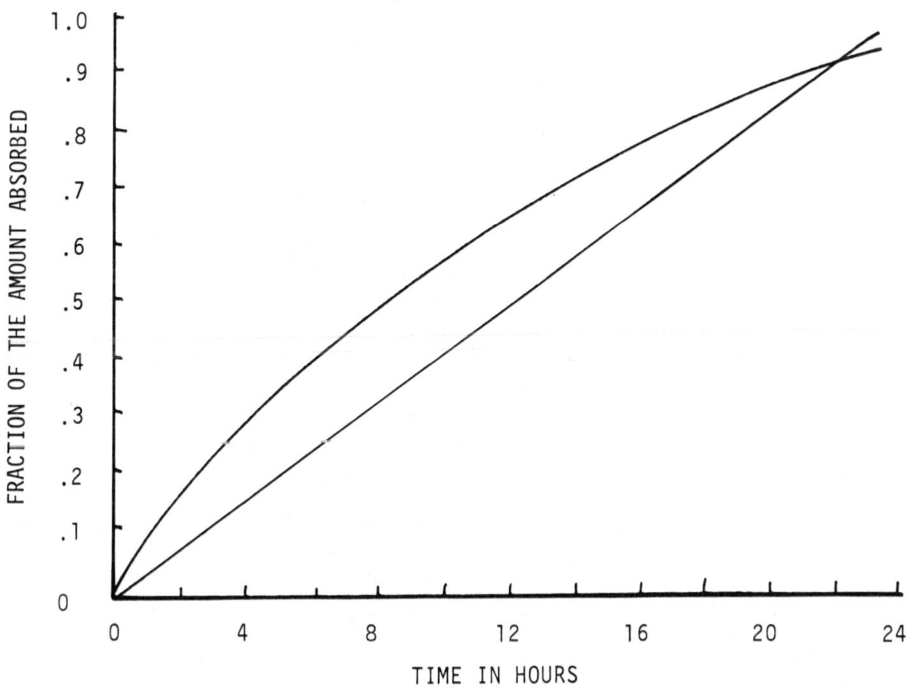

Fig. 3 Fraction of the amount absorbed plot of drug associated with acceptable C_{min} steady-state variation. Fraction of the amount absorbed plot calculated by the Wagner-Nelson Method. Note that, in this simulation based on real data, 95% of the drug dosed is absorbed within the 24-hr dosage interval. The additional 5% will be absorbed within the next dosage interval.

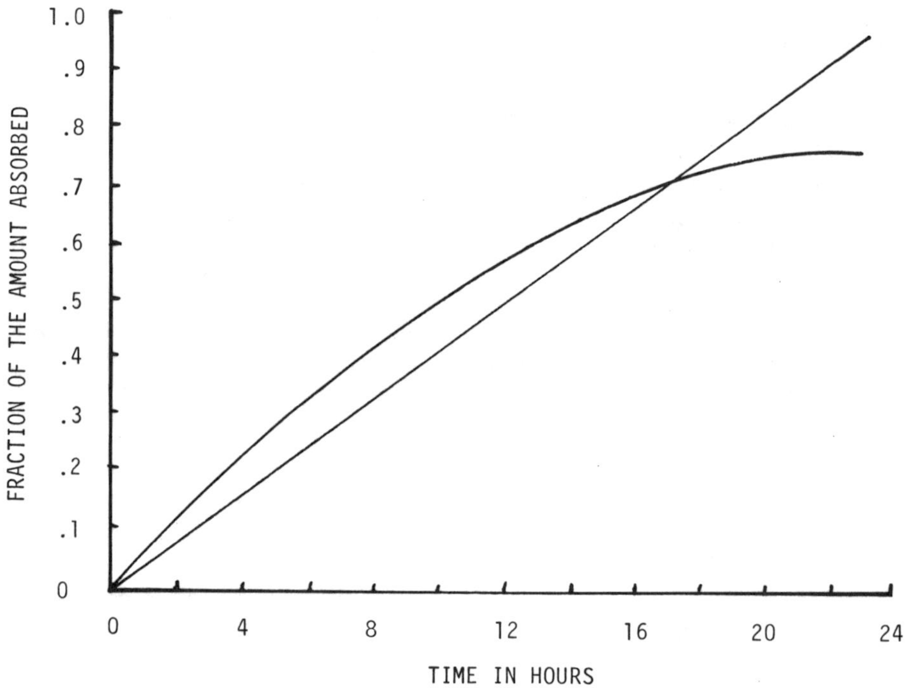

Fig. 4 Fraction of the amount absorbed plot of drug associated with large C_{min} steady-state variation. Fraction of the amount absorbed plot calculated by the Wagner-Nelson Method. Note that, in this simulation based on real data, only 75% of drug dosed is absorbed within the 24-hr dosage interval. The additional 25% will be absorbed in the next two dosage intervals.

the next dose is given), it can contribute to the variability of the dosage form, or decreased bioavailability. While not requiring the use of the Wagner-Nelson [16] and/or Loo-Reigelman [17] calculation as a condition of new drug approval, it is recommended that these or other methods (e.g., deconvolution) be used for calculation of the fraction of the amount absorbed versus time in hours. This enables the determination of the percentage of gut residual remaining to be absorbed during the next dosing interval (or in some cases the next two dosage intervals) (Fig. 3 and 4). The larger the percentage of gut residual, the greater will be the potential for day-to-day variation of blood levels.

VII. DISSOLUTION RATE--ASSESSMENT

In conventional (i.e., immediate release) preparations, drug absorption is usually quite rapid and most often dependent upon the concentration of the drug dissolved in the gastrointestinal fluids. Elimination is usually slower, such that the elimination rate constant K_e is considerably smaller than the absorption rate constant K_a. The purpose of a controlled release preparation, on the other hand, is to deliver drug over a longer time interval so as to maintain sustained drug plasma levels. In fact, for controlled release products, the drug dosage system is designed such that the rate of absorption will be slower than the rate of elimination by reducing the release rate in order to prolong absorption. Models such as this have been called "flip-flop" by pharmacokineticists. Thus, for most controlled release dosage forms, the *in vivo* dissolution and release from erodible tablets, coated beads, undissolving matrices, hydrostatic pumps, etc., becomes the most important, rate-limiting step.

Since controlled release drug dosage forms are exposed to a milieu of varying pH in the gastrointestinal tract (pH approaching 1 in the acid-secreting stomach to a pH approaching 8.0 in the distal section of the intestinal tract), pH becomes a major variable that must be considered in both the design and evaluation process. In addition, since controlled release dosage forms will usually be dosed in the presence of food as well as under fasting conditions, dramatic pH changes as well as the solubilizing influences of both bile and the highly buffered pancreatic secretions, should be considered in the dosage form design and evaluation.

Obviously, these variables can greatly influence the dissolution rate of a controlled release dosage form and present a much more complex situation than that observed with conventional preparations. For example, two quinidine gluconate formulations—one of the innovator brand (BE) and the other a generic version (B-1) which was formulated and marketed without FDA approval—were found to be bio-inequivalent despite identical dissolution characteristics in a dissolution system used by the innovator (Fig. 5) [18]. As shown in Table 4, the unapproved marketed product was only 35% as bioavailable based on peak height (C_{max}) and only 41% based on area under the curve (AUC) [19].

However, using a discriminating dissolution procedure developed by the FDA's Division of Biopharmaceutic's Research Laboratory, this firm formulated a new product (B-2), which was found to provide a dissolution profile virtually identical to the innovator (Fig. 6). Bioavailability studies conducted on this revised formulation showed the product to be bioequivalent to the innovator (Table 5).

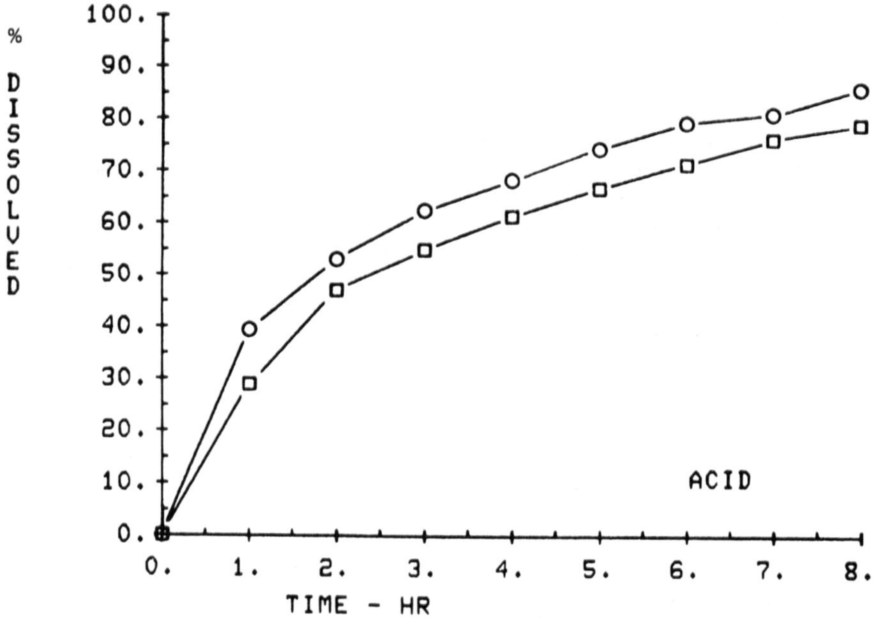

Fig. 5 Dissolution of quinidine gluconate. Dissolution profile of two quinidine gluconate sustained release products in 0.1N HCl dissolution media. Each data point is the mean of 12 tablets. —○— Innovator—Berlex Quniaglute. —□— Dosage form marketed withoud FDA approval.

Table 4 *In Vivo* Data for Quinidine Gluconate Tablet Products[a]

Parameter (BO-1/BE × 100)	BE	Unapproved dosage form (B-1)
Dose	648 mg	648 mg
C_{max} (mcg/ml)	1.26 ± 0.34	0.47 ± 0.13 (35%)[b]
T_{max} (hr)	3.18 ± 1.20	3.51 ± 0.67
AUC (mcg/ml × hr)	15.5 ± 4.81	6.38 ± 2.35 (41%)[b]

[a]Each value is the mean ± SD of 12 subjects.
[b]% Bioavailability relative to BE product.

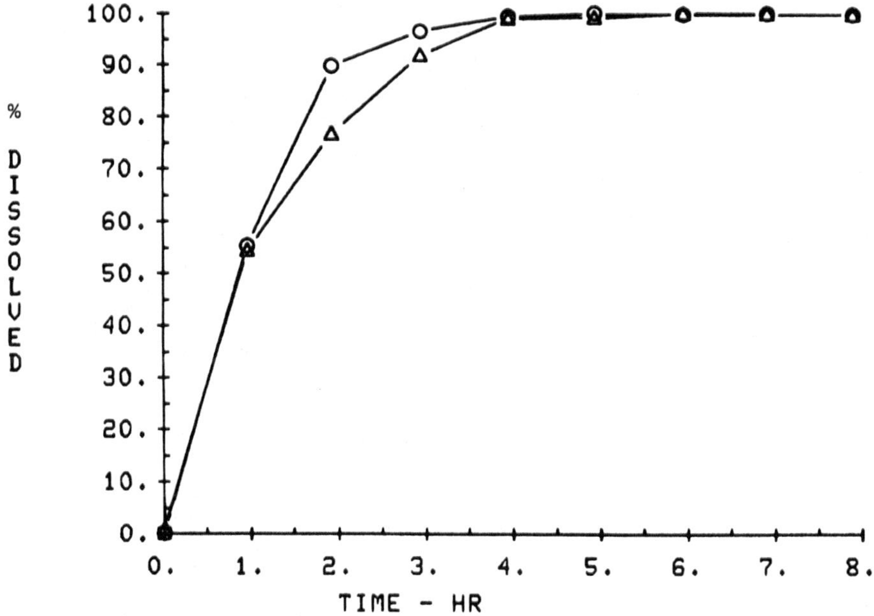

Fig. 6 Dissolution of quinidine gluconate. The dissolution profile of Berlex Quinaglute^R brand of quinidine gluconate and the reformulated generic quinidine gluconate in pH 5.4 acetate buffer (paddle method at 100 rpm). —△— Reformulated approved generic version of quinidine gluconate. —○— Berlex' Quinaglute brand of quinidine gluconate.

Table 5 *In Vivo* Data for Quinidine Gluconate Tablet Products

Parameter	BE	B-2 FDA approved dosage form
Dose	324 mg	324 mg
C_{max} (mcg/ml)	0.52 ± 0.22	0.56 ± 0.18
T_{max} (hr)	6.1 ± 1.65	5.5 ± 1.27
AUC (mcg/ml × hr)	6.23 ± 2.87	6.37 ± 2.67

Each value is the mean ± SD of 20 subjects.

Controlled release products which have virtually the same rate of dissolution over time in the same media are not necessarily equivalent when tested *in vivo*, and in fact may have quite different bioavailability profiles. At that time, it was our conclusion that conventional dissolution testing was not a reliable predictor for all controlled release products. We propose, however, that if the rate of dissolution had been also plotted as a function of pH, the possible lack of equivalence could have been recognized. this is shown as a three-dimensional topographical plot in Figure 7 [20,21].

After an initial rapid dissolution phase, Berlex' Quinaglute exhibits the same gradual increase in the percent dissolved over time previously observed in Figure 5. Since the rate of dissolution was determined at pH 1.0, pH 5.4, pH 6.0, and pH 7.4, the dissolution rate effectively has been characterized as a function of pH. The slight decrease in the rate of dissolution at about pH 4.0, however, is in stark contrast to the topographical dissolution characterization of the unapproved marketed brand (Fig. 8). Although the two products show somewhat similar dissolution characteristics in two dimensional plots in pH 1 for 1 hr followed by pH 7.4 media for

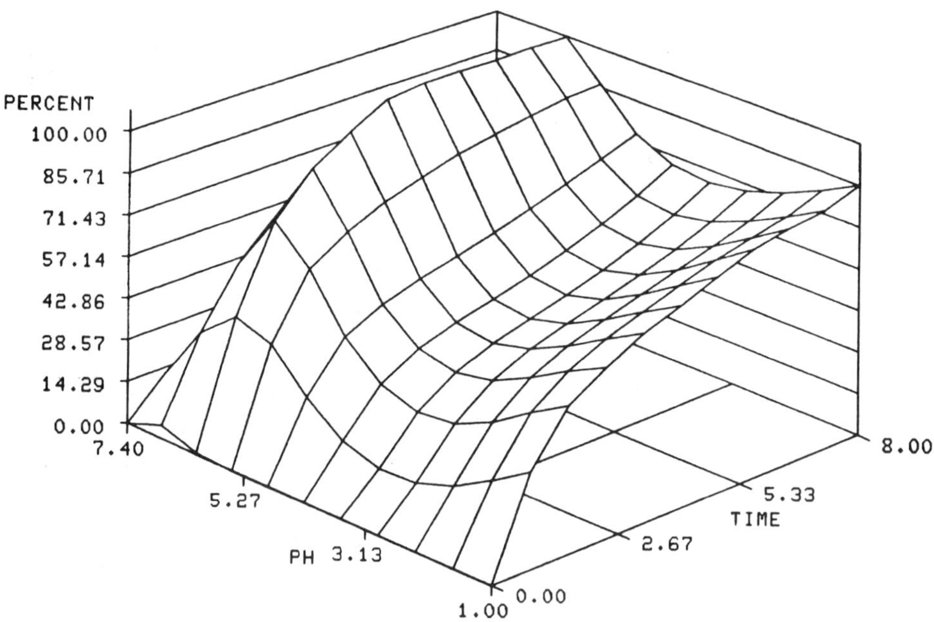

Fig. 7 Topographical dissolution characterization of quinidine gluconate. Topographical dissolution characterization of Berlex' Quinaglute® brand of quinidine gluconate, as a function of time and pH.

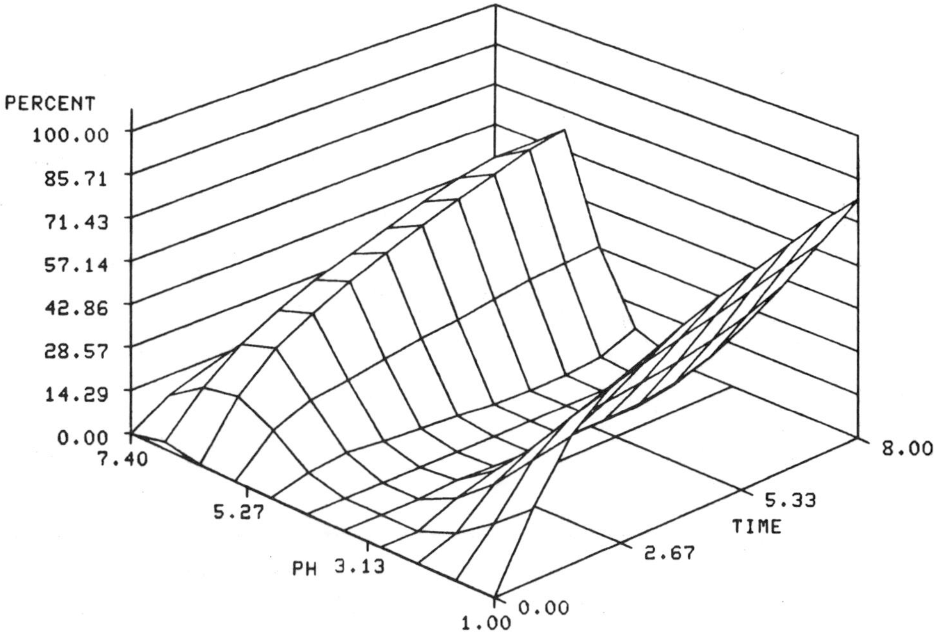

Fig. 8 Topographical dissolution characterization. Topographical dissolution characterization (of an unapproved marketed quinidine controlled release preparation) as a function of time and pH.

7 additional hours (Fig. 5 and Fig. 9), they are clearly not comparable at the intermediate pH values.

It is even possible that for some controlled release dosage forms a good correlation between the rate of *in vitro* release and *in vivo* absorption could be obtained under a specific set of conditions, but not under any other conditions. For instance, the dissolution procedure, which was predictive for drug administered under fasting conditions, would not necessarily be predictive for drug administered with food. Thus, although it is possible to obtain such a correlation for fasted drug administration using 0.1 N HCl as the dissolution medium. This correlation would not hold for drug administered with certain types of food, such as a high fatty meal, because of the effect of bile salts, buffered pancreatic secretions, changes in intragastric pH, and gastric emptying, etc.

Figure 10 shows a topographical dissolution characterization of a controlled release theophylline formulation, which has been shown in single dose studies to have a greater rate and extent of bioavailability when administered with food than when administered under fasted

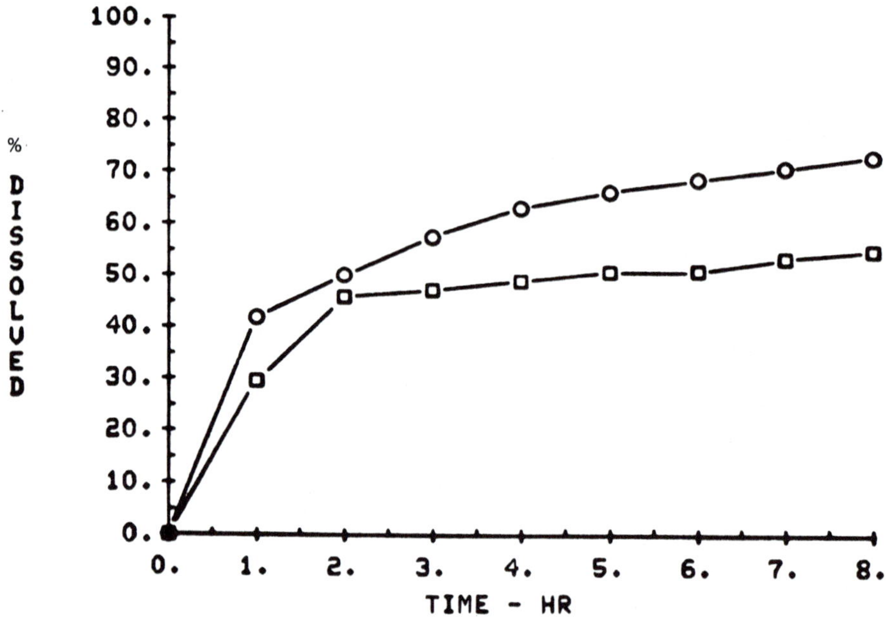

Fig. 9 Dissolution of quinidine gluconate. Dissolution of Berlex's Quinaglute® brand of quinidine gluconate and the 35% bioavailable unapproved, marketed product. Dissolution was conducted in pH 1 media for one hour followed by an additional seven hours in pH 7.4 phosphate buffer using Method 2 at 100 rpm. —○— BE in acid and 7.4 phosphate buffer. —□— BO in acid and 7.4 phosphate buffer.

conditions [14]. The data show that although reproducible 12-hr dissolution profiles were obtained in media with pH less than 6.6, increased rates of dissolution in 8 hr were obtained as the pH of the media was raised incrementally from pH 6.6 to pH 8.0 [22]. This contrasts with the topographical dissolution characterization of another formulation (Theodur® tablets) shown not to be affected by drug administration with food (Fig. 11) [10]. This product shows no significant change in the rate of dissolution as a function of pH. Additional work will be required to determine if these effects can be extrapolated to other products and whether the differences in *in vitro* dissolution-pH profiles is directly related to observed differences in food effects. However, a pH-dissolution profile with a steep gradient such as shown in Figure 10, is diagnostic of potential variability due to the great variability of pH *in vivo*.

The increased complexity of the *in vivo*/*in vitro* association for controlled release drug products compared to conventional release is obvious. While for conventional release solid oral dosage forms *in vivo/in vitro* relationship is usually adequately described by a two dimensional type plot (i.e., the percent dissolved at a time interval versus the amount absorbed), the relationship for controlled release often must be viewed as being multidimensional with pH being one important factor (in the case of orally administered drug).

Such data may be illustrated by Figure 12. Note that increasing dissolution as a function of the speed of paddle rotation (agitation) is not correlated with the absorption process in this example. On the other hand, the *in vitro* rate of dissolution increased as the pH of the media increased. The extent of *in vivo* absorption correspondingly, dramatically increased (reflective of the greater amount in solution at higher pH). Products in which dissolution profiles are rather insensitive to either dissolution RPM or media pH changes may be illustrated by Figure 13 where the rate of dissolution would not be expected to be affected by such change. In employing dissolution results to predict probable *in vivo* bioavailability it would be hazardous to rely upon a single dissolution test. One needs to

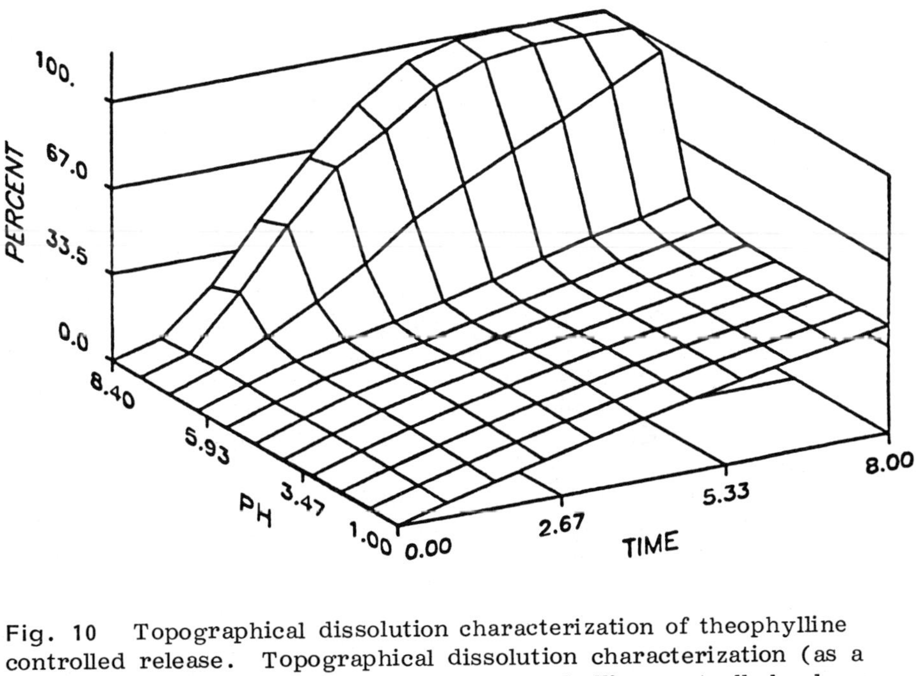

Fig. 10 Topographical dissolution characterization of theophylline controlled release. Topographical dissolution characterization (as a function of time and pH) of Theo-24, a theophylline controlled release preparation, which has been shown to have a greater rate and extent of bioavailability when dosed after a high fat meal than when dosed under fasted conditions.

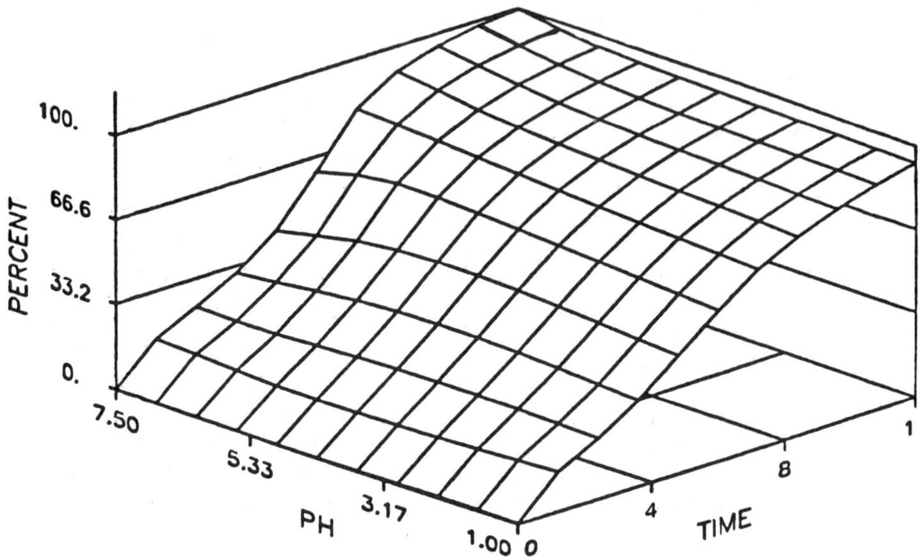

Fig. 11 Topographical dissolution characterization of theophylline controlled release. Topographical dissolution characterization (as a function of time and pH) of Theodur a theophylline controlled release preparation, the bioavailability of which was essentially the same whether administered with food or under fasted conditions.

perturb the system so as to ascertain whether the topographic surface of the important variables is flat or sloping. If the slope is steep, a slight change in dissolution could yield quite unexpected *in vivo* results.

Figure 14 illustrates a more complex relationship wherein the fluctuation within the therapeutic window is related to the apparent half-life of absorption. In the example selected, the rate of dissolution does not change as a function of pH and therefore the media pH affects neither the half-life of absorption or the fluctuation within the therapeutic window. On the other hand, as the half-life of absorption increases from 0 to 24 hr, a bioavailability associated with minimum fluctuation is reached such that a population with specified clearance could be easily maintained within the therapeutic window. As the half-life of absorption is gradually increased above that optimum, the degree of fluctuation within the therapeutic window increases. The relationship between fluctuation and absorption half-life involves a complex interaction between the elimination half-life, the dosage interval, gastric and intestinal transit time, and the half-life of absorption.

Based on the above examples, it is clear that a multifactorial graphical characterization of relevant dissolution variables is a better predictor of *in vivo* performance of a controlled release product than a single dissolution test conducted in a single medium. While not providing the assurance of a single dose or steady-state bioavailability study, this type of characterization can provide reasonable and adequate assurance of lot-to-lot uniformity and bioequivalence characterization of a formulation whose bioavailability and controlled release characteristics have been fully defined. On the other hand, relying on dissolution data obtained from a single medium, as seen in the quinidine gluconate case, can be very misleading.

Once the *in vivo/in vitro* relationship is fully characterized, one should be able to employ dissolution testing in lieu of *in vivo* data for certain regulatory processes, e.g., minor equipment changes, changes of manufacturing process or manufacturing site, etc. If one is operating on a plateau as depicted in Figure 13, assurance is provided that minor changes in one variable are likely to have only a negligible effect on other variables. On the other hand, if one is

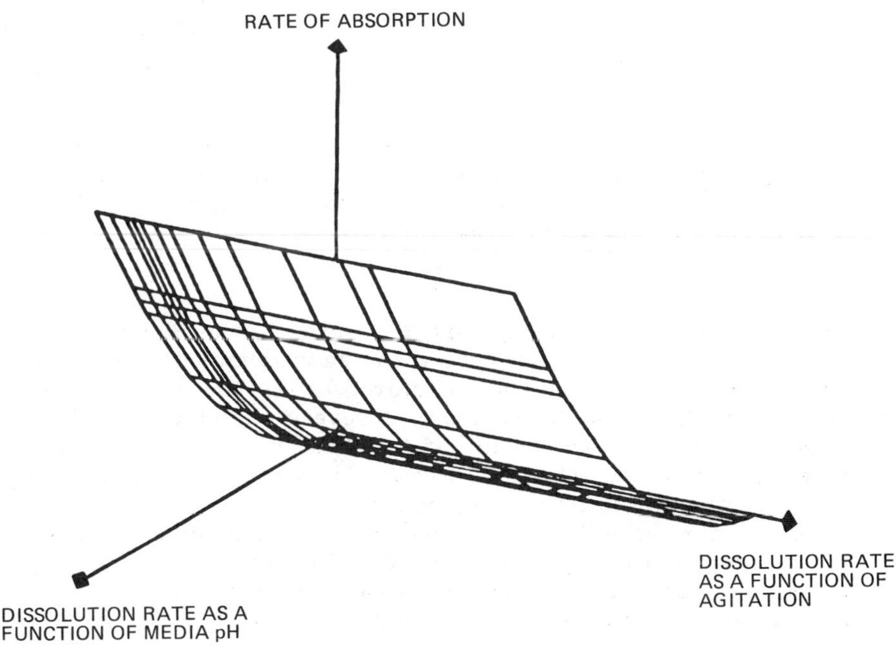

Fig. 12 *In vivo/in vitro* association. An example of a three dimensional *in vivo/in vitro* association for an oral controlled release dosage form where the dissolution rate varies as a function of the pH of the dissolution media.

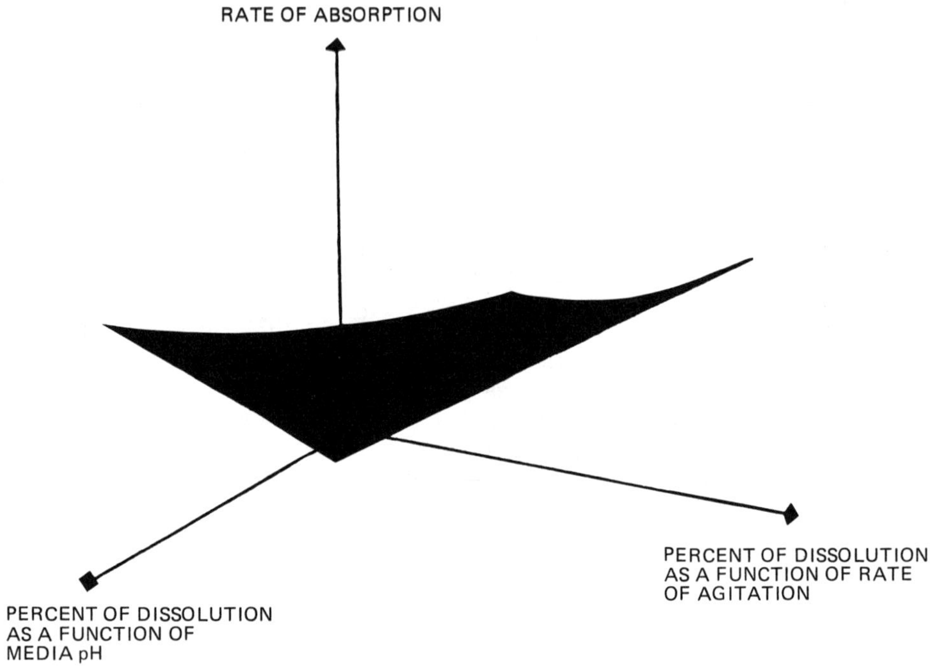

Fig. 13 *In vivo/in vitro* association. An example of a three dimensional *in vivo/in vitro* association for an oral controlled release dosage form where the dissolution rate is independent of both the rate of agitation and the pH of dissolution media.

operating on a slope, as depicted in Figure 12, then duplicative testing of dosage forms (employing the same manufacturing processes and identical formulations) manufactured at the two different sites (e.g., New York and Puerto Rico) at several dissolution media pHs would be required. Obviously, if the dissolution system had not been previously characterized, several tests may be necessary to determine the appropriate, sensitive variables.

Dissolution specifications should be developed for each controlled release product employing the most discriminating media and pH as determined from the topographical dissolution characterization. A dissolution window at one hour should be included in the specification to detect possible dose dumping. Two or three other windows should be provided to assure the controlled release characteristics of the drug. A minimum dissolution specification (about 75 or 80%) should also be provided at the last sampling window. The FDA recommended dissolution specification for phenytoin extended release is a good example [23].

Recently, the USP proposed in its modified release proposal, that dissolution windows be established at 25, 50, and 75% of the dosage interval. Although the authors concur in the desirability of designing such characteristics into new dosage forms, they are aware that many good controlled release dosage forms presently approved for marketing would fail that specification. The USP allows for this by permitting drug products which cannot meet these (case 1) specifications to fall into USP case 2 or 3, which provide for different methods and/or more individualized specifications. Moreover, in a few instances the specification of 25% of a 24-hr dosage interval (i.e., 6 hr) would not necessarily provide assurance against dose dumping. Figure 15 shows that a specification of 20 to 50% dissolved at 25% of the dosage interval for a BID preparation would allow up to 50% of the drug dosage to be dissolved and available for absorption within minutes of dosing.

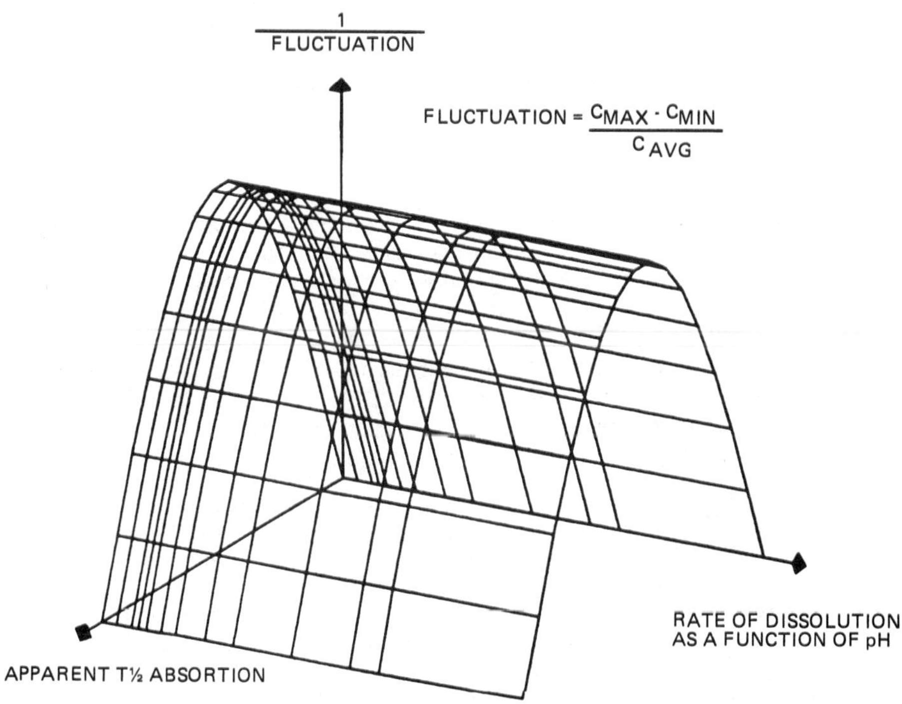

Fig. 14 *In vivo/in vitro* association. An example of a three dimensional *in vivo/in vitro* association for an oral controlled release dosage form where the rate of dissolution is independent of the pH of the dissolution media. Note that the apparent half-life of absorption is related to the *in vitro* dissolution rate and the fluctuation of the drug concentration within the therapeutic window.

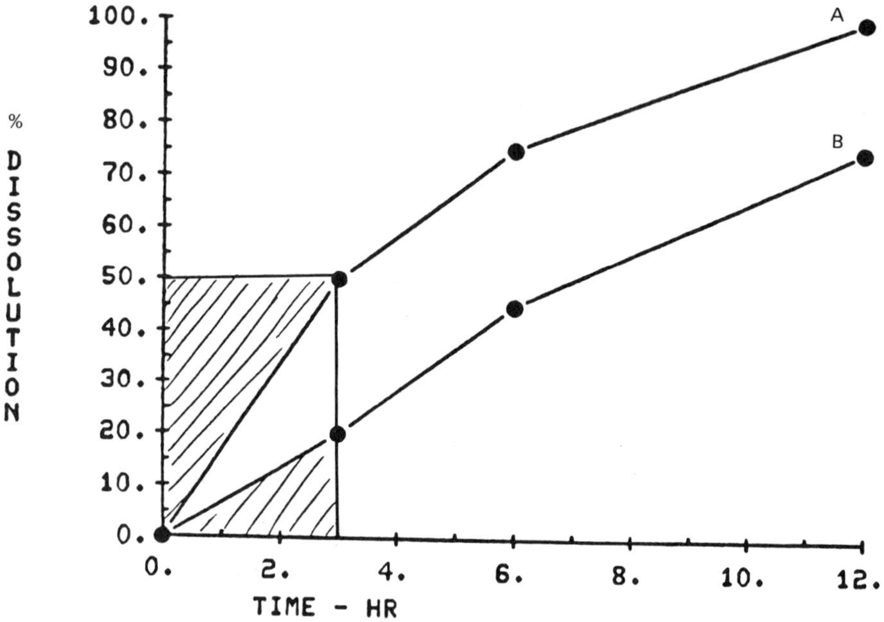

Fig. 15 First interval USP limit on controlled release dissolution. The USP provides for a dissolution specification window which is to be selected on the basis of the dosage interval "Tau." Their specification provides for the first sampling window at 25% of Tau. In this example for a b.i.d. dosage form with a first sampling point window of 20–50% dissolved, note that up to 50% may be dissolved immediately and be available for absorption. (A) USP low, (B) USP HI; dissolution range: Q1 to Q2 (e.g., 20–50).

To ensure against this possibility, the FDA requires that a 1-hr dissolution window should be employed for all controlled release dosage forms.

The USP proposal, as modified, provides for continued testing through three levels unless the results conform at L_1 or at L_1 and L_2 using the following acceptance table (Table 6). This requirement is an important step forward in providing assurance if lot to lot reproducibility.

One of the major problems inherent in present official dissolution methodology, i.e., USP Method I (USP basket), or USP Method II (the former FDA paddle method) for controlled release drug products is that they lack any erodible component. It may be desirable to develop a procedure which allows both erosion and dissolution to be

Table 6 USP Acceptance table

Level	No. tested	Criteria
L_1	6	No individual value lies outside the stated range and no individual values is less than the stated amount at final test time.
L_2	6	The average value of the 12 units ($L_1 + L_2$) lies within the stated range and none is more than 10% of labeled content outside of the stated range; and none is less than the stated amount at the final test time.
L_3	12	The average of the 24 units lies within the stated range and not more than 2 of the 24 units are more than 10% of the labeled content outside of the stated range; not more than 2 of the 24 units are less than the stated amount at final test time, and none of the units is more than 20% of labeled content outside of the stated range, or less than 20% of the stated amount.

tested simultaneously, e.g., for some matrix type tablets which do not readily dissolve, but which are known to release drug in the gastrointestinal tract.

VIII. BIOPHARMACEUTIC CONSIDERATIONS IN THE REGULATORY ASSESSMENT OF CONTROLLED RELEASE PRODUCTS

In order to gain FDA approval of New Drug Applications for a new chemical entity initially marketed in Controlled Release Dosage Forms (as with all other similar products), clinical studies in patients establishing the safety and efficacy of each particular dosage form are required. In addition, as a result of the FEDERAL REGISTER publication of January 7, 1977 on Drug Bioavailability, it is required that the bioavailability of each new dosage form be determined. The pharmacokinetic description of the absorption, distribution, metabolism and elimination of that particular chemical entity in that dosage form, and justification of the dosage regimen recommended in the labeling needs to be submitted.

As with new drugs in conventional dosage forms, data need to be submitted for regulatory approval of a controlled release drug product (or drug delivery system) to substantiate the clinical safety and efficacy (if not otherwise known), of the controlled release product and demonstration of its controlled drug release characteristics.

A. Demonstration of Safety and Efficacy of Controlled Release Drugs

1. For drugs that have been approved by the FDA as safe and effective in conventional dosage forms, the Food and Drug Administration has taken the position that controlled clinical studies may be required to demonstrate the safety and efficacy of the drugs (already approved for use in conventional forms) in the controlled release formulation. For drugs like theophylline where the pharmacolinetic and pharmacodynamic relationship is well defined, they have accepted pharmacokinetic data in lieu of clinical trials. The need for clinical trials is addressed in Section IV. In any case, bioavailability data for the drug)s) in the controlled release formulation are required.
2. For drugs that have been previously approved as safe and effective in controlled release dosage forms, data are required to establish bioavailability comparability to an approved controlled release drug product. In this case, the labeling must be identical to the reference standard with regard to effectiveness and side effects. Without appropriate clinical studies to justify the change, the labeling cannot be modified to make any different claims in clinical effectiveness or side effects.
3. Single dose bioavailability studies are acceptable for determining the fraction of the amount absorbed, lack of dose dumping, lack of food effects, etc. Pharmacokinetic studies, performed under steady-state conditions, are acceptable to demonstrate comparability to an approved immediate release drug product, occupancy time within a therapeutic window, percent fluctuation, etc., and are acceptable for supporting dosage administration labeling.
4. The optimum single dose study would be a three-way crossover comparing a rapidly available dosage form (i.v. solution, oral solution, or a well-characterized FDA approved conventional dosage form), and the controlled release dosage form under fastin conditions with the controlled release dosage form administered immediately after the ingestion of a high fat meal. If there are no significant differences in AUC and PEAK concentrations as a function of the meal, no further food effect studie are necessary. If significant differences were found, it is nece sary to define the cause of the food effect, i.e., does food affect drug release from the dosage form and/or absorption and/o disposition changes (distribution and/or elimination independent of absorption). This may be determined in the absence of liter

ture data by conducting a fed/fasting single dose study employing a solution or immediate release dosage form. The effect of time on the food-drug effect should be tested by conducting a four way, single dose crossover under the following treatment conditions: fasting, drug with a high fat meal, drug one hour before a high fat meal and drug two hours after a high fat meal.

The optimum multiple-dose steady-state design depends on whether data exist to establish that the conventional drug follows linear pharmacokinetics. When existing data establish that the immediate release product follows linear pharmacokinetics, a steady-state study with the controlled release product at one dosage rate (preferably at the high end of usual dose rate range), using an immediate release formulation as the control, must be conducted. Plasma concentrations over at least one dosage interval of the controlled release product should be measured in each leg of the crossover, although it may be preferable to measure concentrations over the entire day in each leg. The controlled release product would be acceptable if it produced the same equivalent AUC (using accepted FDA criteria) as the immediate release product and the degree of fluctuation for the controlled release was comparable to or less than that for the immediate release product. The appropriate measurements would include, of course, unchanged drug and/or major active metabolites.

Where steady-state comparison of the immediate release product at different dose rates is not available or where nonlinearity is exhibited, steady-state crossover studies comparing the controlled release product with the immediate release product at two different dose rates should be conducted (one at the low end of the recommended dosing range and a second at the high end of the dosing range). For each of the comparisons the controlled release product must meet the same criteria in regard to AUC and fluctuation as specified above. If there are significant differences between the controlled release product and the immediate release product at either the high end or the low end of a dosing rate, this data alone would not serve as a basis of drug product approval.

With drugs having a narrow therapeutic index, it might be necessary to carry out more extensive plasma concentration measurements in patients to determine the potential for unusual drug release patterns. In these studies more than one measurement would be made to assess patient variability with both the controlled release and immediate release dosage forms.

B. Submitted Data

Submitted data should provide assurance that:

1. The drug product meets the controlled release claims made for it. If zero-order absorption is claimed, then an appropri-

ately calculated input function should be provided to substantiate that the majority of the input function is zero-order.
2. The bioavailability profile established for the drug product rules out the occurence of dose dumping (especially when dosed with a fatty meal).
3. The drug product's steady-state performance is equivalent to a currently marketed conventional release, or a specified controlled release drug product containing the same active drug ingredient or therapeutic moiety, which is subject to an approved new drug application. Daily dosage must be comparable.
4. The drug product's formulation provides consistent pharmacokinetic performance between individual dosage units.

C. Recommended Reference Standard for Comparative Studies

1. Either an intravenous solution or an oral solution or suspension of the same active drug ingredient or therapeutic moiety. If a suspension is used care must be taken that the suspension itself has adequate bioavailability.
2. A currently marketed, approved, conventional release drug product with defined bioavailability and reproducibility, containing the same active drug ingredient or therapeutic moiety, or
3. A specified currently marketed controlled release drug product with defined reproducible bioavailability, subject to an approved new drug application containing the same active drug ingredient or therapeutic moiety.
4. In some instances (1) or (2) and (3) above may be required.
5. In order to avoid selection of an inappropriate reference, the Director, Division of Biopharmaceutics (or in the case of generic drugs, Director, Division of Bioequivalence), should be consulted before initiating studies.

Bioavailability data consisting of blood levels and/or urinary excretion rate profiles performed under steady-state conditions may be acceptable in lieu of clinical trials, if it can be demonstrated that the blood levels and/or urinary excretion rates are comparable to multiple doses of the same drug in appropriate conventional dosage forms, or to an equivalent dose of the same drug in appropriate controlled release dosage forms. In these cases, the labeling must clearly indicate that the recommended dosing regimen and the claims of effectiveness and side effects are identical with the reference dosage form. Because of the difficulty that may be encountered in frequent urine collection and the validity of urine data, urinary excretion rate profiles, as a condition for bioavailability comparability, should be cleared with the Division Director before protocol approval.

Any labeling claims of clinical advantage, such as greater effectiveness and/or reduced incidence of side effects, must be substantiated by appropriate well-controlled clinical studies. Clinical testing may be required unless there is substantial evidence that the drug's effectiveness is related to the absolute blood level achieved at steady state, rather than the rate of change of drug level.

D. Demonstration of a Product's Controlled Release Nature

It is necessary (where possible) to demonstrate the controlled release nature of a drug from a controlled release formulation by both *in vitro* and *in vivo* methods. Formulators of controlled release drug products are urged to develop reproducible and sensitive *in vitro* methods to characterize the release mechanisms of the controlled release drug products. The *in vitro* test developed should be utilized to access the bioavailability of the controlled release dosage form by "red flagging" possible lot-to-lot *in vivo* performance differences.

1. Biopharmaceutic considerations

While it is generally accepted that the present state of technology does not permit meaningful *in vitro* versus *in vivo* correlations for extended release dosage forms, adequately validated *in vitro* dissolution testing can be developed to facilitate process control and to enable the determination of some of the final product specifications. The Controlled Release Workshop recommended that "to determine the suitability of this *in vitro* test, the relationship of the results obtained with this test to the actual *in vivo* absorption characteristics of the test products should be established in a small group of human subjects."

It recommended that the *in vitro* test was desirable for the purposes of (a) providing necessary process control and stability determinations of the relevant release characteristics, and (b) facilitating certain regulatory determinations and judgments, concerning minor formulation changes, site of manufacturing changes, etc. It recommended: (a) Preparation of at least three dosage formulations with different biopharmaceutic charcteristics (changes in *in vitro* dissolution of these test dosage forms being accomplished by changing only thsse process and component variables that are likely to be varied under normal manufacturing conditions); (b) Development of an appropriate *in vitro* test capable of distinguishing between these formulations; and (c) Determinaation of the absorption characteristics of these formulations in a small group of human subjects. The *in vitro* drug release kinetics of the dosage form intended to be marketed should be characterized as a function of medium pH, rate of agitation, and possibly also medium composition (such as surfactants and bile salts). Since the knowledge of controlled release product *in vitro/in vivo* correlation development and testing is still evolving, alternative approaches to this problem should be explored and should be considered by the Agency on their merits.

The key elements for dissolution are:

(1) Reproducibility of the method
(2) Proper choice of media
(3) Maintenance of sink conditions
(4) Control of solution hydrodynamics
(5) Dissolution rate as a function of pH ranging from pH 1 to pH 8, including several intermediate values, preferably as topographic dissolution characterization.
(6) Selection of the most discriminating variables (media, pH, rotation speed, etc.) as the basis for the dissolution test and specification.

c. The dissolution procedure should establish:
   (1) Lack of dose dumping—indicated by a narrow limit on the one hour dissolution specification.
   (2) Controlled release characteristics—by employing additional sampling windows over time. (Narrow limits with an appropriate Q value system will control the degree of first order release.)
   (3) Complete drug release—indicated by a 75–80% minimum release specification at the last sampling interval.
   (4) Dosage form pH dependence/independence indicated by percent dissolution in water, appropriate buffer, gastric,* and simulated intestinal* fluid.

2. *In vivo* bioavailability data:
   a. General
      (1) Pharmacokinetic profile, including profile of fraction of amount absorbed (Wagner-Nelson, Loo-Reigelman, etc.).
      (2) Bioavailability data—demonstrating either comparability to the reference dosage form(s) with the same labeling, indications, and side effects; or lack of comparability to the reference dosage form. In the latter case data demonstrating safety and efficacy as well as different labeling will be required.
      (3) Where a therapeutic window exists, determination of percent of time the blood level remains in the therapeutic range, i.e., the "therapeutic occupancy time."

---

*Minus enzymes.

(4) Percent of fluctuation $\dfrac{C_{max} - C_{min}}{\left(\dfrac{C_{max} + C_{min}}{2}\right)}$

(5) Reproducibility of *in vivo* performance.

(6) Lack of *in vivo* dose dumping.

(7) Lack of significant food effect.

The controlled release formulation developed should aim to accomplish two important objectives: (1) It should allow a maximum possible percentage of the dose in the formulation to be absorbed; and (2) it should be capable of minimizing patient-to-patient variability.

b. Specific types of *In Vivo* studies

(1) Fasted single-dose studies

(a) For a controlled release dosage form the major concern is the fraction of drug absorbed and the rate of release (i.e., the input function).

(b) The Wagner-Nelson or Loo-Reigelman equation needs to be applied to single dose study data, so as to obtain the fraction of the amount absorbed per unit time where appropriate.

(2) Postprandial study

The conditions of the postprandial study should be the same as for the fasted study except for drug dosing. In this instance, the controlled release product should be administered immediately after the ingestion of a standard breakfast. We recommend 2 medium-sized eggs, 2 strips bacon, toast with butter, 2–4 oz hash brown potatoes, and a glass of whole milk. Subjects should then fast for 4 hr.

(3) Multiple-dose steady-state studies

It is not really possible for a controlled release drug product to be properly evaluated by single dose administration alone. For prescription products there is a need to determine whether the controlled release dosage can achieve well-defined therapeutic plasma levels or that the plasma levels obtained are comparable to those generated by an immediate release dosage form administered to healthy volunteers or patients as labeled.

It should be emphasized that bioequivalence employing exact superimposition of plasma levels need not be domonstrated for purposes of product approval; for by definition, the rate of absorption for a controlled release dosage form will differ appreciably relative to immediate release dosage forms, and may differ from other controlled release dosage forms.

What needs to be established is satisfactory bioavailability and pharmacokinetics to support drug labeling. The following criteria should be met:

(a) Satisfactory steady-state plasma levels should be obtained with the test drug and reference drug in sufficient patients or volunteers to warrant a comparability determination.

(b) Determination of steady state should be established by comparison of C_{min} (trough values) on three or more consecutive days. Fluctuation greater than 15% should be closely examined for food effect, diurnal variation, achievement of steady-state, etc.

(c) Failure to achieve satisfactory steady-state in a large percentage of subjects tested may indicate possible lack of patient compliance, failure of dosage form performance, etc.

(d) Comparison of pharmacokinetic parameters, e.g., C_{min}, AUC values, etc., should be limited only to subjects who achieve steady-state conditions.

(e) Comparison of AUC during a dosing interval is only proper if both the test drug and reference drug are at steady-state.

(f) Where it exists, consideration must be given to the "therapeutic window." One is concerned, at steady state, as to what percentage of time the drug concentration lies within the therapeutic window. The "occupancy time" for each subject and for mean data should be determined.

E. Consideration for Specialized Controlled Release Drug Delivery Systems

In recent years, novel drug delivery systems have evolved which are designed to deliver drugs at pre-defined rates over a prolonged period of time. Included among these are Ocusert®, Oros®, copper and progesterone releasing IUDs, and transdermal systems. All such new drug delivery systems are considered new drugs requiring full new drug applications (NDA) as a basis of drug approval. The studies described previously (omitting food studies for non-oral forms) are appropriate for alternate routes of administration unless an altered biotransformation pattern of active metabolite is observed.

In addition to safety and efficacy considerations, which includes an understanding of the drug input function, plasma blood level oscillation, and the drugs pharmacodynamics, there are biopharmaceutic and pharmacokinetic issues that need to be addressed by the manufacturer such as:

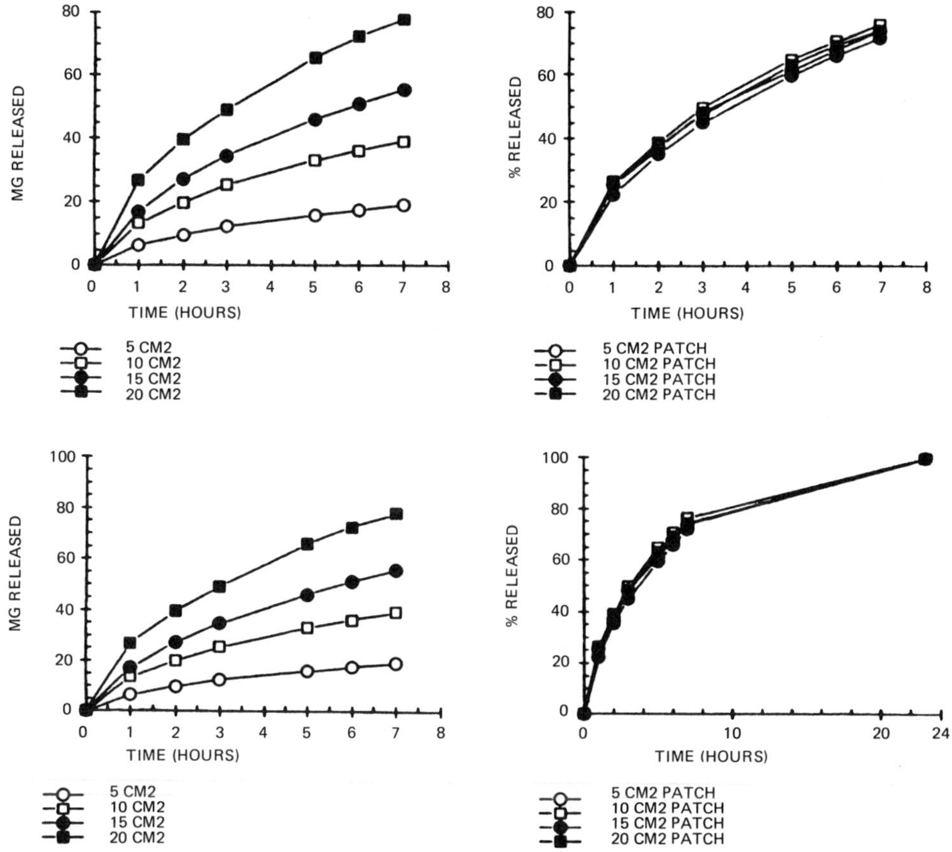

(a)

Fig. 16 (a) Nitroglycerine release from Key patch. (b) Nitroglycerine release from Ciba patch. (c) Nitroglycerine release from Searle patch.

1. Reproducibility of the new drug delivery system by *in vivo* or *in vitro* studies.
2. A defined bioavailability profile which rules out dose dumping.
3. Demonstration of reasonably good absorption relative to an appropriate standard and which considers important elements, e.g., obviating of first pass gut or liver metabolism.
4. A well-defined pharmacokinetic profile to support drug labeling.
5. *In vitro* characterization (where possible).

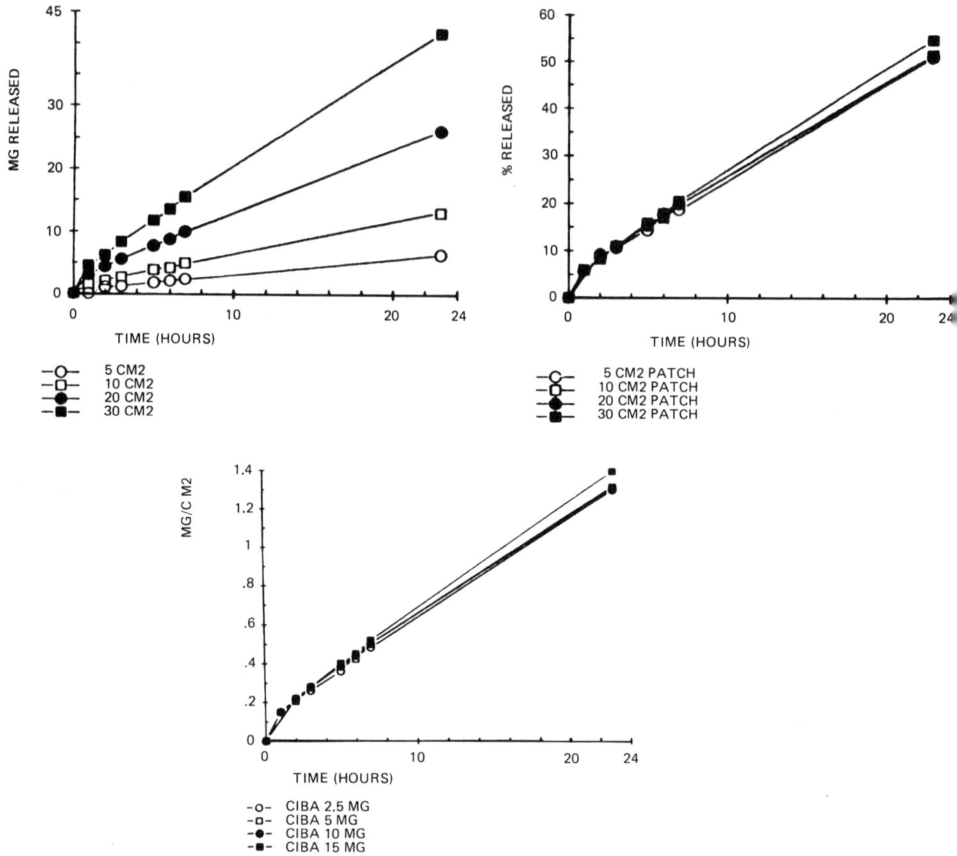

(b)

Fig. 16 (Continued)

The toxicological and clinical requirements for systemically effective dermal-transdermal drugs should parallel other systemic drugs of the same pharmacological class. From a biopharmaceutic point of view, there is a need to define the bioavailability/pharmacokinetics relative to an intravenous dose, ideally, or an oral dose if an I.V. dose is not feasible. As well as defining the pharmacokinetic profile of a new drug delivery system, it is necessary to demonstrate the reproducibility of such systems. This involves both demonstrating the reproducibility of the dosage form as well as drug delivery to the patient. The latter can be achieved by comparison of the blood level profiles of different batches of a new drug delivery system in the same patients or by *in vitro* dissolution testing be used to define

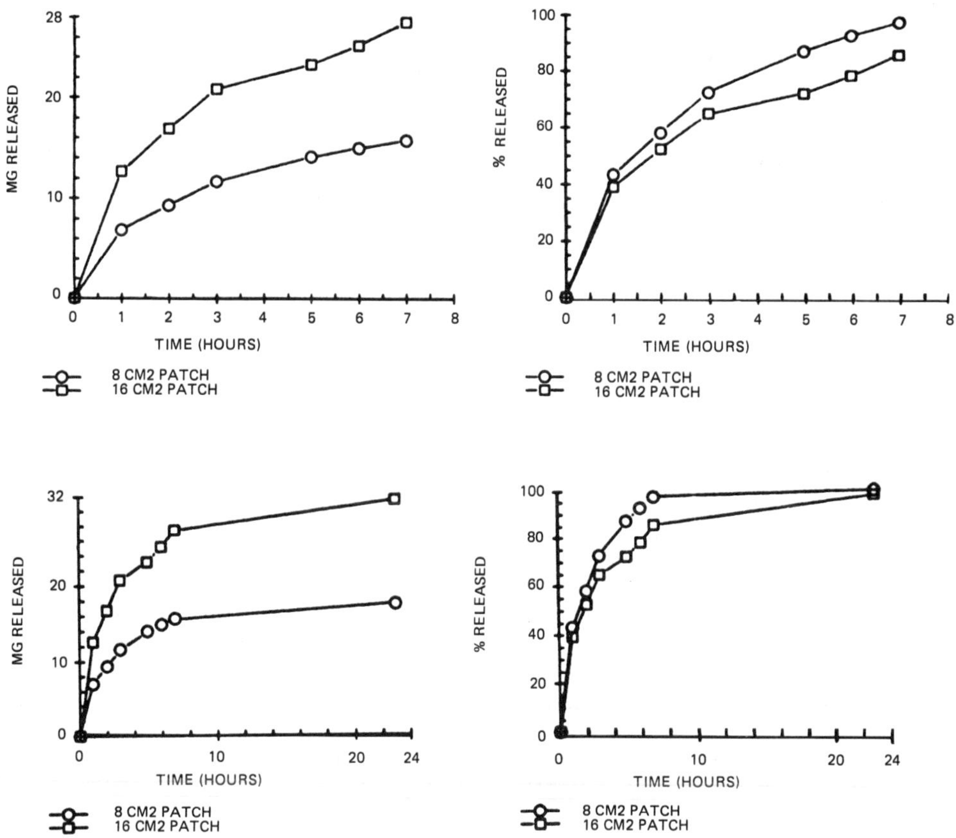

(c)

Fig. 16 (Continued)

reproducibility. FDA's Division of Biopharmaceutics has studied this with its Baltimore District Office and developed satisfactory dissolution procedures for nitroglycerine transdermal patches (Fig. 16a,b,c). The data show consistent dissolution performance among product lines and even establish dose proportional dissolution within the same product line [24].

In summary, the justification for regulatory approval of controlled release formulations of established and new drug entities should be based solely on the scientific documentation for that drug in terms of safety and efficacy. Regulatory approval of a controlled release drug product in terms of bioavailability needs demonstration of the controlled release nature of the product and in many cases may be used in lieu of clinical studies.

ACKNOWLEDGMENT

The authors gratefully acknowledge the contribution of Edward Purich, Ph.D. (formerly Chief, Pharmacokinetics Branch), Vinod P. Shah, Ph.D. (Chief, Science, Management Operations and Policy Branch), and Lawrence A. Yamamoto, Ph.D., all of the Division of Biopharmaceutics, in the preparation of various aspects of this chapter.

REFERENCES

1. USP Modified Release Dosage Form Policy. United States Pharmacopeial Convention publication; 1985-USP XXI, Published by USP, Rockville, MD, 1984.
2. J. P. Skelly and W. H. Barr; Short course in controlled release dosage forms; biopharmaceutic considerations in designing and evaluating novel drug delivery systems, Academy of Pharmaceutical Sciences National Meeting Symposium, Miami Beach, Florida, November, 1983.
3. Controlled Release Dosage Forms "Issues and Controversies" (Sept. 29–Oct. 1, 1985) Cosponsored by Food and Drug Administration, Academy of Pharmaceutical Science, and American Association for Clinical Pharmacology & Therapeutics, Washington, DC.
4. W. H. Barr, Bioavailability of solid oral dosage forms and clinical response to drug therapey, in J. Swarbrick, ed., *Current Concepts in the Pharmaceutical Sciences; Dosage Form Design and Bioavailability*. Lea & Febiger, Philadelphia, 1973.
5. S. S. Davis, Principles and pharmacokinetic applications of external visualization techniques—Use of scintography in the development and optimization of dosage forms; 24th International Industrial Pharmaceutical Conference, Tapatio Springs, Boerne, TX, 1984.
6. J. Gummitt, and R. J. Sawchuk, FDA contract number 223-76-3019,
7. United States Pharmacopeial Convention publications; 1985-USP XXI, published by USP; Rockville, MD.
8. M. A. Osman, R. B. Patel, D. S. Irwin, and P. G. Welling, Absorption of theophylline from enteric coated and sustained release formulations in fasted and non-fasted subjects, *Biopharm. Drug Dispos. 4*, 63–72 (1983).
9. A. P. Sips, R. M. Edelbroek, S. Kulstad, F. A. de Wolff, and J. H. Dijkman, Food does not affect bioavailability of theophylline from Theolin Retard, *Eur. J. Clin. Pharmacol. 26*, 405–407 (1984).

10. N. H. Leeds, P. Gal, A. A. Purohit, and J. B. Water, Effect of food on the bioavailability and pattern of release of a sustained release theophylline tablet, *J. Clin. Pharmacol.* 22, 196–200 (1982).
11. M. Lagas and J. H. G. Jonkman, Greatly enhanced bioavailability of theophylline on postprandial administration of a sustained release tablet, *Eur. J. Clin. Pharmacol.* 24, 761–767 (1983).
12. S. Pedersen and J. Moeller-Petersen, Influence of food on the absorption rate and bioavailability of a sustained release theophylline preparation, *Allergy* 37, 531–534 (1982).
13. S. Pedersen and J. Moeller-Petersen, Erratic absorption of a slow release Theophylline Sprinkle product, *Pediatrics* 74, 534–538 (1984).
14. L. Hendeles, M. Weinberger, G. Milavetz, M. Hill, and L. Vaughan, Food induced "dose dumping" from a once-a-day theophylline product as a cause of theophylline toxicity, *Chest* 87, 758–765 (1985).
15. A. Karim, University of Maryland Third Annual Conference on Current Concepts in Biopharmaceutics and Clinical Trials, Pharmacokinetic and pharmacodynamic considerations in designing bioavailability and clinical efficacy studies, Baltimore, MD, October 2–4, 1984.
16. J. G. Wagner, Wagner-Nelson equation, *J. Pharm. Sci.* 52, 610 (1963).
17. J. G. Wagner, Pharmaceutic absorption plots from oral data alone or oral intravenous data and an exact Loo-Reigelman equation, *J. Pharm. Sci.* 72, 838 (1983).
18. V. K. Prasad, V. P. Shah, P. Knight, H. J. Malinowski, B. E. Cabana, and M. C. Meyer, Importance of media selection in establishment of *in vitro/in vivo* relationships for quinidine gluconate, *Int. J. Pharm.* 13, 1–7 (1983).
19. M. C. Meyer, A. B. Straughn, P. Lieberman, and J. T. Jacob, Serious bioavailability problem with a generic prolonged release quinidine gluconate product, *J. Clin. Pharmacol.* 22, 131–134 (1982).
20. J. P. Skelly, L. A. Yamamoto, V. P. Shah, M. K. Yau, and W. H. Barr, Topographical dissolution characterization for controlled release products—A new technique. *Drug Dev. Ind. Pharm.* 12, 1159–1175 (1986).
21. J. P. Skelly, M. K. Yau, J. S. Elkins, L. A. Yamamoto, V. P. Shah, and W. H. Barr, *In vitro* topographical characterization as a predicator of *in vivo* controlled release quinidine gluconate bioavailability, *Drug Dev. Ind. Pharm.* 12, 1177–1201 (1986).
22. J. P. Skelly, Bioavailability of sustained release dosage forms—relationship with *in vitro* dissolution, Academy of Pharmaceutical Sciences Meeting, Minneapolis, MN, 1985.

23. V. Shah, V. K. Prasad, C. Freeman, J. P. Skelly, and B. E. Cabana, Phenytoin II: *In vitro/in vivo* bioequivalence standard for 100 mg phenytoin sodium capsules, *J. Pharm. Sci. 72*, 309–310 (1983).
24. V. P. Shah, N. Tynes, L. A. Yamamoto, and J. P. Skelly, *In vitro* dissolution profile of transdermal nitroglycerin patches using paddle method, *Int. J. Pharm. 32*, 243–250 (1986).

II

Design and Fabrication of Technology Based Controlled Release Drug Delivery Systems

8

Novel Chemical Approaches for Sustained Drug Delivery

NICHOLAS BODOR and THORSTEINN LOFTSSON* / University of Florida, Gainesville, Florida

I. INTRODUCTION

Optimization of drug delivery by means of chemical modifications of known drugs or their analogs has gained increasing interest during recent years. Commonly two general approaches have been used to

---

*On leave of absence from the University of Iceland, Rekjavik, Iceland.

attain this goal: (a) the design of an analog, which is basically a new drug with new pharmacological and pharmacokinetic characteristics, or (b) the design of a prodrug, which essentially has the same pharmacological features as the lead drug but possesses different pharmacokinectic properties [1-4]. Thus, the promoiety gives the drug new physiochemical properties which may result in increased membrane permeability and higher concentration of the active agent at its site of action. Some of the classical prodrugs have been designed to provide sustained release forms through modification of physical properties, such as solubility and lipophilicity [5,6]. Although originally aimed to improve currently marketed and known drugs, the prodrug approach should become an integral part of early drug design.

The main objective in designing an improved chemical delivery form of a drug should be improvement of its therapeutic index (TI). The therapeutic index (TI) of a drug reflects its selectivity and margin of safety by expressing the ratio between activity and toxicity. It is often defined as the ratio between median toxic dose and median effective dose (TD_{50}/ED_{50}) in which the effective dose refers to its characteristic and most desired therapeutic effect. This apparently simple difinition is, however, much more complex since toxicity is a much more complicated term than activity. Toxicity results from a number of processes and factors. This includes not only all the other pharmacological effects of the drug itself, but the various effects of its metabolites, its reactive intermediates, and various structures resulting from direct interaction between the drug and/or all these other compounds with the cell components. In order to introduce logical steps into a drug design process based on drug toxicity considerations, we must analyze the variety of processes a drug undergoes after its administration as summarized in Scheme 1.

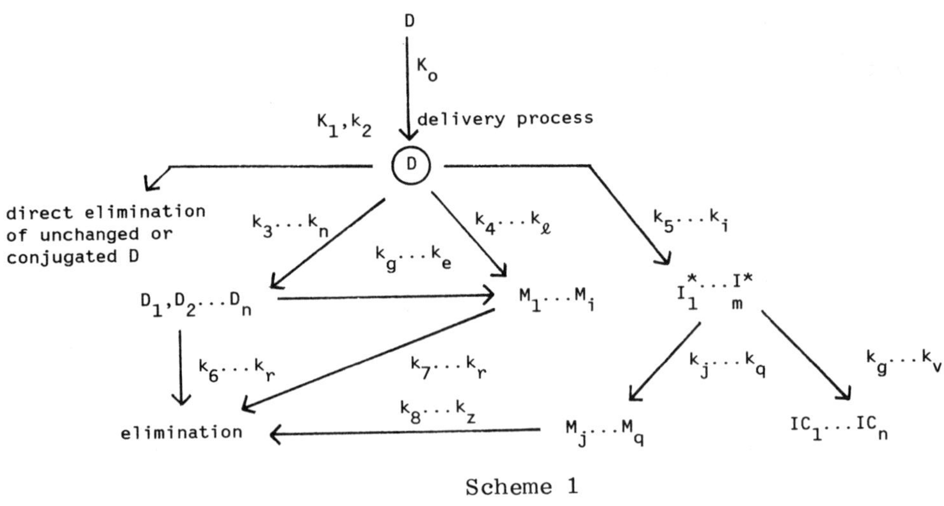

Scheme 1

Thus, following administration a drug (D) can undergo a variety of processes including (a) direct elimination of its unchanged or conjugated form; (b) transformation into structurally close analogs represented by $D_1 \ldots D_n$, which are active metabolites having similar type of activity as the drug itself but with altered pharmacokinetic properties; (c) transformation into metabolites $M_1 \ldots M_i$ having different types of biological activities; and (d) transformation into reactive intermediates represented by $I_1^* \ldots I_i^*$ which can be further metabolized to $M_j \ldots M_g$ or form toxic species like $IC_1 \ldots IC_n$ by reacting with cellular components. The overall toxicity (T) of the drug (D) can now be described as a combination of (a) toxicity due to the drug itself which is essentially its lack of selectivity or intrinsic toxicity (T_i) and (b) toxicity due to various metabolic products. This obviously includes the different selectivities of the active metabolites $D_1 \ldots D_n$, the possible different types of activities of the metabolites $M_1 \ldots M_i$, and toxicities such as carcinogenicity and mutagenicity of the reactive intermediates $I_1^* \ldots I_m^*$. Thus the overall toxicity is

$$T(D) = T_i + T(D_1 \ldots D_n) + T(M_1 \ldots M_i) + T(I_1 \ldots I_m)$$

Intrinsic toxicity is a molecular property and, in most cases, is attempted to be improved by structure-activity (or rather structure-receptor binding) studies. Since intrinsic toxicity includes primarily the selectivity aspect of the compound, it is very much affected by site-specific delivery manipulations, the simplest of which is the obvious alteration of the route of administration. In recent years, however, a number of novel chemical approaches were developed for sustained drug delivery. These methods involve careful design of inactive transport form(s) to be subject to chemical and/or enzymatic processes, resulting ultimately in a rate controlled release of the active drug. The two main directions are prodrugs and the more recent site-specific chemical delivery systems.

II. PRODRUGS

Simple prodrug approaches might alter toxicity-selectivity by changing the pharmacokinetic aspects of drug delivery and by preventing formation of some toxic metabolites. Ideally, a prodrug (PD) is inactive and is transformed into the active drug *in vivo* without substantial direct elimination or unwanted metabolism (Scheme 2). Essentially, prodrugs are designed in such a way that their major, and preferably only, metabolic transformation is the one leading to the active drug ($k_2 >> k_1 + k_3$). The simple prodrug approach, however, even in the best cases, can only optimize the delivery and elimination processes and indirectly affect some other toxicities which are due to specific rate dependent processes, such as saturation of enzymatic reactions.

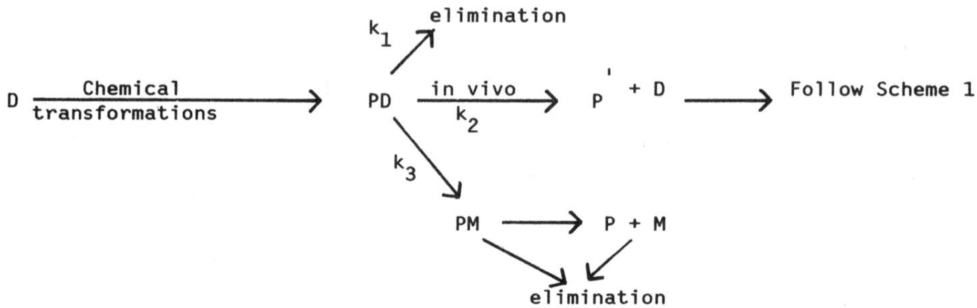

Scheme 2

Prodrugs might effectively reduce some toxicities by protecting the drug from certain unwanted degradations, particularly ones which occur in the gastrointestinal tract prior to and during absorption or possibly during first passage through liver. Several recent reviews on prodrugs discuss these aspects [1,2,7]. It is clear, however, that prodrug manipulations will not substantially influence the formation of active or highly reactive species. Furthermore, simple manipulations cannot affect site specificity of drugs in most cases, although prodrugs can be used to sustain drug release. On the other hand, site-specific, sustained delivery via chemical delivery systems, has great potential to improve the therapeutic index of drugs.

III. CLASSICAL PRODRUGS AS CHEMICAL DELIVERY SYSTEMS

The application of the classical prodrug approach in the design of sustained drug delivery forms has in the past been limited due to various toxicological considerations. There are, however, a few examples where this type of approach has been applied with considerable success, such as injectable suspensions of complexes or salts of penicillins, cyanocobalamin, and insulin, as well as long acting ester-type prodrugs of steroids [5,6].

Many steroids have short biological half-lives and undergo extensive first-pass metabolism when given orally. Esterification of steroids bearing one or more hydroxyl groups has been found to enhance their duration of activity greatly [8]. When such steroid esters are given as intramuscular injections in the form of suspensions or oil solutions, a depot is formed at the site of injection. The rate of drug release from the depot to the general circulation is determined by the physicochemical characteristics of the steroid ester and vehicle composition. Testosterone cypionate (duration of activity 2–4 weeks), estradiol cypionate (duration of activity about 1 week), and medroxyprogesterone acetate (duration of activity about 3 months) are a few examples of such sustained release prodrug delivery systems. These kinds of systems were reviewed recently [6] and will not be discussed in detail in the present paper.

Theophylline is a fairly water soluble compound with good bioavailability when given orally, but theophylline has a rather short biological half-life and narrow therapeutic range (10–20 μm/ml in plasma), which makes plasma concentration monitoring essential. In an effort to overcome these shortcomings, several sustained release prodrugs of theophylline have been designed [9].

Theophylline has only one atom available for reversible modification, the nitrogen in the 7-position. The slow release approach is based on decreasing aqueous solubility and hence dissolution rate by increasing lipophilicity and by decreasing intermolecular forces in the crystals of theophylline by acylating at the 7-position. Unlike other aliphatic and arylamides, 7-acetyltheophylline, the only carefully studies member of this series, hydrolyzes quickly.

The rapid hydrolysis of the 7-acyltheophyllines ensure rapid release of theophylline from the solvated 7-acyltheophyllines. Simultaneously, by using lipophilic acyl portions in the theophylline derivatives, their solubility in water is decreased. Thus, the slow dissolution of the derivatives due to their hydrophobic nature, followed by quick hydrolysis of the theophylline derivatives once they are in solution, results in a slowly released theophylline.

To confirm this hypothesis, some 7-acyltheophyllines were prepared and their dissolution rates were determined. Based on dissolution rates, active component content, toxicity, and stability, the derivative, 7,7-succinylditheophylline (1) was tested further *in vivo*, and some interesting aspects of its chemistry were explored.

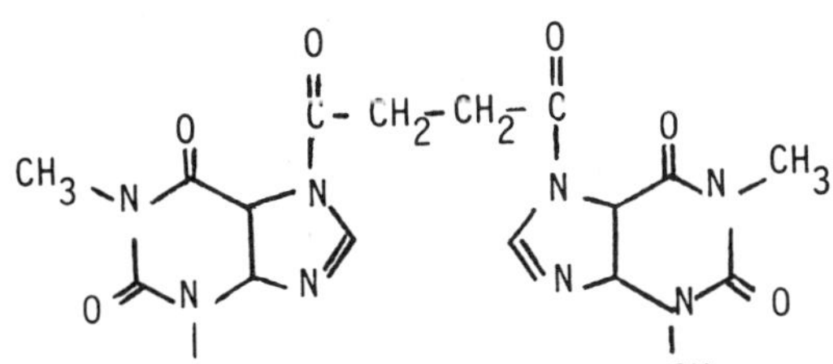

(1)

The dissolution rate of 1 was independent of pH in the range of 2 to 7. Its hydrolysis in solution under these circumstances has a half-life of about 10 sec. Thus, the release of theophylline from the prodrug in the GI tract was independent of pH and only controlled by the dissolution of the solid compound. Dissolution rate with a half-time ranging from 1 to 22 hr was obtained by changing the size of the crystals. After oral administration of the crystalline form with a dissolution half-time of ∿ 4 hr to dogs, therapeutic blood levels of theophylline were observed over 12 hr were observed. Twice a day dosing for four days maintained the plasma levels within the therapeutic range. Despite its very fast hydrolysis rate, prodrug 1 was stable over several years.

Since sustained release is, in this case, a molecular property, the sometime dangerous "dose dumping" observed in formulations based on physical sustained release would not occur. Moreover, due to its low water solubility, a freshly made suspension of 1 is tasteless, providing good patient acceptability.

It should be mentioned that this case is one of the very few prodrug approaches involving chemical and not enzymatic instability of the prodrug. In general, approaches based on chemical reactivity fail to yield successful prodrugs, due to problems of stability in the formulations.

IV. SUSTAINED CHEMICAL DELIVERY SYSTEMS

Chemical delivery systems (CDS) is a more advance step forward from prodrugs in that the drug is transformed into an inactive derivative which will then undergo sequential enzymatic transformations to deliver a drug at its site of action. The emphasis on the several, successive steps will result in optimization of not only drug delivery to a specific site of action, but also of the therapeutic index by effectively isolating the site of action from the rest of the body. By introducing sustained release into the delivery system the therapeutic index can be optimized even further (Scheme 3).

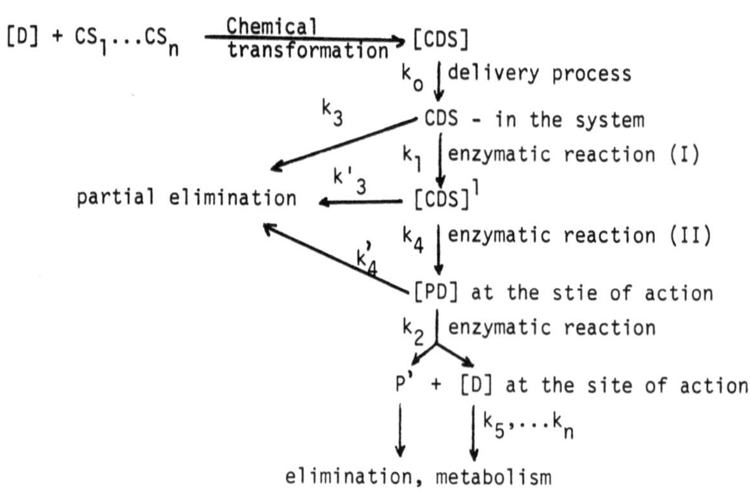

Scheme 3

This rather oversimplified scheme illustrates a chemical delivery system where $CS_1 \ldots CS_n$ represent certain chemical carriers or transient derivatizing groups which are successivley hooked to the drug (D). The resulting chemical delivery system will then, via a succession of enzymatic reactions, release the drug at the desired site of action while the intermediate transient derivatives are all inactive and will effectively result in the ultimate separation of activity and toxicity. By careful manipulation of the steric and electronic features of the chemical delivery system, the rate of various enzymatic reactions can be controlled. Thus, site specificity can be obtained when the rate of elimination from the general circulation (k_3 and k'_3) is faster than the rate of elimination of the precursor (PD) at the site (k_2 and k_4) of action ("lock-in" mechanism). The concentration of drug at the site of action and the duration of pharmacological effect are controlled by k_2,k_4 and k_5. Specific examples which will clarify this general approach will follow.

V. SUSTAINED DELIVERY OF NATURAL SOFT DRUGS

Endogenous substances, such as steroid hormones (hydrocortisone, progesterone, testosterone, estradiol) or neutotransmitters (dopamine, GABA and others) can be considered natural soft drugs [10–12], since the body has developed efficient and fast metabolic systems for their elimination without going through highly reactive intermediates. Thus, their metabolism is predictable and, if they are used at concentrations close to their normal levels, they will not cause unexpected toxicity. The metabolism of these compounds is often so fast that they cannot be used efficiently as drugs. This situation can possible be controlled by a prodrug-soft drug or CDS-soft drug combination. Although hydrocortisone is an endogenous glucocorticoid, its topical applications that result in higher than normal *in vivo* levels of hormone frequently cause side effects such as dermal atrophy, thymus involution, and separation of adrenal, hypothalamus and pituitary functions [14]. Formulations of hydrocortisone or its derivatives that merely increase the efficiency of their delivery cannot realistically be expected to alleviate these side effects. Improved separation of activity from toxicity (improved selectivity) should result from a derivative of hydrocortisone that is inactive itself, i.e., a prodrug, but accumulates in the skin and hydrolyzes slowly to give the parent drug at such a rate that the rate of systemic metabolism of the parent drug to inactive, easily excreted substances more closely matches the rate of release of the parent drug from the skin. These objectives were achieved using 3-spirothiazolidine derivatives such as the compounds described by formula 2 in Table 1 [15].

Table 1 Synthesized Hydrocortisone 3-Spirothiazolidines

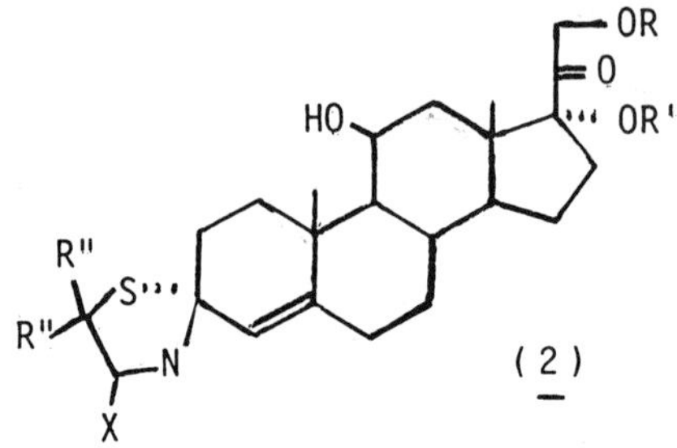

(2)

CH	X	R	R'	R''
2a	$CO_2C_2H_5$	$COCH_3$	H	H
2b	H	$COCH_3$	H	H
2c	H	H	H	H
2d	$CO_2C_2H_5$	H	H	H
2e	$CO_2C_2H_5$	H	COC_4H_9	H
2f	$CO_2C_2H_5$	H	COC_2H_5	H
2g	H	H	COC_3H_7	H
2h	H	H	COC_2H_5	H
2i	H	H	$COCH_3$	H
2j	$CO_2C_2H_5$	H	$COCH_3$	H
2k	$CO_2CH_2CH_2OH$	$COCH_3$	H	H
2l	$CO_2C_2H_5$	$COCH_3$	H	CH_3
2m	$CO_2C_{10}H_{21}$	$COCH_3$	H	H
2n	$CO_2C_6H_{13}$	$COCH_3$	H	H
2o	$CO_2C_4H_9$	$COCH_3$	H	H
2p	CO_2CH_3	$COCH_3$	H	H

These types of compounds, by eliminating the 2,3-unsaturated 3-ketone group, lack specific hydrocortisone binding and affinity properties. Several derivatives of hydrocortisone 21-acetate (4), were tested for their topical antiinflammatory activity, and the results of their relative potency to hydrocortisone are given in Table 2. Hydrocortisone 17-butyrate (5) was included to confirm the relative potencies.

It is evident that spirothiazolidines of hydrocortisone acetate are about 3–4 times more potent than hydrocortisone or six- to eightfold over the corresponding hydrocortisone acetate, implying that hydrocortisone itself is somehow better released locally at the site of action and in a more sustained fashion. The thymus involution studies on selected compounds such as the simple 2a indicate that the spirothiazolidine derivative has less systemic side effect than hydrocortisone or hydrocortisone acetate, as shown in Table 3, implying a lower systemic delivery of the active species. In other words, the chemical delivery system of this type somehow enhances local but reduces systemic delivery of the active species. Indeed, as shown in Table 4, significantly less hydrocortisone is delivered transdermally when using the spirothiazolidine (2a) than with hydrocortisone or hydrocortisone 21-acetate. The overall result using this chemical delivery system for hydrocortisone is a three- to fourfold decrease in the anitiinflammatory ED_{50} and about a twofold reduction in the toxicity-selectivity (thymus involution). Even local toxicity, as reflected by skin atrophy, was reduced, as shown in Table 5. The improvement in the therapeutic index can thus be considered to be about 10-fold. The activity enhancement observed in the animal studies was also confirmed in the blanching studies using human volunteers [15].

Based on these results as well as the mechanism of stepwise hydrolysis of the thiazolidone ring to deliver the active 3-keto derivative [16,17], the enhanced local activity and reduced systemic toxicity can be explained by binding of the intermediate 6, through a disulfide bond, to skin components. This is shown in Scheme 4. The bound 7 which now serves as the final form of the delivery system will release the active hydrocortisone upon hydrolysis. This local binding in the skin was confirmed by a similar type of behavior of the thiazolidine of progesterone (see below).

Similar types of derivatives for testosterone and progesterone were also synthesized (see Table 6) [18]. In both cases, the double bond initially situated between carbons 4 and 5 can migrate during synthesis and thus some of the 5–6 double-bond analogs were also obtained. It was found that the rate of hydrolysis and the regeneration of the active species are significantly slower from the 5–6 analogs than from the 4–5. Also, in the case of progesterone, bisthiazolidines, as represented by 9, were also obtained besides the 3-spirothiazolidines 10.

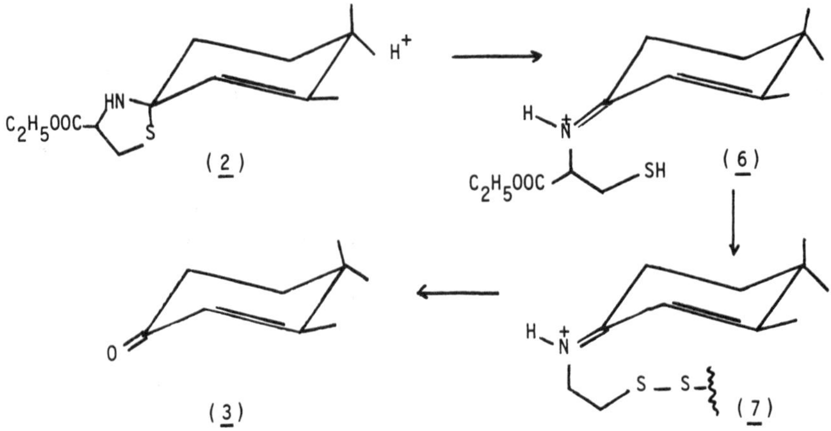

Scheme 4

Pharmacological studies indicate that none of the progesterone derivatives, when given orally or subcutaneously, had more than one-tenth the activity of a subcutaneous dose of progesterone in the Clauberg test. In contrast, one derivative of testosterone, 8i, was found to be more active than the parent steroid as shown in Table 7.

The lack of activity of the progesterone derivatives can be attributed to their relatively slow plasma hydrolysis. The associated half-lives ranged from 15 hours for the mono and up to 160 hours for the bisthiazolidines. However, these derivatives have other potential use, for instance, as a possible antiacne preparation (19). For this reason, 9a was applied topically to hairless mice, and the residence time of the steroid in the skin was studied as compared to progesterone which has shown activity in controlling acne [20]. The results of the *in vivo* study indicate the remarkable tendency of the thiazolidine 9a to increase the relative amount of labelled steroid in the skin. Probably, disulfide bond formation involving the intermediate iminium salt enhances residence time and concentration of the progesterone derivative in the skin and simultaneously reduces transdermal drug delivery. The results are shown in Table 8.

Very interesting results for the distribution of the thiazolidine derivatives were obtained when two of the progesterone derivatives were injected into the tail veins of rats. As shown in Table 9, a very significant portion of the dose was concentrated in the lung as compared to the distribution of progesterone. The reason for the high concentration can be related to the fact that in a number of species (rabbit, rat, and hamster), the mixed function oxygenase activity is at least one order of magnitude higher in the lung than in the liver—the proposed disulfide bond-type binding of these compounds involves oxidation.

Table 2 Relative Antiinflammatory Activity of Selected Cystein Based 3-Spirothiazolidine Derivatives of Hydrocortisone[a]

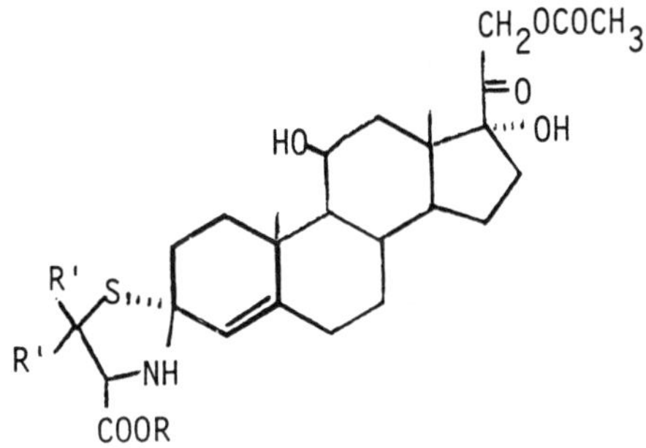

Nr	R	R'	$ED_{50}(M)$[b]	Relative potency to hydrocortisone
2p	CH_3	H	0.0035	3.1
2a	CH_2H_5	H	0.0033	3.2
2o	CH_4H_9	H	0.0027	4.0
2n	C_6H_{13}	H	0.0039	2.7
2m	$C_{10}H_{21}$	H	0.0036	3.0
2h	C_2H_5	CH_3	0.0055	1.9
3	Hydrocortisone		0.0107	1.0
4	Hydrocortisone 21-acetate		0.0203	0.5
5	Hydrocortisone 17-butyrate		0.0011	10.0

[a]The test compounds were applied in acetone solution containing 2% croton oil on the anterior and posterior surfaces of the right ear of mice. Three hours later, the mice were sacrificed and both ears were removed. Circular sections were punched out and drug effect expressed as percent inhibition inflammation compared to the control.

[b]Linear regression analysis of data obtained at 3×10^{-5}, 3×10^{-4}, 3×10^{-3}, and 3×10^{-2} M.

Table 3 Thymus Involution in Rats after Topical Application of Steroids[a]

Compound	mg of thymus / 100 g of rat ± S.D.	% Reduction in thymus[b]
Blank[c]	268 ± 25	–
Vehicle	257 ± 59	–
Hydrocortisone	168 ± 30	35
Hydrocortisone 21-acetate	167 ± 18	35
2a	204 ± 20	21
5	206 ± 20	20

[a]All compounds were administered in a total of 50 μl as a 0.03 M acetone/isopropyl myristate (90:10) solution to 10 rats, each.

[b]Compared to vehicle.

[c]Untreated rats.

Table 4 Steroid Diffusion Through Fresh Hairless Mouse Skin

Compound[a]	Mole % hydrocortisone[b] diffused ± S.D.[c] (hr after application)				
Hydrocortisone (3)		2.1 ± 0.8 (4)	4.1 ± 1.3 (9)	7.5 ± 1.8 (18)	8.4 ± 3.0 (24)
Hydrocortisone 21-acetate (4)		1.7 ± 0.6 (4)	3.5 ± 1.3 (9)	6.2 ± 1.3 (18)	14.1 ± 5.9 (24)
Thiazolidine (2a)	0.1 ± 0.05 (2)	0.6 ± 0.1 (4)	1.2 ± 0.2 (7.5)	1.8 ± 0.3 (12)	3.2 ± 0.7 (24)

[a] 50 μl of 0.03 M acetone isopropyl myristate 90:10 was applied to the membranes.

[b] Only hydrocortisone was found on the receptor side of the membrane under HPLC conditions where hydrocortisone 21-acetate could have been detected. Samples for thiazolidine 2a were split and one-half was analyzed directly while the other half was treated with acid to hydrolyze any intact thiazolidine; there was no observable difference in the two results.

[c] $n = 3$.

Table 5 Ear Thinning in Mice after Application of Steroids[a]

Compound	Concentration (M)	Ear thickness ± S.D.[b]				% Reduction in ear thickness[c]
		First day		Fifth day		
		Left	Right	Left	Right	
Hydrocortisone	3×10^{-3}	86 ± 5	86 ± 5	70 ± 4	89 ± 4	18.6
	1×10^{-3}	86 ± 5	86 ± 5	76 ± 4	88 ± 3	11.6
	3×10^{-4}	88 ± 6	88 ± 7	83 ± 6	91 ± 3	5.7
Hydrocortisone 21-acetate	3×10^{-3}	90 ± 7	87 ± 5	81 ± 6	86 ± 5	10.0
	1×10^{-3}	87 ± 4	84 ± 3	79 ± 5	83 ± 3	9.2
	3×10^{-4}	88 ± 3	87 ± 4	80 ± 5	83 ± 6	9.1
Thiazolidine (2a)	3×10^{-3}	88 ± 6	90 ± 6	82 ± 4	87 ± 6	6.8
	1×10^{-3}	87 ± 4	86 ± 5	78 ± 3	88 ± 7	10.3
	3×10^{-4}	89 ± 7	90 ± 7	84 ± 5	88 ± 6	5.6

Hydrocortisone 17-butyrate (5)	1×10^{-3}	90 ± 4	92 ± 5	69 ± 4	86 ± 4	23.3
	3×10^{-4}	91 ± 5	90 ± 7	75 ± 4	87 ± 5	17.6
	1×10^{-4}	90 ± 5	89 ± 6	78 ± 5	90 ± 3	13.3
	3×10^{-5}	89 ± 6	89 ± 7	83 ± 7	89 ± 4	6.7
Hydrocortisone 17-valerate	3×10^{-3}	89 ± 5	88 ± 6	68 ± 3	82 ± 4	23.6
	1×10^{-3}	87 ± 5	89 ± 5	72 ± 4	88 ± 6	17.2
	3×10^{-4}	88 ± 5	88 ± 8	75 ± 7	89 ± 7	14.8
Triamcinolone acetonide	3×10^{-4}	87 ± 4	89 ± 6	66 ± 3	86 ± 5	24.1
	1×10^{-4}	84 ± 4	88 ± 6	70 ± 5	85 ± 5	16.7
Vehicle		90 ± 7	92 ± 5	91 ± 4	88 ± 4	–

[a] Left ears treated for 4 days with 10 μl of the steroid solution.

[b] 1×10^{-4} inches.

[c] $\% \text{ Reduction in thickness} = \dfrac{100 \times \text{thickness of left ear (day 1)} - \text{thickness of left ear (day 5)}}{\text{thickness of left ear (day 1)}}$

Table 6a Thiazolidines of Testosterone

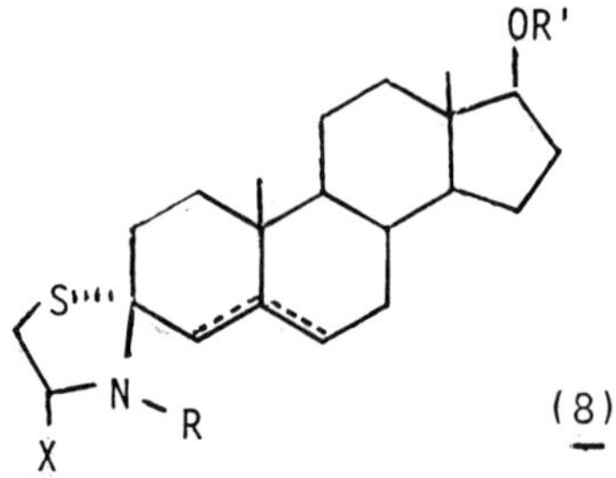

(8)

Compound	X	R	R'	Δ
8a	$CO_2C_2H_5$	H	COC_2H_5	5,6
8b	$CO_2H_2H_5$	H	COC_2H_5	4,5
8c	$CO_2C_2H_5$	H	H	5,6
8d	$CO_2C_2H_5$	H	H	4,5
8e	$CO_2CH_2CH_2OH$	H	COC_2H_5	5,6
8f	$CO_2CH_2CH_2OH$	H	H	5,6
8g	H	H	COC_2H_5	5,6
8h	H	H	H	5,6
8i	H	CH_3	H	5,6

Table 6b   Thiazolidines of Progesterone

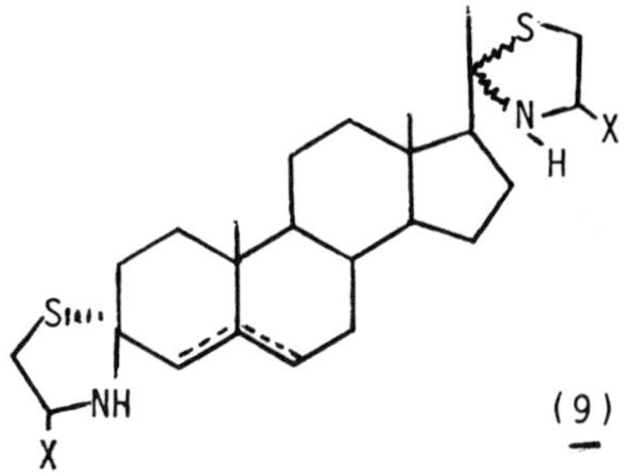

(9)

Compound	X	Δ
9a	$CO_2C_2H_5$	5,6
9b	$CO_2C_2H_5$	4,5
9c	$CO_2C_4H_9$	4,5
9d	$CO_2C_6H_{13}$	4,5:5,6(1:1)
93	$CO_2C_{10}H_{21}$	4,5

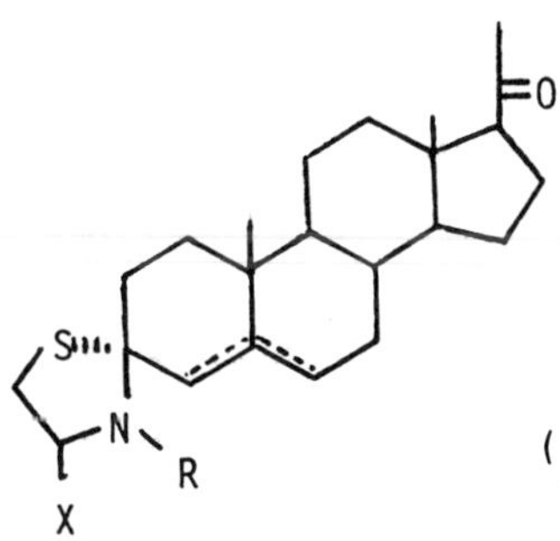

(10)

Compound	X	H	Δ
10a	$CO_2C_2H_5$	H	5,6
10b	$CO_2C_2H_5$	H	4,5
10c	H	H	5,6
10d	H	COCH	5,6
10e	H	$COCH_3$	5,6
10f	H	$COCH_2NHCO_2CH_2C_6H_5$	5,6
10g	H	CH_3	5,6

Table 7 Androgenic Test[a]

Compound	Total dose (mg)	Seminal vesicle weight (mg)	Ventral prostate weight (mg)
Testosterone	16.0	14.0 ± 2.0	38.5 ± 2.5
2i	32.0	13.4 ± 1.2[b]	45.7 ± 2.0
	64.0	28.9 ± 3.2	67.1 ± 2.5
	4.0	8.2 ± 0.4	39.9 ± 1.9
8i	8.0	8.9 ± 0.6	45.7 ± 2.5
	16.0	15.8 ± 0.8	50.9 ± 3.4
Vehicle		6.4 ± 0.3	8.3 ± 0.5

[a]The compounds were given orally as a suspension in sesame oil daily for 10 days starting on day of castration using 10 rats/dose.

[b]Unusually low value compared to data at same concentration in all other control experiments (17.0 ± 1.7 mg).

Table 8 Dermal Delivery of Progesterone and Its Derivative (9a)

	% Dose, mean ± SE[a]	
	Progesterone[b]	9a[c]
Feces	16.55 ± 1.75	0.95 ± 0.13
Urine	7.00 ± 1.14	0.40 ± 0.09
Skin circle[d]	1.98 ± 0.10	4.52 ± 1.18
Intestine/fat	2.28 ± 0.47	0.09 ± 0.00
Liver	0.75 ± 0.06	0.08 ± 0.01
Blood	0.08 ± 0.02	0.28 ± 0.04
Kidney/spleen	0.06 ± 0.01	0.03 ± 0.01
Lung	0.04 ± 0.02	0.01 ± 0.00
Subtotal	28.74	6.36
Patch[e]	54.06 ± 1.6	83.46 ± 1.4
Total	82.80	89.82

[a] $n = 6$.

[b] 75 µl of a solution of 0.9 mg in 675 µl in ethanol-isopropyl myristate (90:10).

[c] 75 µl of a solution of 1.85 mg in 675 µl ethanol-isopropyl myristate (90:10).

[d] 2-cm diameter plug of epidermis taken directly under the bandage patch (3 cm^2).

[e] Includes the contents of an ethanolic wash of the skin after the bandage patch was removed.

Table 9 Distribution of [4-^{14}C] Progesterone, 9a and 9d in Rats[a] 1 Hr After Intravenous Administration

Compound	Dose (mg/kg)[b]	Equivalents of progesterone (mg/kg)	Organ	% Dose/organ (Mean ± SE)
Progesterone	0.98	0.98[c]	Liver	16.25 ± 1.33
			Lung	0.50 ± 0.07
			Blood	2.91 ± 0.39
			Feces	35.15 ± 2.97
9d	2.21	1.01[c]	Liver	14.22 ± 1.13
			Lung	79.22 ± 4.14
			Blood	3.55 ± 0.51
			Feces	0.24 ± 0.06
9a	1.96	1.07[c]	Liver	14.39 ± 1.38
			Lung	60.73 ± 1.12
			Blood	2.07 ± 0.49
			Feces	2.39 ± 0.27
9a	0.135	0.074[c]	Liver	40.57 ± 1.56
			Lung	22.15 ± 1.62
			Blood	18.56 ± 2.68
			Feces	16.18 ± 4.5
9a	0.143	0.078[d]	Liver	34.41 ± 2.14
			Lung	20.20 ± 1.76
			Blood	5.49 ± 0.56
			Feces	5.69 ± 0.94

[a] $n = 6$.

[b] 5 μl benzyl alcohol vehicle.

[c] Activity of progesterone, 1 μCi/mg.

[d] Activity of progesterone, 9.47 μCi/mg, $n = 4$.

VI. BRAIN-SPECIFIC SUSTAINED CHEMICAL DELIVERY SYSTEMS

The delivery of drugs to the brain is often actively limited by transport and metabolic factors intrinsic to the blood-brain barrier (BBB) [21]. Roughly speaking, the ability of a given molecule to penetrate the blood-brain barrier is a function of its partition coefficient. Due to this and to the fact that the rate of entry is much slower than the rate of elimination from the cerebral spinal fluid, highly ionized and/or lipophobic compounds fail to achieve a cerebral spinal fluid/plasma ratio of unity, unless actively transported [22]. The problem of delivering drugs to the CNS is, therefore, a good candidate for prodrugs. Note that although one can improve delivery of various compounds to the brain, this could lead to simultaneous improved transport to other tissue and depots, increasing the possibility of systemic side effects. In addition, these prodrugs may be kept at therapeutic useful concentration in the CNS only if their concentration in the general circulation is also kept at constantly high levels.

Clearly, delivery of drugs exclusively or preferably to the brain is very difficult. Until recently, no simple and general method to achieve this goal was known. A general method based on a dihydropyridine-pyridinium type redox delivery system for brain specific sustained release of drugs was recently developed [23]. Scheme 5 illustrates this approach.

According to this scheme, a given drug [D] is either coupled to a tertiary carrier and the quaternized or coupled to a quarternary carrier $[QC]^+$ directly, and the product obtained $[D\text{-}QC]^+$ is reduced chemically to the dihydro form [D-QHC]. Alternatively, the drug can directly be coupled with the dihydro carrier [QHC]. After *in vivo* administration of this lipophilic dihydro form, it is quickly distributed (k_0) throughout the body, including the brain. The dihydro form [Q-DHC] is then oxidized in the brain (k_1^1) and in the body (k_1^2) (i.e., the NAD-NADH system) to the original $[D\text{-}QC]^+$ (ideally inactive) quaternary salt. (Superscript 1 refers to the processes in the brain, while superscript 2 indicates similar processes in the body. These latter processes are given an overall rate [i.e., k_1^2 for oxidation], although the actual process takes place with different rates in the various organs.) $[D\text{-}QC]^+$, due to its ionic hydrophilic character, should be rapidly eliminated from the body, while the BBB should prevent its elimination from the brain. Enzymatic cleavage of the $[D\text{-}QC]^+$ that is "locked in" brain will result in a sustained delivery of the drug species [D], following its normal elimination (k_5^1). A properly selected carrier, $[QC]^+$, will also be eliminated rapidly from the brain ($k_6^1 >> k_3$). Due to facile elimination of $[D\text{-}QC]^+$ from the general circulation, only small amounts of drugs are released in the body ($k_2 >> k_4^2$), and [D] will be released primarily in the brain

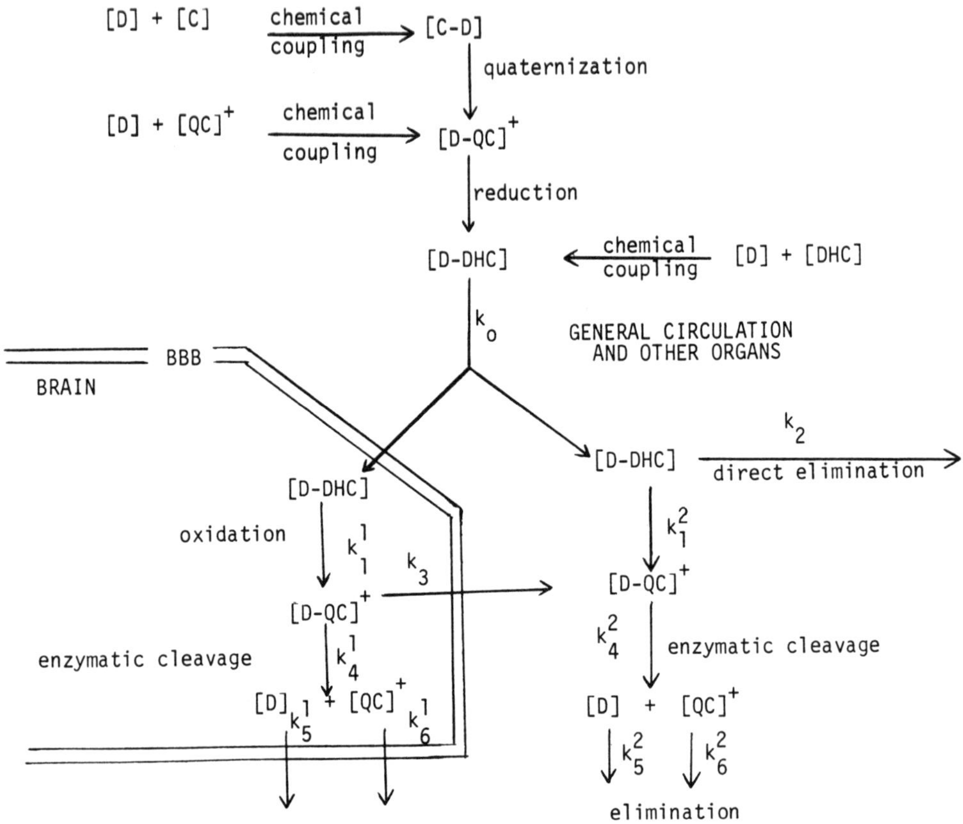

Scheme 5

($k_4^1 > k_3$). The overall result, ideally, will be a brain-specific sustained release of the target drug.

Thus, this method can potentially provide the desired level of a drug in the CNS, without requiring high circulatory concentrations. The drug blood level has virtually no effect on the brain levels, after the last oxidation step and the "lock-in" process take place. This is expected to significantly reduce systemic toxicity by accelerating the elimination of the drug-quaternary carrier system from the general circulation. Moreover, central toxicity should also be reduced by providing a low level, sustained release of the active species in the brain. One main factor in this whole picture is the choice of the quaternary carrier, which must be of low toxicity alone and in combination with the drug.

This general approach was first applied for phenylethylamine 11 which was transformed into the chemical delivery system 12 in which the redox carrier is the dihydrotrigonelline-trigonelline redox system [24].

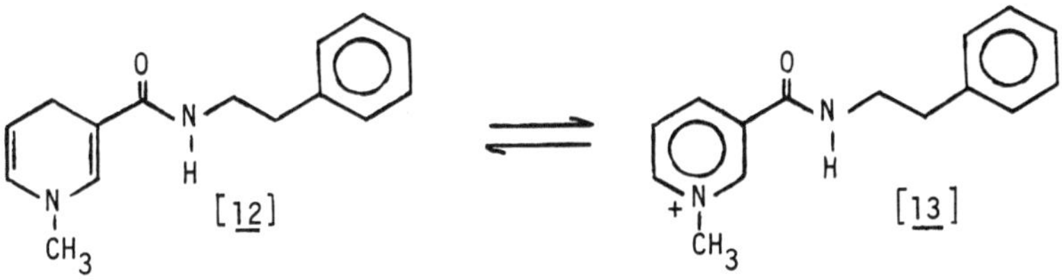

[12] [13]

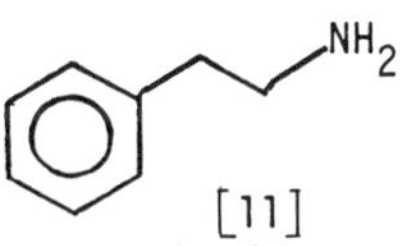

[11]

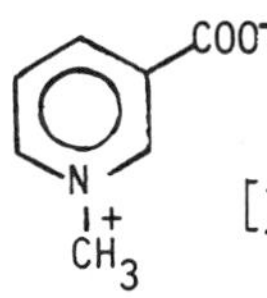

[14]

The lipoidal form 12 is oxidized to the quaternary form 13 with relative ease in various biological fluids as shown in Table 10. The corresponding *in vivo* oxidation assured not only a "lock-in" of this oxidized form in the brain but also a continuous buildup of its brain concentration with a simultaneous decline in blood concentration. As illustrated in Figure 1, at about 1 hr after i.v. administration, a very high brain concentration of the precursor 13 was achieved in the brain and drug was almost completely eliminated from the blood. The descending portion of the brain concentrations in Figure 1

Table 10 Rate of Oxidative Conversion in Biological Fluids[a] of 1-Methyl-3-(*N*-Phenethyl-Carbamoyl)-1,4-Dihydropyridine 12 to the Corresponding Quaternary Pyridinium Salt 13

		12 → 13	
Medium	*n*	$k \times 10^4$, s^{-1}	$t_{1/2}$, min
Human plasma	13	1.80 ± 0.34	64.2 ± 12.1
Whole blood	5	8.40 ± 0.94	13.7 ± 1.9
Brain homogenate	8	4.12 ± 0.28	28.2 ± 2.0
Liver homogenate	7	8.13 ± 0.96	14.2 ± 2.1

[a]At 37°C, undiluted heparinized human whole blood, 20% fresh human plasma, and 2% rat brain and liver homogenates were used. The conversions of 12 to 13 was followed by the changes in their characteristic UV spectra (λ_{max} ≅ 350 nm 12; 262 nm for 13) against appropriate reference samples.

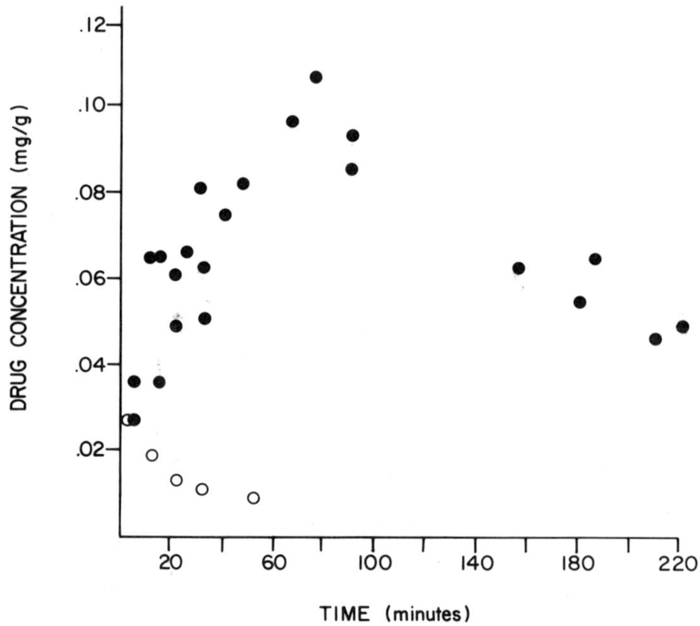

Fig. 1 The concentration of 1-methyl-3-(*N*-phenethylcarbamoyl) pyridinium (ion) (13) in the brain (•) and the blood (○) of rats following administration of 1-methyl-3-(*N*-phenethyl-carbamoyl)-1,4-dihydropyridine (17). Protocol: A group of 22 male Sprague-Dawley rats, average weight 300 ± 50 g, was anesthetized with Innovar-vet and the freshly prepared dihydro compound (12) (0.5 g/ml in dimethyl sulfoxide) was injected through the external jugular at a dose of 125 mg/kg. After appropriate time periods, the blood and brain were analyzed for 13 by HPLC.

corresponds to a half-life of 2.35 hr. The rate of disappearance of 13 in freshly prepared rat brain homogenate had a half-life of 3 hours, phenylethylamine (11) and trigonelline (14) being the main products. Thus, all criteria set forth in the previous scheme were met. One i.v. injection of a drug coupled to a dihydropyridine carrier system resulted in accumulation of the corresponding drug-quaternary carrier species in the brain, followed by sustained release of the drug in the brain, while the drug-quaternary carrier system was rapidly eliminated from the blood. In contrast, when the quaternary derivative 13 was administered at equivalent dose levels, no drug could be detected in the brain of rats.

A similar type of delivery system was then used for the sustained delivery of dopamine (15) to the brain and/or the anterior pituitary while providing much lower concentrations in the peripheral circulation and other tissues (25). Following i.v. administration of 16b to rats, high concentration of 17a could be detected in the brain. The loss of the compound from the brain was slow with a half-life of 3.2 hr. If the quaternary derivative 17b was administered peripherally, compound 17a could not be detected in the brain and the half-life of elimination from the systemic circulation was found to be 27 min. This locked-in form 17a then resulted in sustained slow release of dopamine to the anterior pituitary, leading to very substantial and prolonged inhibition of prolactin release, as shown in Figure 2. It is important to note that the carrier precursor form 17a does not have intrinsic dopaminergic activity. However, when injected as such it causes only very brief reduction in the prolactin release, which returns to the normal value within 1 hr.

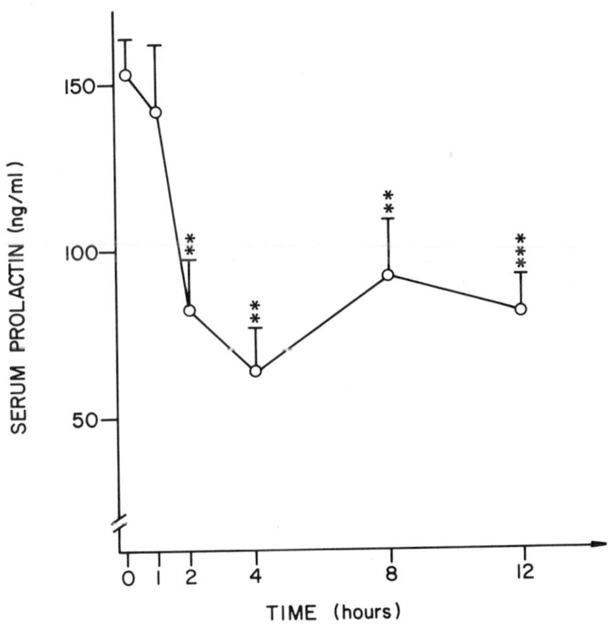

Fig. 2 Effect of compound 16b administered i.v. at a 1 mg/kg dose level on serum prolactin levels in rats. Error bars represent standard error of mean, $*p < 0.025$; $**p < 0.01$; $***p < 0.005$ vs. control. Each point represents the average of six (6) animals. For details see Ref. 32.

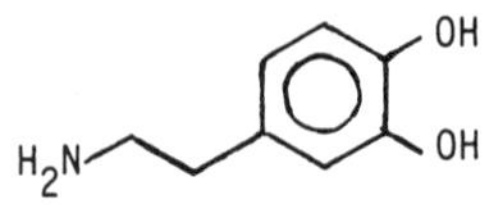

(15)

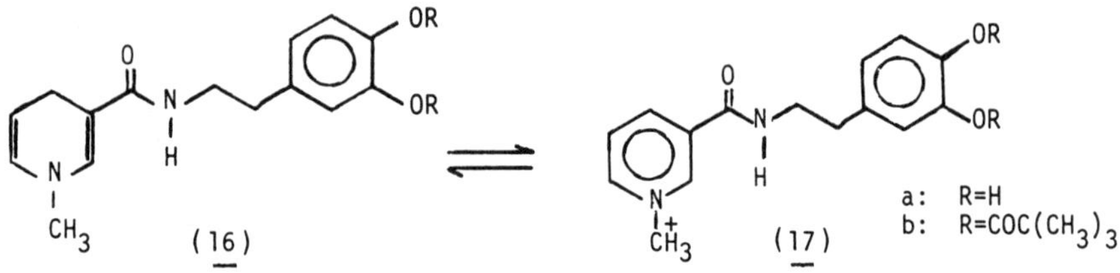

(16) (17)

The redox-type chemical delivery system to the brain has also been applied to steroids. There are a number of clinical situations in which the delivery of sex hormones to the brain is desirable. These include contraception and sexual dysfunctions like impotence. The first compound in this class was testosterone. In developing a CDS for testosterone, another factor was considered, namely, drug delivery across the blood-testes barrier (BTB) [26–29]. Like the BBB, this barrier acts to exclude compounds from the seminiferous tubules but, unlike the BBB, it is not the result of a vascular component. Most recent theories indicate that this impermeable barrier is due to tight junctions in the Sertoli cells which surround the spermatogenic apparatus. In principle, the dihydropyridine-pyridinium salt redox system should be effective in concentrating testosterone in the testes just as it does in the brain. The testosterone-CDS 19 was obtained [30] and adminstered systemically to female rats. The quaternary compound 20 was found in high concentrations in the brain. It was actually locked in as the half-life of efflux was 5.7 hr. In addition, the quaternary salt after systemic injections was rapidly lost from the peripheral circulation, with a half-life of elimination in the order of 50 minutes. The system was also capable to slow delivery of testosterone itself in the brain. The testosterone formed *in situ* shows elimination which is very slow with a half-life of about 20 hours. This may be due to its sustained formation from the precursor or due to testosterone binding to high-affinity globulins. When testosterone itself is given in equimolar amounts, it is rapidly lost from both the brain and the blood. These data are summarized in Figure 3.

Other types of analogous chemical sustained delivery systems have been developed. One of these makes use of the endocyclic

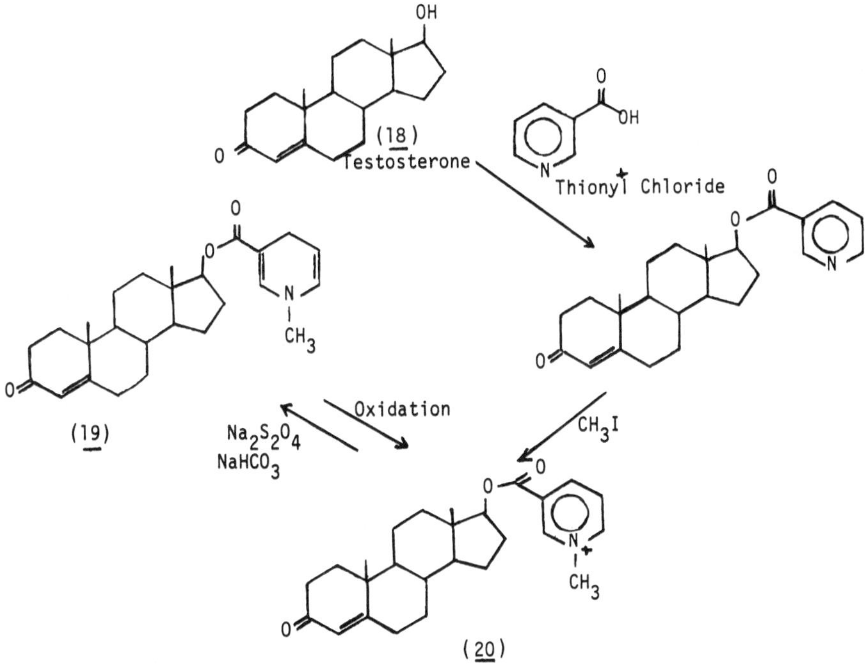

nitrogen atom of nicotinamide. In this chemical delivery system the rate of oxidation of the dihydro form (21) and the rate of drug release are controlled by the electronic and steric properties of the drug and its link to the carrier. The basic principles of this approach were first tested using phenylethylamine [31]. The oxidative conversion of the dihydro (21) form to the corresponding quaternary salt (23) in rat brain homogenate was highly dependent on the number of methylene groups separating the drug from the carrier with half-lives of 130, 27, and 19 min for methylene, propylene, and n-propylene derivatives, respectively. After a single i.v. injection of 22a-c to rats, the quaternary salts (23) disappeared quickly from the blood, while relatively high levels were maintained in the brain (Table 11). Not surprisingly, 22c, which had the shortest oxidative

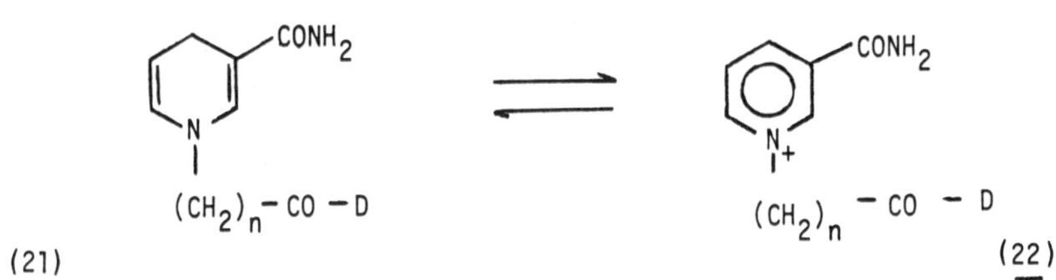

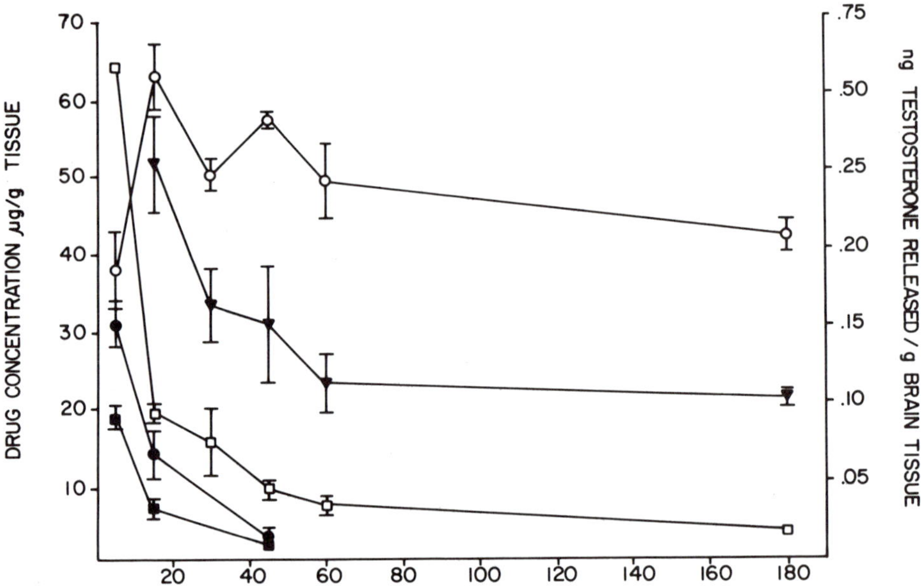

Fig. 3 Concentrations, with standard errors, against time for testosterone-17-nicotinate-*N*-methyl cation (20), calculated as iodide, in brain (○) and in blood (□) and concentration of released testosterone (µg/g) in brain (▼) all following administration of corresponding dihydropyridine derivative (19). Also, concentrations of testosterone in brain (■) and blood (●) following administration of testosterone. Female Sprague-Dawley rats were used.

half-life in rat brain homogenate, shows the highest brain availability, while 23a, which had the longest oxidative half-life, shows the lowest brain availability.

A similar approach was applied to testosterone [32]. After i.v. administration of the dihydro (24a-c) derivatives to rats, high concentrations of 25a-c could be detected in the brain (Table 12).

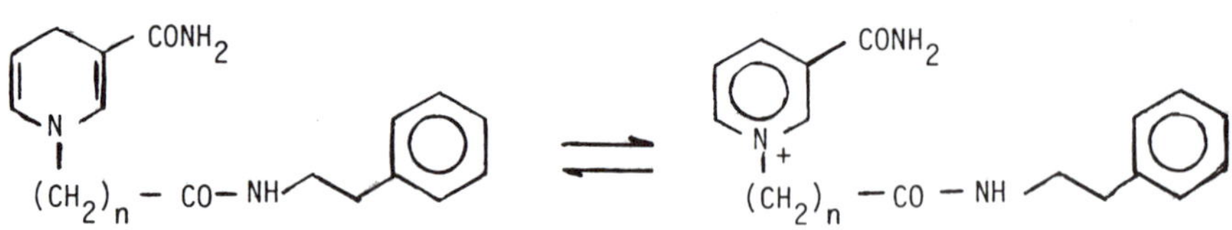

(22)

a: n=1
b: n=2
c: n=3

(23)

Table 11 Concentrations with Standard Errors Against Time of 3-Carbamoyl-1-{*N*-[β-(Phenyl)-ethyl]carbamoylalkyl}pyridinium Cations 23a, 23b or 23c in Brain, Blood, Kidney, Liver, and Testes After Administration of 3-Carbamoyl-1-{*N*-[β-(Phenyl)ethyl]carbamoylalkyl}-1,4-dihydropyridines 22a, 22b, or 22c

Time (min)	Organ	Concentration ± S.E. (μg/g blood or wet organ) 23a	23b	23c
5	Brain	11.95 ± 1.14	9.93 ± 0.65	24.28 ± 2.06
	Blood	78.25 ± 2.60	99.46 ± 3.37	155.20 ± 2.29
	Kidney	167.47 ± 16.75	238.44 ± 15.49	440.14 ± 2.07
	Liver	a	9.92 ± 1.81	65.09 ± 0.92
	Testes	Female	5.86 ± 1.29	8.18 ± 0.50
30	Brain	3.20 ± 0.34	6.20 ± 1.13	19.57 ± 1.25
	Blood	5.15 ± 0.29	6.10 ± 0.84	6.99 ± 1.35
	Kidney	47.70 ± 1.67	64.20 ± 1.86	196.53 ± 50.01
	Liver	a	a	103.14 ± 36.47
	Testes	Female	4.21 ± 0.29	8.76 ± 1.05
60	Brain	4.79 ± 0.18	13.36 ± 0.92	14.56 ± 1.22
	Blood	3.23 ± 1.82	5.19 ± 0.55	a
	Kidney	30.43 ± 11.49	376.95 ± 17.23	84.11 ± 9.98
	Liver	1.36 ± 1.60	14.33 ± 3.97	7.73 ± 1.18
	Testes	Female	5.03 ± 1.06	6.36 ± 0.75
120	Brain	6.64 ± 0.57	1.28 ± 0.008	21.06 ± 1.56
	Blood	1.77 ± 0.15	1.37 ± 0.22	a
	Kidney	21.43 ± 0.15	30.77 ± 0.95	11.39 ± 31.24
	Liver	a	a	13.16 ± 21.11
	Testes	Female	a	4.44 ± 0.39

[a]Below detection limit.

Table 12 Concentrations with Standard Errors Against Time of 17β-{[(3'-Carbamoyl-1'-Pyridinium)acyl]oxy}androst-4-en-3-ones 25a, 25b or 25c in Brain, Blood, and Kidney After Administration of 17β-{[(3'-Carbamoyl-1',4'-Dihydropyridinyl)Acyl]oxy}androst-4-en-3-ones 24a, or 24c

Time (min)	Organ	Concentration ± S.E. (μg/g blood or wet organ[a]) 25a	25b	25c
5	Brain	48.71 ± 10.12	2.21 ± 3.08	11.05 ± 1.07
	Blood	30.45 ± 6.70	33.91 ± 0.24	41.58 ± 3.82
	Kidney	425.80 ± 52.50	606.02 ± 56.23	689.26 ± 60.98
30	Brain	13.58 ± 3.19	15.35 ± 2.82	12.85 ± 1.16
	Blood	5.07 ± 0.51	12.04 ± 1.78	5.14 ± 0.84
	Kidney	135.50 ± 10.00	275.21 ± 15.96	216.19 ± 12.55
60	Brain	8.82 ± 0.76	3.22 ± 0.76	6.11 ± 0.50
	Blood	2.57 ± 0.61	5.72 ± 1.70	0.29 ± 0.21
	Kidney	43.00 ± 5.70	190.68 ± 4.49	88.61 ± 8.53
120	Brain	3.02 ± 0.37	1.90 ± 1.29	4.70 ± 0.22
	Blood	1.03 ± 0.40	b	2.88 ± 0.76
	Kidney	25.08 ± 3.27	71.81 ± 3.40	43.43 ± 5.69
240	Brain	2.49 ± 0.36	b	2.91 ± 0.92
	Blood	b	b	0.17 ± 0.19
	Kidney	16.00 ± 1.44	20.16 ± 3.55	10.21 ± 0.73

[a]Calculated with hydroxide as the counter ion.
[b]Below detection limit.

Table 13 Concentrations with Standard Errors Against Time of the Released Testosterone in Brain, Blood, Kidney Following Administration of 17β-{[(3'-Carbamoyl-1', 4'-Dihydropyridinyl) acyl]oxyl}androst-4-en-3-ones 24a, 24b, or 24c

Time (min)	Organ	Concentration ± S.E. (μg/g blood or wet organ) of testosterone after administration of		
		24a	24b	24c
5	Brain	19.15 ± 1.51	12.08 ± 0.27	6.16 ± 0.52
	Blood	13.82 ± 0.69	9.83 ± 0.70	7.16 ± 0.68
	Kidney	55.60 ± 0.40	69.08 ± 4.75	61.29 ± 3.24
30	Brain	12.39 ± 0.77	14.97 ± 1.41	6.07 ± 0.47
	Blood	5.32 ± 0.43	9.23 ± 0.53	3.99 ± 0.36
	Kidney	33.02 ± 5.67	98.62 ± 4.73	27.83 ± 1.56
60	Brain	7.80 ± 0.91	6.00 ± 0.31	7.43 ± 0.28
	Blood	3.90 ± 0.51	4.78 ± 0.38	4.41 ± 0.19
	Kidney	25.02 ± 2.63	22.92 ± 1.58	26.79 ± 1.22
120	Brain	6.72 ± 0.72	4.40 ± 0.20	4.52 ± 0.18
	Blood	2.22 ± 0.10	2.80 ± 0.24	2.60 ± 0.42
	Kidney	18.32 ± 1.26	10.65 ± 0.69	11.45 ± 1.49
240	Brain	4.90 ± 0.23	2.62 ± 0.13	2.32 ± 0.11
	Blood	1.76 ± 0.52	1.43 ± 0.008	0.40 ± 0.07
	Kidney	9.20 ± 0.38	4.75 ± 0.20	1.11 ± 0.84

The loss of the quaternary compounds from the brain was faster than in the case of the trigonelline delivery system (compound 20), due to facile hydrolysis of the ester linkage. The rate of oxidation of 24a-c and subsequent "lock-in" the brain of the corresponding quaternary carrier-drug species 25a-c, as well as the rate of the hydrolytic release of the drug, depend on the length and branching of the alkyl chain separating the carrier moiety from the drug. Thus, 24a was oxidized fastest in the brain *in vivo* and 25a consequently showed the highest brain availability, while 25b released testosterone at a faster rate (Table 13). Compound 24a gives the highest brain availability of testosterone (the highest overall concentration of testosterone in the brain) while the more hindered 24c-25c derivative pair gave the most consistent sustained brain release for testosterone (most favorable brain/blood concentration ratio).

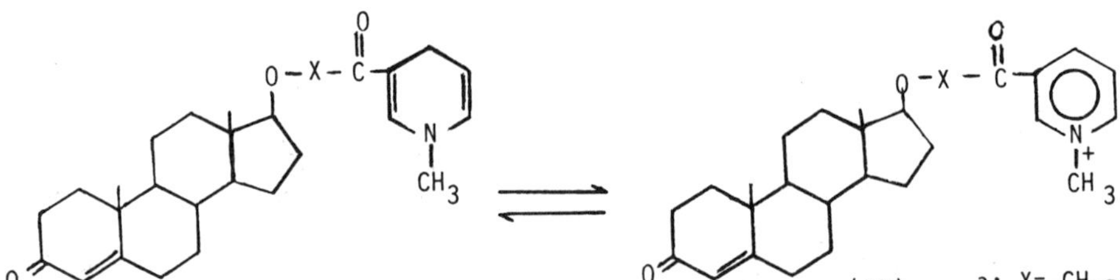

(24) (25)

a: X=$-CH_2-$
b: X=$-CH_2-CH_2-$
c: X=$-CH(CH_3)-$

VII. CONCLUSIONS

Various novel chemical approaches to achieve sustained drug release were developed. The classical prodrug approach was used successfully in some cases, such as the sustained release of theophylline. The more sophisticated "chemical delivery systems" (CDS) approach has shown great promise in site-specific and sustained drug release, as exemplified by drug delivery to the skin, special segment of the eye, and the brain.

The most successful methods are based on controlling enzymatic reactions and manipulating metabolism through structural design. Successive enzymatic reactions can specifically optimize the presence and activity of the active species at or around the site of action. Rather than looking for the elusive (and most likely nonexistent) organ and site-specific enzyme systems which will possibly activate certain precursors only at the site of action, the examples given strongly suggest that a combination of the basics of physical chemistry, enzyme activity and kinetics as well as drug metabolism would be useful in achieving successful sustained site-specific drug delivery.

REFERENCES

1. A. A. Sinkula and S. H. Yalkowsky, Rationale for design of biologically reversible drug derivatives: Prodrugs, *J. Pharm. Sci. 64*, 181 (1975).
2. N. Bodor, Novel approaches in prodrug design, *Drugs of Future, 6*, 165 (1981).
3. N. Bodor, Novel approaches for the design of membrane transport properites of drugs. In, *Design of Bio-Pharmaceutical Properties Through Pro-Drugs and Analogs* (E. B. Roche, Ed.), APhA, Washington, DC, 1977, Chap. 7, pp. 98–135.
4. V. Stella, Prodrugs: An overview and definition. In, *Prodrugs as Novel Drug Delivery Systems* (T. Higuchi and V. Stella, Eds.), ACS Symposium Series, vol. 14, American Chemical Society, Washington, DC, 1975, pp. 1–115.
5. A. A. Sinkula, Methods to achieve sustained drug delivery: The chemical approach. In, *Sustained and Controlled Release Drug Delivery Systems* (J. R. Robinson, Ed.), Marcel Dekker, New York, 1978, pp. 411–555.
6. A. A. Sinkula, The chemical approach to achieve sustained drug delivery. In, *Optimization of Drug Delivery* (H. Bundgaard, A. B. Hansen, and H. Kofod, Eds.), Alfred Benzon Symposium 17, Munksgaard, Copenhagen, 1982, pp. 199–210.
7. N. Bodor, Novel approaches in prodrug design. In, *Optimization of Drug Delivery* (H. Bundgaard, A. B. Hansen, and H. Kofod, Eds.), Alfred Benzon Symposium 17, Copenhagen, 1982, pp. 156–174.
8. K. Miescher, A. Wettstein, and E. Tschopp, The activation of the male sex hormones, *Biochem. J. 30*, 53 (1982).
9. N. Bodor, K. B. Sloan, Y.-N. Kuo, and T. Higuchi, Controlled delivery of theophylline: Chemistry of 7-acyl-and 7,8'-acyldi-theophylline derivatives, *J. Pharm. Sci. 67*, 1045 (1978).
10. N. Bodor, Soft drugs: Strategies for design of low toxicity drugs, Proceedings of the Centre de Recherchers Clin Midy Symposium on Drug Metabolism and Drug Design: Quo Vadis?, Montpellier, November 26–27, 1981.
11. N. Bodor, Soft drugs: Strategies for design of safer drugs. In, *Strategy in Drug Research*, Vol. 4 (J. A. K. Buisman, Ed.), Elsevier Scientific Company, Amsterdam, 1982, pp. 137–164.

12. N. Bodor, Designing safer drugs based on the soft drug approach, *Trends Pharmacol. Sci. 3*, 53 (1982).
13. N. Bodor, The soft drug approach, *Chemtech 14*, 28 (1984).
14. A. M. Kligman and K. H. Kaidbey, Hydrocortisone revisited: An historical and experimental evaluation, *Cutis 22*, 232 (1978).
15. N. Bodor, K. B. Sloan, R. J. Little, S. H. Selk and L. Caldwell, Soft drugs 4: 3-spirothiazolidines of hydrocortisone and its derivatives, *Int. J. Pharm. 10*, 307 (1982).
16. K. B. Sloan, N. Bodor, and R. J. Little, ^{13}C NMR spectroscopy of 4,5 and 5,6-double bond isomers of spiro-3-steroidal ketone derivatives: The determination of the structures of steroidal thiazolidines, *Tetrahedron 37*, 3467 (1981).
17. K. B. Sloan, N. Bodor, and J. Zupan, Acylation of the 4,5- and 5,6-double bond isomers of 3-steroidal thiazolidines, *Tetrahedron 37*, 3463 (1981).
18. N. Bodor and K. B. Sloan, Soft drugs V: Thiazolidine-type derivatives of progesterone and testosterone, *J. Pharm. Sci. 71*, 514 (1982).
19. N. Bodor and K. B. Sloan, Thiazolidine prodrugs for the improved delivery of anti-inflammatory corticosteroids, U.S. Patent, 4,239,757, December 16, 1980.
20. J. Girard, A. Barbier, and C. Lafille, Inhibition of testosterone metabolism and lipogenesis in animal sebaceous glands by progesterone, *Arch. Dermatol. Res. 269*, 281 (1980).
21. S. E. Rappoport, *Blood Brain Barrier in Physiology and Medicine*, Raven Press, New York, 1976.
22. R. A. Fishman, Carrier transport of glucose between blood and cerebrospinal fluid, *Am. J. Physiol. 206*, 836 (1964).
23. N. Bodor, H. H. Farag, and M. E. Brewster, Site-specific sustained release of drugs to the brain, *Science 214*, 1370 (1981).
24. N. Bodor and H. H. Farag, Improved delivery through biological membranes II: A redox chemical drug-delivery system and its use for brain-specific delivery of phenylethylamine, *J. Med. Chem. 26*, 313 (1983).
25. N. Bodor and H. H. Farag, Improved delivery through biological membranes 13: Brain-specific delivery of dopamine with dihydropyridine pyridinium salt type redox delivery system, *J. Med. Chem. 26*, 528 (1983).
26. M. Kormano, Distribution of injected L-3,4-dihydroxyphenylanine (L-dopa) in the adult rat testis and epididymis, *Acta Physiol. Scand. 71*, 125 (1967).
27. M. Kormano, Dye permeability and alkaline phosphatase activity of testicular capillaries in the postnatal rat, *Histochemie 9*, 327 (1967).

28. D. W. Fawcett, L. V. Leav, and P. M. Heidger, Electron microscopic observation of the structural components of the blood-testis barrier, *J. Reprod. Fertil. 10 (Suppl.)*, 105 (1970).
29. N. Dym and D. W. Fawcett, The blood-testis barrier in the rat and the physiological compartmentation of the seminiferous epithelium, *Biol. Reprod. 3*, 308 (1970).
30. N. Bodor and H. Farag, Improved delivery through biological membranes XIV: Brain-specific sustained delivery of testosterone using a redox chemical delivery system, *J. Pharm. Sci. 73*, 385 (1984).
31. N. Bodor and A. M. AbdelAlim, Improved delivery through biological membranes XIX: Novel redox carriers for brain-specific chemical delivery systems, *Int. J. Pharm.* (in press).
32. N. Bodor and A. M. AbdelAlim, Improved delivery through biological membranes XX: Nicotinamide dihydronicotinamide based ester-linked redox carrier systems, *Int. J. Pharm.* (in press).

9

Design and Fabrication of Oral Controlled Release Drug Delivery Systems

HO-WAH HUI* and JOSEPH R. ROBINSON / University of Wisconsin, Madison, Wisconsin

VINCENT H. L. LEE / University of Southern California, Los Angeles, California

I. INTRODUCTION

Oral ingestion has long been the most convenient and commonly employed route of drug delivery. Indeed, for sustained-release systems, the oral route of administration has by far received the most attention with respect to research on physiological and drug constraints

---

**Current affiliation:* Abbott Laboratories, North Chicago, Illinois

as well as design and testing of products. This is because there is more flexibility in dosage form design for the oral route than there is for the parenteral route.

As is the case for systems for nonoral routes, the design of oral sustained release delivery systems is subject to several intercalated variables of considerable importance. Among these are the type of delivery system, the disease being treated, the patient, the length of therapy, and the properties of the drug.

This chapter will review oral controlled release systems, with particular emphasis on the practical aspects of design and fabrication. The majority of these systems are either tablets or capsules although a few liquid products are also available. The paucity of liquid sustained release products is related to the nature of the sustained release mechanisms employed. These usually rely on diffusion or dissolution so that when in contact with water the drug will leach out by the controlling mechanism. While attempts have been made to minimize the water content of liquid products by using combinations of honey, glycerin, and viscosity-inducing agents, thereby retarding drug release while in storage, the drug still leaches out in time and thus presents a potentially toxic dose in a product.

Sustained release tablet and capsule dosage forms usually consist of two parts: an immediately available dose to establish the blood level quickly and a sustaining part that contains several times the therapeutic dose for protracted drug levels. Several approaches are available to add the immediately available portion to the sustaining part. Simple addition of a nonsustained dose of drug to a capsule or tablet is the most direct method; placement of the initial dose in the tablet coat with the sustaining portion in the core represents an alternate approach. The heart of the system, nevertheless, resides with the sustaining portion of the dosage form [1]. Potential physical methods that can be used to retard drug release are summarized below and all but the last two will be discussed in this chapter.

1. Capsules of polymeric material filled with a solid or liquid drug or with a suspension of drug in a fluid, in which drug release is controlled by diffusion through the capsule wall
2. A heterogeneous dispersion of drug particles in a solid matrix which can be either biodegradable or nonbiodegradable and which controls drug release by diffusion through the matrix, by erosion of the matrix, or by a combination of both diffusion and erosion
3. A laminate of agent and polymeric material made by coating a film of biodegradable or nonbiodegradable material with solid drug and then by forming the film into a sealed "sandwich" or "jellyroll", in which drug release is by diffusion, erosion, or both

4. A heterogeneous dispersion or solution of drug in a water-swellable hydrogel matrix, which controls drug release by slow surface-to-center swelling of the matrix by water and subsequent diffusion of the drug from the water-swollen part of the matrix
5. Liquid-liquid encapsulation of the drug in a viscous solution of polymer, which controls drug release by slow diffusion through dilution of the media
6. Pumps that either mechanically or chemically (osmotic pressure) provide drug in a controlled manner.
7. Drug coated micropellets which have an apparent density lower than that of gastric juice. Thus, the final product floats on gastric juice for an extended period, while slowly releasing drug
8. Drug-containing bioadhesive polymer that adheres to the mucin coating of the GI tract and which is retained on the surface epithelium to extend GI transit time of the drug. Drug is released at a constant rate from the bioadhesive polymer for subsequent absorption
9. Chemical bonding of a drug to a polymer backbone by pendent amide or ester linkages, which controls drug release by hydrolysis
10. Formation of macromolecular structures of the drug via ionic or covalent linkages, which controls drug release by hydrolysis, thermodynamic dissociation, or microbial degradation

II. DESIGN AND FABRICATION OF ORAL SYSTEMS

The majority of oral controlled release systems rely on dissolution, diffusion, or a combination of both mechanisms, to generate slow release of drug to the gastrointestinal milieu. Starting with limited data on a drug candidate for sustained release, such as dose, rate constants for absorption and elimination, some elements of metabolism and some physical-chemical properties of the drug, one can estimate a desired release rate for the dosage form, the quantity of drug needed, and a preliminary strategy for the dosage form to be utilized.

Some consideration of the *in vitro* systems that can be used to assess drug release kinetics is necessary. Several systems have been designed and used [2–6]. In the absence of *in vitro/in vivo* correlations for any one system it does not seem to matter which system is employed. Consequently, the rotating flask [7] and the USP basket arrangement [8,9] would be equally useful in this regard. The formulator will merely design a dosage form based on *in vitro* studies, test it in a human or animal model, and then modify the system according to these results. This iteration to the final dosage form is inefficient but in the absence of a predictable *in vitro* system is the only approach possible.

A. Dissolution Controlled Release

Sustained release oral products employing dissolution as the rate-limiting step are in principle the simplest to prepare. A drug with a slow dissolution rate is inherently sustained. Some examples of these drugs include digoxin, griseofulvin, and salicylamide. Others, such as aluminum aspirin, ferrous sulfate, and benzphetamine paomate, produce such forms when in contact with the absorption pool contents [10]. Steroids have been reported to undergo transformation into less soluble polymorphs during dissolution in the absorption pool [11].

For those drugs with high water-solubility and therefore high dissolution rate, one can decrease solubility through appropriate salt or derivative formation. Unfortunately, forms such as these do not meet the criterion of constant availability rate because their surface area decreases with time. Nevertheless, sustained drug release can be achieved by coating drug particles or granules with materials of varying thickness or by dispersing them in a polymeric matrix.

The basic principle of dissolution control is as follows [12]. If the dissolution process is diffusion layer controlled, where the rate of diffusion from the solid surface through an unstirred liquid film to the bulk solution is rate limiting, the flux J is given by:

$$J = -D(dc/dx) \tag{1}$$

where D is the diffusion coefficient and dc/dx is the concentration gradient from the solid surface to the bulk solution. The flux can also be defined as the flow rate of material (dm/dt) through a unit area (A), thus one has the equation:

$$J = (1/A)dm/dt \tag{2}$$

If the concentration gradient is linear and the thickness of the diffusion layer is h,

$$dc/dx = (Cb - Cs)/h \tag{3}$$

where Cs is the concentration at the solid surface and Cb is the concentration in the bulk solution. By combining the above equations, the flow rate of material is given by

$$dm/dt = -(DA/h)\ (Cb - Cs) = kA(Cs - Cb) \tag{4}$$

where k is the intrinsic dissolution rate constant.

The above equation predicts constant dissolution rate if the surface area, diffusion coefficient, diffusion layer thickness, and concentration difference are kept constant. However, as dissolution proceeds, all of the parameters, the surface area especially, may change.

A useful expression to describe the dissolution of dosage forms of various geometry is available [11]. Thus,

$$Mt/M_\infty = 1 - [1 - K_o t/c_o a]^n \tag{5}$$

where Mt is the amount of drug released in time t, M_∞ is the amount of drug released at infinite time, a is the half-thickness of a slab or the radius of a sphere or of a cylinder, and *n* is equal to 3 for a sphere, 2 for a cylinder, and 1 for a slab.

The common forms of dissolution control formulations are shown in Figure 1. Most of the products fall into two categories: (a) encapsulation dissolution control and (b) matrix dissolution control. There is considerable overlap between the two areas and the subdivision is made primarily for organizational purposes.

1. *Encapsulation Dissolution Control*

These methods generally involve coating individual particles or granules of drug with a slowly dissolving material. The coated particles can be compressed directly into tablets as in Spacetabs or placed in capsules as in the Spansule products. Since the time required for dissolution of the coat is a function of its thickness and aqueous solubility, one can obtain repeat or sustained action by employing a narrow or a wide spectrum of coated particles of varying thicknesses, respectively. Ever since the Spansule sustained release dosage form was introduced in the early 1950s, there have been numerous studies on the *in vivo* performance [13–35] as well as clinical effectiveness of these types of products [36–46].

Seed or Granule Coated Products

A wide range of drugs have been formulated as sustained release coated granules and compressed into tablets. These include antispasmodic-sedative combinations [61], phenothiazines [62–65], anticholinesterase agents [66], and aspirin [67,68].

There are several ways to prepare drug-coated beads or granules. A common procedure is to coat nonpareil seeds with the drug followed

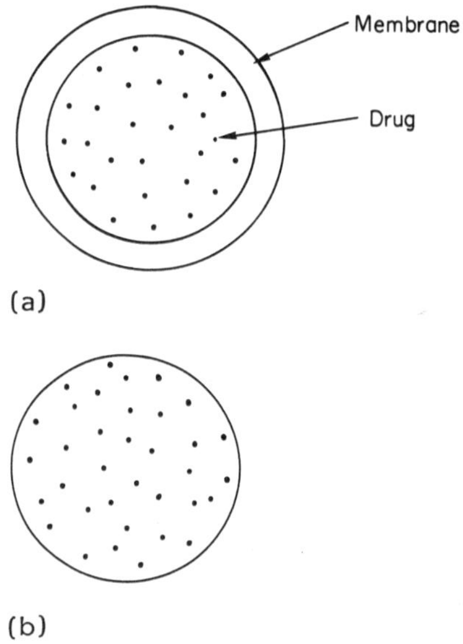

Fig. 1 Schematic representation of dissolution controlled drug release. (a) Dissolution control of drug release via thickness and dissolution rate of the membrane barrier coat. (b) Dissolution control of drug release via polymer core erosion.

by a coat of slowly dissolving material such as carbohydrate sugars and cellulose, polyethylene glycol, polymeric materials, and wax. Colbert [47] and Johnson [48] have compiled a rather complete listing of patents issued between 1960 and 1974 based on these digestible bases. Table 1 is a brief listing of some coating materials and their properties.

It is common practice to employ one-quarter to one-third of the seeds in nonsustained form to provide for immediate drug release, with the remaining three-quarters or two-thirds of the seeds being divided into groups of varying coating thickness to provide for sustained effect over the desired time period.

An illustration of this approach is given in the series of papers by Rosen et al. [26,27], in which they described the release of amobarbital and dextroamphetamine sulfate from both nonsustained and sustained release dosage forms of drug released in each time period is progressively less as the percentage of wax in the coating increases, indicating that drug release rate can be varied quite readily by changing the makeup of the coating material for the drug granules [22,28]. The dashed line in this figure indicates the release pattern when certain granule sizes are combined.

Table 1 Coating Materials and Their Properties

Type of coating	Most suitable dosage form(s)	Examples	Probable release mechanisms	Properties
Barrier coating (including microencapsulation) [49–55]	1. Film-coated tablets	Various shellacs [49]	1. Diffusion and dialysis	1. Slow or incomplete release
	2. Film-coated pellets of granules placed in gelatin capsules	Beeswax [49]	2. Some disintegration possible	2. Coating is subject to fracture during compression
	3. Compressed tablets containing mixtures of barrier coated particles with filler particles	Glyceryl monostearte [49]	3. Also have had pH-dependent dissolution and some enzymatic breakdown incorporated into some films, but these are poor "barriers"	3. Release depends on drug solubility and pore structure membrane
	4. Compressed tablets containing only barrier coated particles forming a matrix	Ethylcellulose [49]		4. Constant release resulted when GI fluid passes through barrier to dissolve drug
		Nylon [49]		
		Acrylic resins [49]		
		Cellulose acetate butyrate [50]		
		dl-Polylactic acid [50]		
		1.6-Hexanediamine [50]		
		Diethylenetriamine [50]		
		Polyvinyl chloride [50]		
		Sodium carboxymethylcellulose [51]		

Table 1 (Continued)

Type of coating	Most suitable dosage form(s)	Examples	Probable release Mechanisms	Properties
Embedment into a fatty coating (similar to embedding in a matrix of fatty materials)	1. Compressed granules into a tablet 2. Compressed granules placed in a gelatin capsule 3. Multi layered tablets 4. Compression coated tablets	Glycerol palmitostearate [49] Beeswax [49] Glycowax [49] Castor wax [49] Carnauba wax [49] Glyceryl monostearate [49] Stearyl alcohol [49]	1. Gradual erosion of the coat, aided by pH and enzymatic hydrolysis of the fatty acid esters 2. Coating may contain portion of the dose for quick release upon hydrolysis with subsequent slow release from erosion of a core	1. Slow or incomplete release 2. Difficult to con- release pattern due to variations in pH and enzyme content of the GI tract
Repeat action coatings	1. Sugar coating of an enteric coated core tablet 2. Compression coating of an enteric coated core tablet	Cellulose acetate phthalate [49] (Many of the examples listed for "Barrier Coating" apply here also)	1. pH dependent dissolution and enzymatic breakdown 2. Outer coating releases first dose rapidly	1. Variations due to changing stomach emptying times 2. Not a "true" sustained form

			in stomach fluids, inner enteric-coated core releases a second dose at some later time in intestinal fluids	
Coated plastic matrix	1. Multilayer tablets 2. Compression coated tablets	Polyethylene [49] Polyvinyl acetate [49] Polymethacrylate [49] Polyvinyl chloride [49] Ethylcellulose [49] Silicone devices [50] Methylmethacrylate [50] 2-Hydroxyethyl methacrylate [50] 1,3-Butylene glycol dimethacrylate [50] Ethylene glycol dimethacrylate [50] Vinyl pyrrolidone [50]	1. Outer coating containing active drug dissolves rapidly to provide drug for immediate absorption 2. Above process is followed by leaching of drug from inert matrix via penetration of GI fluids into pores of the matrix	1. Slow or incomplete release 2. Only water soluble or fairly water soluble drugs can be used 3. Plastic matrix skeleton is excreted in its original shape 4. Drug liberation depends only on solubility in GI completely independent of pH, enzyme activity, concentration or GI motility

Table 1 (Continued)

Type of coating	Most suitable dosage form(s)	Examples	Probable release mechanisms	Properties
Coated hydrophilic matrix	1. Multilayer tablets 2. Compression coated tablets	Carboxymethyl cellulose [49] Hydroxypropylmethylcellulose [49] Methacrylate hydrogels [56] Polyethylene glycols [49] Sodium carboxymethyl cellulose [49]	1. Outer coating containing active drug dissolves rapidly along with rapid dissolution from the surface of the matrix to provide drug for immediate absorption 2. Above process continues until a viscous gelatinous barrier is formed around the matrix surface	1. Drug liberation rate is dependent on type and amount of gum used 2. High water solubility of the drug is absolutely necessary

		3. Once the gelatinous barrier has formed, diffusion and dissolution, via erosion, occur at slow controlled rate	3. Release is controlled by drug diffusivity more than by gum dissolution or water penetrability as long as hydrated gelatinous layer remains intact

Source: J. M. Conrad and J. R. Robinson, Sustained drug release from tablets and particles through coating. In, *Coating* (L. Lachman and H. Lieberman, Eds.), Marcel Dekker, New York, 1982, Chap. 4, with permission.

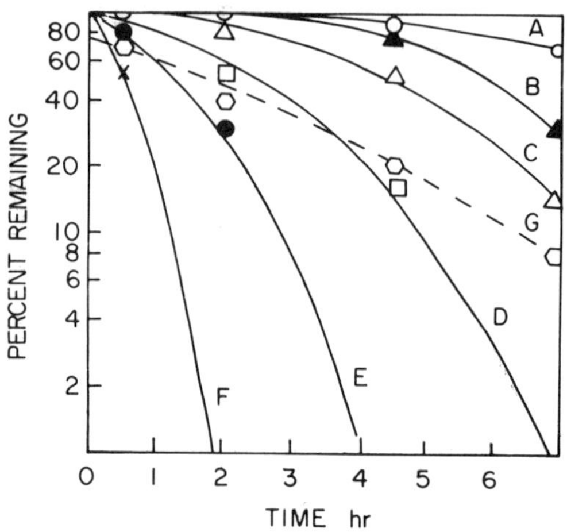

Fig. 2 *In vitro* release patterns of [14C]dextroamphetamine sulfate pellets pan-coated with various amounts of a fat-wax coating. A, 17% coating; B, 15% coating; C, 13% coating; D, 11% coating; E, 9% coating; F, 7% coating; G, selected blend of uncoated and coated pellets. (Reproduced with permission from Ref. 57.)

Coated granules or seeds can be placed in a capsule for administration to patients. Feinblatt and Ferguson [58,59] photographed the disintegration and dispersal of coated granules *in vivo*. They demonstrated that after 10–12 hr the coated granules were well dispersed in the GI tract and the active ingredient dissolved.

With tablet dosage forms, there are the added concerns of the influence of excipients and compression on the release rate. However, the role of excipients in the dissolution pattern of compressed coated granules has not been fully elucidated. In contrast, the problem of granular fracture or fusion has been studied by Green [60]. This investigator found that, in microencapsulated sustained release aspirin, a small amount of the microcapsules was fractured thereby producing greater amounts of immediately available aspirin than anticipated. However, the amount of drug from fracture is usually so small that it can be incorporated into the immediately available dose.

Microencapsulation

We have placed microencapsulation in this section because from most of the microencapsulation reports it appears that a portion of drug becomes embedded in the coating material and thus drug is provided in a sustained fashion as the coat dissolves. It is clear that other forms of microencapsulation can be used for pulsed dosing

Table 2 Classification of Microencapsulation Processes

Process	Types of material for coating
1. Coacervation/phase separation technique	Water-soluble polymer
2. Interfacial polymerization	Water-insoluble and water soluble monomers
3. Electrostatic method	Oppositely charged aerosols
4. Precipitation	Water or solvent-soluble polymers
5. Hot melt	Low molecular weight lipids
6. Salting out	Water-soluble polymers
7. Solvent evaporation	Solvent-soluble polymers

or for providing drug through a diffusion process, but to organize this material concisely we elect to discuss the process here. Microencapsulation can be used to encase liquids, solids or gases [69–75], using any of the processes listed in Table 2.

Coacervation heads the list because this appears to be the earliest process used to make an encapsulated product. This process utilizes the interaction of two oppositely charged polyelectrolytes in water to form a polymer-rich coating solution called a coacervate [76]. This coacervate encapsulates the liquid or solid to form an embryo capsule. When the system is cooled, the coating solution gels due to network formation of the gelatin. The gelled coacervate is then crosslinked to form the capsule wall. Both water soluble and insoluble drugs can be microencapsulated using a gelatin-gum arabic coacervate system provided that, prior to microencapsulation, the drug is protected from the aqueous environment by coating with carnauba wax or polymers such as ethylcellulose and cellulose acetate phthalate [77]. A pictorial representation of this microencapsulation method is shown in Figure 3.

Interfacial polymerization technique involves dispersing the organic phase containing drug particles into the aqueous phase containing monomers, whereby the monomers react at a liquid/liquid interface to form a capsule wall [78,79]. A cross-linking agent may be added to the continuous phase to effect polymerization at the interface. Drugs best encapsulated with this method are low-melting solids or poorly soluble organic liquids.

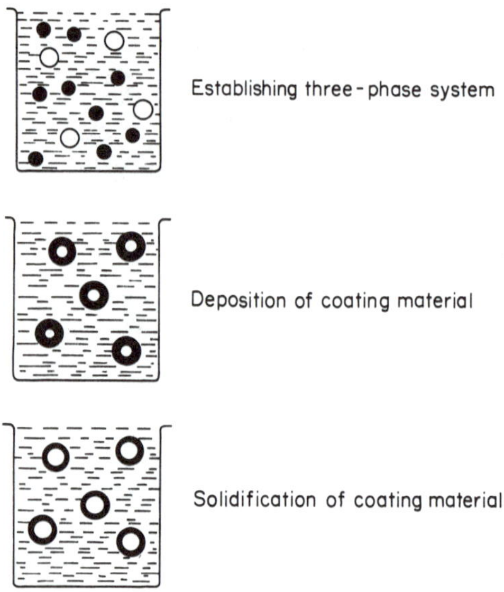

Fig. 3 Schematic representation of microencapsulation process. ○, drug; ●, coating material; ---, liquid material.

The electrosatic method is useful when the coating material and drug to be encapsulated are both aerosols and oppositely charged [80]. The drug and coating material are atomized resulting in the formation of microcapsules, which are then cooled and collected by an appropriate aerosol collection system.

The precipitation process covers many techniques. Examples include the precipitation of ethylcellulose from cyclohexane by cooling, gelation of sodium alginate with aqueous calcium salt solutions, and the desolvation of water-soluble polymers with water-miscible solvents. The objective of this method is to precipitate or congeal a preformed polymer around the drug being encapsulated.

Hot melt techniques involve mechanical drop formation at an elevated temperature followed by a cooling step. The hot melt coatings are composed of relatively low molecular weight lipids. These coatings have low melt viscosities at reasonable operating temperatures and can be readily sprayed. Drugs to be encapsulated by this method must be thermally stable.

The salting-out method involves the addition of salt to an aqueous polymer solution thereby separating the polymer from solution. One concern with this approach is the possibility of incorporating a relatively high concentration of salt into the capsule wall.

The last process in Table 2 is solvent evaporation. In this approach, the drug and capsule wall material are dissolved in a water-immiscible volatile organic solvent and then dispersed into an aqueous solution to form an emulsion. Next the solvent is evaporated, thus forming solid microcapsules.

The thickness of a microcapsule coat can be adjusted from less than 1 μm to 200 μm by changing the amount of coating material from 3 to 30% of the total weight. Wall thickness can be calculated theoretically from known capsule size [81]. Figure 4 represents theoretical thickness versus capsule size at various core material contents.

The coating material can be selected form a wide variety of natural and synthetic polymers, depending on the material to be coated and the release characteristics desired. For example, Sears [82] applied synthetic phopholipids, which are resistant to phosphorylase C hydrolysis, as a coating material to achieve sustained release of insulin from microcapsules.

Microorganism cells were also used as microcapsules. Yeast, molds or other fungi which synthesize fat within themselves can

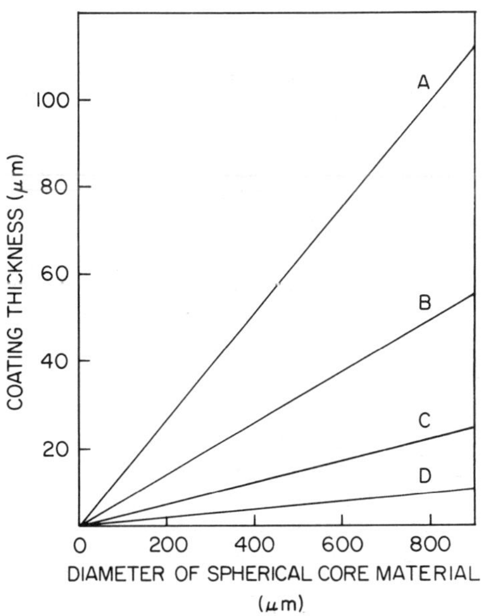

Fig. 4 Coating thickness versus particle size at various core material contents. A, 80% coating; B, 30% coating; C, 15% coating; and D, 3% coating. (Reproduced with permission from Ref. 81.)

absorb fat-soluble drugs and prolong the potency of the drugs. This technology has been applied to sustain the release of aspirin [83].

Microencapsulation has the additional advantage that sustained drug release can be achieved with taste abatement and better GI tolerability. Good examples are microencapsulated aspirin [84] and potassium chloride [85]. In both cases drug effects from the microencapsulated dosage forms were more prolonged with less gastric irritation than the same amount taken as ordinary tablets.

2. *Matrix Dissolution Control*

It was noted earlier that reduced drug solubility plus larger particle size can be used to modify availability rates. However, these approaches, alone or in combination, are limited in their usefulness. There is an upper restriction on the size of particles one can employ for the oral route while the low solubility approach will produce a changing dissolution rate as the area for dissolution decreases.

An alternate approach is to compress the drug with a slowly dissolving carrier of some sort into a tablet form. Here, the rate of drug availability is controlled by the rate of penetration of the dissolution fluid into the matrix. This, in turn, can be controlled by porosity of the tablet matrix, the presence of hydrophobic additives, and the wettability of the tablet and particle surface.

The porosity of the tablet, i.e., surface area available, can be altered in a compressed tablet by compression force, adhesion between adjacent particles as well as size and shape of the particles [102]. In addition, hydrophobic fillers can be added to decrease the effective porosity by limiting the number of pores that can be penetrated by the eluting fluid.

Numerous illustrations exist in the literature for this approach. Becker and his associates throughly investigated the formulation and release characteristics of sulfaethylthiadiazole impregnated in wax [86–91]. Two general methods of preparing wax-drug particles exist: aqueous dispersion and congealing. The aqueous dispersion method simply involves spraying or placing the wax-drug mixture in water and collecting the resulting particles. In the congealing method, drug is mixed with the wax material and either spray congealed or congealed and screened. Kawashima et al. [92] used a modified spherical agglomeration technique as an alternative to the spray-congealing method. In this technique, drug particles are dispersed in distilled water and the system is heated gradually to 90°C while agitating. The wax for a particular formulation is added to the system and agitation is continued for 10 min at this temperature. The molten wax collects about the dispersed drug and yields spherical agglomerates. The system is cooled to room temperature under stirring to allow the agglomerates to harden. The resultant agglomerates are then filtered and dried for 24 hr at 40°C. The average size of the agglomerates decreases as the agitation speed increases.

Not surprisingly the method of preparation influences the release characteristics obtained. In particular, the aqueous dispersion method provides higher release rates of all waxes, perhaps due to increased area and physical entrapment of water. Becker and coworkers [86–91] also found that the size of the microcapsule, physical properties of the various wax coating materials, and addition of surfactant all had a profound effect on release rates. Compression of the spray-congealed particles gave a release pattern that appeared to be due to erosion, solubilization, and leaching of drug from the tablet. No one model is adequate to describe the release characteristics, however,

A slow release procainamide tablet, releasing drug through matrix dissolution, has been compared to intravenous dosing by Graffner et al. [95]. The rates of absorption from the tablet were well correlated to the *in vitro* dissolution properties. As can be seen from Figure 5, administration of slow release tablets every 8 hr provides about the same mean plasma level at steady state as ordinary tablets given every 4 hours, and the availability was the same from both preparations.

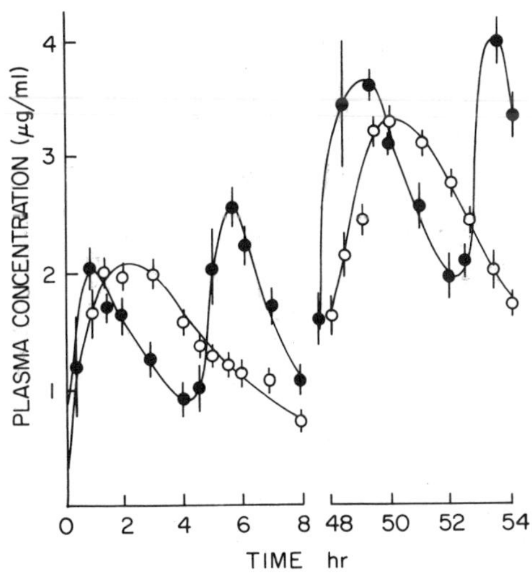

Fig. 5 Plasma concentrations of procainamide after repeated doses of slow release tablets every 8 hr (○) and conventional tablets every 4 hr (●) (mean and SEM). (Reproduced with permission from Ref. 95.)

DeRitter [96] evaluated Roches's Roniacol Timespan matrix tablets. The immediate release portion of the dose is provided by a drug-containing coating while the sustaining portion is provided by erosion of the matrix in the GI tract. The results indicate good correlation of *in vitro* and *in vivo* release rates and the drug is as available in this form as in conventional tablets.

A major disadvantage of matrix devices is that drug release rate continuously decreases with time. This is a consequence of increased diffusional distance and decreased surface area at the penetrating solvent front. Consequently, to achieve zero order release from matrix devices, it will be necessary to select a geometry that compensates the increase in diffusional distance with a corresponding increase in surface area for dissolution. In a pioneering study, Rippie and Johnson [97] investigated various geometries of the dissolving solid including triangular, cross, and star shaped to seek a suitable shape whose change in effective surface area was minimized. They found that thin wafers and thin-walled cylinders provided a more constant dissolution rate. However, the high surface-to-volume ratio was judged to yield unacceptably large dissolution rates.

In a subsequent study, Brook and Washkuhn [98] developed a cylindrical device which had a single aperture leading to a matrix that was pie-wedged. Through this aperture the dissolution medium diffused towards the matrix and released the drug. Shortly thereafter, Hsieh et al. [99] reported a more elegant version of this device which utilized an inward releasing hemisphere. This hemisphere was coated with an impermeable barrier everywhere except in a small aperture in the center of the circular face. Such a device has been applied to the polypeptide hormone insulin and, when implanted in diabetic rats, has been found to achieve sustained lowering of blood glucose over 100 days [100].

Recently, Lee reported a novel approach to achieve zero order drug release that was based on nonuniform drug distribution in a matrix instead of constant drug activity in a reservoir [101]. Here, nonuniform drug distribution was achieved by controlled extraction of drug from an initially dry, drug-loaded hydrogel with a solvent, followed by rapid removal of the solvent by lyophilization. The hydrogel used, 2-hydroxyethyl methacrylate, possessed the characteristic of being glassy in the dry state with the capability of being transformed to an elastic gel upon imbibing water.

Although zero-order release is a desirable feature of most systems, there are systems that would benefit more from release that is controlled by the composition of the releasing medium, such as pH. Heller and Trescony [93] synthesized methyl vinyl ether/maleic anhydride copolymer whose erosion rate, hence drug release rate, is extraordinarily sensitive to the pH of the aqueous environment.

These polymer systems show a characteristic pH above which they are completely soluble and below which they are completely insoluble. The pH depends on the size of the alkyl group in the copolymer ester. Thus, polymer dissolution and drug release can be strictly controlled to fit any desired pH environment.

A similar study by Alhaique et al. [94] demonstrated that a derivative of the polysaccharide scleroglucan, obtained by oxidizing 75% of its glucopyranose side chains to free carboxylic acid, underwent reversible sol-gel transformation depending on the pH of the medium. A 2% solution of this derivative behaved as a viscous liquid at pH above 6 but as a compact gel at pH below 3.5. This sol-gel transformation was found to affect the *in vitro* release characteristics of the model compounds, salicylic acid and Orange II. However, its applicability *in vivo* has yet to be investigated. In principle, these systems can be used in oral controlled delivery where absorption at the specific site in the intestine is desired.

B. Diffusion Controlled Release

The principles of diffusion controlled drug release have been extensively discussed in the literature. A particularly comprehensive article in this regard is the review by Flynn et al. [103], in which the various conditions for diffusion release of drug are presented, together with the appropriate equations for data treatment.

There are basically two types of diffusion controlled systems which have been developed over the past two decades: reservoir devices and matrix devices.

1. *Reservoir Devices*

In this system, a water-insoluble polymeric material encases a core of drug. Drug will partition into the membrane and exchange with the fluid surrounding the particle or tablet. Additional drug will enter the membrane, diffuse to the periphery, and exchange with the surrounding media. A schematic description of the process is shown in Figure 6.

The flux of drug, J (in amount/area-time), across a membrane in the direction of decreasing concentration is given by Fick's first law:

$$J = -D\ dC/dx \tag{6}$$

where D is the diffusion coefficient in area/time and dC/dx is the change of concentration C with distance x. Assuming steady state, Eq. (6) can be integrated to give

$$J = -D\Delta C/\ell \tag{7}$$

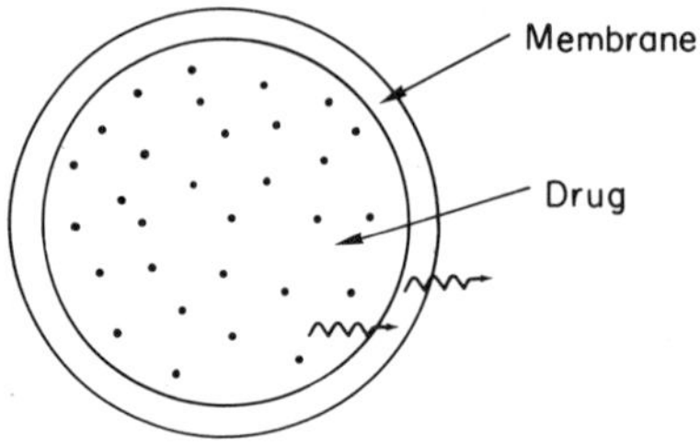

Fig. 6 Diffusion control of drug release by a water-insoluble polymer.

In terms of the amount of drug released, the release rate dM/dt is given by

$$dM/dt = ADK\ \Delta C/\ell \qquad (8)$$

where A is the area, D is the diffusion coefficient, K is the partition coefficient of drug between the membrane and drug core, ℓ is the diffusional pathlength (thickness of coat in the ideal case), and ΔC is the concentration difference across the membrane.

An important parameter in Eq. (8) is the partition coefficient which is defined as the concentration of drug in the membrane over the concentration of drug in the core. If the partition coefficient is high, the core will be depleted of drug in a short time so that zero order release will be observed only over a short segment of the time course of drug release.

Indeed, to obtain a constant drug release rate from a reservoir device it is necessary to maintain constant area, diffusional pathlength, concentration, and diffusion coefficient. In other words, all of the terms on the right hand side of Eq. (8) must be held constant. It is common in many oral sustained release products that one or more of the above terms will change in the product, thus giving rise to non-zero-order release. Examples of this will be shown subsequently.

Methods that have been used to develop reservoir type devices are as follows. Both the press-coating [116–118] and air suspension techniques [119–122] have been used to apply insoluble polymeric materials to enclose drug containing cores in tablets, while the microencapsulation process is a commonly used procedure to coat drug particles to be incorporated into tablets or capsules [57,67,104–114]. In most cases, drug is incorporated in the coating film as well as in the core of the microcapsule so as to provide the initial and sustaining doses, respectively. Generally, slowly soluble films and coating are applied via pan coating techniques or by some form of polymerization resulting in coated pellets, granules or microcapsules that could then be compressed into tablets or placed in a capsule. Care must be taken during placement into tablet or capsule dosage forms to minimize fragmentation or fusion of the particles since both effects will alter release characteristics [115].

There have been several studies which evaluated polymers and/or copolymers for their potential use as coating materials for encapsulated diffusion controlled dosage forms [119–122]. For example, Borodkin and Tucker [123] examined the release of methapyrilene, pentobarbitral, and salicylic acid from cast films of hydroxypropylcellulose by a diffusion-controlled process. By laminating a blank film to the releasing side of the film, good *in vitro* zero order release characteristics have been obtained. This is shown in Figure 7, in which the release profile of salicylic acid from hydroxypropylcellulose with and without a membrane layer is compared. In this system, the nondrug layer functioned as a rate-controlling membrane and the drug-containing film served as the reservoir.

Several of the parameters that are crucial in maintaining a constant rate of drug release are as follows.

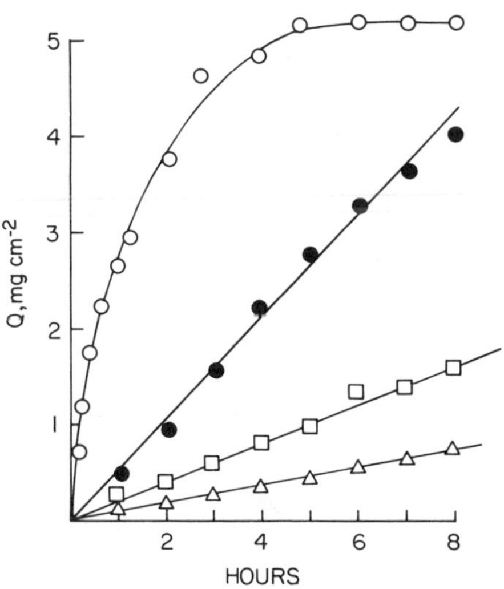

Fig. 7 Drug release from films containing 20% salicylic acid in hydroxypropyl cellulose as the reservoir layer. ○, no membrane layer; ●, 0.164-mm hydroxypropyl cellulose-polyvinyl acetate (8:2) membrane; □, 0.204-mm hydroxypropyl cellulose-polyvinyl acetate (6:4) membrane; △, 0.164-mm hydroxpyropyl cellulose-polyvinyl acetate (4:6) membrane. (Reproduced with permission from Ref. 121.)

Table 3 Effect of Polyethylene Glycol-Ethylcellulose Ratio on the Drug Release Rate Constant (k') for 20% (w/w) Salicylic Acid and 10% (w/w) Caffeine Films

Drug	Proportion of polyethylene glycol	Film thickness (mm)	k' ($mg/36\ cm^2/min^{0.5}$)
Salicyclic acid	0	0.057	0.518
	10	0.057	0.793
	20	0.073	1.24
	30	0.087	1.80
	40	0.082	2.69
Caffeine	0	0.085	0.301
	10	0.069	0.491
	20	0.106	0.851
	30	0.102	1.44
	40	0.130	2.51

Source: Ref. 119.

Polymer Ratio in the Coating

Samuelov et al. examined the release of various drugs from polyethylene glycol-ethylcellulose films [119]. Increasing the proportion of polyethylene glycol in the film at constant drug concentration was found to markedly increase the release rate for all drugs studied (Table 3), in part because this polymer leached out of the system very rapidly, resulting in the formation of large pores. With an increase in porosity, the external solvent would diffuse into the film more readily thereby facilitating drug release. Thus, by selecting the proper mix of polymer and leachable material in the membrane, it is possible to achieve constant drug release [120].

Film Thickness

The drug release rate from an insoluble membrane is expected to increase as the membrane thickness decreases. Madan [124] shows that this is true for microcapsules of clofibrate, prepared by simple coacervation using gelatin-sodium sulfate. Figure 8 shows that increasing the wall thickness retarded drug release for longer than 12 hr.

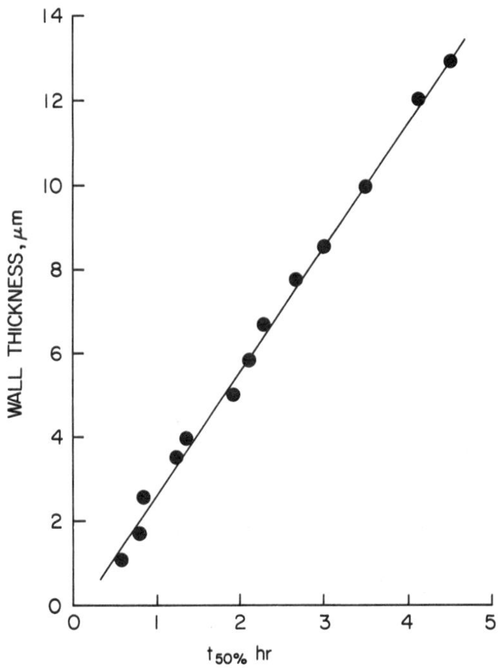

Fig. 8 Wall thickness of microcapsules as a function of *in vitro* $t_{50\%}$ release time. (Reproduced with permission from Ref. 124.)

Hardness of Microcapsule

Luzzi et al. [125] investigated the effect of tablet hardness of tabletted nylon microcapsules on the release of sodium pentobarbital. The results are shown in Figure 9. As expected, increasing the microcapsule hardness prolongs the time of drug release. The mechanism of release in this system probably involves leaching of sodium pentobarbital through a network of nylon fibers constituting the microcapsule.

A combination of dissolution and diffusion may be involved in drug release from microencapsulated material. However, if the material used for encapsulation is chosen properly, diffusion control will predominate. Table 4 summarizes the work that has been done in developing and evaluating reservoir type devices.

2. *Matrix Devices*

In this system, a solid drug is dispersed in an insoluble matrix (Fig. 10). The rate of drug release is dependent on the rate of

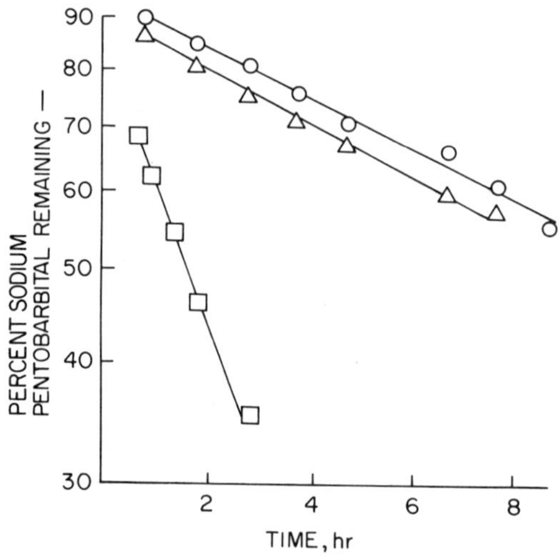

Fig. 9 A comparison of the release relationship of microcapsular tablets of three different hardnesses in 0.1 M phosphate media. ○, 8 hardness; △, 5 hardness; □, 2 hardness. (Reproduced with permission from Ref. 125.)

drug diffusion but not on the rate of solid dissolution. The appropriate equation describing drug release from this system has been derived by T. Higuchi [133].

$$Q = [D\varepsilon/T(2A - \varepsilon C_s)C_s t]^{1/2} \qquad (9)$$

where Q = weight in grams of drug released per unit surface area; D = diffusion coefficient of drug in the release medium; ε = porosity

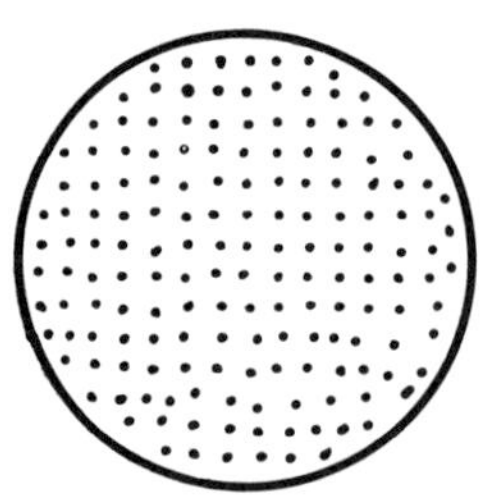

Fig. 10 Diffusion control of drug release by solid drug dispersed in an insoluble matrix.

Table 4 Preparation and Evaluation of Reservoir Type Devices

Coating material and drug investigated	Method of preparation	Method of evaluation	Results and comments
Polyethylene glycol/ethylcellulose [119] Drugs investigated Salicylic acid Caffeine Tripelennamine	A chloroform solution containing drug and polymers was placed on Teflon coated plates. The solvent was allowed to evaporate and the film was removed from the plate and air-dried.	The films were adhered to glass plates with a silicone pressure sensitive adhesive and immersed in 500 ml of buffer solution pre-equilibriated at 37°C. The solution was mixed with a peristaltic pump.	The release profile showed a square root of time dependence. The release rates were independent of film thickness and proportional to drug concentrated in pure ethylcellulose films. The logarithm of the rate constant was proportional to the fraction of polyethylene glycol in the film. In mixed films, the release rate was altered by a change in the external fluid pH.
Hydroxypropyl cellulose/polyvinyl acetate [121] Drugs investigated Methapyrilene Pentobarbital Salicylic acid	The films were cast from a solution containing 10% solids (drugs plus polymer), using a methylene chloride-methanol mixture (9:1) as the solvent. Films were cast as various wet thicknesses using a knife on Teflon-coated plate glass.	Exposed surface of the film was placed at an angle into a 250-ml beaker in a 37°C water bath containing 200 ml of pH 7 buffer. A non-agitated system was selected to eliminate	Drug release followed a diffusion controlled model. The release rate was found to increase with increasing hydroxypropyl cellulose-polyvinyl acetate ratios. The release rates were

Table 4 (Continued)

Coating material and drug investigated	Method of preparation	Method of evaluation	Results and comments
		any effect of turbulence on the release rate. Periodic assays were performed.	also shown to be proportional to drug concentrations but independent of film thickness.
Hydroxypropyl cellulose/polyvinyl acetate methylene chloride [123] Drug investigated Methapyrilene Pentobarbital Salicylic acid	The films were cast as in the preceding system except films were laminated by cutting a section of the drug reservoir film and placing it on Teflon-coated plate glass. One side was sprayed with methylene chloride, then another section of membrane layer was pressed on tacky side of the drug film. The system was allowed to dry for 24 hr.	Exposed surface of the film was placed into a 250-ml beaker in a 37°C water bath containing 200 ml of pH 7 buffer. A nonagitated system was used to eliminate any effect of turbulence on the release rate.	Zero order drug release was observed in the laminated films using 18–45% pentobarbital, methapyrilene, or salicylic acid contained in hydroxypropyl cellulose as the reservoir layer and mixtures of hydroxypropylcellulose and polyvinylacetate as the membrane layer. Inverse relationships were observed between the release rate and membrane thickness as well as between the logarithm of the rate and the percentage of polyvinyl acetate in the membrane layer.

Gelatin-sodium sulfate [124] Drug investigated Clofibrate	Microcapsules were prepared by simple coacervation in gelatin-sodium sulfate and then recovered as discrete free-flowing particles.	Modified flask method was used to evaluate the drug release.	Thinner waller microcapsules gave faster release and showed greater deviation from zero-order kinetics. However, release followed the square root of time plots. In contrast, thicker walled microcapsules approximated zero order release but deviated from the square root of time plots.
Ethylcellulose [128] Drug investigated Caffeine Salicylic acid	Ethylcellulose films were made using a Gardner Ultra Applicator. The wet films were then dried at 94°C for 8 min.	Membranes were adhered to the rim of a cylindrical sintered-glass funnel of constant surface area. The inverted funnel was immersed in water at 37°C. Water was circulated through a 1-cm flow cell in a spectrophotometer using a peristaltic pump.	The ethylcellulose films demonstrated timed release of drugs. Mathematical analysis indicated diffusion controlled.
Poly(hydroxy methacrylate) Drug investigated Progesterone [129]	Polymer films were prepared by free radical polymerization using azobis(methyl isobutyrate) as the initiator.	The diffusion coefficients of progesterone in the polymer films were determined in a glass	Progesterone diffusivity, permeability, and partitioning in poly (hydroxymethacrylate) films did

Table 4 (Continued)

Coating material and drug investigated	Method of preparation	Method of Evaluation	Results and comments
		two compartments of equal volume [130].	not change under the following conditions: (a) when the water content in the initial polymerization mixture was varied from 0 to 40% (v/v), (b) when the polymerization solvent was changed from water to ethanol or t-butyl alcohol, and (c) when the alcohol concentration was changed from 20 to 40%.
2-Hydroxy methacrylate, diethylene glycol dimethacrylate, trimethylolpropane trimethacrylate, glycidyl methacrylate, and hydroxyethyl acrylate were the glass forming monomers. Methyl methacrylate was the nonglass forming monomer. Polymethyl methacrylate,	Drops of polymer, monomer, and drug mixtures were allowed to fall into a cold precipitation medium (−78°C). The solid globules were irradiated for specified time intervals with ^{60}CO-rays. After irradiation, the polymerized spheres were removed and	The dissolution test was carried out with the dissolution apparatus based on USP XIX. The basket was immersed in the vessel containing 1000 ml of dissolution medium at 37°C.	The drug release profiles from polymerized particles were changed by varying the glass-forming monomer and the precipitation medium.

polyethylene glycol 600, and polystyrene were the polymers used [131]. Drug investigated Potassium chloride	dried. The original *n*-hexane precipitation medium was then replaced by cooled 1,4-butanediol, and polymerization was continued at room temperature.		
Dimethylpolysiloxane [132] Drug investigated Butamben	Dimethyl polysiloxane sheeting of medical grade, with a thickness of 0.127 mm was used.	A quasi steady-state diffusion cell was utilized which was shaken mechanically.	The effects of caffeine, β-cyclodextran and povidone on the permeation of butamben from saturated solutions of these complexing agents through a dimethylpolysiloxane membrane were investigated. It was concluded that for a fixed total amount of drug available for release, sustained release is associated with systems containing more stable complexes.
Various polymers and waxes were investigated for microencapsulation of potassium chloride [77]	Polymer coating was done by spray-coating. Wax coating was done by dispersing drug into molten wax, then cooled. For	The *in vitro* dissolution was studied at pH 2 using 2 liters of dissolution medium at 37°C. The stirring speed was 100 rpm.	The gelatin-gum arabic coacervate system offers an effective controlled release system for potassium chloride.

Table 4 (Continued)

Coating material and drug investigated	Method of preparation	Method of evaluation	Results and comments
Drug investigated Potassium chloride	the microencapsulation of coated crystals, equal volumes of acacia and gelatin were prepared. The drug was added to a warmed acacia solution followed by the addition of warmed gelatin solution. After satisfactory coating, formaldehyde was added, and the system was cooled. The microcapsules were then filtered and dried.		
Gelatin [127] Drug investigated Clofibrate	Sperical droplets of clofibrate prepared by a capillary jet method were encapsulated in gelatin by simple coacervation. Sodium sulfate was used as the coacervating agent. The microcapsules were hardened by immersing in a 10% solution of formaldehyde in 2-propanol.	Drug release was evaluated by the modified flask method. A solution of 30% 2-propanol was used as the dissolution medium	Following an initial burst effect, release of drug followed apparent zero order kinetics until nearly 90% of the drug was released.

of the matrix; T = tortuosity of the matrix; C_s = solubility of drug in the release medium; and A = concentration of drug in the tablet, expressed as g/ml.

The assumptions made in deriving Eq. (9) are as follows.

1. A pseudo-steady state is maintained during release.
2. $A \gg C_s$, i.e., excess solute is present.
3. C = 0 in solution at all times (perfect sink).
4. Drug particles are much smaller than those in the matrix.
5. The diffusion coefficient remains constant.
6. No interaction between the drug and the matrix occurs.

For purposes of data treatment, Eq. (9) is usually reduced to:

$$Q = kt^{1/2} \tag{10}$$

Therefore, a plot of amount of drug released versus the square root of time should be linear if drug release from the matrix is diffusion controlled. In this instance, one may control drug release from a homogeneous matrix by varying the following parameters:

1. Initial concentration of drug in the matrix
2. Drug solubility
3. Porosity
4. Tortuosity
5. Leaching solvent composition
6. Polymer system making up matrix

Zero-order release is not commonly achieved *in vivo* using these systems. The most common explanation in this problem is changing diffusional pathlengths.

As in the reservoir device, it is often necessary that a portion of the drug be released quickly for immediate absorption. This is usually accomplished by placing the initial dose in the coat of the tablet. The coat and matrix can be tabletted together by press-coating. In noncoated systems, the initial dose is simply tabletted with the sustaining dose.

The three major types of matrix diffusion control devices are insoluble plastic, fatty, and hydrophilic matrices. Although there has been considerable basic research devoted to developing insoluble matrix devices and although experimentation under idealized conditions suggests that they will work, certain complications do arise when these devices are ingested orally. For example, Ritschel [134] has reported on problems that could arise from chewing an insoluble matrix. If the drug was contained within pores and channels of a polymeric matrix following compression, then upon mastication the drug would be released very quickly. This could be dangerous in the case of drugs with a narrow therapeutic index. Ritschel has described a sandwich tablet that would alleviate this problem somewhat because the drug is dissolved directly in the plastic matrix material and upon mastication will not be released as promptly. A pictorial presentation of Ritschel's tablet is shown in Figure 11.

Essentially fatty matrices consist of waxes and are generally prepared by dispersing the drug and excipients in molten wax. This mixture is then congealed, granulated and compressed into cores. These cores may then be coated as mentioned previously.

Hydrophilic gums were first used to provide sustained drug release in 1962 [135]. The method described involved mining a drug with nondigestible hydrophilic gums such as hydroxypropylmethycellulose or sodium carboxymethylcellulose followed by compressing the mixtures into tablets. When such a tablet is exposed to water or digestive fluids, rapid initial drug release occurs. At the same time,

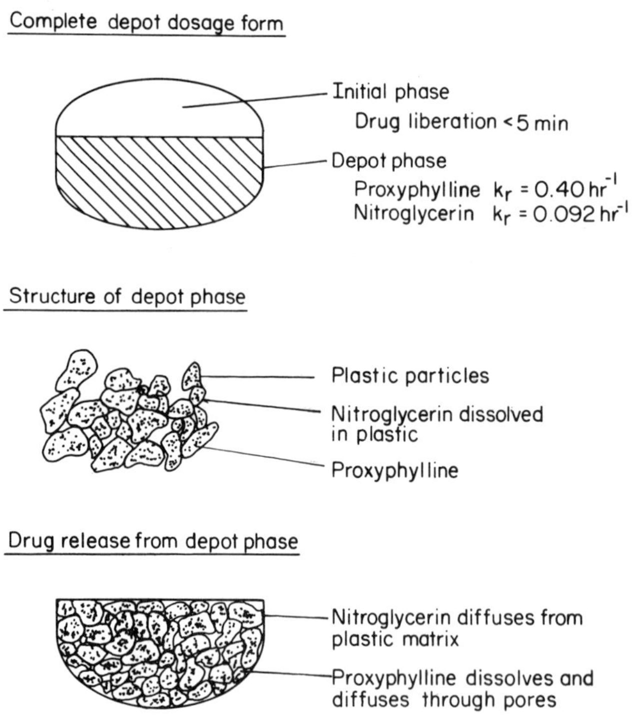

Fig. 11 Diagrammatic structure of the peroral sandwich tablet with timed release and its release characteristics. (Reproduced with permission from Ref. 134.)

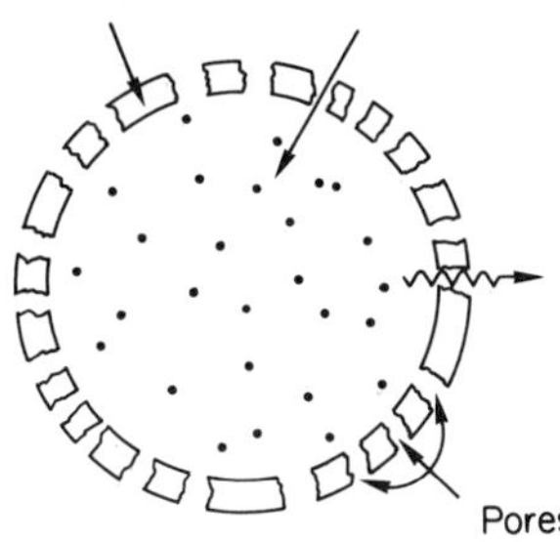

Fig. 12 Diffusion control of drug release by a partially water-soluble polymer. Example: Polymer coating consisting of ethylcellulose and methylcellulose. The latter dissolves leaving the ethylcellulose coat behind.

hydration and gelation of gum at the tablet-liquid interface occurs resulting in a viscous gel barrier which serves to retard further drug release. Studies have shown that release of drugs from some hydrophilic matrices follow Higuchi's diffusion controlled model [136].

Table 5 summarizes the work that has been done in developing the matrix utilizing diffusion as the controlling mechanism.

C. Diffusion and Dissolution Controlled Systems

An example of these systems is shown in Figure 12. The main feature is that the drug core is enclosed with a partially soluble membrane. Dissolution of part of the membrane allows for diffusion of the contained drug through pores in the polymer coat. The release profile of drug from this type of product can be described by the following equation:

$$\text{Release rate} = AD(C_1 - C_2)/\ell \tag{11}$$

where A,D and ℓ are the surface area, diffusion coefficient of drug through pore, and diffusion pathlength, respectively; C_1 is the concentration of drug in the core and C_2 is that in the dissolution medium. The fraction of soluble polymer in the coat will be the dominant factor controlling drug release. Such a system has been demonstrated to provide zero order release of KCl from a tablet and in so doing minimize the gastointestinal irritating effects of this compound [120].

An interesting modification of the matrix tablet approach, using diffusion and dissolution, has been discussed by Javaid et al. [144,

Table 5 Fabrication and Evaluation of Matrix Devices

Matrix material and drug investigated	Fabrication procedure	Method of evaluation	Results and comments
Matrix material Hydrated methylcellulose [136] Drug investigated Chlorpheniramine maleate	The tablets were prepared by mixing hydroxypropyl methylcellulose, ether and drug, followed by granulating with ethanol. The granulation was then dried, screened, and compressed.	The tablet was inserted into a cylindrical tube so that drug release could be measured from only one face of the tablet. The tablet in its holder was placed in a flow cell in which a constant flow of solvent was maintained past the the tablet with no turbulence. The total volume of circulating fluid was 155 ml and the temperature was 37°C.	Drug release appeared to follow Higuchi's model and therefore was diffusion rather than dissolution controlled.
Matrix material Carnauba wax and stearyl alcohol [137] Drug investigated Tripelennamine hydrochloride	Various surface-active ingredients and the drug were mixed in a molten mixture of carnauba wax and stearyl alcohol. The mixture was then congealed, granulated, and compressed into cores.	The USP rotating basket method was used to measure dissolution rate in simulated intestinal fluid while particle-size distribution, tablet hardness, and tablet weight were controlled.	Water-soluble surface active agents increased dissolution rate, probably by creating more channels for contact with the dissolution fluid.

Matrix material Carnauba wax and stearyl alcohol [137] Drug investigated Tripelennamine hydrochloride	Two fabrication methods were used. The first method was that described in the preceding system. In the second method, the materials were blended in a rotary mixer. The mixture was compressed into slugs and passed through air oscillating granulator. The tablets were then compressed.	The rate of drug release in simulated intestinal fluid at 37°C was measured with the USP rotating basket method.	The addition of povidone as a channeling agent increased the rate of drug release significantly.
Matrix material Carbopol 934 [139] Drug investigated Mepyramine maleate	Aqueous solution of mepyramine was added to a constantly stirred equal volume of aqueous dispersion of Carbopol 934 using a mechanically stirrer. Stirring was continued for a few minutes to allow complete entrapment. The gummy product was separated and washed with water, then spread on a glass slab and dried. The dried mass was ground and a 200–500 μm fraction was used.	Each sample was placed in a capped bottle containing 50 ml of 0.1 N HCl. The bottle was rotated at 40 rpm in a thermostatically controlled water bath at 37°C. Every 30 min, half of the dissolution fluid was withdrawn for analysis, and replaced with an equal volume of dissolution fluid.	A linear relationship was obtained in the first 2.5 hr, after which time, there was a negative deviation. This linearity established that an intact hydrated layer was maintained over the first 2.5 hr of the test, therefore, diffusion was the most important factor contributing to drug release during this time interval. Negative deviation might be due to the maximum gelation occuring in the time interval between 2.5 and 3.5 hr.

Table 5 (Continued)

Matrix material and drug investigated	Fabrication procedure	Method of evaluation	Results and comments
Matrix material Silicone [138] Drug investigated Morphine sulfate	Simethicone fluid was added to polydimethylsiloxane elastomer followed by mixing with various powders to be added. Cylindrical pellets were then prepared from the mixture. To polymerize the mixture, stannous octanoate was added followed by placing the mixture rapidly in a plastic tablet mold.	Release rate of drug from the pellets was studied in screw-capped vials containg 15 ml of phosphate beffer. These vials were maintained at 37°C and rotated end over end at 15 rpm.	The release rate of morphine sulfate from silicone polymer was very slow. However, addition of water-soluble carriers to the formulation caused the pellets to swell in aqueous media and the release rate was increased. The release mechanism appears to involve the creation of pores or pathways through the matrix secondary to the swelling.
Matrix material Glyceryl tristearate [87] Drug investigated Sulfaethylthiadiazole	The drug was dispersed in melted glyceryl tristearate. Distilled water containing a dispersant was heated and added to drug-wax dispersion with stirring. The drug-wax particles were separated from the aqueous phase and product was air-dried.	A rotating bottle dissolution apparatus was used. Both simulated intestinal fluid and simulated gastric fluid were used as the media.	Over 50% of total drug was released in the simulated gastric fluid at equilibrium, and this amount was released quite rapidly during the first 15 minutes. However, in the alkaline pancreatic solution, drug continued to be released

			not only due to diffusion but also due to a gradual disintegration of the wax matrix. Sodium monooleate, a dispersing agent, increased the release rate whereas polysorbate, a surfactant, decreased it.
Matrix material Methyl acrylate-methyl methacrylate [140] Drug investigated Sodium pentobarbital Methrapyrilene HCl Ephedrine HCl Dextromethorphan HBr	Uniform mixtures of drug and plastic were prepared, and tablets were compressed to various hardnesses.	Drug release was studied using a resin-kettle flask with four ground glass openings in the cover. Tubes containing one tablet were inserted into three openings. A stirrer was placed into the fourth opening. The flask contained 600 ml of solvent maintained at 37°C.	Drug release followed square root of time dependence. Table hardness appears to have little effect on the release rate.
Matrix material Polyvinyl chloride Polyethylene Halogenated fluorocarbon Drug investigated Sodium salicylate	Tablets were prepared by compressing a uniform drug-plastic mixture. The tablets were then embedded in wax by coating lateral surface and one of the flat sides with molten beeswax. Thus, only one flat surface	Tablet was immersed in 500 ml of solvent contained in a jacketed glass beaker maintained at 30°C. The solution was stirred continuously and samples were withdrawn at specified time intervals.	In all cases, the release profile followed Higuchi's model. The release rates were significantly altered when: (a) the amount of drug in the matrix was varied, (b) drug solubility was changed,

Table 5 (Continued)

Matrix material and drug investigated	Fabrication procedure	Method of evaluation	Results and comments
	of the tablet was exposed for drug release.		(c) different plastics were used as matrix material, and (d) different solvents were used. Drug release rate was increased when surfactants were added to the medium.
Matrix material Polyethylene [142]	Tablets were prepared by compressing a uniform drug-plastic mixture. The	Tablets were placed in a jacketed glass beaker containing 500 ml of sol-	Release rate follows Higuchi model for all drugs studied. More-

Drug investigated Sulfanilamide Caffeine Potassium acid phthalate	tablets were then embedded in wax by coating the lateral surface and one of the flat sides with molten beeswax. Thus, only one flat surface of the tablet was exposed for drug release.	vent maintained at 30°C. The solution was stirred continuously. Samples were obtained at specified time intervals.	over, for all drugs examined, addition of surfactants caused a general increase in release rate.
Matrix material Polyvinyl chloride [143]	Tablets were prepared in the same fashion as in preceding system except that	Release rate was determined as in the preceding system.	The amount of drug released versus square root of time plot was S
Drug investigated Sodium salicylate	polyvinyl chloride was used as the matrix material		shaped. Such a result may be ascribed to a slow release of air from the tablets

145]. They employed a lipase-lipid-drug system to provide sustained release where matrix erosion was due to the lipolytic action of lipase on the substrate. Incorporation of lipase activity accelerators, such as calcium carbonate or glyceryl monostearate, provides flexibility in drug release rates. *In vivo* studies of this system in dogs [145] showed that tablets containing lipase consistently gave higher, more uniform blood levels of drug than those without.

D. Ion-Exchange Resins

The principle of ion exchange has been used for a long time in analytical and protein chemistry. It is an attractive method for sustained drug delivery because, in theory, drug release characteristics rely only on the ionic environment of the resin containing drug and should therefore be less susceptible to environmental conditions, such as enzyme content and pH, at the site of absorption. Because this approach of sustained release requires the presence of ions in solution, it would not be applicable to the skin, the external ear canal, or other areas with limited quantities of eluting ions. In contrast, the subcutaneous and intramuscular routes, where the pool of available ions is more controlled, would appear better suited for this approach. However, the resin may undergo biodegradation with an attendant alteration in the "preprogrammed" release rate. While the GI tract appears to possess a rather constant ionic content, the variability in diet, water intake, and GI content composition make this constant ionic content unlikely. Nevertheless, oral product employing this principle which provide prolonged drug release are available.

Resins are water-insoluble materials containing anionic or cationic groups in repeating positions on the resin chain. The drug-charged resin is prepared by mixing the resin with drug solution either by repeated exposure of the resin to the drug in a chromatographic column or by keeping the resin in contact with the drug solution for extended periods of time. The drug-resin is then washed to remove contaminant ions and dried to form particles or beads.

When a high concentration of an appropriately charged ion is in contact with the ion-exchange group, the drug molecule is exchanged and diffuses out of the resin to the bulk solution according to the following scheme.

$$\text{Resin } [N(CH_3)]^+X^- + Z^- \text{ -----> Resin } [N(CH_3)]^+Z + X^-$$

or

$$\text{Resin } (SO_3^-)A^+ + B^+ \text{ -----> Resin } (SO_3^-)B^+ + A^+$$

where X^- and A^+ are drug ions.

Before the eluted ion can diffuse out, the eluting ions must diffuse into the resin matrix and establish equilibrium with the ionic resin group. As with all diffusion processes, the area of diffusion and diffusional pathlength are important to the rate of diffusion. In addition, the amount of solvent in the matrix of the resin, as well as the structural rigidity of the resin, i.e., cross-linking, also influences the drug diffusion rate. For this reason, the porosity of the resin and the size of the bead or particle must be carefully controlled during the formulation process.

The release rate can be further controlled by coating the drug-resin complex using one of the microencapsulation processes described earlier [147,148] (Fig. 13). Coated and uncoated drug-resin complexes can be mixed in certain ratios and filled into capsules with excipients or suspended in a palatable flavored vehicle containing suitable suspending agents. This has been shown to be a reliable technique to obtain desired release profiles. The release of drug from uncoated resin beads is expected to begin immediately while release from the coated form would be delayed depending on the type and thickness of coat. Thus, drug-resin complex of phenylpropanolamine administered once every 12 hr for 2 weeks provided the same plasma concentrations as a solution of the drug administered once every 5 hr [149].

Further improvement of this ion-exchange type drug delivery system is illustrated by the development of the Pennkinetic system (Fig. 14). In this system, the drug-containing resin granules are first treated with an impregnating polymer such as PEG 4000 to retard the rate of swelling in water and further coated with a water-permeable polymer such as ethyl cellulose to act as a rate-limiting barrier to control drug release.

E. pH-Independent Formulations

As discussed in Chapter 1, the GI tract presents some unusual features that are not found in other routes of drug administration.

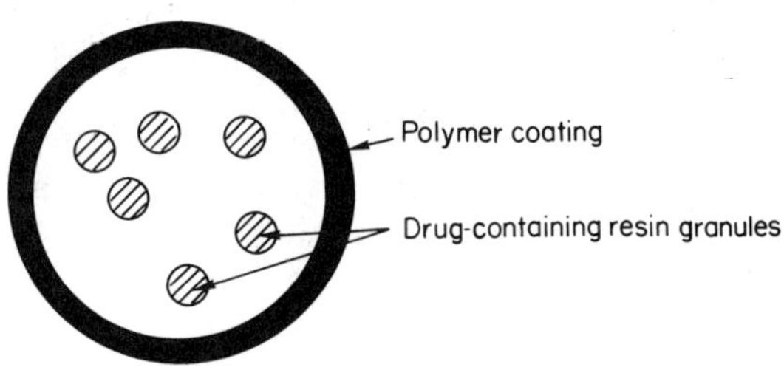

Fig. 13 Polymer-coated drug-resin design (U.S. patent #2,246,037).

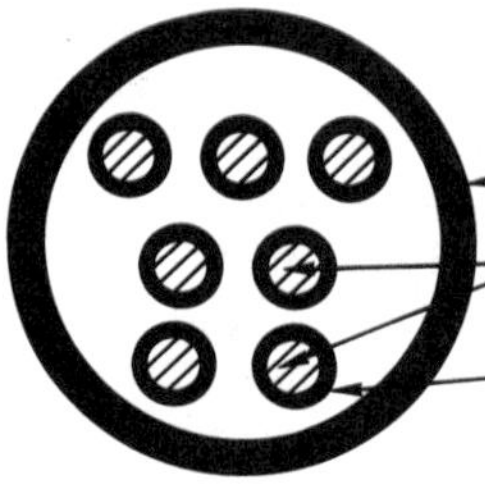

Fig. 14 Polymer-coated drug-resin dispersion (U.S. patent #4,221,778).

The relatively brief transit time through the GI tract constrains the length of prolongation. The variable nature of the chemical environment throughout the length of the GI tract is a further constraint on dosage form design. Indeed, drugs administered orally would encounter a spectrum of pH ranging from 7 in the mouth, 1 to 4 in the stomach, and 5 to 7 in the small intestine. Conceivably, since most drugs are either weak acids or weak bases, their release from sustained release formulations is pH dependent.

The pH dependency of drug release from sustained release formulations has been demonstrated [119,150]. For instance, papaverine hydrochloride was preferentially released in the gastric region than in the intestine because its higher solubility in the upper part of the GI tract. However, buffers can be added to the formulation to help maintain a constant pH thereby rendering pH-independent drug release [115]. To this end, salts of amino acids, citric acid, phthalic acid, phosphoric acid or tartaric acid are commonly used because of their physiological acceptability. Indeed, the rate of availability of propoxyphene from a bufferred controlled release formulation showed significantly increased reproducibility [152].

Further refinements of this approach are exemplified by the so-called pH-independent controlled release granules [153]. The granules are designed for the oral controlled release of basic or acidic drugs at a rate that is independent of the pH in the GI tract [153]. They are prepared by mixing a basic or acidic drug with one or more buffering agents, granulating with appropriate pharmaceutical excipients, and finally, coating with a gastrointestinal fluid permeable film-forming polymer. When the GI fluid permeates through the membrane, the buffering agents adjust the fluid inside to a suitable constant pH, thereby rendering a constant rate of drug release.

F. Osmotically Controlled Release

In this type of drug delivery systems, osmotic pressure is the driving force that generates constant drug release. As shown in Figure 15, this system is fabricated by applying a semipermeable membrane around a core of an osmotically active drug or a core of an osmotically inactive drug in combination with an osmotically active salt. A delivery orifice is drilled in each system by laser or by a high-speed mechanical drill [154–157]. The optimum size of the orifice can be calculated by the following equation.

$$A_s = (LV/t)(8\pi)(\eta/P)^{1/2} \tag{12}$$

where A_s is the cross sectional area of the orifice, V/t is the volume released per unit time, L is the diameter of the orifice, π is 3.14, η is the viscosity of the solution moving from the inside to the outside of the device, and P is the hydrostatic pressure difference. When the osmotic device has more than one orifice, A_s is the total cross sectional area of the orifices [154].

When an osmotic system is exposed to water or any body fluid, water will flow into the core due to an osmotic pressure difference across the coating membrane. Under this osmotic pressure gradient, the volume flow of water into the core reservoir, dV/dt, is expressed as:

$$dV/dt = (Ak/h)\ (\Delta\pi - \Delta P) \tag{13}$$

where A, k and h are the area, membrane permeability, and thickness, respectively, $\Delta\pi$ is the osmotic pressure difference, and ΔP is the hydrostatic pressure difference. If the orifice is sufficiently large, the hydrostatic pressure difference will be small compared to the osmotic pressure difference, and Eq. 13 becomes:

$$dV/dt = (Ak/h)\Delta\pi \tag{14}$$

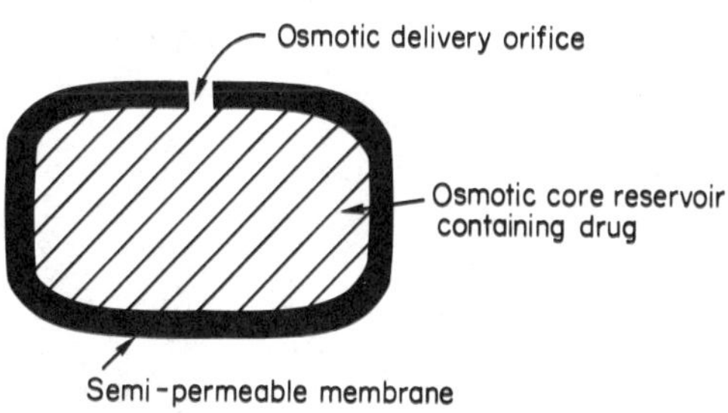

Fig. 15 The elementary osmotic pump.

The drug will be pumped out of the system through the orifice at a controlled rate, dM/dt, which is equal to the volume flow rate of water into the core multipled by the drug concentration, Cs. Thus,

$$dM/dt = (dV/dt)Cs \tag{15}$$

In principle, this delivery system dispenses drug continuously at a zero-order rate until the concentration of the osmotically active salt in the system is below saturation solubility, whereupon a non-zero-order release pattern results. In the case of indomethacin, all three systems investigated were found to release 70% of their contents in a zero order fashion [156].

By design, the coating membrane is rigid and non-swelling so that it is able to maintain the structural integrity of the system during the course of drug release. It is impermeable to drug solutes, but is permeable to gastrointestinal fluid. Examples of polymers used as semi-permeable membranes are listed in Table 6. The permeability of the rate controlling membrane is a composite quantity being a function of the diffusion coefficient and solubility of water in the polymeric membrane, structure of the polymer, relative pressure difference across the membrane, thickness of the membrane, as well as temperature. The flux of water through a semipermeable membrane can be determined and be expressed as water vapor transmission rate (WVTR) [158]. Representative WVTR values of several polymeric membranes are listed in Table 6.

To further regulate the availability of GI fluid for permeation through the semipermeable membrane, a layer of bioerodible polymer can be applied to the external surface of the semi-permeable membrane [159]. Several other modifications of the osmotic pressure-controlled drug delivery system have been developed [160]. One such system consists of two compartments separated by a movable partition (Fig. 16). The osmotically active compartment imbibes the GI fluid to create an osmotic pressure on the partition, which then moves to reduce the volume of the drug reservoir compartment thereby releasing drug through the delivery orifice.

Another modified system is one in which a delivery orifice is absent. In this sytem, as the GI fluid is imbibed, hydraulic pressure is built up inside until the wall ruptures and the contents are released to the environment [161]. This osmotic bursting device can be employed to control drug release by varying the thickness as well as the area of the semipermeable membrane [162].

In summary, osmotically controlled release systems require only osmotic pressure to be effective and is essentially independent of its environment. In light of the rather harsh and inconsistent conditions of pH and mixing in the digestive tract, this appears to be a good sustained release system for oral dosage forms [163–165].

Table 6 Water-Vapor Transmission Rate Values of Some Polymer Membranes

Polymer	Water vapor transmission rates ($g/100\ in^2/24\ hr/1$ mm thick film)
Cellophane, polyethylene coated	1.2
Cellulose acetate	40–75
Cellulose acetate butyrate	50
Ethylcellulose	75
Ethylene propylene copolymer	0.8
Ethylene vinyl acetate	1–3
Methylcellulose	70
Polycarbonate	8
Polyesters	2
Polyethylene	0.5–1.2
Polypropylene	0.7
Polyurethane	30–150
Polyvinyl alcohol	100
Polyvinyl chloride, cast	10–20
Polyvinyl chloride, excluded	6–15
Polyvinyl chloride, rigid	0.7
Polyvinyl fluoride	3
Polyvinylidene fluoride	1.0

Source: Ref. 158, reproduced with permission.

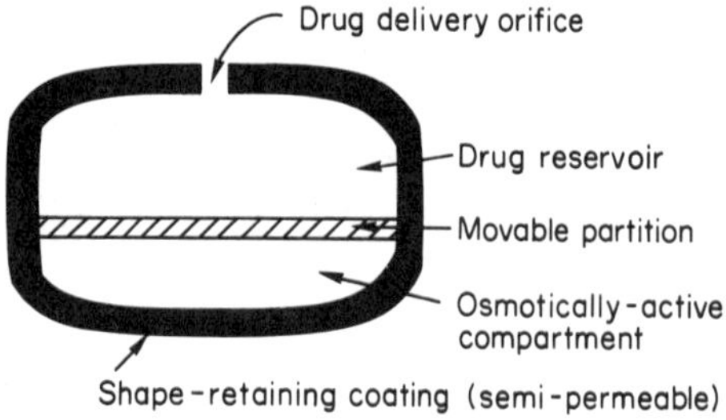

Fig. 16 Osmotic pressure-controlled drug delivery system with two compartments separated by a movable partition.

G. Altered Density Formulations

The GI transit time varies from one individual to another. In most human subjects, it is less than 24 hr, although a range of 8 to 62 hr has been found [169]. Among the factors that influence the GI transit time are the physical properties of the delivery system and the presence of food. A recent publication reported that multiple-unit formulations are less affected by the presence of food than single-unit formulations since their subunits are distributed throughout the GI tract [173]. Moreover, the specific density of these subunits is found to be a more significant factor than their diameter in influencing their GI transit time. Specifically, increasing the density from 1.0 to 1.6 increases the average transit time from 7 to 25 hours [173]. However, subsequent work in non-colostomy patients established that the density of the delivery system in the range of 1 to 3 has minimal influence on G.I. transit time.

It is reasonable to expect that unless a delivery system remains in the vicinity of the absorption site until most, if not all of its drug contents is released, it would have limited utility. To this end, several approaches have been developed to prolong the residence time of drug delivery systems in the GI tract. One such approach is the bioadhesion approach [169–172], which is based on the adherence of bioadhesive polymers to the mucin/epithelial surface of the GI tract.

The other approach is to alter the formulation's density by using either high or low density pellets.

1. High-density approach: In this approach, the density of the pellets must exceed that of normal stomach content and should therefore be at least 1.4 [152]. In preparing such formulations, drug can be coated on a heavy core or mixed with heavy inert materials such as barium sulfate, titanium dioxide, iron powder, and zinc oxide. The weighted pellet can then be covered with a diffusion controlled membrane.

2. Low-density approach: Globular shells which have an apparent density lower than that of gastric fluid can be used as a carrier of drug for sustained release purposes [174]. Polystyrol, poprice, and even popcorn are all candidates as carriers. The surface of these empty shells is undercoated with sugar or with a polymeric material such as methacrylic polymer and cellulose acetate phthalate. The undercoated shell is then coated by a mixture of drug with polymers such as ethylcellulose and hydroxypropylcellulose. The final product floats on the gastric fluid for a prolonged period, while slowly releasing drug.

The above principle can be applied to formulate buoyant tablets or capsules [175,176]. The tablet formulation is prepared by simply granulating a mixture of drug, excipients, and 20–75% w/w of hydrocolloids, such as hydroxyethylcellulose, hydroxpropylcellulose and hydroxypropylmethylcellulose. These granules are then compressed to a hardness of 5–6 SCU [177]. On contact with gastric fluid, the tablet forms a water-impermeable colloid gel barrier around its surface and maintains a bulk density of less than one, thereby allowing it to remain buoyant in the gastric fluid (Fig. 17). However, subsequent work established that low density dosage forms are unable to retain these systems in the stomach unless water is present. This requires that subjects injest a glass of water every hour, an unacceptable procedure under most circumstances.

Alternatively, the buoyant tablet can be modified into a bilayer tablet consisting of one immediate release layer and one sustained release layer. After the initial dose is released, the sustained release layer absorbs the gastric juice and forms a water-impermeable colloid

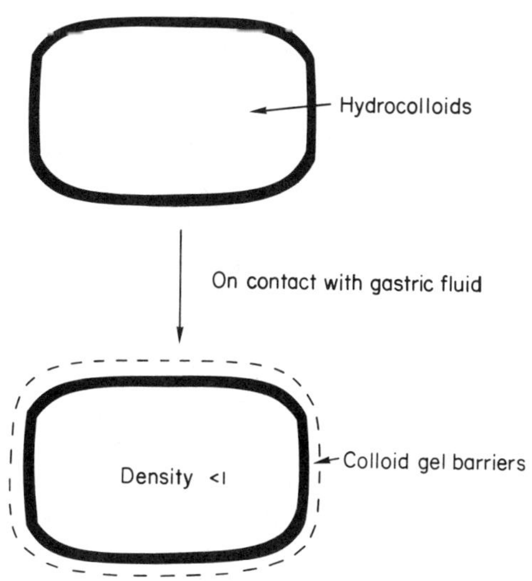

Fig. 17 Intragastric floating tablet.

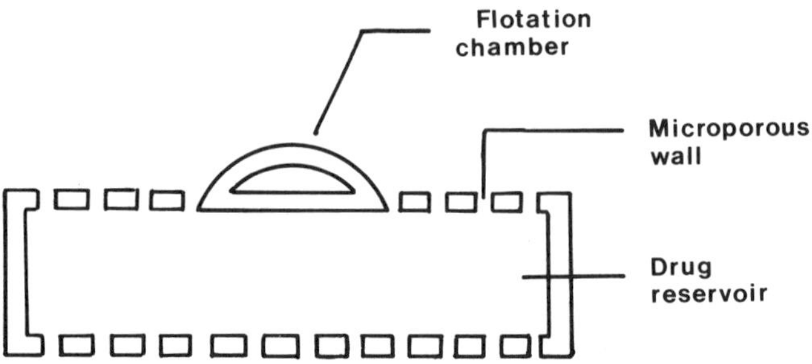

Fig. 18 Drug delivery system with flotation chamber.

gel barrier around its surface. Once again, it maintains a bulk density of less than one and remains buoyant in the stomach [178].

Another application of the buoyancy principle is the incorporation of a gas-filled flotation chamber into a microporous compartment which houses a drug reservoir, as shown in Figure 18 [179]. A feature of this compartment is the presence of apertures along its top and bottom walls through which gastric fluids pass to dissolve the drug. Its peripheral walls are sealed, however, to prevent the undissolved drug from making contact with the stomach.

III. SUMMARY

Over the past 50 years a number of techniques have been developed and employed to sustain the delivery of oral medications to the systemic circulation. By and large, these are based on the principles of diffusion, dissolution, or ion exchange and, only recently, on the principle of osmosis. Regardless of the mechanism of sustained release, however, more and more of these systems are becoming polymer-based. In this light, a thorough understanding of the properties of polymers will be crucial to the design of future oral sustained and controlled release systems for a drug candidate. Unfortunately, few, if any, of these systems are deliberately designed to outlive the GI transit time so that obtaining a period of drug release beyond 12 hr in the general population is an exception rather than the rule. It is imperative that the next level of sophistication in the design of oral sustained delivery systems aim at prolonging the GI transit time of a given system. This would require the incorporation of concepts in engineering and cell biology into the design of oral controlled drug release systems. Presently, there are systems based on the buoyancy principle which prolong the retention of a delivery system in the stomach. There are also those which are based on the bioadhesion principle whose goal is to promote the retention of a delivery system, hence drug release, at a specific region in the GI tract. Finally, with an increasing understanding of the role of peptides in therapy, hence a need to deliver these labile substances to the systemic circulation intact, it is suggested that future research in oral sustained and controlled drug delivery should aim at discovering means to input drug into the body via the oral route without subjecting it to extensive presystemic clearance.

REFERENCES

1. R. D. Cowsar, Introduction to controlled release. In, *Controlled Release of Biologically Active Agents* (A. C. Tanquary and R. E. Lacey, Eds.), Plenum, New York, 1974.
2. The United States Pharmacopeia, 20th rev., Mack Publishing Co., Eaton, PA, 1980, p. 959.
3. A. C. Shah, C. B. Peot, and J. F. Ochs, Design and evaluation of a rotating filter-stationary basket *in vitro* dissolution test apparatus I: Fixed fluid volume system, *J. Pharm. Sci. 62*, 671 (1973).
4. H. Weintraub and M. Gibaldi, Rotating-flask method for dissolution rate determinations of aspirin from various dosage forms, *J. Pharm. Sci. 59*, 1792 (1970).
5. J. E. Tingstad, E. Gropper, L. Lachman, and E. Shami, Dissolution rate studies III: Effect of type and intesity of agitation on dissolution rate, *J. Pharm. Sci. 62*, 293 (1973).
6. E. O. Kruger and E. B. Vliet, *In vitro* testing of timed release tablets and capsules, *J. Pharm. Sci. 51*, 181 (1962).
7. P. B. Chemburkar, R. D. Smyth, D. B. Shah, R. S. Joslin, A. Polk, and N. H. Reavey-Cantwell, Correlations between dissolution characteristics and absorption of methaqualone from solid dosage forms, *J. Pharm. Sci. 65*, 529 (1976).
8. S. Stavchansky, J. T. Doluisio, A. Mastin, C. Martin, B. Cabana, S. Dighe, and A. Loper, Correlation of *in vivo* bioavailability of erythromycin stearate tablets with *in vitro* tests, *J. Pharm. Sci. 69*, 1309 (1980).
9. H. Schneider, C. H. Nightingale, R. Quintriliani, and D. R. Flanagan, Evaluation of an oral prolonged-release antibiotic formulation, *J. Pharm. Sci. 67*, 1620 (1978).
10. S. Eriksen, Sustained action dosage forms. In, *The Theory and Practice of Industrial Pharmacy*, 1st ed. (L. Lachman, H. A. Lieberman, and J. L. Kanig, Eds.), Lea & Febiger, Philadelphia, 1970.
11. H. B. Hopfenberg, Controlled release from erodible slabs, cylinders, and spheres. In, *Controlled Release Polymeric*

Formulations (D. R. Paul and F. W. Harris, Eds.), American Chemical Society, Washington, DC, 1976, p. 26.
12. J. T. Carstensen, Dissolution of solids. In, *Pharmaceutics of Solids and Solid Dosage Forms*, Wiley-Interscience, New York, 1977, p. 63.
13. K. R. Heimlich, D. R. MacDonnell, T. L. Flanagan, and P. D. O'Brien, Evaluation of a sustained release form of phenylpropanolamine hydrochloride by urinary excretion studies, *J. Pharm. Sci. 50*, 232 (1961).
14. S. Benita and M. Donbrow, Coacervation of ethyl cellulose, the role of polyisobutylene and the effect of its concentration, *J. Colloid Interface Sci. 77*, 102 (1980).
15. Y. Takeda, N. Nambu, and T. Nagai, Microencapsulation and bioavailability in beagle dogs of indomethacin, *Chem. Pharm. Bull. 29*, 264 (1981).
16. S. Benita and M. Donbrow, Dissolution rate control of the release kinetics of water-soluble compounds from ethyl cellulose film-type microcapsules, *Int. J. Pharm. 12*, 251 (1982).
17. J. P. Benoit, J. Y. Drouin, F. Puisieux, F. Brunelle, M. Dubois, and M. Beaufils, Selective embolization of the renal artery of the rat by cross-linked serum/albumin microcapsules. In, *Microspheres and Drug Therapy*, Elsevier, Amsterdam, 1983.
18. S. Benita, Microcapsules: New applications and characterization, *Labo-Pharma-Propl. Tech. 32*, 694 (1984).
19. K. R. Heimlich, D. R. MacDonnell, A. Polk, and T. L. Flanagan, Evaluation of an oral sustained release dosage of trimeprazine as measured by urinary excretion, *J. Pharm. Sci. 50*, 213 (1961).
20. J. G. Wagner, O. S. Carpenter, and E. J. Collins, Sustained action oral medication. I. A quantitative study of prednisolone in man, in the dog and *in vitro*, *J. Pharmacol. Exp. Ther. 129*, 101 (1960).
21. J. F. Nash and R. E. Cabtree, Absorption of tritiated d-desoxyephedrine in sustained-release dosage forms, *J. Pharm. Sci. 50*, 134 (1961).
22. E. Rosen and J. V. Swintosky, Preparation of a (35)S-labelled trimeprazine tartrate sustained action product for its evaluation in man, *J. Pharm. Pharmacol. 12*, 237 (1960).
23. L. E. Hollister, Studies of delayed-action medication. I. Meprobamate administered as compressed tablets and as two delayed-action capsules, *N. Engl. J. Med. 266*, 281 (1962).
24. E. Rosen, P. Tannenbaum, T. Ellison, S. M. Free, and A. P. Crosley, Absorption and excretion of radioactively tagged dextroamphetamine sulfate from a sustained-release preparation, *JAMA 194*, 145 (1965).

25. A. A. Sugerman and E. Rosen, Absorption efficiency and excretion profile of a prolonged-action form of chlorpromazine, *Clin. Pharmacol. Ther.* *5*, 561 (1964).
26. E. Rosen, T. Ellison, P. Tannenbaum, S. M. Free, and A. P. Crosley, Comparative study in man and dog of the absorption and excretion of dextroamphetamine-C14 sulfate in sustained-release and nonsustained-release dosage forms, *J. Pharm. Sci.* *56*, 365 (1967).
27. E. Rosen, A. Polk, S. M. Free, P. J. Tannenbaum, and A. P. Crosley, Comparative study in man of the absorption and excretion of amobarbital-C14 from sustained-release and nonsustained-release dosage forms, *J. Pharm. Sci.* *56*, 1285 (1967).
28. S. Khalil and S. Elgamal, *In vitro* release of aspirin from various wax-coated formulations, *J. Pharm. Pharmacol.* *23*, 72 (1971).
29. J. Royal, *In vitro* method for the determination of the rate of release of amphetamine sulfate from sustained release medication, *Drug Standards* *26*, 41 (1958).
30. J. Royal, A comparision of *in vitro* rates of release of several brands of dextroamphetamine sulfate sustained release capsules, *Drug Standards* *27*, (1959).
31. J. Campbell, E. Nelson, and D. G. Chapman, Criteria for oral sustained release medication with particular reference to amphetamine, *Can. Med. Assoc. J.* *81*, 15 (1959).
32. R. A Nash and A. D. Marcus, An *in vitro* method for the evaluation of sustained release products, *Drug Standards* *28*, 1 (1960).
33. E. Vliet, A suggested *in vitro* procedure for measuring the rate of drug release from timed release tablets and capsules, *Drug Standards* *27*, 92 (1959).
34. A. Beckett and G. Tucker, A method for the evaulation of some oral prolonged-release forms of dextroamphetamine in man using urinary excretion data, *J. Pharm. Pharmacol.* *18*, 725 (1966).
35. J. A. Campbell, Evaluation of sustained-action release rates, *Drug Cosmetic Ind.* *87*, 620 (1960).
36. S. Benita and M. Donbrow, Release kinetics of sparingly soluble drugs from ethyl cellulose walled microcapsules. Theophylline microcapsules, *J. Pharm. Pharmacol.* *34*, 77 (1982).
37. M. Donbrow and S. Benita, Release kinetics of sparingly soluble drugs from ethyl cellulose walled microcapsules. Salicylamide microcapsules, *J. Pharm. Pharmacol.* *34*, 547 (1982).
38. M. Oyaalpar and V. Walters, The prolongation of the *in vitro* dissolution of a soluble drug (phenethicillin potassium) by microencapsulation with ethyl cellulose, *J. Pharm. Pharmacol.* *33*, 419 (1981).

39. I. Jalsenjak, J. R. Nixon, R. Senjkovic, and I. Stivic, Sustained-release dosage forms of microencapsulated isoniazid, *J. Pharm. Pharmacol. 32*, 678 (1980).
40. M. A. Green, One years' experience with sustained release antihistamine medication, *Ann. Allergy 12*, 273 (1954).
41. H. L. Rogers, Treatment of allergic conditions with sustained release chlorprophenpyridamine maleate, *Ann. Allergy 12*, 266 (1954).
42. D. Berkowitz, The effect of a long-acting preparation (Spansule) of belladonna alkaloids on gastric secretion of patients with peptic ulcer, *Gastroenterology 30*, 608 (1956).
43. S. Morrison, The use of a sustained release tranquilizer-anticholinergic combination in patients with disturbed digestive function, *Am. J. Gastroenterol. 29*, 518 (1958).
44. H. V. Graham, Antihypertensive effects of reserpine in sustained-release form: a comparative study, *J. Am. Geriatr. Soc. 6*, 671 (1958).
45. S. H. Burness, Clinical evaulation of a sustained release belladonna preparation, *Am. J. Dig. Dis. 22*, 111 (1955).
46. J. Vasconcellos and A. A. Kurland, Use of sustained-release chlorpromazine in the management of hospitalized chronic psychotic patients, *Dis. Nerv. Sys. 19*, 173 (1958).
47. J. C. Colbert, *Controlled Action Drug Forms*, Chemical Technology Review No. 24, Noyes Data Corp., Park Ridge, NJ, 1974.
48. J. C. Johnson, *Tablet Manufacture*, Chemical Technology Review No. 30, Noyes Data Corp., Park Ridge, NJ, 1974.
49. W. A. Ritschel, Peroral solid dosage forms with prolonged action. In, *Drug Design*, Vol. 4 (E. J. Arien, Ed.), Academic, New York, 1973, Chap. 2, p. 37.
50. D. R. Paul and F. W. Harris, *Controlled Release Polymeric Formulations*, ACS Symposium Series 33, American Chemical Society, Washington DC, 1976, p. 27.
51. D. W. Doerr, E. R. Series, and D. L. Deardorff, Tablet coatings: Cellulosic high polymers, *J. Am. Pharm. Assoc. (Sci. Ed.) 43*, 433 (1954).
52. L. P. Gagnon, H. G. DeKay, and C. O. Lee, Coating of granules, *Drug Standards 23*, 47 (1955).
53. S. S. Ahsan and S. M. Blaug, A study of tablet coating using polyvinylpyrrolidone and acetylated monoglyceride, *Drug Standards 26*, 29 (1958).
54. J. R. Nixon and S. E. Walker, The *in vitro* evaluation of gelatin coacervate microcapsules, *J. Pharm. Pharmacol. 23*, 1475 (1971).
55. J. G. Wagner, W. Veldkamp, and S. Long, Enteric coatings. IV. *In vitro* testing of granules and tablets coated with

styrene-maleic acid copolymer, *J. Am. Pharm. Assoc. (Sci. Ed.)* *49*, 128 (1960).

56. J. D. Andrade, *Hydrogels for Medical and Related Applications*, ACS Symposium Series 31, American Chemical Society, Washington, DC, 1976, p. 88.
57. J. A. Bakan and J. L. Anderson, Microencapsulation. In, *The Theory and Practice of Industrial Pharmacy*, 2nd ed. (L. Lachman, H. A. Lieberman, and J. L. Kaing, Eds.), Lea & Febiger, Philadelphia, 1967, Chap. 13, Part III.
58. T. M. Feinblatt and E. A. Ferguson, Timed-disintegration capsules: an *in vivo* roentgenographic study, *N. Engl. J. Med.* *254*, 940 (1956).
59. T. M. Feinblatt and E. A. Ferguson, Timed-disintegration capsules (Tympcaps): A further study. An *in vivo* roentgenographic study, blood level study and relief of anginal pain with pentaerythritol tetranitrate, *N. Engl. J. Med.* *256*, 331 (1957).
60. D. M. Green, Tablets of coated aspirin microspherules: A new dosage form, *J. New Drugs* *6*, 294 (1966).
61. F. Steigmann, L. Kaminski, and S. Nasatir, Clinical-experimental evaulation of a prolonged acting antispasmodic-sedative, *Am. J. Dig. Dis.* *4*, 534 (1959).
62. T. J. Mellinger, Serum concentration of thioridazine after different oral medication forms, *Am. J. Psychiatry* *121*, 1119 (1965).
63. L. E. Hollister, Studies of prolonged-action medication. II. Two phenothiazine tranquilizers (thoridazine and chlorpromazine) administered as coated tablets and prolonged action preparations, *Curr. Ther. Res.*, *4*, 471 (1962).
64. T. J. Mellinger, E. M. Mellinger, and W. T. Smith, Thioridazine blood levels in patients receiving different oral forms, *Clin. Pharmacol. Ther.* *6*, 486 (1965).
65. N. D. Vestre and B. C. Schiele, An evaluation of slow-release and regular thioridazine and two medication schedules, *Curr. Ther. Res.* *8*, 585 (1966).
66. K. R. Magee and M. R. Westerberg, Treatment of myasthenia gravis with prolonged-action Mestinon, *Neurology* *9*, 348 (1959).
67. L. J. Cass and W. S. Frederik, Clinical comparison of a sustained- and a regular-release aspirin, *Curr. Ther. Res.* *7*, 673 (1965).
68. L. J. Cass and W. S. Frederik, A clinical evaluation of a sustained-release aspirin, *Curr. Ther. Res.* *7*, 683 (1965).
69. A. F. Kydonieus, Ed., *Controlled Release Technologies: Methods, Theory, and Applications*, Vol. II, CRC Press, Inc., Boca Raton, FL, 1980.
70. C. Banse, J. J. Bentz, C. Brossard, G. Cognyl, J. C. Crubezy, F. Herbemont, L. Thankh Thuy, and R. Sarfati, Microencapsulation, *Sci. Technol. Pharm.* *7*, 73 (1978).

71. J. A. Bakan and J. A. Anderson, Microencapsulation. In, *Theory and Practice of Industrial Pharmacy*, 2nd ed. (L. Lachman, H. A. Lieberman, and J. L. Kanig, Eds.), Lea & Febiger, Philadelphia, 1967, p. 420.
72. A. Kondo, *Microcapsule Processing and Technology* (J. W. Van Valkenburg, Ed.), Marcel Dekker, New York, 1979, p. 35.
73. C. Thies, Microencapsulation. In, *McGraw-Hill Yearbook of Science and Technology*, McGraw-Hill, New York, 1979, p. 12.
74. C. Thies, Physicochemical aspects of microencapsulation, *Polymer Plast. Technol. Eng.* 5, 1 (1975).
75. A. Watanabe and T. Hayashi, Microencapsulation techniques of Fuji Photo Film Co. Ltd., and their applications. In, *Microencapsulation* (J. R. Nixon, Ed.), Marcel Dekker, New York, 1976, Chap. 2.
76. H. G. Bungenberg de Jong, Complex colloid systems. In, *Colloid Science*, Vol. II (H. R. Kruyt, Ed.), Elsevier, New York, 1949, Chap. 10.
77. M. S. Harris, Preparation and release characteristics of potassium chloride microcapsules, *J. Pharm. Sci. 70*, 391 (1981).
78. T. Kondo, Microcapsules: Their preparation and properties. In, *Surface and Colloid Science*, Vol. 10 (E. Matijevic, Ed.), Plenum Press, New York, 1978, Chap. 1.
79. T. M. S. Change, *Artificial Cells* (T. C. Charles, Ed.), Charles C. Thomas, Springfield, IL, 1972.
80. G. Langer and G. Yamote, U.S. Patent # 3,159,874, 1964.
81. J. A. Bakan, Microcapsule drug delivery systems. In, *Polymers in Medicine and Surgery* (R. L. Kronenthal, Z. Oser, and E. Martin, Eds.), Plenum, New York, 1975, p. 213.
82. B. D. Sears, U.S. Patent # 4,145,410, 1979.
83. J. L. Shank, U.S. Patent # 4,001,480, 1977.
84. V. H. Saggers, I. F. Chasseaud, and A. J. Copper, Plasma concentrations, duration of analgelsia, and bioavailability of microencapsulated aspirin (Levius), *Clin. Trials J. 9*, 36 (1972).
85. L. Kuhns and K. Hospes, Klinische bedeutung and Anwendung eines Kaliumdefizit-Testes unter Berucksrchtigung der Therapie mit Frednison, *Schweiz. Med. Wochenschr. 86*, 783 (1956).
86. E. B. Draper and C. H. Becker, Some wax formulations of a sulfaethylthiadiazole produced by aqueous dispersion for prolonged-release medication, *J. Pharm. Sci. 55*, 376 (1966).
87. I. C. Robinson and C. H. Becker, Sulfaethylthiadiazole release from synthetic wax prolonged-release particles. I. Effect of dispersant concentration, *J. Pharm. Sci. 57*, 49 (1968).
88. P. M. John and C. H. Becker, Surfactant effects of spray-congealed formulations of sulfaethylthiadazole-wax, *J. Pharm. Sci. 57*, 584 (1968).

89. A. G. Cusimano and C. H. Becker, Spray-congealed formulations of sulfaethylthiadazole and waxes for prolonged-release medication: effect of wax, *J. Pharm. Sci. 57*, 1104 (1968).
90. Y. Raghunathan and C. H. Becker, Spray-congealed formulations of sulfaethylthiadazole and waxes for prolonged-release medication: effect of modifiers, *J. Pharm. Sci. 57*, 1748 (1968).
91. I. S. Hamid and C. H. Becker, Release study of sulfaethylthiadazole from a tablet dosage form prepared from spray-congealed formulations of SETD and wax, *J. Pharm. Sci. 59*, 511 (1970).
92. Y. Kawashima, H. Ohno, and H. Takenaka, Preparation of spherical matrices of prolonged-release drugs from liquid suspension, *J. Pharm. Sci. 70*, 913 (1981).
93. J. Heller and P. V. Trescony, Controlled drug release by polymer dissolution II: Enzyme-mediated delivery device, *J. Pharm. Sci. 68*, 919 (1979).
94. F. Alhaique, F. M. Riccierie, E. Santucci, V. Crescenzi, and A. Gamini, A possible pH-controlled drug delivery system based on a derivative of the polysaccharide sceleroglucan, *J. Pharm. Pharmacol. 37*, 310 (1985).
95. C. Graffner, G. Johnson, and J. Sjogren, Pharmacokinetics of procainamide intravenously and orally as conventional and slow release tablets, *Clin. Pharmacol. Ther. 17*, 414 (1975).
96. E. DeRitter, Evaluation of nicotinic alcohol Timespan tablets in humans by urinary excretion tests, *Drug Standards 28*, 33 (1960).
97. E. G. Rippie and J. R. Johnson, Regulation of dissolution rate by pellet geometry, *J. Pharm. Sci. 58*, 428 (1969).
98. D. Brooke and R. J. Washkuhn, Zero-order drug delivery systems: theory and preliminary testing, *J. Pharm. Sci. 66*, 159 (1977).
99. D. S. T. Hsieh, W. D. Rhine, and R. Langer, Zero-order controlled-release polymer matrices for micro- and macromolecules, *J. Pharm. Sci. 72*, 17 (1983).
100. R. A. Siegel and R. Langer, Controlled release of polypeptides and other macromolecules, *Pharm. Res. 1*, 2 (1984).
101. P. I. Lee, Novel approach to zero-order drug delivery via immobilized nonuniform drug distribution in glassy hydrogels, *J. Pharm. Sci. 73*, 1344 (1984).
102. C. Brossard, D. Lefort Des Ylousas, D. Duchene, F. Puisieux, and J. T. Carstensen, Dissolution of a soluble drug substance from vinyl polymer matrices, *J. Pharm. Sci. 72*, 162 (1983).
103. G. L. Flynn, S. H. Yalkowsky, and T. J. Roseman, Mass transport phenomena and models: Theoretical concepts, *J. Pharm. Sci. 63*, 479 (1974).

104. S. Benita and M. Danbrow, Effect of polyisobutylene on ethylcellulose-walled microcapsules: Wall structure and thickness of salicylamide and theophylline microcapsules, *J. Pharm. Sci. 71*, 205 (1982).
105. H. Takenaka, Y. Kawashima, and S. Y. Lin, Polymorphs of spray-dried microencapsulated sulfamethoxazole with cellulose acetate phthalate and colloidal silica, montmorillonita, or talc, *J. Pharm. Sci. 70*, 1256 (1981).
106. F. Lim and R. D. Moss, Microencapsulation of living cells and tissues, *J. Pharm. Sci. 70*, 351 (1981).
107. M. Arakawa and T. Kondo, Preparation of hemolysate-loaded poly(*N*., *N*-*L*-lysinediylterephthaloyl) nanocapsules, *J. Pharm. Sci. 70*, 354 (1981).
108. T. Ishizaka, K. Endo, and M. Koishi, Preparation of egg albumin microcapsules and microspheres, *J. Pharm. Sci. 70*, 358 (1981).
109. J. Krueter and E. Liehl, Long-term studies of microencapsulated and adsorbed influenza vaccine nanoparticles, *J. Pharm. Sci. 70*, 367 (1981).
110. J. W. McGinity, A. Martin, G. W. Cuff, and A. S. Combs, Influences of matrices on nylon-encapsulated pharmaceuticals, *J. Pharm. Sci. 70*, 372 (1981).
111. J. R. Nixon, *In vitro* and *in vivo* release of microencapsulated chlorothiazide, *J. Pharm. Sci. 70*, 376 (1981).
112. Y. Nozawa and S. W. Fox, Microencapsulation of methylylmal and two derivatives, *J. Pharm. Sci. 70*, 385 (1981).
113. H. Takenaka, Y. Kawashima, and S. Y. Lin, Preparation of enteric-coated microcapsules for tableting by spray-drying technique and *in vitro* simulation of drug release from the tablet in GI tract, *J. Pharm. Sci. 69*, 1388 (1980).
114. H. Takenaka, Y. Kawashima, and S. Y. Lin, Micromeritic properties of sulfamethonazole microcapsules prepared by gelatin-acacia coacervation, *J. Pharm. Sci. 69*, 513 (1980).
115. D. M. Green, Tablets of clated aspirin microspherules—A new dosage form, *J. New Drugs 6*, 294 (1966).
116. A. Williams, *Sustained Release Pharmaceuticals*, Nayes Development Corp, Park Ridge, NJ, 1969.
117. J. C. Colbert, *Controlled Action Drug Forms*, Chemical Technology Review No. 24, Nayes Data Corporation, Park Ridge, NJ, 1974.
118. J. C. Johnson, *Tablet Manufacturer*, Chemical Technology Review No. 30, Nayes Data Corporation, Park Ridge, NJ, 1974.
119. Y. Samuelov, M. Donbrow, and M. Friedman, Sustained release of drugs from ethylcellulose-polyethylene glycol films and kinetics of drug release, *J. Pharm. Sci. 68*, 325 (1979).

120. G. Kallstrand and B. Ekman, Membrane-coated tablets: A system for the controlled release of drugs, *J. Pharm. Sci. 68*, 325 (1979).
121. S. Borodkin and F. E. Tucker, Drug release from hydroxypropyl cellulose-polyvinyl acetate films, *J. Pharm. Sci. 63*, 1359 (1974).
122. M. Yoshida, M. Kumakura, and I. Kaetsu, Controlled Drug dissolution by radiation induced polymerization in the presence of dimethylaminoethyl methacrylate-methyl methacrylate copolymer or methacrylic acid-methyl acrylate copolymer, *J. Pharm. Sci. 68*, 860 (1979).
123. S. Borodkin and F. E. Tucker, Linear drug release from laminated hydroxypropyl cellulose-polyvinyl acetate films, *J. Pharm. Sci. 64*, 1289 (1975).
124. P. L. Madan, Clofibrate microcapsules II: Effect of wall thickness on release characteristics, *J. Pharm. Sci. 70*, 430 (1981).
125. L. A. Luzzi, M. A. Zoglio, and M. V. Maulding, Preparation and evaluation of the prolonged release properties of nylon microcapsules, *J. Pharm. Sci. 59*, 338 (1970).
126. N. Mason, C. Thies, and T. J. Ciero, *In vivo* and *in vitro* evaluation of a microencapsulated narcotic antagonist, *J. Pharm. Sci. 65*, 847 (1976).
127. P. L. Madan, D. K. Madan, and J. C. Price, Clofibrate microcapsules: Preparation and release rate studies, *J. Pharm. Sci. 65*, 1476 (1976).
128. M. Donbrow and M. Friedman, Timed release from polymeric films containing drugs and kinetics of drug release, *J. Pharm. Sci. 64*, 76 (1975).
129. G. M. Zentner, J. R. Cardinal, and D. E. Gregonis, Progestin permeation through polymer membranes III: Polymerization solvent effect on progesterone permeation through hydrogel membranes, *J. Pharm. Sci. 68*, 794 (1979).
130. G. M. Zentner, J. R. Cardinal, and S. W. Kim, Progestin permeation through polymer membranes I: Diffusion studies on plasma-soaked membranes, *J. Pharm. Sci. 10*, 1347 (1978).
131. M. Yoshida, M. Kumakura, and I. Kaetsu, Drug entrapment for controlled release in radiation-polymerized beads, *J. Pharm. Sci. 68*, 628 (1979).
132. M. Nakamo, K. Juni, and T. Arita, Controlled drug permeation I: Controlled release of butamben through silicon membrane by complexation, *J. Pharm. Sci. 65*, 709 (1976).
133. T. Higuchi, Rate of release of medicaments from ointment bases containing drugs in suspension, *J. Pharm. Sci. 50*, 847 (1961).
134. W. A. Ritschel, Influence of formulating factors on drug safety of timed-release nitroglycerin tablets, *J. Pharm. Sci. 60*, 1683 (1971).

135. H. E. Huber, L. B. Dale, and G. L. Christensen, Utilization of hydrophilic gums for the control of drug release from tablet formulations I: Disintegration and dissolution behavior, *J. Pharm. Sci. 55*, 974 (1966).
136. H. Lapidus and N. G. Lordi, Some factors affecting the release of a water-soluble drug from a compressed hydrophilic matrix, *J. Pharm. Sci. 55*, 840 (1966).
137. A. Dakkuri, L. D. Butler, and P. P. Deluca, Sustained release from inert wax matrices III: Effect of povidone on tripelennamine hydrochloride release, *J. Pharm. Sci. 67*, 357 (1978).
138. J. W. McGurrity, L. A. Hunke, and A. B. Combs, Effect of water soluble carriers on morphine sulfate release from a silicone polymer, *J. Pharm. Sci. 68*, 662 (1979).
139. N. Salib, S. Abd El-Fattah, and M. El-Massik, Preparation and *in vitro* evaluation of controlled release mepyramine maleate-carbopol 934 entrapped systems, *Pharm. Ind. 45*, 902 (1983).
140. F. W. Goodhart, R. H. McCoy, and F. C. Ninger, Release of a water soluble drug from a wax matrix timed-release target, *J. Pharm. Sci. 63*, 1748 (1974).
141. S. J. Desai, A. P. Simonelli, and W. I. Higuchi, Investigation of factors influencing release of solid drug dispersed in inert matrices, *J. Pharm. Sci. 54*, 1459 (1965).
142. S. J. Desai, P. Singh, A. P. Simonelli, and W. I. Higuchi, Investigation of factors influencing release of solid drug dispersed in inert matrices III: Quantitative studies involving the polyethylene plastic matrix, *J. Pharm. Sci. 55*, 1230 (1966).
143. S. J. Desai, P. Singh, A. P. Simonelli, and W. I. Higuchi, Investigation of factors influencing release of solid drug dispersed in inert matrices. IV: Some studies involving the polyvinyl chloride matrix, *J. Pharm. Sci. 55*, 1235 (1966).
144. K. A. Javaid, J. H. Fincher, and C. W. Hartman, Timed-release tablets employing lipase-lipid-sulfamethizole systems prepared by spray-congealing, *J. Pharm. Sci. 60*, 1709 (1971).
145. K. A. Javaid and C. W. Hartman, Blood levels of sulfamethizole in dogs following administration of timed-release tablets employing lipase-lipid-drug systems, *J. Pharm. Sci. 61*, 900 (1972).
146. S. Eriksen, Sustained action dosage forms. In, *The Theory and Practice of Industrial Pharmacy* 1st ed. (L. Lachman, H. A. Lieberman, and J. L. Kanig, Eds.), Lea & Febiger, Philadelphia, 1970.
147. S. Motycka and J. G. Naira, Influence of wax coatings on release rate of anions from ion-exchange resin beads, *J. Pharm. Sci. 67*, 500 (1978).

148. S. Motycka, C. J. L. Newth, and J. G. Nairn, Preparation and evaluation of microencapsulated and coated ion-exchange resin beads containing theophylline, *J. Pharm. Sci. 74*, 643 (1985).
149. Y. Raghunathan, L. Amsel, O. Hinsvack, and W. Bryant, Sustained-release drug delivery systems I: Coated ion-exchange resin system for phenylpropanolamine and other drugs, *J. Pharm. Sci. 70*, 379 (1981).
150. R. J. Timko and N. G. Lordi, *In vitro* evaluation of three commercial sustained-release papaverine hydrochloride products, *J. Pharm. Sci. 67*, 496 (1978).
151. A. M. Pederson, U.S. Patent #3,917,813.
152. H. Bechgaard and S. Baggesen, Propoxyphene and norpropoxyphene: Influence of type of controlled release formulation on intra- and intersubject variations, *J. Pharm. Sci. 69*, 1327 (1980).
153. A. M. Pederson, German Patent #2,414,868.
154. F. Theeuwes and T. Higuchi, U.S. Patent #3,916,899.
155. F. Theeuwes, Evolution and design of rate-controlled osmotic forms, *Curr. Med. Res. Opin., 8 (Suppl.)*, 220 (1983).
156. F. Theeuwes, D. Swanson, P. Wong, P. Bonsen, V. Place, K. Heimlich, and K. C. Kwan, Elementary osmotic pump for indomethacin, *J. Pharm. Sci. 72*, 253 (1983).
157. F. Theeuwes, Oral dosage form design: Status and goals of oral osmotic systems technology, *Pharm. Int. 5*, 293 (1984).
158. J. C. Johnson, *Sustained Release Medication*, Noyes Data Corporation, Park Ridge NJ, 1980, p. 116.
159. A. Zaffaroni, A. S. Michaels, and F. Theeuwes, U.S. Patent #4,096,238.
160. F. Theeuwes, U.S. Patent #4,111,202.
161. R. W. Baker, U.S. Patent #3,952,741.
162. R. Gale, S. K. Chandrasekaran, D. Swanson, and J. Wright, Use of osmotically active therapeutic agents in monolithic systems, *J. Memb. Sci. 7*, 319 (1980).
163. K. Heilmann, Innovations in drug delivery systems, *Curr. Med. Res. Opin., 8 (Suppl. 2)*, 3 (1984).
164. J. D. Rogers, Osmosin tablets, *Curr. Med. Res. Opin., 8 (Suppl. 2)*, 38–46 (1983).
165. A. R. Phymer, J. A. Sromovsky, C. Dicenta, and C. B. Hart, Osmosin tablets, *Curr. Med. Res. Opin., 8, (Suppl. 2)*, 62–71 (1983).
166. W. Bayne, V. Place, F. Theeuwes, J. D. Rogers, R. B. Lee, R. O. Davies, and K. C. Kwan, Kinetics of osmotically controlled indomethacin delivery systems after repeated dosing, *Clin. Pharmacol. Ther. 32*, 270 (1982).

167. J. D. Rogers, R. B. Lee, P. R. Souder, R. K. Ferguson, R. O. Davies, F. Theeuwes, and K. C. Kwan, Pharmacokinetic evaluation of osmotically controlled indomethacin delivery systems in man, *Int. J. Pharm. 16*, 191 (1983).
168. J. M. Hinton, J. E. Lennard-Jones, and A. C. Young, A New Method for Studying Gut Transit Times Using Radioopaque Markers, *Gut, 10*, 842 (1969).
169. K. Park and J. R. Robinson, Bioadhesive polymers as platforms for oral-controlled drug delivery: Method to study bioadhesion, *Int. J. Pharm. 19*, 107 (1984).
170. K. Park, H. S. Ching, and J. R. Robinson, Alternative approaches to oral controlled drug delivery: Bioadhesive and *in-situ* systems. In, *Recent Advances in Drug Delivery Systems* (J. M. Anderson and S. W. Kim, Ed.), Plenum, New York, 1984, pp. 163.
171. H. S. Ch'ng, H. Park, Kelly, and J. R. Robinson, Bioadhesive polymers as platforms for oral controlled drug delivery II: Synthesis and evaluation of some swelling, water-insoluble bioadhesive polymers, *J. Pharm. Sci. 74*, 399 (1985).
172. M. A. Longer, H. S. Ch'ng, and J. R. Robinson, Bioadhesive polymers as platforms for oral controlled drug delivery III: Oral delivery of chlorothiazide using a bioadhesive polymer, *J. Pharm. Sci. 74*, 406, (1985).
173. H. Bechgaard and K. Ladefoged, Distribution of pellets in the gastrointestinal tract. The influence on transit time exerted by the density or diameter of pellets, *J. Pharm. Sci. 30*, 690 (1978).
174. S. Watanabe, M. Kayano, Y. Ishino, and K. Miyao, U.S. Patent #3,976,197.
175. P. R. Sheth and J. L. Tossounian, U.S. Patent #4,126,672.
176. P. R. Sheth and J. Tossounian, The hydrodynamically balanced system (HBS): A novel drug delivery system for oral use, *Drug Dev. Ind. Pharm. 10*, 313 (1984).
177. P. R. Sheth and J. L. Tossounian, U.S. Patent #4,167,558.
178. P. R. Sheth and J. L. Tossounian, U.S. Patent #4,140,755.
179. R. M. Harrigan, U.S. Patent #4,055,178.

10

Parenteral Products

SAU-HUNG SPENCE LEUNG and JOSEPH R. ROBINSON / University of Wisconsin, Madison, Wisconsin

VINCENT H. L. LEE / University of Southern California, Los Angeles, California

I. INTRODUCTION

The intravenous, subcutaneous, intramuscular, intraperitoneal, and intrathecal routes are all examples of parenteral routes of drug administration. For a variety of reasons, the most notable being physiological and anatomical constraints, not all of these are useful as routes for controlled drug delivery. Up to the present, efforts in developing controlled release parenteral dosage forms seem to have concentrated on the subcutaneous and intramuscular routes, resulting in such products as aqueous and oil suspensions, oil solutions, and implants.

There are currently a number of injectable depot formulations on the market [1], e.g., pencillin G procaine suspensions (Duracillin Squibb); medroxyprogesterone acetate suspensions (Depo-Provera, Upjohn); fluphenazine enanthate and decanoate in oil solutions (Prolixin enanthate and Prolixin decanoate, Squibb); ACTH-Zn tannate/gelatin preparations (H.P. Acthar, Armour); microcrystalline deoxycorticosterone pivalate in oleaginous suspension (Percortan pivalate; Ciba); testosterone enanthate (Delatestryl, Squibb); testosterone enanthate/estradiol valerate in ethyl oleate BP repository vehicle (Ditate-DS, Savage); nandrolone decanoate injection (Decadurabolin, Organon); and insulin-zinc suspensions (Ultralente, Lente, and Semi-lente, Novo).

When these formulations are injected into subcutaneous or muscular tissues, a depot is formed at the site of injection which acts as a reservoir for drug. Drug molecules will be released continuously from the reservoir at a rate determined by the characteristics of each formulation. This continuous release of drug molecules will result in a prolonged drug blood level. The rate of drug absorption and hence duration of therapeutic activities will be determined by the nature of the vehicle, the physiocochemical characteristics of the drug or its derivatives, and the interactions of drug with vehicle and tissue/fluids. One example of preparing prolonged-action dosage forms is by preparing slightly soluble forms of a drug. For example, the duration of action of a regular insulin injection is increased by approximately four times when it is complexed with protamine to form the slowly dissolving protamine insulin.

In addition to oil solutions and aqueous and oil suspensions, recent efforts have been made to develop controlled and sustained release parenteral delivery systems via encapsulation, carrier, and magnetic systems. Before discussing the various parenteral controlled drug delivery systems, it is worthwhile to list the desirable characteristics of an ideal parenteral drug carrier. These are as follows [1]:

1. Versatility in that the carrier can deliver a variety of agents
2. High capacity to carry a sufficient quantity of drug per unit carrier to release therapeutic concentrations to the target site without excessively loading the host with the carrier
3. Restricting drug distribution to the desired target tissue
4. Uniform distribution within the capillary vasculature of the target tissue
5. Affording drug ready access to the parenchyma of the target tissue
6. Restricting drug activity at the target site over a prolonged period
7. Minimizing systemic drug release during intravascular transit
8. Protecting drug from inactivation by plasma enzymes
9. Being biocompatible and minimally antigenic
10. Undergoing biologic degradation with prompt elimination and minimal toxicity of the breakdown products

II. MAJOR ROUTES OF PARENTERAL ADMINISTRATION

The subcutaneous and intramuscular routes are the major routes of administration for the majority of sustained/controlled parenteral delivery systems, although the intravenous and peritoneal routes have also been used.

A. Subcutaneous

Adipose and connective tissues are poorly perfused with blood. This route is generally limited to non-irritating, water-soluble drugs that are well absorbed, e.g., insulin. It is important that the injection site be rotated for chronically administered drugs to avoid local tissue damage and accumulation of unabsorbed drug. The volume of subcutaneous injection is usually restricted to 0.5–1.5 ml.

B. Intramuscular

The best sites for intramuscular injection are the gluteal, deltoid, and vastus lateralis muscles. It is important that the injection be deep in the muscle and away from major nerves and arteries. To avoid tissue damage, the volume of intramuscular injection should not exceed 2 ml. A polymeric membrane that is either impregnated with drug or surrounds a drug reservoir can be used as the drug delivery device. A slightly soluble form of the drug can also serve as the drug source, thereby generating the desired constant rate of release. In the case of butorphanol tartrate, the subcutaneous and intramuscular routes of administration were found to be bioequivalent [2].

C. Intravenous

The intravenous route is occasionally used as a route of administration for sustained/controlled dosage forms such as liposomes, nanoparticles, erythrocytes, and polypeptides. When drug particles are injected intravenously, particles larger than about 1 μm are trapped in the lung, whereas particles with diameter between 0.1 and 7 μm are trapped or taken up primarily by the liver or spleen. Only small particles with a diameter less than 0.1 μm accumulate in bone marrow [3].

D. Intraperitoneal

Lymphatic channels are frequently the route by which tumors metastasize [4]. Macromolecules administered intraperitoneally can gain access to the lymphatic system and return slowly to the vascular compartment [5]. Thus, a macromolecule may be used as a carrier to target antineoplastic agents into the lymphatic system.

With subcutaneous and intramuscular injections, local trauma to the tissue occurs each time an injection is made. The trauma can be either chemical due to the pH or tonicity of the drug solution, mechanical due to puncture of tissue by needle and sudden distention of the tissue, or both. Thus, use of a sustained/controlled release dosage form which maintains therapeutic concentrations for a prolonged period of time is expected to produce greater tissue insult and injury. Therefore, irritating substances should be excluded from sustained/controlled-release parenteral dosage forms. The subject of injection injury has been reviewed by Gray [6].

III. BIOPHARMACEUTICS OF SUSTAINED/CONTROLLED RELEASE PARENTERAL DRUG PRODUCTS

When a sustained/controlled drug formulation is administered parenterally into a tissue space, muscle, or adipose tissue, a depot is formed. Before the drug can exert its therapeutic action, it must first be released from the formulation into the general circulation and then to the site of drug action. A possible sequence of events is depicted in Scheme 1:

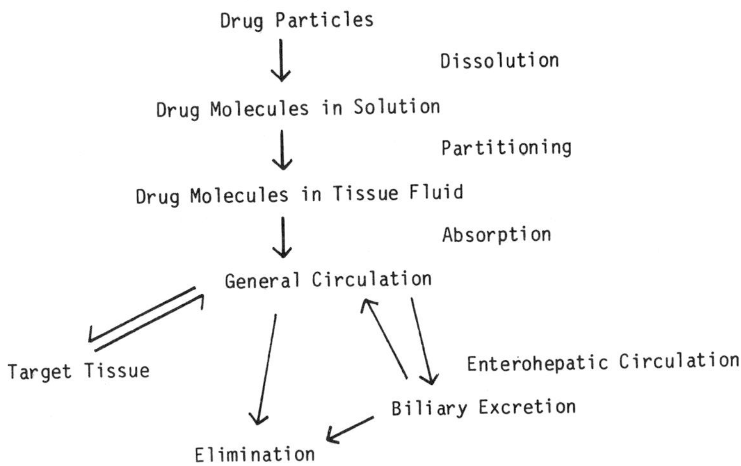

Scheme 1

Generally, the release rate of a drug is affected by the dissolution, partitioning, or absorption step. However, in many cases, the rate-limiting step is dissolution of drug particles in the formulation and/or partitioning of drug molecules from the vehicle to the surrounding tissue fluid. Thus, factors that affect the dissolution step and/or the partitioning step will affect parenteral drug absorption.

As an example, subcutaneous absorption from an aqueous suspension of practically water insoluble drug in rats was found to increase with decreasing particle size, probably due to an increased dissolution rate [7]. In contrast, subcutaneous absorption of a suspension of this drug in oil was governed predominantly by the distribution coefficient between the oily vehcile and the aqueous subcutaneous medium while unaffected by vehicle viscosity [8].

Besides particle size, polymorphism can be used to modify drug solubility, hence drug dissolution. Most organic substances exist in more than one crystal form called polymorphs. The drug molecules in each polymorph are the same, only the packing of the molecules differs. For a drug with two polymorphic forms, one of which is stable and the other metastable, the metastable form will show higher solubility and, hence, a higher dissolution rate. Consequently, the metastable form provides more rapid drug absorption.

Another factor that may affect drug absorption is the pH of the vehicle. For strongly acidic or strongly basic drugs, the vehicle pH will have little, if any, effect on the degree of ionization and therefore solubility of the drug. In contrast, the vehicle pH has a significant effect on the degree of ionization of a weakly acidic or basic drug, as summarized in the Henderson-Hasselbalch equation. Specifically, for a weakly acidic drug,

$$HA \underset{}{\overset{Ka}{\rightleftharpoons}} H^+ + A^-$$

$$Ka = [H^+]\,[A^-]/[HA]$$

$$pH = pKa + \log\,[A^-]/[HA]$$

Similarly, for a weakly basic drug,

$$B + H^+ \underset{}{\overset{Kb}{\rightleftharpoons}} HB^+$$

$$Kb = [HB^+]/[B]\,[H^+]$$

$$pH = pKa + \log\,[B]/[HB^+]$$

Clearly, a weakly acidic or weakly basic drug can exist in either the ionized or unionized form depending on the pKa of the drug and pH of the medium. For acidic drugs, the degree of ionization increases at pH values above the pKa and the drug will exist predominately in the ionized form. In contrast, basic drugs will exist predominately in the unionized form at pH's above their pKa. Thus, the solubility of these drugs, hence dissolution rate, can be altered by changing the pH of the formulation.

The viscosity of the medium can also alter drug dissolution by affecting the diffusion coefficient of a drug molecules in accordance with the Stokes-Einstein equation,

$$D = kT/6\pi\eta r$$

where D is the diffusion coefficient of the drug, k is the Boltzmann constant, T is the absolute temperature, η is the vehicle viscosity, and r is the molecular radius. Therefore, an increase in the vehicle's viscosity will decrease the drug's diffusion coefficient as well as dissolution rate. As an illustration, a thixotropic suspension, on standing or after intramuscular (or subcutaneous) injection, becomes highly structured and shows a nearly infinite viscosity, resulting in a compact depot. But upon shaking, the structure breaks, and fluidity of the formulation increases enough to pass through a hypodermic needle. Thixotropic behavior has been demonstrated in penicillin G procaine suspension [9]. The depot effect of penicillin G procaine suspension in gelled vegetable oils appears to be related to the combined effects of a reduction in aqueous solubility of penicillin G and a decrease in intramuscular drug absorption. The reduction in solubility of penicillin G is the result of formation of a procaine salt with low aqueous solubility. The decrease in drug absorption is caused by formation of a depot in the tissue, hence increase in vehicle viscosity, when the suspension is injected.

After the drug has dissolved in the vehicle, it will be in contact with the physiological fluid bathing the depot. The degree of ionization of the drug will then be affected by physiological pH, which in turn determines partitioning of the drug from the bathing fluid into tissue cells. It is generally accepted that the unionized form of a molecule partitions into the tissue more rapidly and extensively than the charged form. Thus, if the degree of ionization of the drug molecule is high, then the partitioning step in Scheme 1 will be rate limiting.

Hansch and Dunn [10] and Fujito et al. [11] have shown that for many body tissues, e.g., the gastrointestinal tract, skin, and blood-aqueous barrier of the eye, the optimum partition coefficient at which maximum flux occurs is approximately 1000/1 in n-octanol/water.

Since a drug must enter the systemic circulation before reaching its target tissue, the onset and magnitude of drug response oftentimes are affected by blood flow through the sites of injection. Coadministration of agents that affect blood flow through the injection site have been found to influence the absorption rate. For example, epinephrine causes constriction of the vascular bed and decreases blood flow, thereby delaying subcutaneous absorption of drugs. In contrast, hyaluronidase enhances drug absorption by spreading the drug solution over a large surface area in connective tissue [12]. In addition, an increase in muscular activity, which increases blood flow to muscles, may enhance absorption of drug from the site of injection. Thus, the duration of drug action in ambulatory patients is expected to be shorter than in bedridden patients.

IV. BIOCOMPATIBILITY OF POLYMERIC MATERIALS

Sustained/controlled drug delivery systems are different from conventional drug dosage forms in that they reside at a body location for an extended period of time. With the ever increasing emphasis on polymers in parenteral drug delivery, the issue of biocompatibility of these materials is becoming important. In general, biocompatibility of a given polymeric material with tissue is described in terms of acute and chronic local inflammatory responses and the subsequent fibrous capsule that may form following implantation of the polymeric material [13]. Langer et al. [14] examined tissue compatibilities of five different polymeric materials in the rabbit cornea. They found that poly(hydroxyethyl methacrylate) and alcohol-washed ethylene-vinyl acetate copolymer were non-inflammatory, whereas polyacrylamide and poly(vinyl pyrrolidone) produced significant inflammation. In a separate study, Ratcliffe et al. [15] found that polybutylcyanoacrylate, polymerized gelatin, and polylactic acid caused joint inflammation whereas polymerized albumin did not. On this basis, these investigators recommended that polymerized albumin was the most acceptable polymer to use intraarticularly to sustain drug release.

Besides inflammatory responses, the biocompatibility of implants can be measured in terms of sensitivity reactions and infections. Merritt [16] discovered that the majority of sensitivity reactions were caused by metal implants. He also found that the rough or porous surface of implants is more prone to cause infection in agreement with the findings of Sprinel et al. [17]. In addition, Bobyn et al. [18] reported that the strength of collagenized fibroconnective tissue attachment to implants increased with increasing pore size range as well as with increased implant time.

The events occurring at the tissue/implant interface include an initial adhesion of macrophages, followed by phagocytosis of wound debris and erosion, invasion, and phagocytosis of the polymer by macrophages and giant cells [19]. Salthouse [20] found that macrophages were in close contact with the implant surface within 24 hr postimplantation. Thereafter, fibroblasts and connective tissue proliferated and encapsulated the implant. It is suggested that the presence of macrophages is required for activation of collagen synthesis by fibroblasts [20]. Macrophage behavior is affected by the shape and surface of the implant in that smooth, well-contoured implants with no acute angles have superior tissue compatibility. Furthermore, the composition and degree of ionization of the polymer affect the amount of thrombus formed on the surface of implants [21].

In intravascular administration, thrombus formation can substantially limit the duration of therapy that can be achieved. Local vascular constriction and thrombus formation can cause venous statis and lead to drug being infused into essentially nonperfused veins, which often results in venous phlebitis that is erroneously attributed to infusion solution components [22].

The properties of a surface which control its interaction with blood are complex and difficult to define. The minimum interfacial, free-energy hypothesis and the optimum polar/apolar ratio hypothesis have been postulated to explain the observed blood-materials interactions [23]. The minimal interfacial, free-energy hypothesis says that the driving force for protein adsorption decreases as the interfacial free energy approaches zero. On the other hand, the hydrophilic/hydrophobic ratio hypothesis says that suitable proteins will be adsorbed and remain adherent if there is a proper balance between the polar and apolar surface characteristics. Coleman et al. [23] tested these two hypotheses and concluded platelet adhesion is not a good indicator of "hemocompatibility" and should not be used as the only test to screen polymers. However, Baier et al. [24] found the mean apparent volume of fibroblast cells counted around the subdermal implant was dependent on the initial surface energy and cleanliness of the implants. A high-energy surface has greatest cellular adhesion.

One potential method of improving the compatibility of polymers in the blood is to impregnate these polymers with heparin [25,26]. The polymeric materials that are combined with heparin can be divided into two basic categories [25]: those that release heparin at a controlled manner at the blood/polymer interface by an ion-exchange or simple diffusion mechanism and those that immobilize heparin at the surface.

There are various ways of heparinizing polymer surfaces [25–31] (Fig. 1):

1. Ionically bound heparin on positively charged surfaces
2. Ionically bound heparin to polymer and used as a coating on a substrate polymer
3. Cross-linked heparin on the surface
4. Immobilized heparin directly on the surface
5. Immobilized heparin on the surface via a spacer arm
6. Heparin dispersed on hydrophobic polymer
7. Heparin-albumin conjugate coated surfaces

After finding a polymer that is biocompatible, it is necessary to determine whether this biopolymer can be used as a sustained/controlled drug delivery system. Heller et al. [32], for instance, found that water-soluble macromolecules can be entangled in a bioerodible hydrogel successfully to provide a reasonably linear macromolecule release rate from the hydrogel. This release rate is

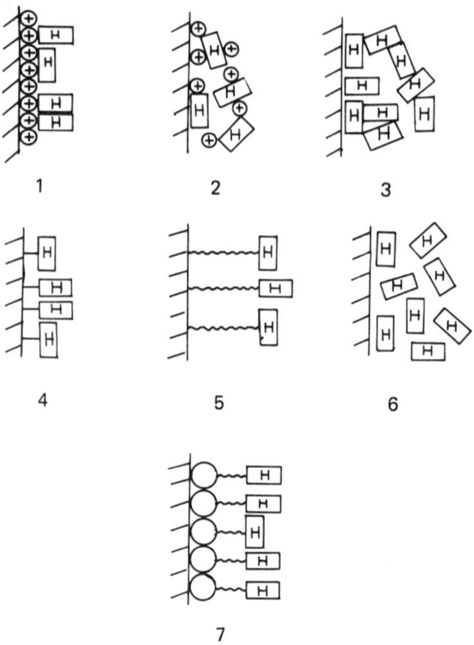

Fig. 1 Various ways of heparinization of polymer surfaces. (From Ref. 25.)

controlled by erosion and can be manipulated by simple structural variations of the hydrogel. As Kopecek pointed out, it is possible to further regulate molecular weight as well as biodegradability of carrier molecules by connecting synthetic polymeric chains via oligopeptide bridges [33].

V. SUSTAINED/CONTROLLED RELEASE PARENTERAL DOSAGE FORMS

Numerous approaches have been used to achieve sustained and/or controlled release of drug via parenteral administration. Scheme 2 illustrates the rate-limiting step in drug release with several of these approaches.

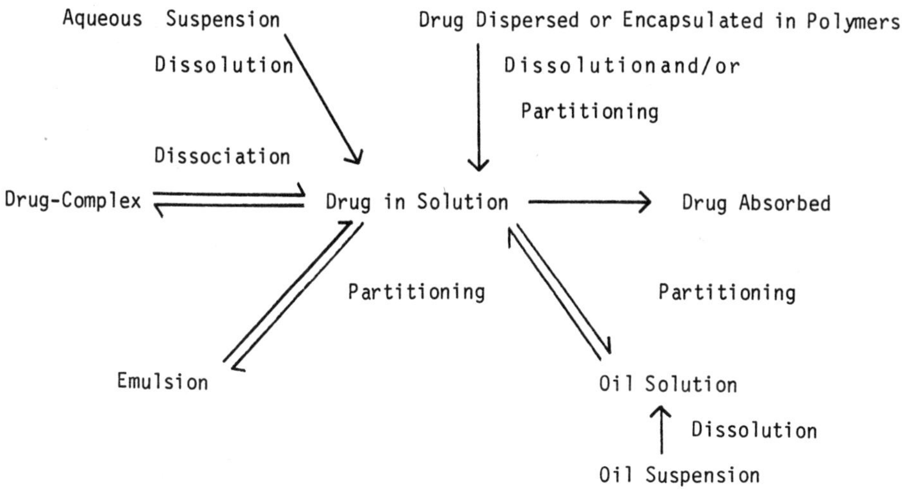

Scheme 2

A. Aqueous Solutions

1. *High Viscosity Products*

Earlier in this chapter it was mentioned that by increasing viscosity of the vehicle, the diffusion coefficient of the drug will be reduced, thereby delaying drug transfer. Examples of such viscosity agents are methylcellulose, sodium carboxymethycellulose, and polyvinylpyrrolidone. Delay in drug absorption also occurs if a water-soluble drug undergoes complexation with these macromolecules.

It is conceivable and likely that increased viscosity of the medium not only decreases molecular diffusion but also localized the injected volume. Thus, the absorptive area is reduced and the rate of drug transfer is better controlled. In fact, this is one of the reasons for incorporating gelling agents like aluminum monostearate into oil solutions [34,35]. Diffusion of low molecular weight drugs, i.e., up to about 750, is not impeded significantly by aqueous viscous solutions. Thus, while the apparent viscosity of such systems may be high, the actual viscosity is close to that of water, thus offering little diffusion resistance.

2. *Complex Formation*

The role of plasma protein and tissue binding in prolonging drug action is well known [36–39]. In principle, the same result can be achieved by forming a dissociable complex of a drug with such macromolecules as methylcellulose, sodium carboxymethylcellulose, and polyvinylpyrrolidone, for intramuscular administration. Assuming that a constant fraction of drug is complexed and that only free drug is absorbed, the absorption rate d[C]/dt may be expressed as:

$$d[C]/dt = -k\ f\ [C] \qquad (1)$$

where k is the absorption rate constant, f is the fraction of drug that is free, and [C] is the total concentration of drug at the absorption site. In terms of the apparent association constant K and the equilibrium concentration of macromolecule [M], it can be shown that:

$$f = 1/(1 + Ka[M]) \qquad (2)$$

which, if Ka is very much larger than 1, simplifies to:

$$f = 1/Ka[M] \qquad (3)$$

Thus, various degrees of control can be exercised by selecting the appropriate type and concentration of macromolecule since each drug-macromolecule pair has a characteristic association constant and since the free drug concentration is inversely proportional to the macromolecule concentration. As expected, the extent of binding is dependent on the relative concentrations of drug and macromolecule. This has been shown by Higuchi and Kuramato [40,41]. Consideration must also be given to the rate at which dissociation of the complex occurs. This is especially important in the period immediately following dosing because the drug-macromolecule complex is exposed to a relatively large pool of interstitial fluid, favoring dissociation. Equations (2) and (3) are the correct forms for f in Eq. (1) only if the dissociation rate is large relative to the intrinsic absorption rate. For most complexes of this type, dissociation is probably instantaneous.

There are many reports in the literature [42–49] pointing to the potential of complex formation as a means of achieving controlled drug delivery. The majority of these investigations are clinical in nature or are carried out with the objective of finding a suitable complexing agent without elucidating the fundamental processes involved. This immediately suggests that there is a need for a systematic approach to evaluate the number of binding sites per molecule, the magnitude of the association constant, and the nature of the intermolecular forces which are responsible for interaction and to correlate these physical parameters with clinical response.

In addition to complexes between drug molecules and macromolecules, complexes can also be formed between drug molecules and other small molecules such as caffeine. In contrast to complexes with macromolecules, complexes with small molecules can be absorbed. Levy and his co-workers have published a series of papers on the effect of complex formation on drug absorption [50–58]. In particular, they examined this phenomenon from the standpoint of alteration of physiochemical properties of the drug molecule upon complexation, the effect of the complexing agent on the barrier, and the stability constant of the molecular complex. The intuitive disadvantage to this approach is the small association constant that usually exists between small molecules. Thus, a substantial portion of the drug will exist in the non-complexed form. Consequently, this approach does not appear to hold much potential for development of prolonged-action intramuscular products.

There is yet a third class of complexes which controls the release of drug, not by dissociation but by decreasing solubility of the parent drug. Chow and Repta [59] reported that acetaminophen formed 1:1 complexes with theophylline and caffeine, which had lower solubilities and therefore lower dissolution rates than the parent compound. Complexes formed between large drug molecules, such as peptide hormones, and small complexing agents, such as tannic acid, fall into the same category. Notable examples are protamine zinc insulin [60], ACTH zinc tannte [61], and cyanocobalamin zinc tannate [34].

B. Aqueous Suspensions

A suspension usually gives a longer duration of action than an aqueous solution when given intramuscularly or subcutaneously. In the case of suspensions, the drug is continuously dissolving to replenish what is being lost, a situation that is not possible with aqueous solutions. To appreciate how suspensions can be utilized to control drug delivery, it is necessary to examine factors influencing the dissolution rate.

The dissolution rate of a drug can be described by a modified form of the Noyes-Whitney equation:

$$\text{Mean dissolution rate} = ADC_s/L \qquad (4)$$

where A is the mean surface area available for dissolution, D is the drug's diffusion coefficient, Cs is the saturation solubility of the drug, and L is the thickness of the diffusion layer. From a formulation standpoint, the parameters that are accessible to change are A (i.e., particle size), D, and, to an extent, Cs. These parameters are subject to constraints imposed by stability, syringeability, pain upon injection, and minimum effective concentration, among others.

The main problem in stability of suspensions is sedimentation. The factors influencing the rate at which it occurs, dx/dt are summarized by Stoke's law:

$$dx/dt = 2Rr(d - d_o)g/9\eta \qquad (5)$$

The parameters that are of interest here are the radius of the particle R (strictly speaking, the average radius in a particle size distribution) and viscosity of the medium η. Upon comparing Eqs. (4) and (5), the following picture emerges. Considering particles as spheres with radius R and density d, for a given amount of drug M, the following relationship holds:

$$N\ (4\pi/3)\ R^3 d = M \tag{6}$$

where N is the total number of particles. Upon rearrangement, one obtains:

$$3M/4\pi d = NR^3 \tag{7}$$

The left-hand side of Eq. (7) is a constant and can be denoted by K so that:

$$K = NR_3 \tag{8}$$

The total surface area is then given by:

$$A = N4\pi Rr = 4\pi K/R = K'/R \tag{9}$$

Here K' is a constant. Substituting Eq. (9) into Eq. (4), one obtains:

$$\text{Mean dissolution rate} = (DCs/L)\ (K'/R) \tag{10}$$

Thus, increasing particle size as a means to decrease dissolution rate causes an increase in the sedimentation rate resulting in an unstable suspension. This means that a compromise in particle size is necessary if this approach is sought to achieve controlled drug release.

To appreciate the influence of viscosity η on the dissolution rate, one may substitute the Stokes-Einstein relation for the diffusion coefficient D into Eq. (10), bearing in mind that this relation strictly applies to non-interacting spheres. In so doing, the following expression is obtained:

$$\text{Mean dissolution rate} = (kT/6\pi\eta r)\ (Cs/L)\ (K'/R) \tag{11}$$

where k is the Boltzmann constant, T is the absolute temperature, r is the hydrodynamic radius of the drug molecule, and the other symbols are as defined previously. It follows from Eqs. (5) and (11) that changing the viscosity of the medium affects rates of sedimentation and dissolution in a similar fashion. This suggests that by

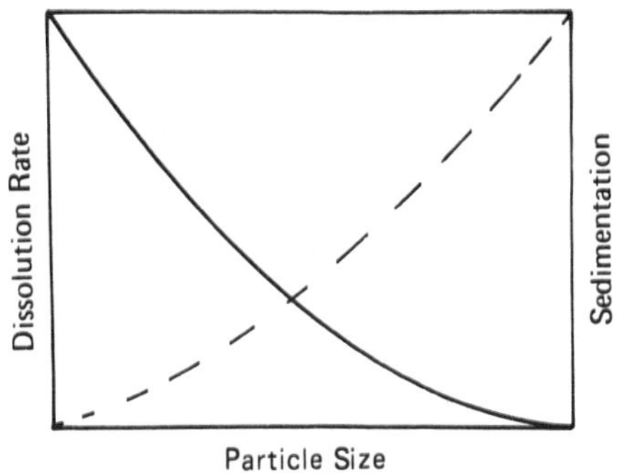

Fig. 2 Expected variation of dissolution rate (——) and sedimentation rate (---) with particle size for a given amount of a hypothetical drug. The relative position of the curves is arbitrary. (From Robinson, J. R., Ed., *Sustained and Controlled Release Drug Delivery Systems*, 1st ed., Marcel Dekker, Inc., New York, 1978.)

appropriately varying viscosity and particle size, a stable suspension that offers controlled release can be produced. Figures 2 and 3 illustrate variation of sedimentation and dissolution rates with particle size and viscosity.

A few general comments on particle size and solids content are in order. As a working rule the content of solids in parenteral

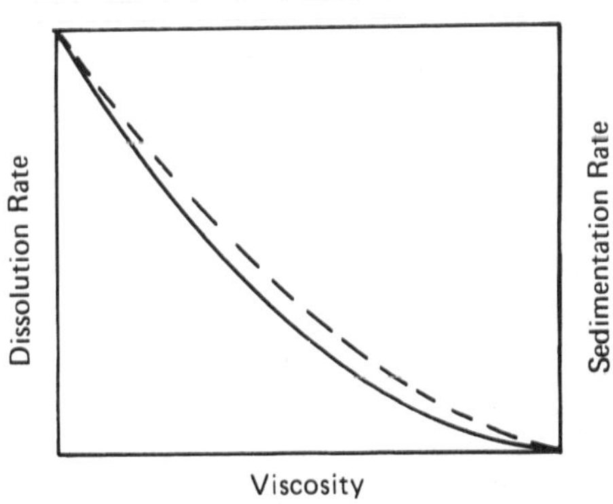

Fig. 3 Expected variation of dissolution rate (——) and sedimentation rate (---) with viscosity of the medium for a given amount of a hypothetical drug. The relative position of the curves is arbitrary. (From Robinson, J. R., Ed., *Sustained and Controlled Release Drug Delivery Systems*, 1st ed., Marcel Dekker, Inc., New York, 1978.)

suspensions should fall between 0.5 and 5% [62]. To minimize pain and tissue irritation, it is recommended that the particle size should be below 10 μm [63]. Depending on the drug, there is an upper limit on particle size beyond which therapeutic drug levels are not attained even though prolonged release is achieved [64]. Below this limit, the duration of action is proportional to particle size [65,66].

In addition to particle size, prolonged release can be achieved by altering solubility of the drug. The most direct approach in this regard is with salt and derivative formation, although using polymorphic forms can sometimes be effective. Mullins and Macek [67] reported that the amorphous form of novobiocin was approximately 10 times more soluble than the crystalline form. Based on the free energy of transition determined by Aguiar and Zelmer [68], it was found that there was a three- to fivefold difference in solubility between the most and the least stable polymorphs of chloramphenicol palmitate. Such differences in equilibrium solubilities are reflected in the dissolution rate and therefore the rate at which the drug is available for absorption [67–70]. The reader is referred to an excellent review article by Haleblian and McCrone [71] for a discussion on the pharmaceutical application of polymorphism.

Modification of duration of action by controlling the dissolution rate via the influence of crystallinity on solubility and via the influence of particle size on surface area is illustrated by insulin zinc suspensions USP. Insulin precipitates as an insoluble complex in the presence of zinc chloride, and depending on the pH, either an amorphous or a crystalline form is obtained. Prompt insulin zinc suspension USP consists of an amorphous zinc complex, while extended insulin zinc suspension USP consists of crystalline zinc complex. The former formulation has a shorter duration of action than the latter, not only because the amorphous form is more soluble but also because it is made up of smaller particles than the crystalline form [71].

1. *Use of a Viscosity Builder*

The use of a viscosity builder to increase vehicle viscosity and reduce the diffusion coefficient of the drug molecules can also be applied to aqueous suspensions. The net result is that the dissolution rate is diminished in proportion to the reduction in diffusion coefficient [Eq.(9)]. Using the dialysis rate as a measure of dissolution rate, Shah and Sheth [72] found that in a methylcellulose solution with a viscosity of 1300 cps, the dialysis rate constant was reduced by 50%. Seager [73] and Florence et al. [74] reported similar findings.

2. *Microspheres*

Microspheres are solid, spherical particles containing dispersed drug molecules either in solution or crystalline form (Fig. 4). This

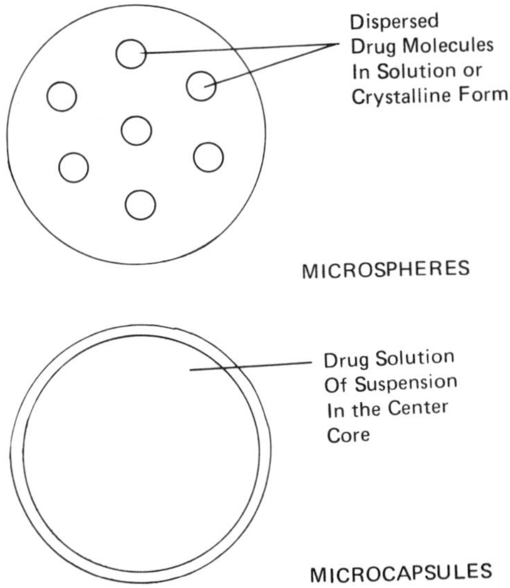

Fig. 4 Pictorial representation of microspheres and microcapsules.

delivery system has been applied to narcotic antagonists and antieoplastic agents [75–79]. The method consists of suspending the drug in a biodegradable/bioerodible polymer, followed by reducing the mixture to particles of the order of 600 μm, which are then injected as a suspension in carboxymethylcellulose solution. Some examples of biodegradable/bioerodible polymers are polyglactin 910 [19], poly(isobutyl cyanoacrylate) [80], poly(2-hydroxyethyl-*L*-glutamine) [81], and poly(lactic acid) [79]. This system is essentially a large collection of small matrices so that the mathematics and kinetics governing drug release from matrices apply here. Since drug release from this system is rate limited by dissolution of the matrix, it is not surprising to find that small polymer particles released drug at a faster rate than the larger ones. Yolles [79] described two other systems of injectable sustained drug delivery. The first system involves incorporating a drug into a polymer matrix, which was then shaped into small particles. The release rate of these matrices was diffusion controlled. The second system consisted of combining the drug with the polymer matrix via covalent bonds and shaping them into small particles. The release mechanism was by hydrolysis followed by diffusion of the drug through the polymer.

A cited advantage of this form of drug delivery over that of an implant is that surgical implantation is unnecessary [75]. In principle, by using polymer particles with a characteristic distribution of sizes in a fashion similar to that employed in Spansules,® various degrees of controlled release can be achieved.

3. *Microcapsules*

Microcapsules are spherical particles containing drug concentrated in the center core (Fig. 4). Microencapsulation can be used to encase particles of liquids, solids, or gases. The coating material can be selected from a wide variety of natural and synthetic polymers, depending on the material to be coated and the characteristics desired. Examples of these polymers include nylon [82], dl-polylactic acid [83,84], albumin [85,86], and cross-linked starch [87]. The amount of coating material used ranges from 3 to 30% of total weight, which corresponds to a dry film thickness of less than 1–200 μm, depending on the surface area to be coated. The possible mechanisms of release can be divided into dissolution control, diffusion control, and dissolution and diffusion control. Detailed descriptions of the mechansisms and theory underlying the release of drugs can be found in Chapter 11. Among the factors which affect drug release are the microcapsule size [88,89] and the thickness of the microcapsule wall [90–92]. Madan [91] demonstrated that microcapsules having thick walls released their contents slowly approximating zero order kinetics whereas those with thinner walls released their contents rapidly demonstrating square root dependence.

A variety of drugs have been microencapsulated. These include antineoplastic drugs [93,94], narcotic antagonists [83], methylglyoxal and its derivatives [95], chlorothiazide [96], fluphenazine embonate [97], gold sodium thiosulfate [98], potassium chloride [99], phenacetin [93], steroid hormones [100], micronized sulfamethoxazole [101], fine hydrophilic particles [85], luteinizing hormone-release hormone analogs [102], invertase [103], hemoglobin [104–106], macromolecules [107–110], and proteins [87].

Even vaccine [111], living cells, and tissues [112,113] have been microencapsulated. In tissue culture media, microencapsuated rat pancreatic islets were found to continue releasing insluin and to respond to glucose and theophylline stimulation with a typical physiological biphasic insulin-release pattern for over 2 months [112]. In experimental animals, a single intraperitoneal transplant of encapsulated islets reversed the diabetic state for 650 days [114], in part the result of protection of the transplanted cells from the host's immune system. Microencapsulation of red blood cells, hepatoma cells, and sperm cells was also successful [112].

Like other microparticulate carriers such as liposomes and serum albumin beads, the usefulness of microcapsules/microspheres in targeted drug delivery is limited by their failure to exit the vasculature as well as by their efficient clearance by the reticuloendothelial system. After intravascular administration, these carriers are taken up by the mononuclear phagocytes of the reticuloendothelial system [115–117], a process which is highly dependent on particle size, surface charge, and surface hydrophobicity. Illum and Davis [3] demonstrated that particles greater than 7 μm in diameter were trapped in the lung, whereas those with diameter between 0.1 and 7 μm were trapped or taken up by the liver and spleen. Only small particles less than 0.1 μm were found in the bone marrow. After an intravenous injection, over 60–80% of acrylic microspheres were found in the liver and spleen and a much smaller amount was found in the bone marrow [118]. At this low dose, there were no signs of acute toxicity to the cells of the reticuloendothelial system which phagocytized the microspheres [119]. Similarly, polystyrene microspheres phagocytized by lymphocytes were found not to stimulate an immune response [120]. However, very large doses of microparticles (100–200 mg/kg body weight) caused transient hepatosplenomegaly in mice lasting 4–8 weeks [119].

Besides particle size, the charge carried by the particles significantly affects their fate. By coating small polystyrene microspheres with a non-ionic surfactant, polyoxyethylene-polyoxypropylene, the zeta potential on the particles is reduced. This causes a significant reduction in liver uptake and an increase in lung uptake [3].

A third factor affecting uptake of microparticles by the reticuloendothelial system is their surface hydrophobicity. Hydrophobic particles are taken up by macrophages directly, whereas hydrophilic particles must be coated with immunoglobulin G before they can be engulfed [3].

Numerous methods have been explored to localize the release of therapeutic agents from microparticles to particular sites. These include varying degrees of blockade of the reticuloendothelial system before administering the carrier [117–121] and the incorporation of cell-surface specific ligands onto the surface of the carrier [122–124]. Thus far, neither approach has been met with much success. Other approaches include the use of magnetic microspheres, which will be discussed next, and a procedure called transcatheter embolization, which has been utilized to deliver microencapsulated mitomycin C to the corticomedullary region of the kidney, thereby sparing the rest of the body from the toxic effect of this cytotoxic drug [125–127].

4. *Magentic Microspheres*

Magnetic microspheres were developed to minimize reticuloendothelial clearance and to increase target site specificity [1,128–134]. They can be used to entrap a wide variety of drugs. This system has great potential in the treatment of localized tumors in regions of well-defined blood supply. Indeed, target site enhancement by this carrier is significantly greater than that achieved by any other targeting techniques reported to date [1].

Magentic microspheres can be prepared from albumin and magnetite (Fe_3O_4) [1]. They are about 1.0 μm in size, which is small enough to allow them to be injected intravenously without occluding the microvasculature. These microspheres are relatively nontoxic and nonreactive with blood components. They can be stabilized by heating or chemically cross-linking albumin to achieve a wide spectrum of drug release kinetics [128].

Typically, magnetic microspheres are infused into an artery supplying a given target site. A magnet of sufficient field strength is then placed externally over the target area to localize the microspheres at the capillary bed in this region. In order to localize microspheres in a fastmoving arterial system, generally a greater field strength is required. Widder and Senyei [1] found that localization of the microspheres at the target site increased with intensity of the magnetic field. These investigators also suggested that long-term retention of microspheres at the target site possibly was the result of movement of microspheres from the vascular space to the interstitial environment. When the microspheres were first pushed against the endothelial cells by the magnetic field, an endocytotic response was triggered. With continuous magnetic influence over certain periods of time the microspheres migrated from endothelial cells into the interstitial compartment and formed a depot for sustained drug release over an extended period of time.

The kinetics of magnetically targeted low-dose doxorubicin were studied by Senyei et al. [132]. They reported that as late as 60 min post-injection, 1% of a free intravenous dose of doxorubicin magnetically localized resulted in almost twice the local tissue concentration than was achieved by a 100-fold higher intravenous dose. The specificity of magnetic microspheres can be enhanced further by incorporating a cell surface specific ligand, such as staphlycococcal protein A, which can bind specifically to a given cell type in a heterogeneous cell population [135].

C. Oil Solutions

A less elegant mechanism to achieve parenteral controlled release is through the use of oil solutions. In this case, drug release is controlled by partitioning of drug out of the oil into the surrounding aqueous medium (see Scheme 2). This process can be thought of as a dynamic equilibrium between drug in the oil phase and that in the aqueous phase with a characteristic constant, the apparent partition coefficient K, given by:

$$K = \text{Drug concentration in oil/drug concentration in water} = [Do]/[Dw] \tag{12}$$

where drug concentration in water refers to both ionized and union-ized species of drug. In terms of the volume of the oil phase Vo and that of aqueous phase Vw, the total amount of drug Dt in the system at any time can be represented by:

$$Dt = (Dw)\,(KVo + Vw) \tag{13}$$

If the equilibrium is established sufficiently fast to replenish what is absorbed, the fractional amount of drug, f, that is in the aqueous phase can be calculated according to:

$$f = 1/(K\alpha + 1) \tag{14}$$

where α is Vo/Vw. Since absorption is driven by concentration (or to be precise, activity), not amount, an expression for the fractional concentration of drug that is in the aqueous phase, f', is more appropriate. Assuming additivity of volumes, this corresponds to:

$$f' = (1 + \alpha)/(1 + K\alpha) \tag{15}$$

Three limiting cases of Eq. (15) can be distinguished:

Case 1. For $\alpha << 1$, one obtains:

$$f' = 1/(1 + K\alpha)$$

Case 2. For $\alpha >> 1$, one obtains:

$$f' = \alpha/(1 + K\alpha)$$

Case 3. Provided K is sufficiently large, one obtains from Case 2:

$$f' = 1/K$$

These equations indicates: (a) that the fraction of drug that is available for absorption is controlled by the partition coefficient and the ratio of the volumes of the two phases, α, and (b) that it remains constant as long as α is constant. In the usual case, Vw is constant since it is a physiological parameter so that the value of α is controlled solely by the volume of solution injected, Vo. As is evident in Case 3, its influence of f' is removed only when K is sufficiently large.

Provided that drug absorption occurs via the aqueous phase, an expression describing the absorption rate d[C]/dt similar to that for the complex formation case can be written:

$$d[C]/dt = -k_a f'[C] \tag{16}$$

For a given absorption rate, $k_a f'$ can be obtained from this relationship. Usually an estimate of k_a is available so that f' can be determined. Then, for a given value of α, K can be estimated from the rearranged form of Eq. (15):

$$K = [(1 - f')/Vo](f'/Vw) + 1/f' \tag{17}$$

Two limitations of this method in evaluating K are immediately obvious. Both of them reside in the ratio α. First, the volume of interstitial fluid at the injection site is ill defined. Second, oils can be absorbed so that Vo is continuously changing with time [136,137]. This change, albeit small, has a definite influence on the magnitude of A which, in turn, causes a change in calculated K. Table 1 shows the variation of calculated K with A and f'.

From the above discussion, it is obvious that the success of this approach hinges on the magnitude of K, which is a function of the drug involved and the oil selected. The number of oils that are acceptable for intramuscular injection is rather limited. They include sesame oil, olive oil, arachis oil, maize oil, almond oil, cottonseed oil, and castor oil. In short, the "oily solution" approach is limited

Table 1 Some Examples Showing the Variation of K with A and f'

	K		
A	f' = 0.01	f' = 0.1	f' = 0.5
0.01	10,000	910	102
0.05	2,080	190	22
0.1	1,090	100	12
0.25	496	46	6
0.5	298	28	4
0.75	232	22	3.3
1.0	199	19	3

Source: Robinson, J. R., *Sustained and Controlled Release Drug Delivery Systems*, 1st ed., Marcel Dekker, Inc., New York, 1978.

to those drugs which are appreciably oil soluble and have the optimum partition coefficient.

D. Oil Suspensions

Drug release from oil suspensions combines the principles involved in aqueous suspensions and oil solution. With the suspended particles acting as a drug reservoir, the process of drug availability consists of dissolution of drug particles followed by partitioning of drug from the oil solution to the aqueous medium. In contrast to the case of oil solutions where concentration is equal to or less than equilibrium solubility is possible, the drug concentration in the oil phase containing the suspended particles is close to equilibrium solubility. However, as can be seen in Eq. 15, this has no bearing on the fractional concentration of drug that is in the aqueous phase. Intuitively, one would expect that the duration of action obtained from oil suspensions would be longer than that from oil solutions.

E. Emulsions

Besides use in topical drug delivery, emulsions have been used as drug vehicles both orally and parenterally [138–142]. While not matching topical emulsions, more progress has been made with parenteral than with oral emulsions. For example, emulsions have been administered intravenoulsy in parenteral nutrition [143,144]. Fortner et al. [145] obtained satisfactory results with an intravenous emulsion of a water-soluble antineoplastic agent.

One of the major limitations of cancer chemotherapy is systemic drug toxicity on normal replicating cells. To reduce drug toxicity, low density lipoproteins (LDL) have been studied as novel carrier system for antineoplastic drugs [146,147]. This is because of the greater uptake [148] and metabolism [149] of LDL by tumors than normal cells. Lipid-soluble antineoplastic agents such as methotrexate diester were incorporated into microemulsions which act as readily obtainable synthetic, protein-free analogues of LDL [147]. However, *in vitro* activity of the microemulsion against L1210 murine leukemia cells was found to be low [147]. More studies in this area are required.

1. Oil-in-Water and Water-in-Oil Emulsions

In immunology, water-in-oil emulsions find popularity as adjuvants, and the literature on this subject has been reviewed by Hilleman [150]. Freund and Bonato [151] were among the first to demonstrate the elevation and prolongation of antitoxin levels obtained by dispersing diphtheria toxoid in oily vehicles before injection. Using emulsified influenza vaccine, Salk et al. [152] found a 10-fold increase in antibody titer with persistence of high titers up to 4 years after injection. According to Freund [153] and Davenport [154], one mechanism by which the adjuvant action is brought about is the slow, continuous release of antigen from the emulsion.

The release of drugs from oil-in-water emulsions has been treated by Higuchi and his associates [155], while that from water-in-oil emulsions has been treated by Windheuser et al. [156].

In the case where the drug makes up the entire oily phase, Higuchi et al. [155] showed that release at steady state can be described by:

$$\text{Rate} = 4P(ao^2 + 2D\Delta Ct/d)^{1/2}\, D\Delta C \tag{18}$$

where ao is the initial radius of the droplet, D is the diffusion coefficient, d is the density of the solute, and ΔC is the difference in concentration between the surface of the droplet and the bulk phase. In the case of solute making up part of the oil phase, appropriate corrections for the distribution coefficient of solute between oil and water phases and for the partial molal volume of the solute in the droplet must be made.

In the treatment by Windheuser et al. [156], the water-in-oil emulsion is imagined as a uniform dispersion of water droplets containing the drug throughout an external oil phase. To simplify the mathematics, only a small segment of the system was considered as shown in Figure 5. Assuming that drug release proceeds via diffusion rather than by breaking of the emulsion and that the body fluid

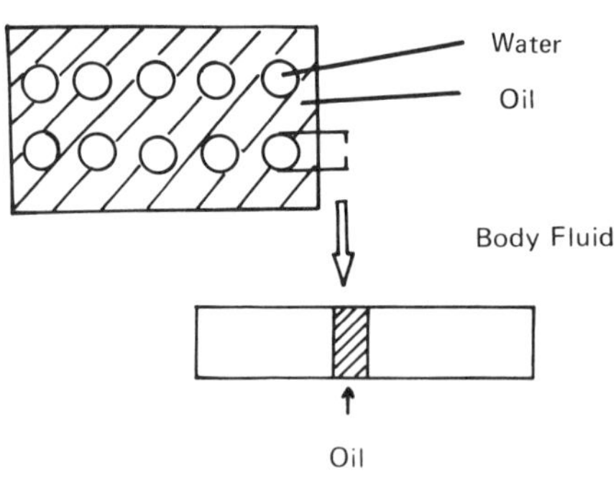

Fig. 5 Model of water-in-oil emulsion. The mathematical analysis of drug release is based on events occurring in the shaded area. (From Robinson, J. R., Ed., *Sustained and Controlled Release Drug Delivery Systems*, 1st ed., Marcel Dekker, Inc., New York, 1978.)

acts as a perfect sink, the rate of disappearance of drug from the aqueous phase (d[C]/dt) in the two-dimensional diffusion model can be described by:

$$d[C]/dt = -k\ [Co]\ \exp(-kt) \tag{19}$$

where [Co] is the initial concentration in the aqueous phase, and k is the rate constant of disappearance of drug from the aqueous phase and is given by:

$$k = ADK/VL \tag{20}$$

where A is surface area of the droplet, D is the diffusion coefficient of the drug, K is the partition coefficient of the drug between oil and water, V is the volume of the aqueous phase, and L is the effective thickness of the oil phase. For a given drug, a fast rate of release is favored by a large K, small droplets (i.e., large A for a fixed V), and a phase volume ratio favoring the oil phase. Since difusion is three-dimensional rather than two-dimensional, the above treatment should only be used to estimate the values of K, A, and phase volume ratio for optimum controlled release.

If the body fluid is not a perfect sink, one can estimate the fraction of drug that is there by using arguments analogous to those for the oil solution case. Specifically,

$$f1 = (1 + V2/V1 + Vo/V1)/[1 + (Vo/V1)K1 + (V2/V1)(K1/K2)] \tag{21}$$

where K1 is the partition coefficient between the oil phase and body fluid; K2 is that between the oil and the aqueos phase of the emulsion; Vo, V1, and V2 are the volumes of the oil phase, body fluid, and aqueous phase, respectively; and f1 is the fractional concentration of total drug in the body fluid. Usually K1 and K2 are approximately equal so that Eq. (21) reduces to:

$$f1 = (1 + V2/V1 + Vo/V1)/[1 + (Vo/V1)K1 + V2/V1] \tag{22}$$

A further simplification can be made if V1 is much larger than V2, which is a likely situation. Under this condition V2/V1 is approximately zero, and Eq. (22) becomes:

$$\begin{aligned} f1 &= (1 + Vo/V1)/[1 + (Vo/V1)K1] \\ &= (1 + \alpha)/(1 + K1\alpha) \end{aligned} \tag{23}$$

where $\alpha = Vo/V1$. Equation (23) is identical to Eq. (15), which was obtained for the oil solution case. Thus, the three limiting cases as well as their implications in controlled drug release apply. Based on this argument alone, no apparent advantage is gained by administering a water-in-oil emulsion rather than an oil solution as far as controlled release is concerned. Finally, similar results can be obtained for drug release from oil-in-water emulsions.

It must be pointed out that with the exception of the treatment of Higuchi et al. [155], all preceding studies ignore the role of the emulsifying agent at the interface in drug transport. They are therefore unrealistic in this sense. Consequently, only rough estimats of parameters such as K and the phase volume ratio can be made. Complicating the picture further is the stability of the emulsion at the injection site, which has definite influence on drug availability. Unfortunately, little is known of this phenomenon at the present time.

Concomitant with the growing interest in using water-in-oil and oil-in-water emulsions as vehicles for parenteral drug delivery is the development of multiple emulsions for controlled drug release [157]. The basic idea of this system is to introduce an additional reservoir into which drug can partition. Using water-oil-water emulsions prepared by dissolving the drug in the internal water phase, Benoy et al. [158] observed a prolongation of action of the chemotherapeutic agents methotrexate and vinblastine sulfate, while Yoshioka et al. [159] observed a prolongation in the release of another chemotherapeutic agent, bleomycin, following intramuscular injection in the rabbit. Collings and Schneider [160] suggested that the rate of drug release can be controlled by varying three basic parameters of the internal phase of the primary water-in-oil emulsion; namely, internal phase volume, concentration of emulsifier, and the osmolarity of the dispersed phase. Multiple emulsions are undoubtedly more complex than their two-phase counterparts from the standpoint of formulation, stability, and drug release [161]. Whether they are a useful tool in achieving controlled drug delivery for the parenteral route has yet to be established.

2. *Magnetic Emulsions*

In cancer chemotherapy, it is ideal to deliver the anticancer agents only to the localized tumor tissue such that there is a sufficiently high concentration of anticancer agent in the localized area to eradicate the tumor cells and at the same time cause minimal side effects to the host. Besides magnetic microcapsules/microspheres mentioned earlier in this chapter, magnetic emulsions have also been tried by Akimoto and Morimoto as a drug carrier for chemoptherapeutic agents [162].

The emulsion described is a magnetically responsivie oil-in-water type emulsion with the capacity to localize the chemotherapeutic agent

1-(2-chloreothyl)-3-(trans-4-methylcylohexyl)-1-nitrosourea (methyl-CCNU) by magnetic means to a specified target site [162]. The magnetic emulsion consists of ethyl oleate-based magnetic fluid as the dispersed phase and casein solution as the continuous phase. The anticancer agent, methyl-CCNU, was trapped in the oily dispersed phase.

Akimoto and Morimoto [162] reported that the magnetic emulsion had high retention by a magnetic field *in vitro*, and after intravenous injection in the rat, the magnetic emulsion was localized at the lungs by application of an electromagnet over the chest. Therefore, magnetic emulsions appear to have potential in conferring site specificity to certain chemotherapeutic agents.

F. Biocompatible Carriers

1. *Erythrocytes*

When erythrocytes are lysed and then resealed, exchange of intracellular and extracellular solutes will occur. A drug present in the medium during the lysis procedure will therefore be encapsulated within the membrane envelope of the erythrocyte upon resealing. Drugs, including ethanol [163], enzymes, and other biological substances such as amino acids [164,165], carbohydrates [166], nucleosides [166], and human factor IX [167] can be encapsulated in erythrocytes by hypo-osmotic lysis, dielectric breakdown, endocytosis, or simple incubation of the erythrocytes in drug solution for various periods of time without disrupting the membrane [168].

There are several advantages of resealed erythrocytes [169]:

1. Erythrocytes are biodegradable.
2. Erythrocytes are nonimmunogenic since the patient's own erythrocytes are used.
3. Resealed erythrocytes can circulate intravascularly for prolonged periods of time or can be quickly sequestered by the reticuloendothelial system depending on the degree of damage on the cell membrane of erythrocytes [168].
4. Erythrocytes protect the entrapped drug from immunological detection and enzymatic inactivation.
5. The entrapment of drug within erythrocytes does not require that the drug be chemically modified.

The major sites of removal of damaged erythrocytes are the phagocytic cells located in the liver and spleen. It is possible to target drugs to these specific cells by using erythrocytes. The release of drug from the erythrocyte carriers may occur following phagocytosis, via simple diffusion, or transport out of the cell by some specific transport system [168].

Erythrocytes can be coupled with other drug carrier systems to achieve controlled and sustained drug release. These include DNA, albumin, polysacchardies, polymers, or proteins. Transport proteins have been inserted into membranes of resealed erythrocytes [170]. The entrapped proteins are protected by the erythrocytes from antibodies or other plasma proteins. Fiddler et al. [171] demonstrated that the tissue distribution of these proteins was not altered even in the sensitized mice. Moreover, entrapped protein in erythrocytes do not elicit a strong immune response, whereas the same protein in liposomes was immunogenic [171–173].

2. *Biological and Synthetic Macromolecules*

A variety of biological macromolecules have been tried as carriers for drug delivery. Serum albumin can be polymerized and cross-linked to form microbeads to entrap steroid hormone, anticancer drugs, dyes, and peptides [174]. Such beads containing progesterone was found to elicit no adverse immunological reactions *in vivo* while releasing drug at a sustained rate for 20–30 days following an initial burst of drug release [175,176]. Similar beads containing insulin when implanted subcutaneously were found to sustain the release of this hormone in diabetic animals for longer than 2 months [177]. The subsequent reduction in insulin release rate was attributed to the formation of a fibrous capsule around the implant.

Other examples of biological carriers are DNA, lipoproteins, antibodies, and dextrans [175]. Some of these substances are called lysosomotropic agents since they are directed to the lysosomes following entry into cells by endocytosis, pinocytosis, or phagocytosis (Fig. 6). Lysosomes are vacuoles 0.2–0.3 μm in diameter containing over 40 hydrolytic enzymes in an acidic milieu (pH 4–5) [178], where the drug, typically a chemotherapeutic agent such as doxorubicin [179,180], that is complexed or conjugated to its carrier is liberated [181].

Besides biological macromolecules, a number of synthetic polypeptides and polymers have been studied as carriers for drug delivery [175]. These include polymers of ethylene glycol, lysine, and glutamic acid. Before a synthetic polymeric material can be used as a parenteral drug carrier, however, its acute, chronic, local, and systemic toxicity should be assessed carefully.

G. Liposomes

Liposomes are hydrated liquid crystals formed when phospholipids are allowed to swell in an aqueous media. When suitably dispersed, they consist of a series of concentric bilayers alternating with aqueous compartments [182,183]. Water- or lipid-soluble substances can be entrapped [184] within their aqueous or lipid phase, respectively.

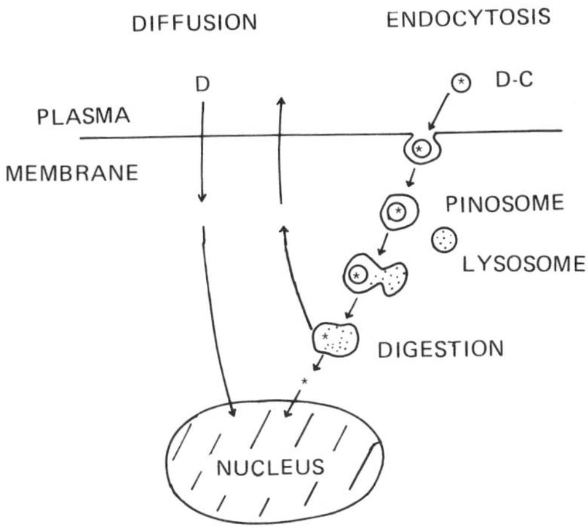

Fig. 6 Uptake of low molecular weight drugs (D) and drugs bound to macromolecular carriers (D-C). (From Ref. 33.)

Depending on the phopholipids used and the ionic composition of the medium, liposomes of various sizes and shapes can be obtained [182, 185,186]. Furthermore, antibodies can be covalently coupled to liposomes to enhance their cell specificity [187].

There are several reasons why liposomes offer great potential in parenteral therapy [188]:

1. Versatility in terms of size and electrical charge
2. Ability to encapsulate both hydrophilic and lipophilic drugs
3. Relative nontoxicity as compared to other carrier systems
4. Ability to protect labile drugs from inactivation in the blood by isolating them from the surrounding medium.

A great deal of attention has been directed toward using liposomes as intravenous carriers for enzymes such as amylogycosidase, β-fructofuranosidase, and neuraminidase [189–193] as well as drugs such as penicillin G [194], actinomycin D [194], colchicine [195], and thaliblastine [196]. When delivered in this fashion, the rate at which drug is cleared from the blood is controlled by the rate of disappearance of the liposomes in which it is housed. The elimination and distribution of liposomes have been shown to be controlled by the size, surface charge, and composition of the liposome [197]. Juliano and Stamp [195] found that small unilamellar liposomes were cleared less rapidly than were large multilamellar ones and that neutral and positively charged unilamellar liposomes were cleared less rapidly than were negatively charged unilamellar ones. Because of their affinity for the phagocytic cells of the liver and spleen, liposomes have been investigated to target drugs to those phagocytic cells which have been infested with parasites [187,198]. However, in spite of their affinity for the reticuloendothelial system, it is possible to maximize the retention of liposomes at sites such as the lung by manipulating the size and phospholipid composition of the liposomes [199].

H. Nanoparticles

Nanoparticles are transport carrier compartments for drugs or other active molecules of non-liposomal character in the nanometer size range [10 nm–1 μm) [178.200]. The advantage of nanoparticles as drug delivery systems are that they are biodegradable, nontoxic, and capable of being stored for a period up to 1 year. Since they are mainly taken up by the reticuloendothelial system following intravenous administration, nanoparticles are useful in delivering drugs to the liver and to cells that are active phagocytically. As such, nanoparticles can be used as lysosomotropic carriers [201,202]. Furthermore, by modifying the surface characteristics of nanoparticles by coating them with substances such as surfactants [203,204], it is possible to enhance delivery of nanoparticles to the spleen relative to the liver.

Methods of incorporating drugs into nanoparticles are as follows [172]:

1. Colloidal coacervation of macromolecules
2. Adsorption on the surface of solid colloidal macromolecular carriers
3. Coating of the particles by polymerization, polycondensation, or coacervation
4. Solidifying spherical micelles under nanocompartmentation by polymerization or polycondensation
5. Interfacial polymerization technique using electrocapillary emulsification [205].

I. Implants

Implants are typically placed subcutaneously to sustain drug release via the mechanisms of drug diffusion, polymer dissolution, or a combination of both. Nonbiodegradable polymers, as exemplified by polydimethylsiloxane, deliver drug by simple diffusion at a rate dependent on drug solubility in the polymer and the surface area of the implant. Biodegradable polymers, such as poly(caprolactone), poly(lactic acid), poly(glycolic acid), and poly(ortho esters), deliver drug by diffusion and/or polymer erosion. Provided the bioerosion rate is constant, drug release rate will be directly proportional to its physical dimensions.

J. Infusion Devices

A variety of infusion devices can be used to sustain and control drug delivery. Typically, these systems consist of a drug reservoir, a rate controlling unit (a pump), an energy source, and a safety device for possible failure of the system. A variety of pumps, differing primarily in the energy source, are available on the market. The simple gravity-fed pump relies on gravity as an energy source. The syringe pump uses a synchronous motor to drive a plunger to meter drug into the body. The nonvolumetric peristaltic pump forces drug solution by external pressure through a tubing to achieve continuous drug delivery. All three pumps are cumbersome to use thus severely limiting mobility of the patient. Consequently, implantable pumps such as the osmotic pump [206,207] and the electro-osmotic pump [208] have been developed [209–211]. All these implantable pumps have been found to possess the following desirable features.

1. The system is capable of maintaining a zero order drug release rate by virtue of an inexhaustible energy source.
2. The system is biocompatible and allows easy adjustment postimplantation.
3. The drug reservoir is small enough for easy implantation but is large enough to minimize frequency of refill, which can be performed readily.

K. Prodrugs

Prodrugs are agents that undergo biotransformation before exhibiting their therapeutic action. Naturally, a prodrug which is converted back to its parent compound in its target tissue or organ can be used to achieve site-specific drug delivery. Examples of these prodrugs as discussed in Chapter 8.

Historically, the impetus for designing prodrugs is to improve some unfavorable physical, chemical, or biological characteristics of the parent drug. For instance, a 3-(hydroxymethyl)-5,5-diphenylhydantoin disodium phosphate ester was synthesized to improve the aqueous solubility of phenytoin [212–214], thereby overcoming the precipitation problem of parenteral phenytoin [215].

For a parent drug that is incompletely absorbed after intramuscular or subcutaneous administration, the prodrug approach can be used to improve bioavailability. If poor bioavailability is due to poor dissolution characteristics, it can be improved by forming a more water-soluble prodrug, as exemplified by the prodrugs for phenytoin just mentioned [212–214,216]. On the other hand, if poor bioavailability is due to unfavorable partitioning characteristics, it can be improved by forming a more lipophilic prodrug. Examples of prodrugs with higher lipophilicity than their parent drugs are oxazolidines for β-amino alcohols and carbonyl-containing compounds [217] as well as 4-imidazolidinones for peptides [218].

When the parent drug has poor therapeutic action due to degradation or metabolism of the parent drug, a prodrug can be formed by protecting the functional group that is susceptible to inactivation [219]. Finally, the prodrug approach can be used to provide sustained, parenteral drug delivery by controlling its release rate from the formulation or by controlling its reconversion rate [220].

VI. SUMMARY

A variety of mechanisms differing in the degree of sophistication are available to control and sustain drug release via the parenteral route. These include the simple oil solutions and aqueous and oil suspensions, the somewhat more complex two- and three-phase emulsions, the technologically more advanced microcapsules, microspheres, nanoparticles, and implantable pumps, as well as those based on biocompatible natural materials such as liposomes, erythrocytes, albumin microspheres, and conjugates with DNA and monoclonal antibodies. These systems have been highlited in this chapter and will be discussed in greater detail in the remaining chapters of this text (Chapters 11–15). To date, with the possible exception of magnetic microspheres, magnetic emulsions, and monoclonal bodies, none of these delivery systems is able to achieve targeted drug delivery. Nonetheless, this goal can be achieved eventually given the increased understanding of the cell biology of target sites and of the biochemical basis of disease states. It is anticipated that the first generation of these site-specific systems would rely on intravenous administration for systemic drug entry, while future generations of these systems would probably be able to traverse epithelial and endothelial barriers from nonintravenous routes to deliver drugs to their sites of action. Realistically, these sophisticated systems are expected to be few in number. For the time being, given the intense efforts in establishing the therapeutic roles of peptides and given the enzymatic lability of these substances, there will be a great demand on parenteral carriers as vehicles for peptides [221], at least until the usefulness of unconventional routes including the nasal [222], rectal [223], and vaginal [224] routes as ports of peptide delivery is confirmed.

REFERENCES

1. K. J. Widder and A. E. Senyei, Magnetic microspheres: A vehicle for selective targeting of drugs, *Pharmac. Ther. 20*, 377 (1983).
2. M. Pfeffer, R. D. Smyth, K. A. Pittman, and P. A. Nardella, Pharmacokinetics of subcutaneous and intramuscular butorphanol in dogs, *J. Pharm. Sci. 69*, 801 (1980).
3. L. Illum and S. S. Davis, The targeting of drugs parenterally by use of microspheres, *J. Parent. Sci. Tech. 36*, 242 (1982).
4. J. Zeidman. In, *Cancer Biology Reviews, Metastasis, an Overview* (I. J. Marchalonis, M. G. Hanna, et al., Eds.), Raven, New York, 1982, pp. 1–27.
5. J. M. Yoffey and F. C. Courtice, *Lymphatics, Lymph and the Lymphomyeloid Complex*, Academic Press, New York, 1970.
6. J. E. Gray. In, *Sustained and Controlled Release Drug Delivery Systems* (J. R. Robinson, Ed.), Marcel Dekker, New York, 1978, pp. 351–410.
7. K. Hirano and H. Yamada, Studies on the absorption of practically water-insoluble drugs following injection VI: Subcutaneous absorption from aqueous suspensions in rats, *J. Pharm. Sci. 71*, 500 (1982).
8. K. Hirano, T. Ichihashi, and H. Yamada, Studies on the absorption of practically water-insoluble drugs following injection V: Subcutaneous absorption in rats from solutions in water immiscible oils, *J. Pharm. Sci. 71*, 495 (1982).
9. S. S. Ober, H. C. Vincent, D. E. Simon, and K. J. Frederick, A rheological study of procaine penicillin G depot preparations, *J. Am. Pharm. Assoc. Sci. Ed. 47*, 667 (1958).
10. C. Hansch and W. J. Dunn, III, Linear relationships between lipophilic character and biological activity of drugs, *J. Pharm. Sci. 61*, 1 (1972).
11. T. Fujita, J. Iwasa, and C. Hansch, A new substituent constant derived from partition coefficients, *J. Am. Chem. Soc. 86*, 5175 (1964).
12. S. Feldman, Physiochemical factors influencing drug absorption from the intramuscular injection site, *Bull. Parent. Drug Assoc. 28*, 53 (1974).
13. D. L. Coleman, R. N. King, and J. D. Andrade, The foreign body reaction: A chronic inflammatory response, *J. Biomed. Mater. Res. 8*, 199 (1974).
14. R. Langer, H. Brem, and D. Tapper, Biocompatibility of polymeric delivery systems for macromolecules, *J. Biomed. Mater. Res. 15*, 267 (1981).

15. J. H. Ratcliffe, I. M. Hunneyball, A. Smith, C. G. Wilson, and S. S. Davis, Preparation and evaluation of biodegradable polymeric systems for the intra-articular delivery of drugs, *J. Pharm. Pharmacol. 36*, 431 (1984).
16. K. Merritt, Role of medical materials, both in implant and surface applications, in immune response and in resistance to injection, *Biomaterials 5*, 47 (1984).
17. L. Sprincl, M. Kuskova, J. Roda, and J. Kralicek, The biocompatibility of polyvinylpyrrolidone in test implantation, *J. Biomed. Mat. Res. 16*, 95 (1982).
18. J. D. Bobyn, G. J. Wilson, D. C. MacGregor, R. M. Pilliar, and G. C. Weatherly, Effect of pore size on the peel strength of attachment of fibrous tissue to porous-surfaced implants, *J. Biomed. Mat. Res. 16*, 571 (1982).
19. B. F. Matlaga and T. N. Salthouse, Ultrastructural observations of cells at the interface of a biodegradable polymer: Polyglactin 910, *J. Biomed. Mat. Res. 17*, 185 (1983).
20. T. N. Salthouse, Some aspects of macrophage behavior at the implant interface, *J. Biomed. Mat. Res. 18*, 395 (1984).
21. M. N. Helmus, D. F. Gibbons, and R. D. Jones, The effects of surface charge on arterial thrombosis, *J. Biomed. Mat. Res. 18*, 165 (1984).
22. R. G. Buckles, Biomaterials for drug delivery systems, *J. Biomed. Mat. Res. 17*, 109 (1983).
23. D. L. Coleman, D. E. Gregonis, and J. D. Andrade, Blood-materials interactions: The minimum interfacial free energy and the optimum polar/apolar ratio hypotheses, *J. Biomed. Mat. Res. 16*, 381 (1982).
24. R. E. Baier, A. E. Meyer, J. R. Natiella, R. R. Natiella, and J. M. Carter, Surface properties determine bioadhesive outcomes: Methods and results, *J. Biomed. Mat. Res. 18*, 337 (1984).
25. S. W. Kim, Heparinized polymers for improving blood compatibility, *MD&DI*, 99 (1984).
26. V. L. Gott, J. D. Whiffen, and R. C. Datton, Heparin bonding on colloidal graphite surfaces, *Science 142*, 1297 (1963).
27. M. F. A. Goosen and M. V. Sefton, Properties of a heparin-poly (vinyl alcohol) hydrogel coating, *J. Biomed. Mat. Res. 17*, 359 (1983).
28. N. A. Peppas and E. W. Merrill, Development of semicrystalline PVA hydrogels for biomedical applications, *J. Biomed. Mat. Res. 11*, 423 (1977).
29. H. R. Lagerren and J. C. Eriksson, Plastics with a stable surface monolayer of cross-linked heparin: Preparation and evaluation, *TASAIO 17*, 10 (1971).
30. G. Schmer, The biological activity of covalently immobilized heparin, *TASAIO 18*, 321 (1972).

31. I. Danishefsky and F. Tzeng, Preparation of heparin-linked agarose and its interaction with plasma, *Thromb. Res. 4*, 237 (1974).
32. J. Heller, R. F. Helwing, R. W. Baber, and M. E. Tuttle, Controlled release of water-soluble macromolecules from bioerodible hydrogels, *Biomaterials 4*, 262 (1983).
33. J. Kopecek, Controlled biodegradability of polymer—a key to drug delivery systems, *Biomaterials 5*, 19 (1984).
34. R. E. Thompson and R. A. Hecht, Studies on a long-action vitamine B-12 preparation, *Am. J. Clin. Nutr. 7*, 311 (1959).
35. M. J. Romansky and G. E. Rittman, A method for prolonging the action of penicillin, *Science 100*, 196 (1944).
36. E. Kruger-Thiemer, W. Diller, L. Dettli, P. Bunger, and J. Seydel, Demonstration des einfluses der eiveissbindung and der ionisation duf die pharmacokonetik am kombineirten gaskinetischen modell nach van't Hoff und Langmuir, *Antibiot. Chemother. 12*, 171 (1964).
37. E. Kruger-Thiemer and P. Bunger, The role of therapeutic regimen in dosage design. Part I, *Chemotherapia 10*, 61 (1965–1966).
38. E. Kruger-Thiemer and P. Bunger, The role of therapeutic regimen in dosage design. Part II, *Chemotherapia 10*, 129 (1965–1966).
39. E. Kruger-Thiemer, P. Bunger, L. Dettli, P. Spring, and E. Wempe, Dosage regimen calculation of chemotherapeutic agents. Part III. Sulfasymazine, *Chemotherapia 10*, 325 (1965–1966).
40. T. Higuchi and R. Kuramoato, Study of possible complex formation between macromolecules and certain pharmaceuticals I, *J. Am. Pharm. Assoc. (Sci. Ed.) 43*, 393 (1954).
41. T. Higuchi and R. Kuramoto, Study of possible complex formation between macromolecules and certain pharmaceuticals II, *J. Am. Pharm. Assoc. (Sci. Ed) 43*, 398 (1954).
42. A. Choay and H. Choay, Prolongation des effets de l'insuline par association a la polyvinypyrrolidone, *Ann. Pharm. Fr. 5*, 520 (1947).
43. K. Eik-nes, A., Sandberg, F. H. Tyler, and L. T. Samuels, Changes in plasma level of 17-hydroxycorticosteroids induced by ACTH. III. Effects of various vehicles and modes of administration, *J. Clin. Endocrinol. Metab. 18*, 882 (1958).
44. M. H. Malone, R. D. Gibson, and T. S. Miya, A pharmacologic study of the effects of various pharmaceutical vehicles on the action of orally administered phenobarbital, *J. Pharm. Sci. 49*, 529 (1960).
45. G. Hangard, K. Kirkeby, and P. Lingjaerde, The potency of repository ACTH preparations, *Acta Med. Scand. 168*, 205 (1960).

46. C. Davison, J. L. Guy, M. Levitt, and P. K. Smith, The distribution of certain non-narcotic analgesic agents in the CNS of several species, *J. Pharmacol. Exp. Ther. 134*, 176 (1961).
47. P. Hedner, On the effect of long-acting corticotrophin preparations, *Acta Endocrinol. 43*, 499 (1963).
48. M. Friedman, Comparison of duration of activity of corticotrophin-gelatin and corticotrophin-carboxymethylcellulose, *Br. Med. J. iii*, 409 (1967).
49. A. Pekkarinen and U. K. Rinne, Comparison of different long-acting corticotrophin preparations in the two-day corticotrophin test in man, *Acta Pharmacol., Suppl. 25*, 1 (1967).
50. G. Levy and R. H. Reuning, Effect of complex formation on drug absorption. I. Complexes of salicylic acid with absorbable and nonabsorbable compounds, *J. Pharm. Sci. 53*, 1471 (1964).
51. G. Levy and T. Matosuzawa, Effect of complex formation on drug absorption. II. Lipid-soluble dye complexes, *J. Pharm. Sci. 54*, 1003 (1965).
52. G. Levy, K. E. Miller, and R. H. Reuning, Effect of complex formation on drug absorption. III. Concentration- and drug-dependent effect of a nonionic surfactant, *J. Pharm. Sci. 55*, 394 (1966).
53. R. H. Reuning and G. Levy, Effect of complex formation on drug absorption. IV. Role of intragastric diffusion in the absorption of free and caffeine-complexed salicylic acid from the rat stomach, *J. Pharm. Sci. 56*, 843 (1967).
54. G. Levy and J. A. Anello, Effect of complex formation on drug absorption. V. Studies on the mechanism of the secobarbital absorption-enhancing effect of polysorbate 80 in goldfish, *J. Pharm. Sci. 57*, 101 (1968).
55. G. Levy and E. J. Mroszczak, Effect of complex formation on drug absorption. VI. Drug permeation through an artificial lipid barrier, *J. Pharm. Sci. 57*, 235 (1968).
56. R. H. Reuning and G. Levy, Effect of complex formation on drug absorption. IX. Determination of the intestinal transfer rate constant of the salicylamide-caffeine complex, *J. Pharm. Sci. 58*, 79 (1969).
57. J. A. Anello and G. Levy, Effect of complex formation on drug absorption. X. Effect of polysorbate 80 on the permeability of biological membranes, *J. Pharm. Sci. 58*, 721 (1969).
58. W. L. Hayton and G. Levy, Effect of complex formation on drug absorption. XIII. Effect of constant concentrations of N,N-di-n-propylpropionamide on prednisolone absorption from the rat small intestine, *J. Pharm. Sci. 61*, 367 (1972).
59. Y. P. Chow and A. J. Repta, Compexation of acetaminophen with methyl xanthines, *J. Pharm. Sci. 61*, 1454 (1972).
60. H. C. Hagerdorn, B. N. Jensen, and N. B. Kramp, Protamine insulinate, *JAMA 106*, 177 (1936).

61. R. E. Thompson, Sustained release of parenteral drug, *Bull. Parent. Drug Assoc. 14*, 6 (1960).
62. R. A. Nash, Formulation of pharmaceutical suspensions I, *Drug Cosmetic Ind. 97*, 843 (1965).
63. R. E. Collard, Formulation and manufacture of corticosteroid preparations, *Pharm. J. 186*, 133 (1961).
64. V. G. Folglia, J. C. Penhos, and E. Montuori, Relation of crystal size to estrogenic activity of parahydroxypropiophenone, *Endocrinology 57*, 559 (1955).
65. R. W. Bates and C. Loury, Effect of particle size of suspension of estrogen crystals on duration of estrus, *Proc. Soc. Exp. Biol. Med. 73*, 576 (1950).
66. F. H. Buckwalter and H. L. Dickison, The effect of vehicle and particle size on absorption by the intramuscular route of procaine penicillin G suspensions, *J. Am. Pharm. Assoc. (Sci. Ed.) 47*, 661 (1958).
67. J. Mullins and T. Macek, Some pharmaceutical properties of novobiocin, *J. Am. Pharm. Assoc. (Sci. Ed.) 49*, 245 (1960).
68. A. J. Aguiar and J. C. Zelmer, Dissolution behavior of polymorphs of chloramphenicol palmitate and mefenamic acid, *J. Pharm. Sci. 58*, 983 (1969).
69. W. E. Hamlin, E. Nelson, B. E. Ballard, and J. G. Wagner, Loss of sensitivity in distinguishing real differences on dissolution rates due to increasing intensity of agitation, *J. Pharm. Sci. 51*, 432 (1962).
70. J. W. Poole, G. Owen, J. Silverio, J. N. Freyhof, and S. B. Roseman, Physicochemical factors influencing the absorption of the anhydrous and trihydrate forms of ampicillin, *Curr. Ther. Res. 10*, 292 (1968).
71. J. Haleblian and W. McCrone, Pharmaceutical applications of polymorphism, *J. Pharm. Sci. 58*, 911 (1969).
72. N. B. Shah and B. B. Sheth, Effect of polymers on dissolution from drug suspensions, *J. Pharm. Sci. 65*, 1619 (1976).
73. H. Seager, The effect of methylcellulose on the absorption of nitrofurantoin from the gastrointestinal tract, *J. Pharm. Pharmacol. 20*, 968 (1968).
74. A. T. Florence, P. H. Elworthy, and A. Rahman, The influence of solution viscosity on the dissolution rate of soluble salts and the measurement of an "effective" viscosity, *J. Pharm Pharmacol. 25*, 779 (1973).
75. J. H. R. Woodland, S. Yolles, D. A. Blake, M. Helrich, and F. J. Meyer, Long acting delivery systems for narcotic antagonists, *J. Med. Chem. 16*, 897 (1973).
76. W. R. Martin and V. L. Snadquist, A sustained release depot for narcotic antagonists, *Arch, Gen. Psychiatry 30*, 31 (1974).
77. S. Yolles, T. D. Leafe, J. H. R. Woodland, and F. J. Meyer, Long acting delivery systems for narcotic antagonists.

II. Release rates of naltrexone from poly(lactic acid) composites, *J. Pharm. Sci. 64*, 348 (1975).
78. S. Yolles, Controlled release of biologically active agents. In, *Polymers in Medicine and Surgery* (R. L. Kronenthal, Z. Oser, and E. Martin, Eds.), Plenum, New York, 1975, pp. 245–261.
79. S. Yolles, Time-release depot for anticancer drugs: Release of drugs covalently bonded to polymers, *J. Parent. Drug Assoc. 32*, 188 (1978).
80. V. Lenaerts, P. Couvreur, D. Christiaens-Leyh, E. Joiris, M. Roland, B. Rollman, and P. Speiser, Degradation of poly-(isobutyl cyanoacrylate) nanoparticles, *Biomaterials 5*, 65 (1984).
81. K. R. Sidman, W. D. Steber, A. D. Schwope, and G. R. Schnaper, Controlled release of macromolecules and pharmaceuticals from synthetic polypeptides based on glutamic acid, *Biopolymers 22*, 547 (1983).
82. J. W. McGinity, A. Martin, G. W. Cuff, and A. B. Combe, Influences of matrixes on nylon-encapsulated pharmaceuticals, *J. Pharm. Sci. 70*, 372 (1981).
83. N. Mason, C. Thies, and T. J. Cicero, *In vivo* and *In vitro* evaluation of a microencapsulated narcotic antagonist, *J. Pharm. Sci. 65*, 847 (1976).
84. S. Benita, J. P. Benoil, F. Puisieux, and C. Thies, Characterization of drug-loaded poly(d,l-lactide) microspheres, *J. Pharm. Sci. 73*, 1721 (198).
85. T. Ishizaka, K. Endo, and M. Koishi, Preparation of egg albumin microcapsules and microspheres, *J. Pharm. Sci. 70*, 358 (1981).
86. J. M. Gallo, C. T. Hung, and D. G. Perrier, Analysis of albumin microsphere preparation, *Int. J. Pharm. 22*, 63 (1984).
87. P. Artursson, P. Edman, T. Laakso, and I. Sjoholm, Characterization of polyacryl starch microparticles as carriers for protein and drugs, *J. Pharm. Sci. 73*, 1507 (1984).
88. Y. Kawashima, S. Y. Lin, A. Kasai, H. Takenaka, K. Matsunami, Y. Nochida, and H. Hirose, Drug release properties of the microcapsules of adriamycin hydrochloride with ethylcellulose prepared by a phase separation technique, *Drug Dev. Ind. Pharm. 10*, 467 (1984).
89. I. Jalsenjak and T. Kondo, Effect of capsule size on permeability of gelatin-acacia microcapsules toward sodium chloride, *J. Pharm. Sci. 70*, 456 (1981).
90. T. Ishizaka and M. Koishi, *In vitro* drug release from egg albumin microcapsules, *J. Pharm. Sci. 72*, 1057 (1983).
91. P. L. Madan, Clofibrate microcapsules II: Effect of wall thickness on release characteristics, *J. Pharm. Sci. 70*, 430 (1981).
92. J. Sjovall, R. Sjoqvist, B. Huitfeldt, and H. Nyqvist, Correlation between the bioavailability of microencapsulated bacampicillin hydrochloride in suspension and *in vitro* microcapsule dissolution, *J. Pharm. Sci. 73*. 141 (1984).

93. M. C. Bissery, F. Valeriote, and C. Thies, *In vitro* lomustine release from small poly (β-hydroxybutyrate) and poly (d, l-lactide) microspheres. In, *11th International Symposium on Controlled Reelase Bioactive Materials*, (W. E. Meyers and R. L. Dunn, Eds.), Controlled Release Society, Inc., 1984, p. 25.
94. P. Edman and I. Sjoholm, Acrylic microspheres *in vivo* VI: Antitumor effect of microparticles with immobilized *L*-asparaginase against 6C3HED lymphoma, *J. Pharm. Sci. 72*, 654 (1983).
95. Y. Nozawa and S. W. Fox, Microencapsulation of methyl glyoxal and two derivatives, *J. Pharm. Sci. 70*, 385 (1981).
96. J. R. Nixon, *In vitro* and *in vivo* release of microencapsulated chlorothiazide, *J. Pharm. Sci. 70*, 376 (1981).
97. A. T. Florence, A. W. Jenkins, and A. H. Loveless, Approaches to the formulation of a long-acting intramuscular injection, *J. Pharm. Pharmacol. Suppl. 25*, 121P (1973).
98. J. D. Scheu, G. J. Sperandion, S. M. Shaw, R. R. Landolt, and G. E. Peck, Use of microcapsules as timed-released parenteral dosage form: Application as radiopharmaceutical imaging agent, *J. Pharm. Sci. 66*, 172 (1977).
99. M. S. Harris, Preparation and release characteristics of potassium chloride microcapsules, *J. Pharm. Sci. 70*, 391 (1981).
100. L. R. Beck, D. R. Cowsar, D. H. Lewis, J. W. Gibson, and C. E. Flowers, New long-acting injectable microcapsule contraceptive system, *J. Obstet. Gynecol. 135*, 419 (1979).
101. H. Takenaka, Y. Kawashima, and S. T. Lin, Micromeritic properties of sulfamethoxazole microcapsules prepared by gelatin-acacia coacervation, *J. Pharm. Sci. 69*, 513 (1980).
102. L. M. Sanders, J. S. Kent, G. I. McRae, B. H. Vickery, T. R. Tice, and D. H. Lewis, Controlled release of a luteinizing hormone-releasing hormone analogue from poly (d,l-lactide-co-glycolide) microspheres, *J. Pharm. Sci. 73*, 1294 (1984).
103. P. Rambourg, J. Levy, and M. C. Levy, Microencapsulation III: Preparation of invertase microcapsules, *J. Pharm. Sci. 71*, 759 (1982).
104. M. C. Levy, P. Rambourg, J. Levy, and G. Potron, Microencapsulation IV: Cross-linked hemoglobin microcapsules, *J. Pharm. Sci. 71*, 759 (1982).
105. T. Konda, M. Arakawa, and B. Tamamushi, Poly(phthaloyl *L*-lysine) microcapsules containing hemoglobin solution: Artificial red blood cells. In, *Microencapsulation* (J. R. Nixon, Ed.), Marcel Dekker, New York, 1976, p. 163.
106. T. M. S. Chang, Semipermeable microcapsules as artificial cells: Clinical applications and perspectives. In, *Microencapsulation* (J. R. Nixon, Ed.), Marcel Dekker, New York, 1076, p. 57.
107. P. Edman and I. Sjoholm, Prolongation of effect of asparaginase by implantation in polyacrylamide in rats, *J. Pharm. Sci. 70*, 684 (1981).

108. P. Edman and I. Sjoholm, Acrylic microspheres *in-vivo*. V. Immunological properties of immobilized asparaginase in microparticles, *J. Pharm. Sci. 71*, 576 (1982).
109. B. Ekman, C. Lefter, and I. Sjoholm, Incorporation of micromolecules in microparticles: Preparation and charcteristics, *Biochemistry 15*, 5115 (1976).
110. M. V. Sefton, L. R. Brown, and R. S. Langer, Ethylene-vinyl acetate copolymer microspheres for controlled release of macromolecules, *J. Pharm. Sci. 73*, 1859 (1984).
111. J. Kreuter and E. Lichl, Long-term studies of microencapsulated and adsorbed influenza vaccine nanoparticles, *J. Pharm. Sci. 70*, 367 (1981).
112. F. Lim and R. D. Moss, Microencapsulation of living cells and tissues, *J. Pharm. Sci. 70*, 351 (1981).
113. T. M. S. Chang, Artificial cells in medicine and biotechnology, *Appl. Biochem. Biotech. 10*, 5 (1984).
114. A. M. Sun, G. M. Oshea, M. F. A. Goosen, and H. Gharapetian, Microencapsulation of living cells as long-term hormone and enzyme delivery system. In, *11th International Symposium on Controlled Release Bioactive Materials* (W. E. Meyer and R. L. Dunn, Eds.), Controlled Release Society Ic., 1984, p. 55.
115. P. Arturson, T. Laakso, and P. Edman, Acrylic microspheres *in vivo* IX: Blood elimination kinetics and organ distribution of microparticles with different surface characteristics, *J. Pharm. Sci. 72*, 1415 (1983).
116. A. W. Segal, E.J. Willis, J. E. Richmond, G. Slavin, C. D. V. Black, and G. Gregoriadis, Morphological observations on the cellular and subcellular destinations of intravenously administered liposomes, *Br. J. Exp. Pathol. 55*, 320 (1974).
117. L. R. McDougall, J. K. Dunnick, M. S. McNamee, and J. P. Kriss, Distribution and fate of synthetic lipid vesicles in the mouse: A combined radionuclide and spin label study, *Proc. Natl. Acad. Sci. USA 71*, 3487 (1974).
118. P. Edman and I. Sjoholm, Acrylic microspheres *in vivo* VIII: Distribution and elimination of polyacryldextran particles in mice, *J. Pharm. Sci. 72*, 796 (1983).
119. P. Edman, I. Sjoholm, and U. Brunk, Acrylic microspheres *in vivo* VII: Morphological studies on mice and cultured macrophages, *J. Pharm. Sci. 72*, 658 (1983).
120. M. Kanke, I. Sniecinske, and P. P. DeLuca, Interaction of microspheres with blood constituents: I. Uptake of polystyrene spheres by monocytes and granulocytes and effect on immune responsiveness of lymphocytes, *J. Parent. Sci. Tech. 37*, 210 (1983).
121. T. Tanaka, K. Taneda, H. Kobayashi, K. Okumura, S. Muranihi, and H. Sezaki, Application of liposomes to the pharamceutical

modification of the distribution characteristics of drugs in the rat, *Chem. Pharm. Bull.* *23*, 3069 (1975).

122. G. Gregoriadis and E. D. Neerunjun, Homing of liposomes to target cells, *Biochem. Biophys. Res. Commun.* *65*, 537 (1975).
123. R. L. Juliano and D. Stamp, Lectin-mediated attachment of glycoprotein-bearing liposomes to cells, *Nature* *261*, 235 (1976).
124. G. Weissman, D. Gloomgarden, R. Kaplan, C. Cohen, S. Hoffstein, T. Collins, A. Gotlieb, and D. Nagle, A general method for the introduction of enzymes by means of immunoglobulin coated liposomes of deficient cells, *Proc. Natl. Acad. Sci. USA* *72*, 88 (1975).
125. T. Kato, R. Nemoto, H. Mori, K. Iwata, S. Sato, K. Unno, A. Goto, M. Harada, M. Homma, M. Okada, and T. Minowa, An approach to magnetically controlled cancer chemotherapy. III. Magnetic control of ferromagnetic mitomycin C microcapsules in the artery, *J. Jpn. Soc. Cancer Ther.* *15*, 28 (1980).
126. T. Kato, R. Nemoto, H. Mori, and I. Kumagai, Sustained-release properties of microencapsulated mitomycin C with ethylcellulose infused into the renal artery of the dog, *Cancer* *46*, 14 (1980).
127. T. Kato, R. Nemoto, H. Mori, M. Takahashi, and Y. Tamakawa, Transcatheter arterial chemoembolization of renal cell carcinoma with microencapsulated mitomycin C, *J. Urol.* *125*, 19 (1981).
128. K. Widder, G. Flouret, and A. Senyei, Magnetic microspheres: Synthesis of a novel parenteral drug carrier, *J. Pharm. Sci.* *68*, 79 (1979).
129. K. J. Widder, A. E. Senyei, and D. G. Scarpelli, Magnetic microspheres: Model system for site specific drug delivery *in vivo*, *Proc. Soc. Exp. Biol. Med.* *158*, 141 (1978).
130. F. Ishiii, A. Takamura, and S. Noro, Magnetic microcapsules for *in vitro* testing as carrier for intravascular administration of anticancer drugs: Preparation and physicochemical properties, *Chem. Pharm. Bull.* *32*, 678 (1984).
131. P. L. Kronick, G. L. Campbell, and K. Joseph, Magnetic microspheres prepared by redox polymerization used in a cell separation based on gangliosides, *Science* *200*, 1074 (1978).
132. A. E. Senyei, S. D. Reich, C. Gonczy, and K. J. Widder, *In vivo* kinetics of magentically targeted low-dose doxorubicin, *J. Pharm. Sci.* *70*, 389 (1981).
133. K. J. Widder, A. E. Senyei, and D. F. Ranney, Magnetically responsive microspheres and other carriers for the biophysical targeting of antitumor agents, *Adv. Pharmacol. Chemo.* *16*, 213 (1979).
134. K. J. Widder, A. E. Senyei, and B. Sears, Experimental methods in cancer therapeutics, *J. Pharm. Sci.* *71*, 379 (1982).

135. K. J. Widder, A. E. Senyei, H. Ovadia, and P. Y. Paterson, Specific cell binding using staphylococcal protein A magnetic microspheres, *J. Pharm. Sci. 70*, 387 (1981).
136. R. Deanesly and A. S. Parkes, Note on the subcutaneous absorption of oils by rats and mice, with special reference to the assay of oestrin, *J. Physiol. 78*, 155 (1973).
137. W. E. Brown, V. M. Wilder, and P. Schwartz, A study of oils used for intramuscular injections, *J. Lab. Clin. Med. 29*, 259 (144).
138. W. G. Waggoner and J. H. Fincher, Influence of HLB values of surfactants on ephedrine release from emulsified liquid systems, *J. Pharm. Sci. 60*, 1830 (1971).
139. K. Kakemi, T. Sezaka, S. Muraniski, H. Ogata, and S. Isemura, Mechanism of absorption of drugs from oil-in-water emulsions I, *Chem. Pharm. Bull. 20*, 708 (1972).
140. P. J. Carrigan and T. R. Bates, Biopharmaceutics of drugs administered in lipid-containing dosage forms. I. GI absorption of griseofulvin from an oil-in-water emulsion in the rat, *J. Pharm. Sci. 62*, 1476 (1973).
141. G. Ln, F. Sadik, W. F. Gilmore, and J. H. Fincher, Influence of hydrophilic-lipophilic balance values of surfactants on ephedrine absorption and release from emulsified systems after oral administration to dogs, *J. Pharm. Sci. 63*, 666 (1974).
142. T. R. Bates and J. A. Sequeira, Bioavailability of micronized griseofulvin from corn oil-in-water emulsion, aqueous suspension and commercial tablet dosage forms in humans, *J. Pharm. Sci. 64*, 793 (1975).
143. D. Hallberg, I. Holm, and A. L. Abel, Fat emulsion for intravenous nutrition, *Postgrad. Med. J. 43*, 307 (1967).
144. H. C. Meng, Use of fat emulsions in parenteral nutrition, *Drug Intell. Clin. Pharm. 6*, 321 (1972).
145. C. L. Fortner, W. R. Grove, D. Bowie, and M. D. Walker, Fat emulsion vehicle for intravenous administration of an aqueous insoluble drug, *Am. J. Hosp. Pharm. 32*, 582 (1975).
146. R. E. Counsell and R. C. Pohland, Lipoproteins as potential site-specific delivery systems for diagnostic and therapeutic agents, *J. Med. Chem. 25*, 1115–1120 (1982).
147. G. W. Halbert, J. F. B. Stuart, and A. T. Florence, The incorporation of lipid-soluble antineoplastic agents into microemulsions—protein-free analogues of low density lipoprotein, *Int. J. Pharm. 21*, 219 (1984).
148. J. Welsh, K. C. Calman, J. F. Stuart, J. Clegg, J. M. Stewart, C. J. Packard, H. G. Morgan, and J. Shepard, Low density lipoprotein uptake by tumors, *Clin. Sci. (London) 63*, P44 (1982).

149. D. Gal, P. E. MacDonald, J. E. Porter, and E. R. Simpson, Cholesterol metabolism in cancer cells in monolayer culture. IV. LDL metabolism, *Int. J. Cancer 28*, 315–319 (1981).
150. M. R. Hilleman, Critical appraisal of emulsified oil adjuvants applied to viral vaccines, *Prog. Med Virol. 8*, 131 (1966).
151. J. Freund and M. V. Bonato, The effect of paraffin oil, lanolin-like substances and killed tubercle bacilli on immunization with diphtheric toxoic and Bact. Typhosum, *J. Immunol. 48*, 325 (1944).
152. J. E. Salk, M. Contakos, A. M. Laurent, M. Sorenson, A. J. Rapalski, I. H. Simmons, and H. Sandbert, Use of adjuvants in studies on influenza immunization, *JAMA 151*, 1169 (1953).
153. J. Freund, Mode of action of mineral oil adjuvants, *Adv. Tuberc. Res. 7*, 130 (1956).
154. F. M. Davenport, Applied immunology of mineral oil adjuvants, *J. Allergy 32*, 177 (1961).
155. W. I. Higuchi, Rate of solute transport out of emulsion droplets in micron size range, *J. Pharm. Sci. 53*, 405 (1964).
156. J. L. Windheuser, M. L. Best, and J. H. Perrin, Evaluation of sustained action parenteral emulsions, *Parent. Drug Assoc. Bull. 24*, 286 (1970).
157. A. F. Brodin, D. R. Kavaliunas, and S. G. Frank, Prolonged drug release from multiple emulsions, *Acta Pharm. Suec. 15*, 1 (1978).
158. C. J. Eenoy, L. A. Elson, and R. Schneider, Multiple emulsions, a suitable vehicle to provide sustained release of cancer chemotherapeutic agents, *Br. J. Pharmacol. 45*, 135P (1972).
159. T. Yoshioka, K. Ikeuchi, M. Hashida, S. Muranishi, and H. Sezaki, Prolonged release of bleomycin from parenteral gelatin sphere-in-oil-in-water multiple emulsion, *Chem. Pharm. Bull. 30*, 1408 (1982).
160. A. J. Collings and R. Schneider, The multiple emulsion formulation for the slow release of drugs, *Br. J. Pharmacol. 38*, 469P (1970).
161. A. T. Florence and D. Whitehill, The formulation and stability of multiple emulsions, *Int. J. Pharm. 11*, 277 (1982).
162. M. Akimoto and Y. Morimoto, Use of magnetic emulsion as a novel drug carrier for chemotherapeutic agents, *Biomaterials 4*, 49 (1983).
163. E. Muler, J. M. Lamers-Stahlhofen, and H. J. Van Der Molen, Interaction between steroids and membranes. Uptake of steroids and steroid sulphates by resealed erythrocyte ghost, *J. Steroid Biochem. 4*, 369 (1973).
164. J. D. Gardner and A. G. Levy, Transport of dibasic amino acids by human erythrocytes, *Metabolism 21*, 413 (1972).

165. W. C. Wise, Maturation of membrane function: Transport of amino acid by rat erythroid cells, *J. Cell Physiol. 87*, 199 (1975).
166. J. M. Oliver, and A. R. P. Paterson, Nucleoside transport. I. A medicated process in human erythrocytes, *Can. J. Biochem. 49*, 262 (1971).
167. J. C. Goldsmith, M. E. S. Roer, and E. P. Orringer, A new treatment strategy for hemophilia B: Incorporation of factor IX into red cell ghost, *Am. J. Hematol. 7*, 119 (1979).
168. G. M. Ihler, Erythrocyte carriers, *Pharmac. Ther. 20*, 151 (1983).
169. G. L. Dale, Resealed erythrocytes as drug carriers. In, *Drug Delivery Systems* (R. L. Juliano, Ed.), Oxford University Press, New York, 1980, pp. 237.
170. G. D. Eytan and E. Eytan, Fusion of proteoliposomes and cells, *J. Biol. Chem. 255*, 4992 (1980).
171. M. B. Fiddler, L. D. S. Hudson, and R. J. Desnick, Immunological evaluation of repeated administration of erythrocyte-entrapped protein to C311/HeJ mice, *Biochem. J. 168*, 141 (1977).
172. L. D. S. Hudson, M. B. Fiddler, and R. J. Desnick, Enzyme therapy. X. Immune response induced by enzyme- and buffer-loaded liposomes in C3H/HeJ Gus mice, *J. Pharmac. Exp. Ther. 208*, 507 (1979).
173. D. A. Tyrrell and B. E. Ryman, The entrapment of therapeutic agents in resealed erythrocyte "ghosts" and their fate *in vivo*, *Biochem. Soc. Trans. 4*, 677 (1976).
174. G. P. Royer, T. K. Lee, and T. D. Sokoloski, Entrapment of bioactive compounds within native albumin beads, *J. Parent. Sci. Tech. 37*, 34 (1983).
175. M. J. Poznansky and L. G. Cleland, Biological macromolecules as carriers of drugs and enzymes. In, *Drug Delivery Systems* (R. L. Juliano, Ed.), Oxford University Press, New York, 1980, pp. 253.
176. T. K. Lee, T. D. Sokoloski, G. P. Royer, Serum albumin beads: An injectable, biodegradable system for the sustained release of drugs, *Science 213*, 233 (1981).
177. M. F. A. Goosen, Y. F. Leung, S. Chou, and A. M. Sun, Insulin-albumin microbeads: An implantable, biodegradable system, *Biomat. Med. Dev. Act. Org. 10*, 205 (1982).
178. O. Vaizolglu and P. Speiser, Intelligent drug delivery systems, *TIPS 3*, 28 (1982).
179. A. Trouet, D. D. De Campeneere, R. Baurain, M. Hybrechts, and A. Zenebergh. In, *Drug Carriers in Biology and Medicine*, Academic Press, London, New York and San Francisco, 1979, p. 87.

180. S. G. Vitals, M. Masquelier, and C. O. Peterson, Low density lipoprotein (LDL) for the targeting of anticancer agents to malignant cells with high LDL receptor activity. In, *11th International Symposium on Controlled Release Bioactive Materials* (W. E. Meyers and R. L. Dunn, Eds.), Controlled Release Society, Inc., 1984, pp. 23.
181. J. Pitha, Nucleic acid and sulfate and phosphate polyanions, In, *Anionic Polymeric Drugs* (L. G. Donaruma, R. M. Ottenbrite, and O. Vogel, Eds.), John Wiley & Sons, Inc., New York, 1980.
182. A. D. Bangham, M. M. Standish, and J. C. Watkins, Diffusion of univalent ions across the lamellae of swollen phospholipids, *J. Mol. Biol. 13*, 238 (1965).
183. D. Papahadjopoulos and J. W. Watkins, Phospholipid model membranes. II. Permeability properties of hydrated liquid crystals, *Biochem. Biophys. Acta 135*, 639 (1967).
184. A. D. Bangham, Membrane models with phospholipids, *Prog. Biophy. Mol. Biol. 18*, 29 (1968).
185. D. Papahadjopoulos and N. Miller, Phospholipid model membrane. I. Structural characteristics of hydrated liquid crystals, *Biochim. Biophys. Acta 135*, 624 (1967).
186. S. M. Gruner, R. P. Lenk, A. S. Janoff, and M. J. Ostro, Novel multilayered lipid vesicles: Comparision of physical characteristics of multilamellar liposomes and stable plurilamellar vesicles, *Biochemistry 24*, 2833 (1985).
187. A. Goundalker, T. Ghose, and M. Mezei, Covalent binding of antibodies to liposomes using a novel lipid derivative, *J. Pharm. Pharmacol. 36*, 465 (1984).
188. L. S. Rao, Liposomal dosage form development-some practical considerations, *J. Parent. Sci. Tech. 37*, 72 (1983).
189. G. Gregoriadis, P. D. Leathwood, and B. E. Ryman, Enzyme entrapment in liposomes, *FEBS Lett. 14*, 95 (1971).
190. G. Gregoriadis and B. E. Ryman, Lysosomal localization of β-fructofuranosidase-containing liposomes injected into rats, *Biochem. J. 129*, 123 (1972).
191. G. Gregoriadis and B. E. Ryman, Fate of protein-containing liposomes injected into rats: An approach to the treatment of storage disease, *Eur. J. Biochem. 24*, 485 (1972).
192. G. Gregoriadis, D. Putman, L. Louis, and E. D. Neerunjun, Comparative effect of non-entrapped and liposome-entrapped neuraminidase injected into rats, *Biochem. J. 140*, 323 (1974).
193. G. Gregoriadis and E. D. Neerunjum, Homing of liposomes to target cell, *Biochem. Biophys. Res. Comm. 65*, 537 (1975).
194. G. Gregoriadis, Drug entrapment in liposomes, *FEBS Lett. 36*, 292 (1973).

195. R. L. Juliano and D. Stamp, The effect of particle size and charge on the clearance rates of liposomes and liposome encapsulated drug, *Biochem. Biophys. Res. Commun. 63*, 651 (1975).
196. G. Deliconstantinos, G. Ramantanis, and D. K. Todorou, Interaction of 99m Tc-labeled liposomes with Walker tumor cells *in vitro*. Liposome-medicated introduction of thaliblastine into resistant Walker tumor cells, *Gen. Pharmacol. 124*, 407 (1983).
197. A. W. Segal, E. J. Wills, J. E. Richmond, G. Slown, C. D. V. Black, and G. Gregoriadis, Morphological observations on the cellular and subcellular destination of intravenously administered liposomes, *Br. J. Exp. Pathol. 55*, 320 (1974).
198. A. Cudd and C. Nicolau, Electron microscope study of the fate of liposomes *in-vivo*. In, *11th International Symposium on Controlled Release Bioactive Materials* (W. E. Meyer and R. L. Dunn, Eds.), Controlled Release Society, Inc., 1984, p. 40.
199. R. M. Abra, C. A. Hunt, and D. T. Lau, Liposome disposition *in-vivo*. VI. Delivery to the lung, *J. Pharm. Sci. 73*, 203 (1984).
200. P. Speiser. In, *Frontiers of Biology*, Vol. 6 (A. Neuberger and E. L. Tatum, Eds.), Elsevier/North Holland Biomedical Press, New York, 1979, p. 653.
201. P. Couvreur, P. Tulkens, M. Roland, A. Trouet, and P. Speiser, Nanocapsules: A new type of lysosomotropic carrier, *FEBS Lett. 84*, 323 (1977).
202. P. Couvreur, B. Kante, V. Lenaerts, Y. Scailteur, M. Roland, and P. Speiser, Tissue distribution of antitumor drugs associated with polyalkylcyanoacrylate nanoparticles, *J. Pharm. Sci. 69*, 199 (1980).
203. L. Illum and S. S. Davis, Effect of the nonionic surfactant poloxamer 338 on the fate and deposition of polystyrene microspheres following intravenous administration, *J. Pharm. Sci. 72*, 1086 (1983).
204. D. Leu, B. Manthey, J. Kreuter, P. Speiser, and P. P. DeLuca, Distribution and elimination of coated polymethyl [2-^{14}C] methacrylate nanoparticles after intravenous injection in rats, *J. Pharm. Sci. 73*, 1433 (1984).
205. M. Arakawa and T. Konda, Preparation of hemolysate loaded poly (*N,N-L*-lysine diterephthaloyl) nanocapsules, *J. Pharm. Sci. 70*, 354 (1981).
206. F. Theeuwes and S. I. Yum, Principles of the design and operation of generic osmotic pumps for the delivery of semisolid or liquid drug formulations, *Ann. Biomed. Eng. 4*, 343 (1976).
207. F. Theeuwes, The elementary osmotic pump, *J. Pharm. Sci. 64*, 1987 (1975).
208. E. L. P. Uhlig, W. F. Graydon, and Dr. W. Zingg, The electroosmotic actuation of implantable insulin micropumps, *J. Biomed. Mat. Res. 17*, 931 (1983).

209. P. J. Blackshear, F. D. Dorman, P. L. Blackshear Jr., R. L. Varco, and H. Buchwald, A permanently implantable, self-recycling, low flow, constant rate multipurpose infusion pump of simple design, *Surg. Forum 21*, 136 (1970).
210. P. J. Blackshear, F. D. Dorman, P. L. Blackshear Jr., R. L. Varco, and H. Buchwald, The design and initial testing of an implantable infusion pump, *Surg. Gynecol. Obstet. 134*, 51 (1972).
211. P. J. Blackshear, T. D. Rohde, F. Prosi, and H. Buchwald, The implantable infusion pump: a new concept in drug delivery, *Med. Prog. Tech. 6*, 149 (1979).
212. S. A. Varia, S. Schuller, and V. J. Stella, Phenytoin prodrugs IV: Hydrolysis of various 3-(hydroxymethyl) phenytoin esters, *J. Pharm. Sci. 73*, 1075 (1984).
213. S. A. Varia and V. J. Stella, Phenytoin prodrugs V: *In vivo* evaluation of some water-soluble phenytoin prodrugs in dog, *J. Pharm. Sci. 73*, 1080 (1984).
214. S. A. Varia and V. J. Stella, Phenytoin prodrugs VI: *In vivo* evaluation of a phosphate ester prodrug of phenytoin after parenteral administration to rats, *J. Pharm. Sci. 73*, 1087 (1984).
215. S. A. Varia, S. Schuller, K. B. Sloan, and V. J. Stella, Phenytoin prodrugs III: Water-soluble prodrug for oral and/or parenteral use, *J. Pharm. Sci. 73*, 1068 (1984).
216. Y. Yamoaka, R. D. Roberts, and V. J. Stella, Low-melting phenytoin pro-drugs as alternative oral delivery modes for phenytoin: A model for other high-melting sparingly water-soluble drugs, *J. Pharm. Sci. 72*, 400 (1983).
217. M. Johansen and H. Bundgaard, Prodrugs as drug delivery systems. XXV: Hydrolysis of oxazolidines—A potential new prodrug type, *J. Pharm. Sci. 72*, 1294 (1983).
218. U. Klixbull and H. Bundgaard, Prodrugs as drug delivery systems. XXX. 4-Imidazolidinones as potential bioreversible derivatives for the α-aminoamide moiety in peptides, *Int. J. Pharm. 20*, 273 (1984).
219. R. A. Lipper, S. M. Machkovech, J. C. Drach, and W. I. Higuchi, Inhibition of drug metabolism by a prodrug: 9-β-D-arabinofuranosyladenine 5'-valerate as an inhibitor of adenosine deaminase. *Mol. Pharmacol., 14*, 366 (1978).
220. V. J. Stella, Drug substances in particular prodrug problems and methods of approach. In, *Formulation and Preparation of Dosage Forms* (J. Polderman, Ed.), Elsevier/North-Holland Biomedical Press, New YOrk, 1977, p. 91.
221. R. A. Siegel and R. Langer, Controlled release of polypeptides and other macromolecules, *Pharm. Res. 1*, 1 (1984).
222. K. S. E. Su, K. M. Campanale, L. G. Mendelsohn, G. A. Kerchner, and G. L. Gries, Nasal delivery of polypeptides I: Nasal

absorption of enkephalins in rats, *J. Pharm. Sci. 74*, 394 (1985).

223. V. Bocci, A. Naldini, F. Corradeschi, and E. Lencioni, Colorectal administration of human interferon-A, *Int. J. Pharm. 24*, 109 (1985).

224. H. Okada, I. Yamazaki, T. Yashiki, T. Shimamoto, and H. Mima, Vaginal absorption of a potent luteinizing hormone-releasing hormone analogue (leuprolide) in rats IV: Evaluation of the vaginal absorption and gonadotropin responses by radioimmunoassay, *J. Pharm. Sci. 73*, 298 (1984).

11

Implantable Therapeutic Systems

YIE W. CHIEN / Rutgers—The State University of New Jersey, Piscataway, New Jersey

I. INTRODUCTION

Lafarge pioneered, in 1861, the concept of implantable therapeutic systems for long-term, continuous drug administration with the development of a subcutaneously implantable drug pellet. The technique was then rediscovered in 1936 by Deanesly and Parkes [1,2], who administered crystalline hormones in the form of solid steroid pellets to mimic the steady, continuous secretion of hormones from an active gland for hormone substitution therapy [3].

The subcutaneous release rate of steroids from the pellet implantation was found to be slowed down and the hormonal activities were prolonged by dispersing the steroids in cholesterol matrix during pellet fabrication [4]. Unfortunately, it was observed that the subcutaneous absorption of steroids from the cholesterol pellets varies greatly from one condition to another. The subcutaneous drug administration by pellet implantation method was then subjected to modifications by several investigators [5,6].

The clinical use of implantable pellets for human health cares has declined in recent years. Currently, there are only a few steroid pellets still commercially available for medication: (a) testosterone (Oreton pellet/Schering), (b) desoxycorticosterone acetate (Percorten pellet/Ciba), and (c) estradiol (Progynon pellet/Schering) [7]. On the other hand, the laboratory use of implantable pellets for experimental purposes has become quite popular [8–17].

Subcutaneous drug administration by pellet implantation is known to have several undesirable drawbacks. The primary one is that release profile of drugs from the pellets is not constant and cannot be readily controlled, in terms of precision of release rate and duration of action. The fact has triggered the research and development of novel, controllable, and implantable therapeutic systems to replace pellets for long-term, continuous subcutaneous administration of drugs.

II. HISTORICAL DEVELOPMENT

Application of biocompatible polymers to the construction of implantable therapeutic systems for achieving a better control of drug release, in terms of duration of drug activity and precision of long-term dosing, was not realized until accidental discovery of the controlled drug permeation characteristics of silicone elastomers.

The story began approximately 20 years ago in the laboratories of U. S. Naval Medical Research Center, where the paths of two unrelated experiments unexpectedly converged [18]. At the time, Dr. Folkman was trying to treat experimental heart block with thyroid hormone pellets that would release a minute dose of the hormone locally at a steady rate; and, at the same time, Dr. Long was experimenting with the heart valves fabricated from silicone elastomer, studying how well these silicone valves performed under stress in turbulent water. For photographic purposes, he attempted to stain the translucent valves with various types of dyes. He observed that certain oil-soluble dyes, such as rhodamine and Sudan III, would penetrate the lipophilic silicone valves and stain them easily, whereas most water-soluble dyes, like methylene blue and chlorazol black, would not. This observation triggered his imagination of applying the reversible sorption of lipophilic dyes into and out of silicone elastomer as a means to control the release of drugs for long-term medication.

To evaluate the potential biomedical application of this finding, a very small capsule-shaped implant was fabricated from silicone polymer tubing to encapsulate thyroid hormone powder. *In vitro* elution studies demonstrated that the silicone capsule released the thyroid hormone at a steady rate, day after day. When it was implanted in the dogs' myocardium with heart block, the controlled release of thyroid hormone was found to produce a localized hyperthyroid myocardium with fast pacemaker activity. Similiar controlled drug release behavior was observed for isoproterenol, digitoxin, and EDTA encapsulated in the silicone capsules [19,20].

One year after this pioneering finding, Bass and his co-workers demonstrated that histamine and atropine can also permeate through silicone capsules for a prolonged period of time [21]. And Powers reported that silicone elastomer can be used for the preparation of pyrimethamine implants to protect chicks from malaria as well as piperazine HCl- and antimony dimercaptosuccinate-implants to provide effective protection in mice against schistosomal infection [22].

Then, in 1966, Dziuk and Cook reported that many steroidal hormones and their synthetic derivatives penetrate readily through the silicone polymer. They also observed that when cattle were implanted with progesterone-releasing silicone capsules, their fertility was inhibited for more than one year [23]. These results were later confirmed by the investigations of Kincl and his associates [24]. Further investigations indicated that radiolabeled steroids penetrate silicone membrane at rates which are substantially greater than the rates of permeation through the membranes fabricated from other synthetic polymers, such as polyethylene. The rate of membrane permeation was found to be controlled by the thickness and surface area of the membrane as well as the polarity of the penetrants. The results later stimulated several clinical studies to evaluate the feasibility of using progestin-releasing silicone capsule to provide a long-term subcutaneous contraception in humans.

All of these historical developments have explored the potential of using silicone capsules as the implantable therapeutic systems to control the duration of drug activity and the precision of long-term, continual dosing. Silicone capsule was later extended to the controlled administration of insecticides, such as proban®, for intraperitoneal control of Louse Polyplax serrata [25], of methoxyflurane for chronic analgesia [26], of nicotine for studying its chronic effect on tobacco smokers [27], of anesthetic agents, like ether, for general anesthesia [28,29], and of *L*-dopa to various focal brain targets [30].

Toward the end of 1960s, a concentrated effort was made to expand the silicone elastomer-based implantable therapeutic system technology to other biocompatible polymers, which can be applied to control the release of water-soluble molecules. Some of the implantable therapeutic systems that have been evolved from this effort include the microporous membrane made from ethylene/vinyl acetate copolymer for the ocular controlled administration of pilocarpine, the biodegradable (lactic/glycolic) copolymer for subcutaneous and intramuscular controlled administrations of narcotic antagonists, the bioerodible polysaccharide polymers for ocular controlled administration of anti-inflammatory steroids, hydrogels for the subcutaneous controlled administration of estrus synchronizing agents, as well as implantable therapeutic systems activated by osmotic pressure, vapor pressure, magnetism and ultrasound etc. energy sources.

III. APPROACHES TO DEVELOPMENT OF IMPLANTABLE THERAPEUTIC SYSTEMS

Historically, the subcutaneous implantation of drug pellets is known to be the first medical approach aiming to achieve prolonged and continuous administration of drugs. This first generation of implantable therapeutic systems was produced by compressing drug crystals, without or with only a small fraction of pharmaceutical excipients, into tiny, cylinder-shaped solid pellets that can be readily implanted into a subcutaneous tissue by means of a Kearns pellet injector or by making a small skin incision. Subcutaneous tissue is essentially a sheet of areolar tissue lying directly underneath the skin. It is rich in fat, but poor in nerve network and hemoperfusion. Therefore, the subcutaneous tissue is an ideal location for implantation and prolonged drug administration because of its ready assess to implantation, slow drug absorption, and low reactivity to the insertion of foreign materials.

Over the years, a number of approaches have been developed to achieve the controlled administration of biologically active agents via implantation or insertion in the tissues. These approaches are outlined as follows:

A. Controlled drug release by diffusion
   1. Membrane permeation-controlled drug delivery using:
      a. Nonporous membranes
      b. Microporous membranes
      c. Semipermeable membranes
   2. Matrix diffusion-controlled drug delivery using:
      a. Lipophilic polymers
      b. Hydrophilic (swellable) polymers
      c. Porous polymers
   3. Microreservoir dissolution-controlled drug delivery using:
      a. Hydrophilic reservoir/Lipophilic matrix
      b. Lipophilic reservoir/Hydrophilic matrix

B. Controlled drug release by activation
   1. Osmotic pressure-activated drug delivery
   2. Vapor pressure-activated drug delivery
   3. Magnetism-activated drug delivery
   4. Ultrasound-activated drug delivery
   5. Hydrolysis-activated drug delivery

In this chapter, the science and engineering behind the development of these approaches will be briefly described.

A. Controlled Drug Release by Diffusion

1. *Membrane Permeation-Controlled Drug Delivery*

In this mode of controlled drug delivery, the drug reservoir is encapsulated within a compartment totally enclosed by a rate-controlling polymeric membrane (Fig. 1). The drug reservoir can be either drug solid particles or a dispersion (or a solution) of drug solid particles in a liquid- or a solid-type dispersing medium. The polymeric membrane can be fabricated from a homogeneous or heterogeneous nonporous polymeric material or a microporous (or a semipermeable) membrane. The encapsulation of drug reservoir inside the polymeric membrane can be accomplished by moulding, capsulation, microencapsulation, or other techniques. Different shapes and sizes of drug delivery devices can be fabricated.

The rate of drug release (dQ/dt) from this type of implantable therapeutic systems should be constant and defined by:

$$\frac{dQ}{dt} = \frac{C_R}{\frac{1}{P_m} + \frac{1}{P_d}} \tag{1}$$

where C_R is the drug concentration in the reservoir compartment; P_m and P_d are, respectively, the permeability coefficients of the

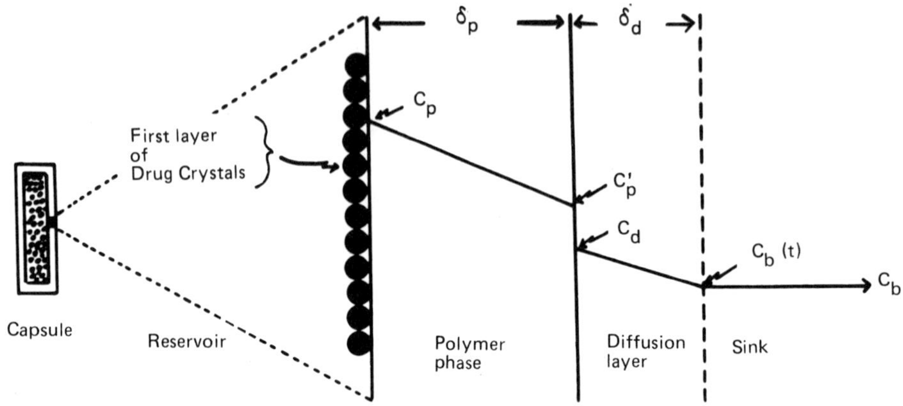

Fig. 1 Schematic illustration of the controlled release of drug molecules from a membrane permeation-controlled drug delivery device filled with solid drug particles. C_p is the solubility of drug in the polymer phase; C_p' is the concentration of drug at the polymer/solution interface; C_d is the concentration of drug at the solution/polymer interface; C_b is the concentration of drug in the bulk of elution solution; δ_p is the thickness of the polymeric membrane; and δ_d is the thickness of the hydrodynamic diffusion layer [From Y. W. Chien, *Chem. Pharm. Bull. 24*, 1471 (1976).]

rate-controlling membrane and of the hydrodynamic diffusion layer existing on the membrane surface and are defined as follows:

$$P_m = \frac{K_{m/r} D_m}{\delta_m} \tag{2}$$

$$P_d = \frac{K_{a/m} D_a}{\delta_d} \tag{3}$$

where $K_{m/r}$ and $K_{a/m}$ are, respectively, the partition coefficients for the interfacial partitioning of drug molecules from the reservoir to the membrane and from the membrane to the aqueous diffusion layer; D_m and D_a are, respectively, the diffusion coefficients in the rate-controlling membrane and in the aqueous diffusion layer; δ_m and δ_d are, respectively, the thicknesses of the rate-controlling membrane and of the aqueous diffusion layer.

Substituting Eq. (2) and Eq. (3) for P_m and P_d in Eq. (1) and then integration to give:

$$\frac{Q}{t} = \frac{K_{m/r} K_{a/m} D_a D_m}{K_{m/r} D_m \delta_d + K_{a/m} D_a \delta_m} C_R \qquad (4)$$

which defines the rate of drug release at steady state from a membrane permeation-controlled drug delivery device. Representatives of this type of implantable therapeutic systems are:

Progestasert IUD

In such a device, the drug reservoir, which is a suspension of progesterone crystals in liquid silicone polymer, is encapsulated in a T-shaped intrauterine device (IUD) enclosed by a non-porous membrane of ethylene-vinyl acetate copolymer (Fig. 2). It is engineered

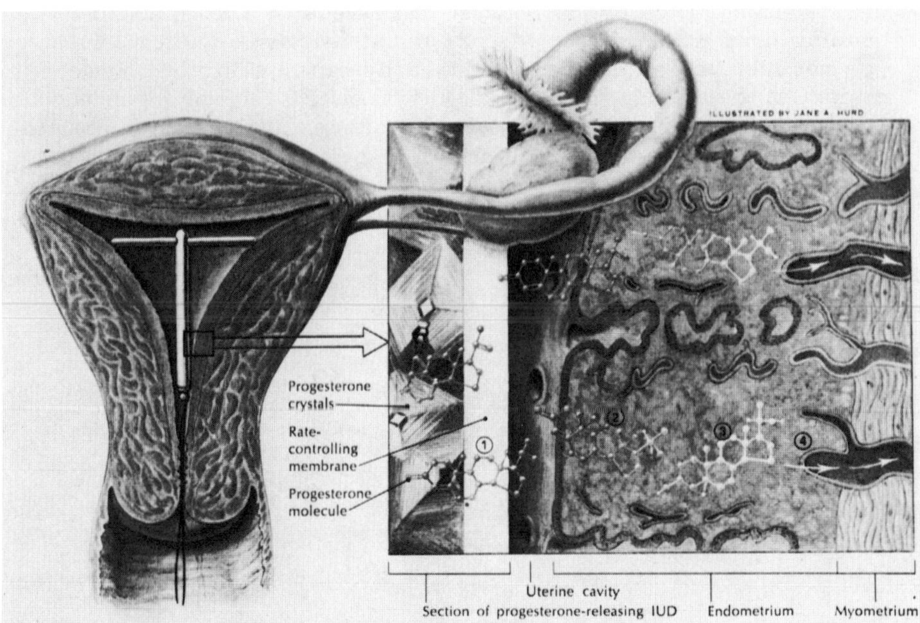

Fig. 2 Illustration of the localized action of progesterone-releasing IUDs. The insert shows progesterone molecules diffusing through the rate-controlling membrane in the vertical bar of the T-shaped IUD (1), penetrating the endometrium, where they exert their pharmacological effects (2), being rapidly metabolized (3), and leaving the endometrium (4) [From R. P. Rao and A. Scommegna, *Am. Fam. Physician 16*, 177 (1977).]

to release 65 mcg/day of progesterone locally in the uterine cavity to achieve contraception for one year (Fig. 3) [31].

Ocusert System

In such a device, the solid drug reservoir, which is a thin disc of pilocarpine alginate, is sandwiched between two transparent sheets of microporous membrane fabricated from ethylene-vinyl acetate copolymer (Fig. 4). It is designed to permit the tear fluid to penetrate the microporous membranes, to dissolve and to carry out pilocarpine at a constant rate of 20 to 40 mcg/hr for weekly management of glaucoma (Fig. 5) [32].

2. *Matrix Diffusion-Controlled Drug Delivery*

In this mode of controlled drug delivery, the drug reservoir is formed by homogeneous dispersion of drug solid particles throughout a lipophilic or hydrophilic polymer matrix (Fig. 6). The dispersion of drug solid particles in the polymer matrix can be accomplished by bending drug solids with a viscous liquid polymer or a semisolid polymer at room temperature, followed by crosslinking of polymer chains, or by mixing drug solids with a melted polymer at an elevated temperature. These drug-polymer dispersions are then extruded to form drug delivery devices of various shapes and sizes. It can also

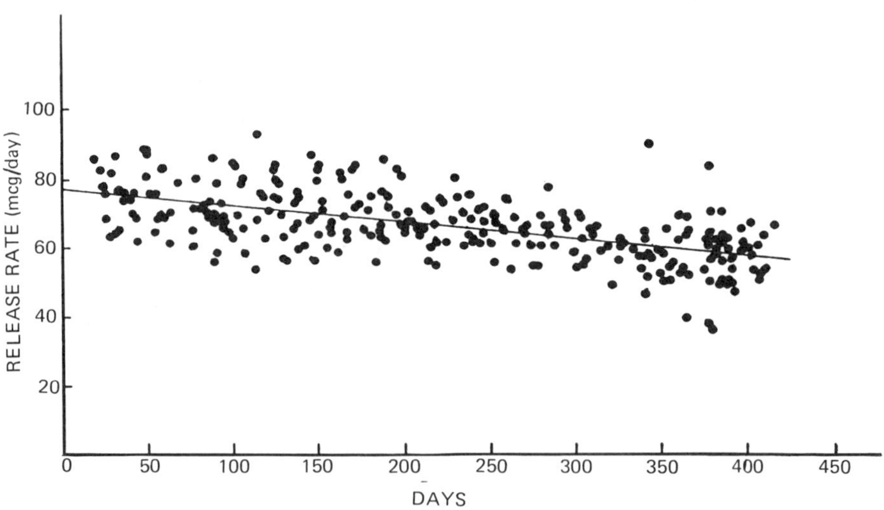

Fig. 3 Intrauterine release rate profiles of progesterone from Progestasert IUD in women for more than 400 days. [From J. Martinez-Manautou, *J. Steroid Biochem.* 6, 889 (1975).]

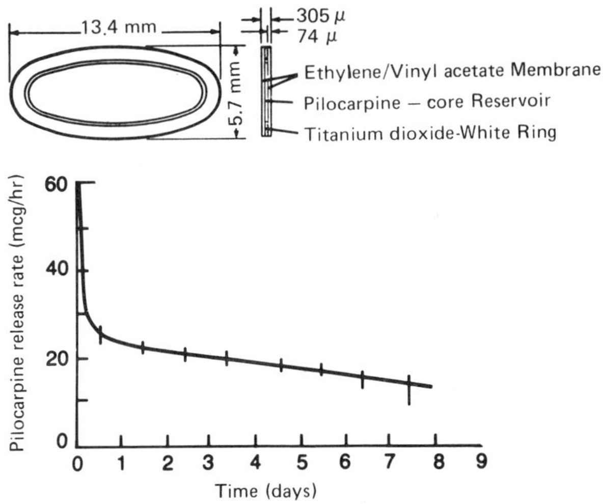

Fig. 4 Upper: Diagrammatical illustration of the Ocusert Therapeutic System—a pilocarpine-releasing ocular insert. Each Pilo-20 unit measured 5.7 × 13.4 mm on its axes and 0.3 mm in thickness and contains 5 mg pilocarpine. Each Pilo-40 unit measured 5.5 × 13 mm on its axes and 0.5 mm in thickness and contains 11 mg pilocarpine. Lower: Ocular release rate profile of pilocarpine from Ocusert Pilo-20 system. [From R. Baker and H. Lonsdale, *Chem. Technol.* 5, 668 (1975).]

be fabricated by dissolving the drug solid and/or the polymer in a common organic solvent followed by mixing and solvent evaporation in a mould at an elevated temperature and/or under a vacuum.

The rate of drug release from this matrix diffusion-controlled drug delivery device is not constant and is defined by:

$$\frac{dQ}{dt} = \left(\frac{ACpDp}{2t}\right)^{1/2} \tag{5}$$

where A is the initial drug loading dose dispersed in the polymer matrix; Cp and Dp are, respectively, the solubility and diffusivity of the drug molecules in the polymer. Integration of Eq. (5) gives:

$$\frac{Q}{t^{1/2}} = (2ACpDp)^{1/2} \tag{6}$$

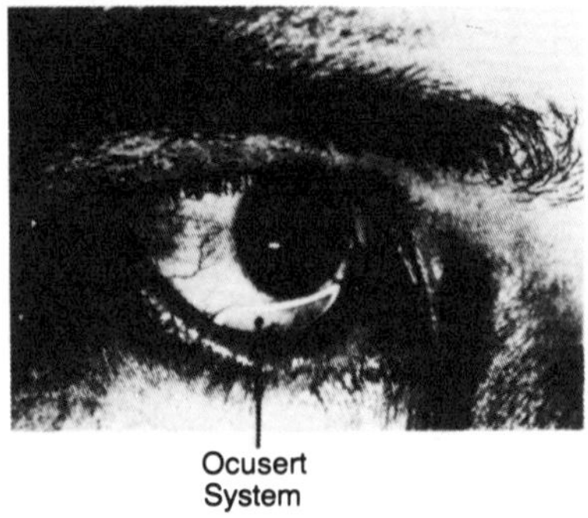

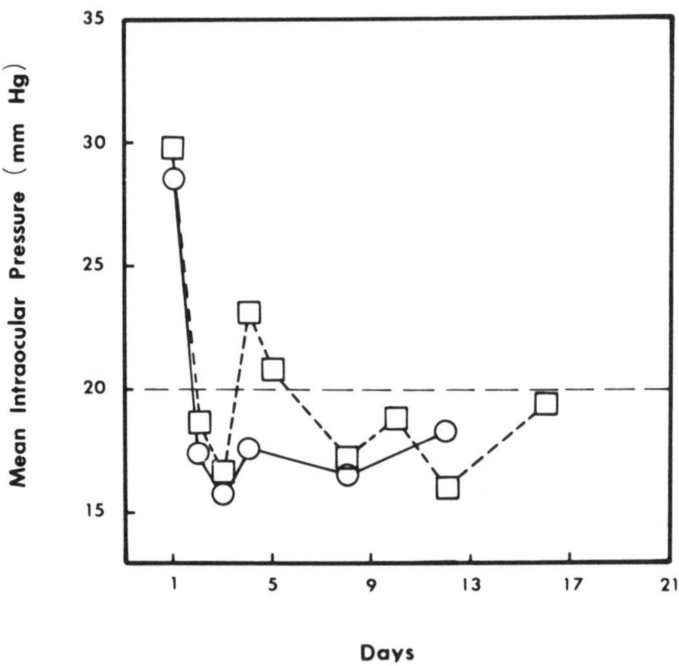

Fig. 5 Upper: A unit of Ocusert System, which releases pilocarpine continuously at constant rate when placed in the upper or lower cul-de-sac of the eye for the relief of intraocular pressure for 7 days. [From R. Baker and H. Lonsdale, *Chem. Technol.* *5*, 668 (1975).] Lower: Duration of intraocular pressure control by consecutive treatment with various pilocarpine-releasing Ocusert systems. ○, insertion of one Ocusert Pilo-20 at Day 1, 4, 8 and 12; □, insertion of one Ocusert Pilo-20 at Day 1 and then one Ocusert Pilo-50 at Day 5, 8 and 12 [From M. F. Armaly and K. B. Rao, *Invest. Ophthalmol.* *12*, 491 (1973).]

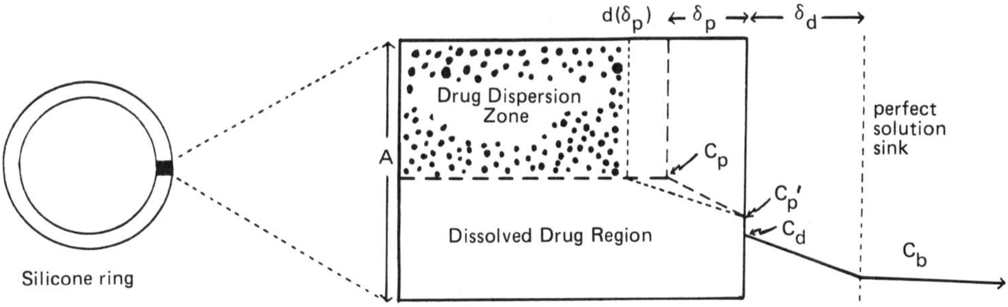

Fig. 6 Schematic illustration of the controlled release of drug molecules from a matrix diffusion-controlled drug delivery device (such as the vaginal ring in Fig. 7). A is the initial amount of drug solids impregnated in a unit volume of polymer matrix; C_p is the solubility of drug in the polymer phase; C_p' is the concentration of drug at the polymer/solution interface; C_d is the concentration of drug at the solution/polymer interface; C_b is the concentration of drug in the bulk of elution solution; δ_p and δ_d are the thicknesses of the drug depletion zone in the matrix and of the hydrodynamic diffusion layer on the immediate surface of the device, respectively; and $d(\delta_p)$ is the differential thickness of the depletion zone formed after more drug solids elute out [From Y. W. Chien, H. Lambert, and T. Lin, *J. Pharm. Sci. 64*, 1643 (1975).]

which defines the flux of drug release at steady state from a matrix diffusion-controlled drug delivery device. Representatives of this type of implantable therapeutic system are:

Contraceptive Vaginal Ring

It is fabricated by dispersing a contraceptive steroid, e.g., medroxyprogesterone acetate, as micronized solid particles in a viscous mixture of silicone elastomer and catalyst and then extruding the steroid-polymer dispersion into a mould to form a donut-shaped vaginal ring (Fig. 7). It is designed to be inserted into the vagina and positioned around the cervix for 21 days to achieve a constant plasma progestin level and cyclic intravaginal contraception (Fig. 8) (33).

Syncro-Mate-B Implant

It is fabricated by dissolving norgestomet crystals in an alcoholic solution of ethylene glycomethacrylate (Hydron S) and then polymerizing the drug-polymer mixture by the addition of a crosslinking agent, such as ethylene dimethacrylate, and an oxidizing catalyst

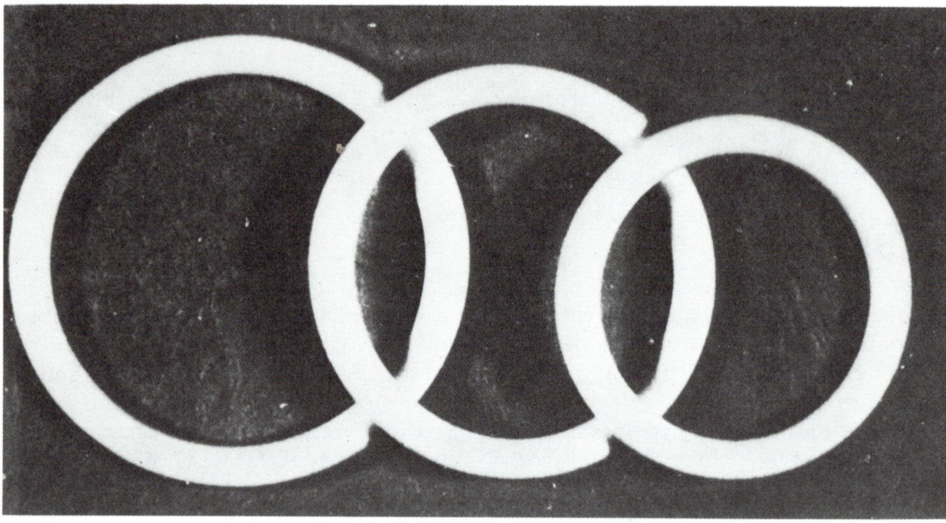

Fig. 7 Contraceptive vaginal rings fabricated from silicone medical grade Elastomer. (From Ref. 33.)

to form a cylinder-shaped insoluble Hydron implant [134]. This tiny subdermal implant is engineered to be inserted into the subcutaneous tissue, using a specially designed implanter (Fig. 9) to release norgestomet at a rate of 504 $mcg/cm^2/day^{1/2}$ for up to 16 days for estrus control and synchronization in livestock (Fig. 10) [35].

Compudose Implant

It is fabricated by dispersing micronized estradiol crystals in a viscous mixture of silicone elastomer and catalyst and then coating the estradiol-polymer dispersion around a rigid silicone rod by extrusion technique to form a cylinder-shaped implant. This subdermal implant is designed for subcutaneous ear implantation in steers for 200–400 days and to release a controlled quantity of estradiol for growth promotion [36].

3. *Microreservoir Dissolution-Controlled Drug Delivery*

In this mode of controlled drug delivery, the drug reservoir, which is a suspension of drug crystals in an aqueous solution of a water-miscible polymer, forms a homogeneous dispersion of millions of discrete, unleachable, microscopic drug reservoirs in a polymer matrix

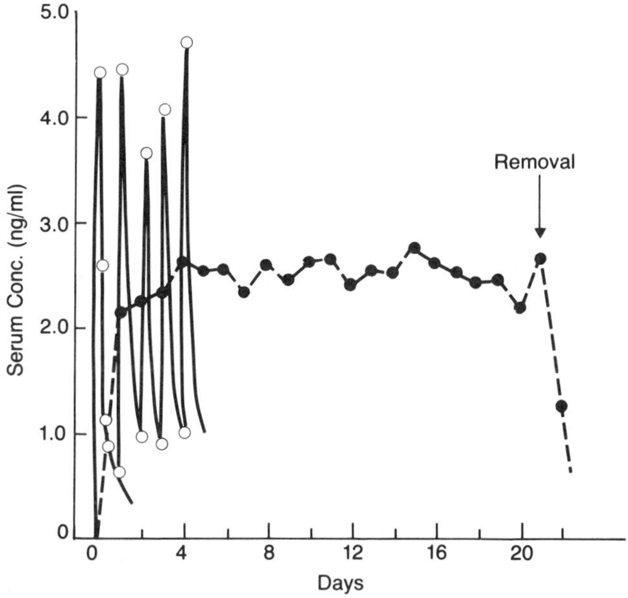

Fig. 8 Comparative serum concentration profiles of medroxyprogesterone acetate in humans resulting from continuous delivery of medroxyprogesterone acetate from the intravaginal administration of one unit of contraceptive vaginal ring (each ring contains 100 mg of medroxyprogesterone acetate) for 21 days (●) and from daily oral intake of one Provera tablet (each contains 10 mg of medroxyprogesterone acetate) for 5 consecutive days (○). [Plotted from the data by Hiroi et al., *Steroids 26*, 373 (1975) and by Thiery et al., *Contraception 13*, 605 (1976).]

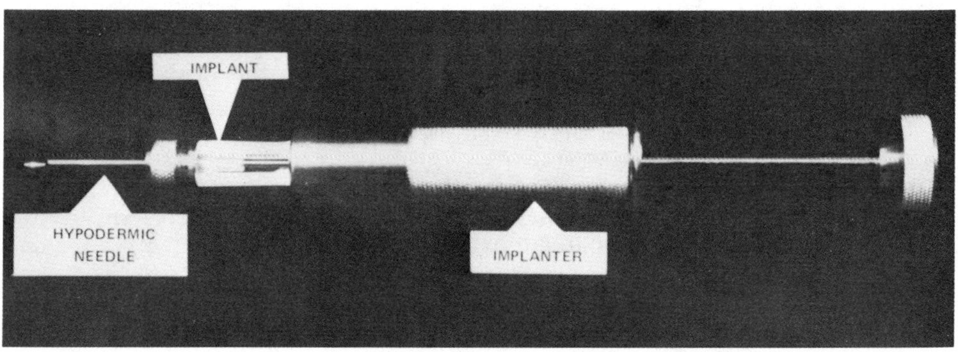

Fig. 9 Implanter, with a Syncro-Mate-B implant in position, designed specifically for the subcutaneous implantation. (From Ref. 35.)

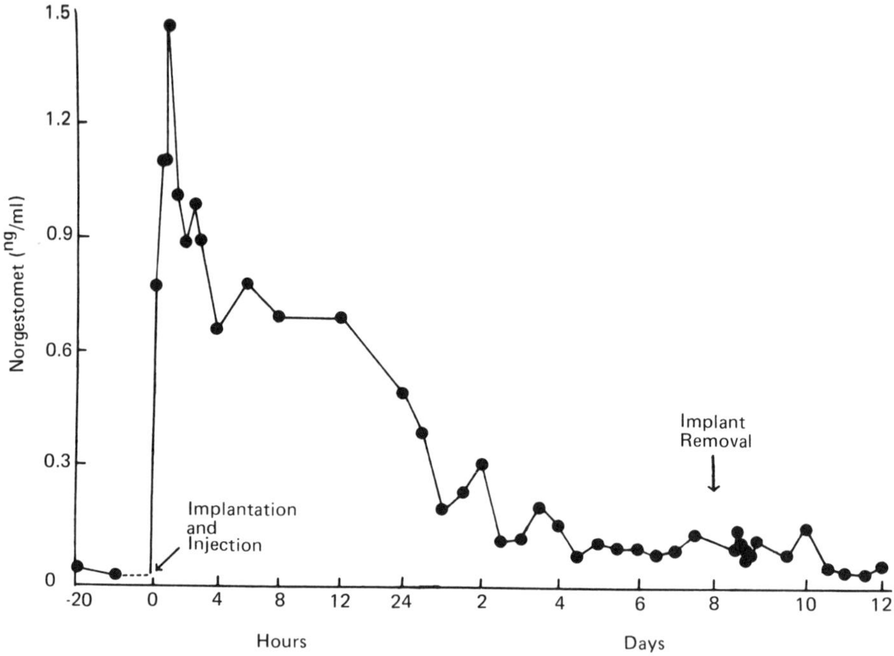

Fig. 10 Plasma levels of Norgestomet following 9-day subcutaneous implantation of one Synchro-Mate-B implant plus an intramuscular injection of 3 mg Norgestomet/5 mg estradiol valerate (in 2 ml of sesame oil) at the first day of implantation. (From Ref. 35.)

(Fig. 11). The microdispersion is accomplished by high-energy dispersion technique [37,38]. Different shapes and sizes of drug delivery devices can then be fabricated from this microresevoir-type drug delivery system by moulding or extrusion technique. Depending upon the physicochemical properties of drugs and the desired rate of drug release, the device can be further coated with a layer of biocompatible polymer to modify the mechanism and the rate of drug release.

Mathematical expression for the rate of drug release (dQ/dt) from this type of drug delivery devices can be derived from the physical model illustrated in Figure 12 and is defined [39] by:

$$\frac{dQ}{dt} = \frac{D_p D_s \alpha' K_p}{D_p \delta_d + D_s \delta_p \alpha' K_p}\left[\beta S_p - \frac{D_l S_l (1-\beta)}{\delta_l}\left(\frac{1}{K_l} + \frac{1}{K_m}\right)\right] \tag{7}$$

where $\alpha' = \partial'/\beta'$. ∂' is the ratio of drug concentration in the bulk of elution solution over drug solubility in the same medium and β' is the ratio of drug concentration at the outer edge of the polymer coating membrane over drug solubility in the same polymer; K_l, K_m, and K_p are the partition coefficients for the interfacial partitioning of drug from the liquid compartments to the polymer matrix, from the polymer matrix to the polymer coating membrane, and from the polymer coating membrane to the elution solution (such as tissue fluids), respectively; D_l, D_p, and D_s are the diffusivities of the

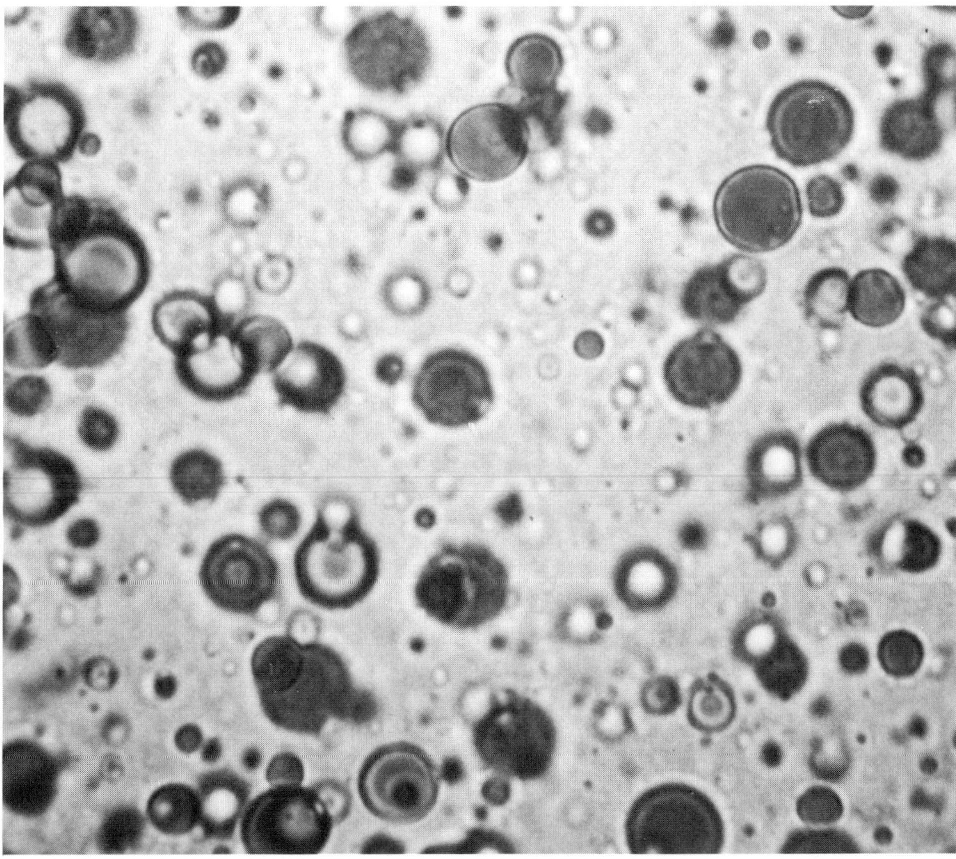

Fig. 11 Photomicroscopic view of a microreservoir-type drug delivery system, which shows the microscopic structure of various components. (From Ref. 39.)

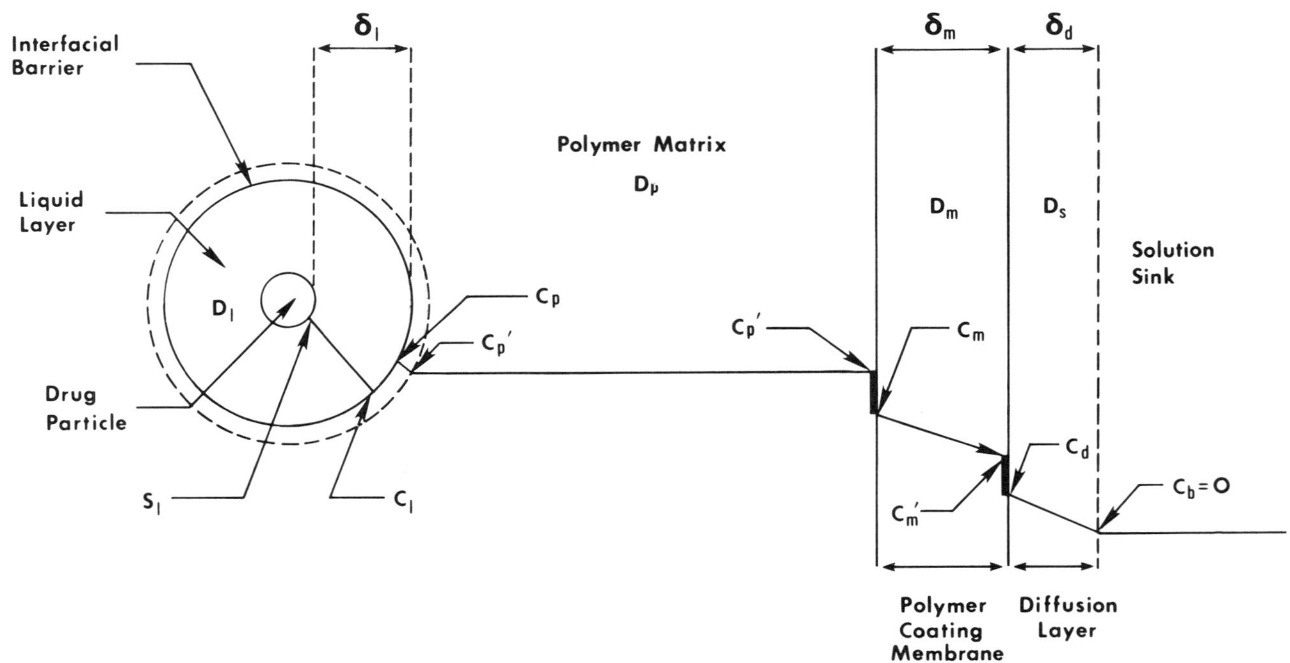

Fig. 12 A theoretical treatment of the controlled release of drug from a microreservoir-type drug delivery system is shown. For simplicity of treatment, a single sphere of drug-containing liquid compartment is analyzed. (From Ref. 40.)

drug in the liquid compartments, polymer coating membrane, and elution solution, respectively: S_l and S_p are the solubilities of the drug in the liquid compartments and in the polymer matrix, respectively; δ_l, δ_p, and δ_d are the thicknesses of the liquid layer surrounding the drug particles, the polymer coating membrane around the polymer matrix, and the hydrodynamic diffusion layer surrounding the polymer coating membrane, respectively; β is the ratio of drug concentration at the inner edge of the interfacial barrier over the drug solubility in the polymer matrix [39,40].

Release of drug from the microreservoir-type drug delivery system can follow either an interfacial partition- or a matrix diffusion-control process depending upon the relative magnitude of S_l and S_p [39]. Representatives of this type of drug delivery device are:

Syncro-Mate-C Implant

It is a cylindrical implant with improvement in both release rate profile and cost saving over the Syncro-Mate-B implant discussed earlier. It is fabricated by dispersing the drug reservoir, which is a suspension of norgestomet in an aqueous solution of PEG 400, to form millions of microscopic drug reservoirs in a viscous mixture of silicone elastomers by high-energy dispersion technique. After the addition of catalyst, the resultant composition is delivered into a silicone medical-grade tubing, which serves as the mould as well as the coating membrane, by extrusion technique and is polymerized *in situ*. The polymerized solid drug-polymer composition is then cut into cylinder-shaped drug delivery device with open ends (Fig. 13). This tiny subdermal implant is designed to be inserted, by a specially designed implanter, and to deliver norgestomet in the subcutaneous tissue in livestock's ear flap for up to 20 days for the control and synchronization of estrus and ovulation. A constant (Q versus t) release profile is achieved (Fig. 14), as compared to the Q vs. $t^{\frac{1}{2}}$ release profile (matrix-control release) for Syncro-Mate-B implant [35,40]. So, a more stable plasma drug profile and greater biological effectiveness are obtained (Fig. 15).

Dual-Release Vaginal Contraceptive Ring

It is fabricated by dispersing the drug reservoir, which is a suspension of a progestin and an estrogen in an aqueous solution of PEG 400, to form many microscopic drug reservoirs in a viscous mixture of silicone elastomers by high-energy mixing technique. After addition of catalyst, the resultant composition is extruded into a mould, by extrusion technique, and is polymerized by heat to form a donut-shaped vaginal ring (Fig. 16). It is designed to permit the users to insert the ring themselves and to release both progestin and estrogen, at a specific rate ratio, in the vagina for 21 days to achieve a cyclic intravaginal contraception.

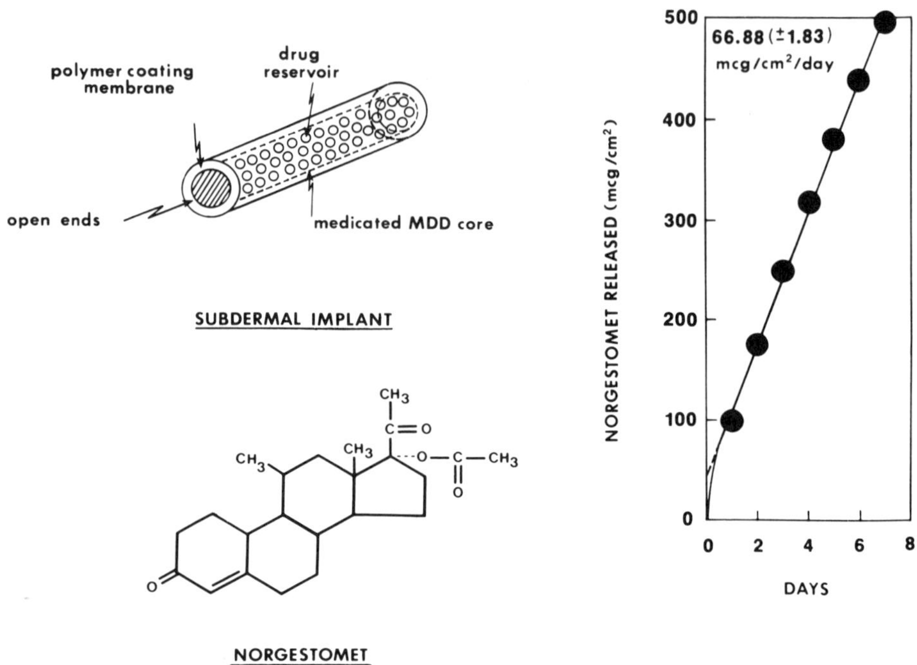

Fig. 13 Subdermal implant fabricated from the microreservoir-type drug delivery system to release norgestomet at constant rate. The open ends on the implant do not affect the zero-order drug release profile. (From Ref. 39.)

B. Controlled Drug Release by Activation

1. Osmotic Pressure-Activated Drug Delivery

In this mode of controlled drug delivery, the drug reservoir, which is a solution formulation, is contained within a semi-permeable housing. The drug is released in solution form at a controlled, constant rate under an osmotic pressure gradient. The rate of drug release (dQ/dt) is constant and is defined by:

$$\frac{dQ}{dt} = \frac{P_w A_m}{h_m} (\pi_s - \pi_e) \tag{8}$$

where P_w, A_m, and h_m are, respectively, the water permeability, the effective surface area, and the thickness of the semipermeable housing; $(\pi_s - \pi_e)$ is the differential osmotic pressure between the drug delivery system, with an osmotic pressure of π_s, and the environment, with an osmotic pressure of π_e. It is exemplified with the development of the Alzet osmotic pump:

Alzet Osmotic Pump

In such a device, the drug reservoir is contained inside a collapsible, impermeable polyester bag, whose external surface is coated with a layer of osmotically active salt. This reservoir compartment is then sealed inside a rigid housing walled with semipermeable polymer membrane (Fig. 17). At the implantation site, the water content in the tissue fluid will penetrate through the semipermeable membrane to dissolve the osmotically-active salt, creating an osmotic pressure in the narrow spacing between the flexible reservoir wall and the

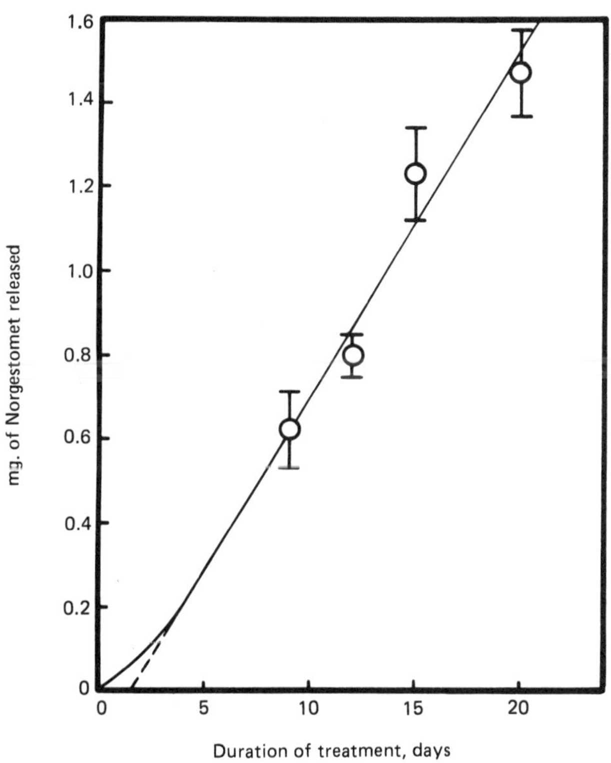

Fig. 14 Subcutaneous release of norgestomet from microreservoir-type subdermal implants in 20 U.S. cows for up to 20 days. The cumulative amount of norgestomet (Q) released is linearly dependent on the length of implantation (in days). (From Ref. 35.)

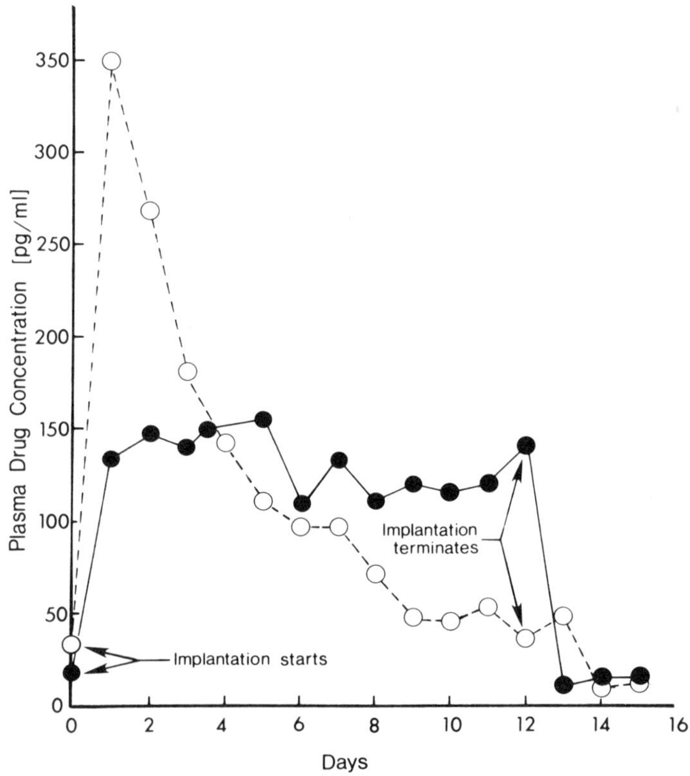

Fig. 15 Plasma profiles of norgestomet in Spanish ewes treated with microreservoir-type subdermal implants (●) or Hydron implants (○) for 12 days. Each data point is the mean of eight determinations conducted in four ewes. (From Ref. 35.)

rigid semipermeable housing. Under the osmotic pressure created, the reservoir compartment is reduced in volume and the drug solution is forced to release at a controlled rate through the flow moderator (Fig. 18). By varying the drug concentration in the solution, different amount of drug can be released at constant rate, following Eq. (8), for a duration of 1–4 weeks [41–43].

2. Vapor Pressure-Activated Drug Delivery

In this mode of controlled drug delivery, the drug reservoir, in a solution formulation, is contained inside an infusate chamber, which is physically separated from the vapor chamber by a freely movable

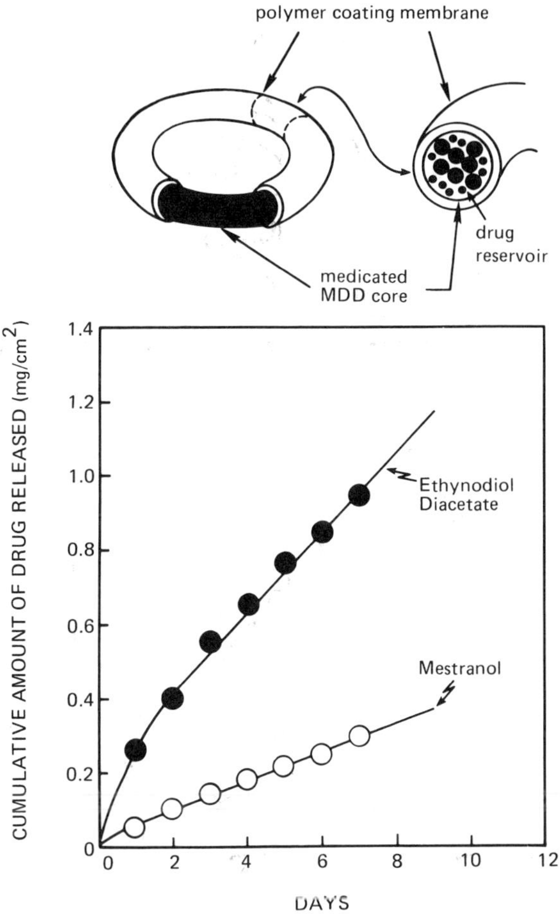

Fig. 16 Vaginal ring fabricated from the microreservoir-type drug delivery system to release ethynodiol diacetate, a synthetic progestin, mestranol, a synthetic estrogen, simultaneously at constant rates with therapeutically effective ratio. (From Ref. 39.)

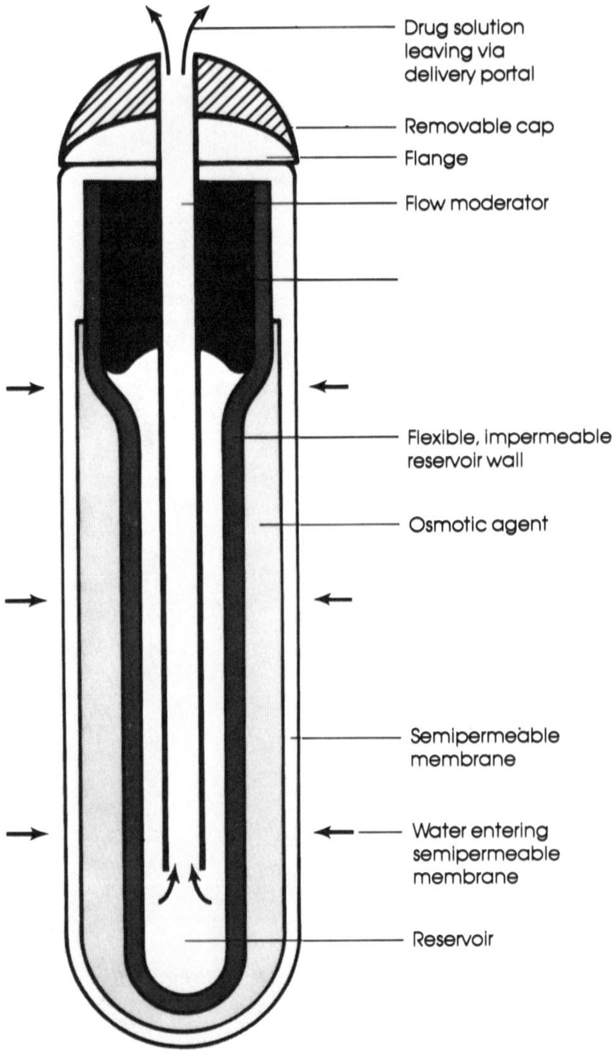

Fig. 17 Cross-sectional view of various structural components of a solution-type osmotic pressure-activated drug delivery system, e.g. Alzet osmotic pump. (From Alza Corp.)

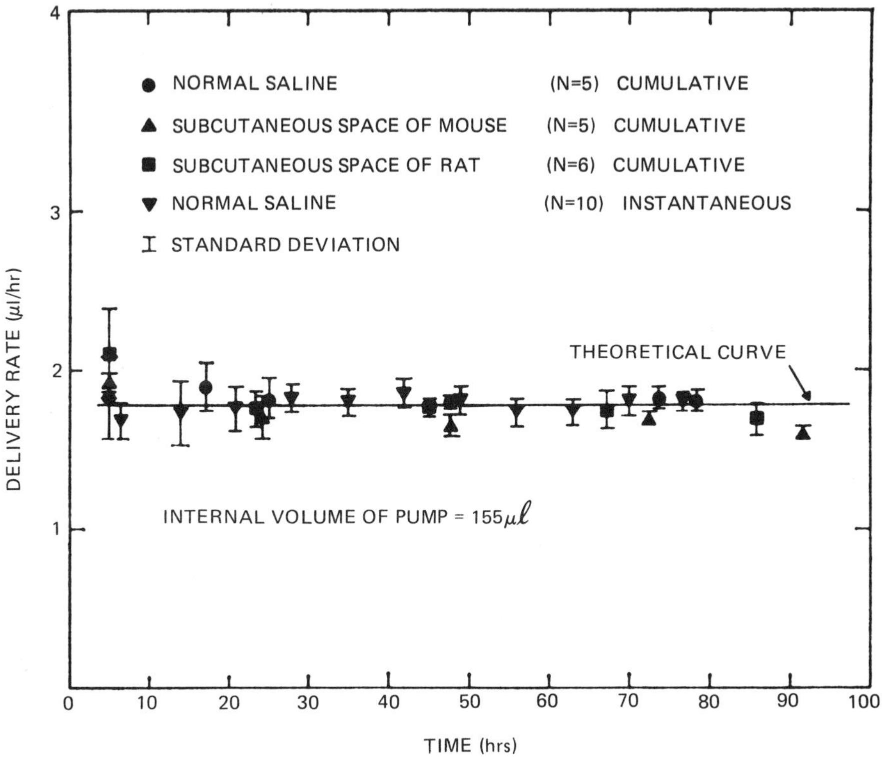

Fig. 18 *In vitro* and *in vivo* pumping rate profiles from the Alzet osmotic pump as a function of time. [From F. Theeuwes and S. I. Yum, *Ann. Biomed. Eng.* 4, 343 (1976.)]

bellows (Fig. 19). The vapor chamber contains a vaporizable fluid, e.g., fluorocarbon, which vaporizes at body temperature and creates a vapor pressure. Under the vapor pressure created, the bellows moves upward and forces the drug solution in the infusate chamber to release, through a series of flow regulator and delivery cannula, into the blood circulation at a constant flow rate [43,44] as defined by:

$$\frac{dQ}{dt} = \frac{3.1416d^4 \Delta p}{128 \mu l} \tag{9}$$

where d and l are the inner diameter and the length of the delivery cannula; Δp is the pressure difference between the vapor pressure

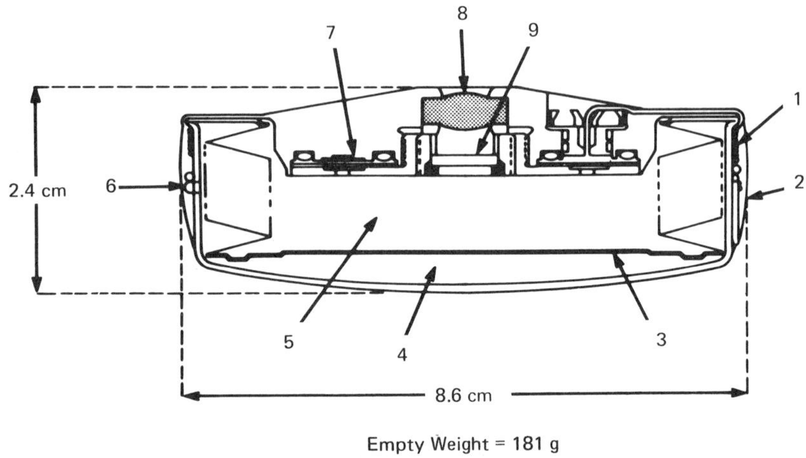

Fig. 19 Cross-sectional view of a vapor pressure-activated drug delivery system, (1) flow regulator, (2) silicone polymer coating, (3) bellows, (4) fluorocarbon chamber, (5) infusate chamber, (6) fluorcarbon fluid filling tube (permanently sealed), (7) filter assembly, (8) inlet septum for percutaneous refill of infusate, (9) needle stop, e.g., Infusaid. (From Ref. 44.)

in the vapor chamber and the pressure at the implantation site; and μ is the viscosity of the drug solution.

A typical example is the development of Infusaid (Fig. 19), an implantable infusion pump, for the constant infusion of heparin for anticoagulation treatment (Fig. 20) [45], of insulin for antidiabetic medication [44], and of morphine for patients suffering from the intensive pain of terminal cancer [46].

3. *Magnetism-Activated Drug Delivery*

Macromolecular drugs, such as peptides, have been known to release only at a relatively low rate from a polymeric drug delivery device. This low release rate has been improved by incorporating a magnetism-triggering mechanism into the polymeric drug delivery device and a zero-order drug release profile has also been achieved by a hemisphere-shaped geometry design [47]. By combining these two approaches, a subdermally implantable, magnetic-modulated hemispheric drug delivery device is developed (Fig. 21). It is fabricated by positioning a donut-shaped magnet at the center of a biocompatible polymer matrix, which contains a homogeneous dispersion of a macromolecular drug at a rather high drug:polymer ratio, to form a

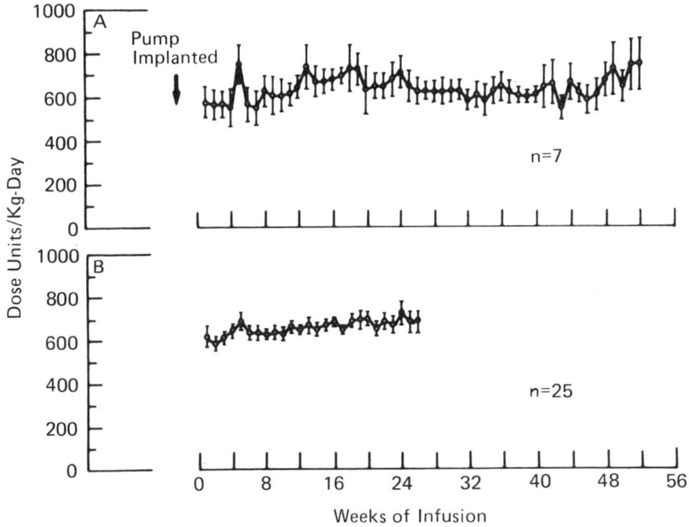

Fig. 20 Calculated daily heparin dose (mean ± S.E.) delivered by the Infusaid pumps to 25 dogs for 6 months (B) and to 7 for 12 months (A). (From Ref. 45.)

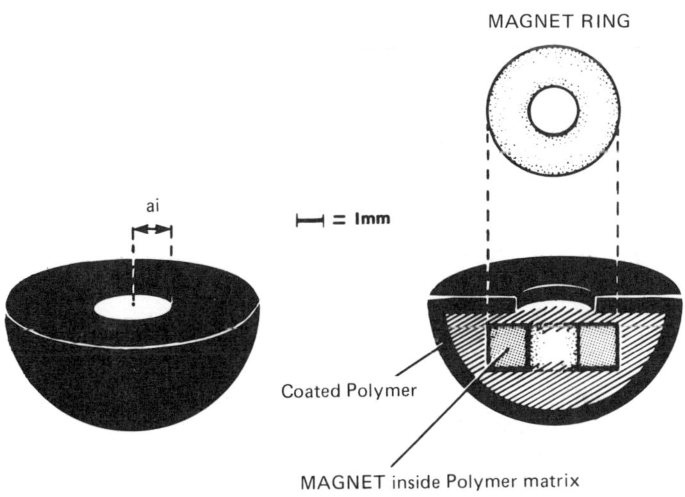

Fig. 21 Diagrammatic illustration of a magnetism-activated drug delivery device, e.g., hemispheric magnetic pellets. (From Ref. 47.)

hemispheric magnetic pellet. The hemispheric pellet is then coated with a pure polymer, e.g., ethylene-vinyl acetate copolymer or silicone elastomers, on all sides, except the cavity at the center of the flat surface, to permit the release of macromolecular drug only through the cavity.

The hemispheric magnetic delivery device can release macromolecular drug at a controlled basal rate, by diffusion process, under nontriggering condition or release the same drug at a much higher rate under the activation from an external magnetic field (Fig. 22).

4. *Ultrasound-Activated Drug Delivery*

It was recently discovered that ultrasonic wave can also be utilized, as an energy source, to facilitate the release of drug at a higher rate from polymeric drug delivery device containing a bioerodible polymer matrix, e.g., poly [bis(*p*-carboxyphenoxy)alkane anhydride] [48]. The potential application of ultrasonic wave for the modulation of drug release is still undergoing evaluation.

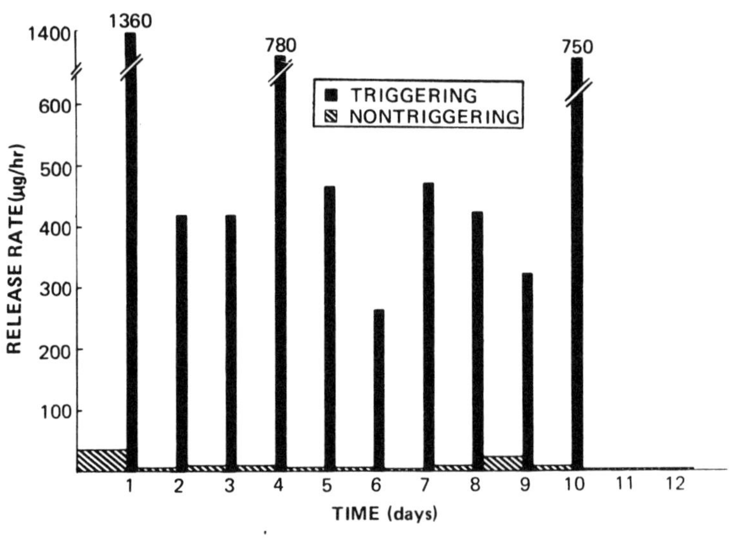

Fig. 22 Magnetic modulation of bovine serum albumin release. Prior to triggering, the pellets were prereleased for 1 day. The pellets were triggered for 5 hr, followed by nontriggering for 19 hr. The cycle of triggering and nontriggering was repeated daily. (■), the quantity of BSA released during the magnetic modulation period; (▨), the quantity of BSA released during the nontriggering period. (From Ref. 47.)

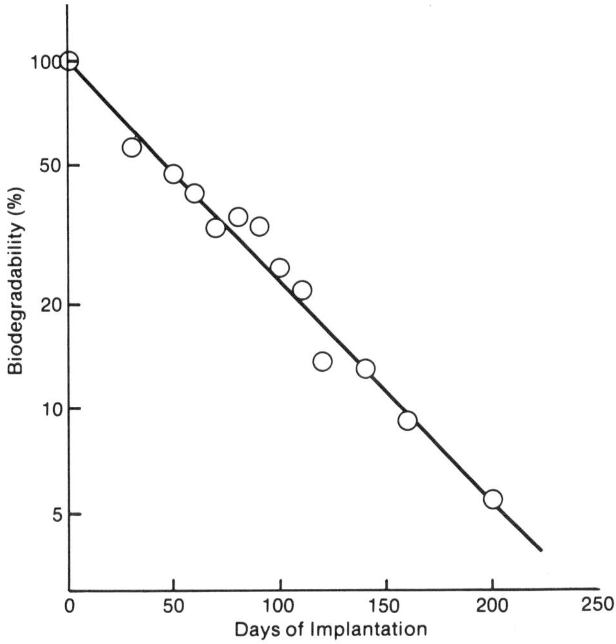

Fig. 23 First-order biodegradation profile of poly(lactide-glycolide) copolymer pellets in mice during long-term subcutaneous implantation. The copolymer was prepared from 90% lactic acid and 10% glycolic acid and had a molecular weight of 90,400. (From Ref. 43.)

5. *Hydrolysis-Activated Drug Delivery*

This type of implantable therapeutic system is fabricated by dispersing a loading dose of solid drug, in micronized form, homogeneously throughout a polymer matrix made from bioerodible or biodegradable polymer, which is then molded into a pellet- or bead-shaped implant. The controlled release of the embedded drug particles is made possible by the combination of polymer erosion through hydrolysis and diffusion through polymer matrix. The rate of drug release is determined by the rate of biodegradation, polymer composition and molecular weight, drug loading, and drug/polymer interactions.

The rate of drug release from this type of drug delivery system is not constant and is highly dependent upon the rate process of polymer matrix erosion (Fig. 23). It is exemplified by the development of biodegradable naltrexone pellets fabricated from poly(lactide/glycolide) copolymer for the antinarcotic treatment of opioid-dependent addicts (Fig. 24).

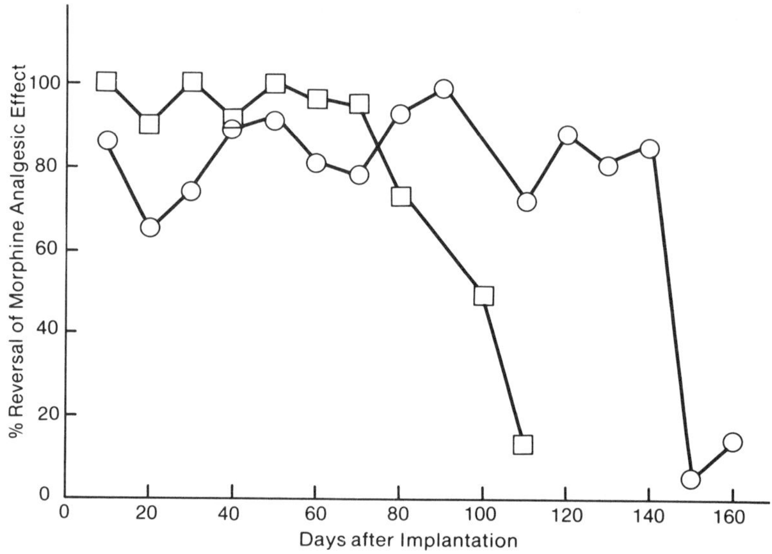

Fig. 24 Narcotic antagonistic activity of naltrexone in mice after subcutaneous implantation of naltrexone pellets fabricated from copolymer of (90% L(+) lactic acid/10% glycolic acid) (○) and polymer of 100% L(+) lactic acid (□). (Both pellets were coated with polylactide polymer.) (From Ref. 43.)

In addition to poly(lactide/glycolide) copolymer, several other biodegradable or bioerodible polymers, such as polysaccharide, polypeptide and homopolymer of polylactide or polyglycolide, can also be used to prepare biodegradable, implantable therapeutic systems. Recently, a new biodegradable polymer, poly(ortho esters), was synthesized and used for the controlled release of contraceptive steroids, e.g., levonorgestrel [51]. This polymer contains linkages in the polymer backbone that are relatively stable at the physiological pH of 7.4, but become progressively unstable as the pH is lowered. The erosion rate of such polymers is controlled by the use of buffering agent, e.g., calcium lactate, which is physically incorporated in the polymer, and, when in contact with water, produces a pH that activates the polymer to hydrolyze at a desirable rate. If the polymer is maintained at a rather high hydrophobicity, then only the buffering agent in the surface layers is exposed to water, and polymer hydrolysis will occur only in the surface layers. So, a constant (zero-order) rate of drug release is obtained.

IV. BENEFITS OF CONTROLLED DRUG ADMINISTRATION VIA IMPLANTATION

The therapeutic benefits of subcutaneous controlled drug administration can be illustrated by comparing the biological activity and duration resulted from the subcutaneous drug administration via a controlled-release drug delivery system with those produced by conventional drug administration through subcutaneous injection.

Subcutaneous controlled administration of megestrol acetate (a very potent antiovulation progestin without any estrogenic or androgenic activities of its own) from silicone capsules was found to be the most efficient way of supplying this progestin [52,53]. The biological potency of megestrol acetate, in terms of delayed implantation, antifertility and antiovulation activities, was found to be enhanced 7–13 times when it was administered at a controlled rate from the silicone capsules as compared to the conventional subcutaneous injection in suspension preparations (Table 1).

It was also reported that progesterone, when administered by silicone capsule, is 13 times more potent than subcutaneous injection

Table 1 Relative Biological Potency of Various Steroid-Releasing Silicone Capsules

Steroid	Biological activity	Relative potency[a]
Estrone	Uterotropic	$\geqslant 2$
Megestrol acetate	Delayed implantation	13.4
	Inhibition of fertility	6.7
Norgestrel	Delayed implantation	32.0
	Compensatory ovarian hypertrophy	41.0
Progesterone	Delayed implantation	12.5
	Deciduoma formation	25.0
19-Norprogesterone	Anti-androgenicity in immature rats	25.0
Testosterone	Parabiotic	
	Gonadotropin inhibition	30.0
	Androgenic activity	30.0
	Androgencity in adult males	15.0

[a] Subcutaneous injection has a biological potency of unity.

Source: Compiled from data in Refs. 52, 54, and 55.

in the delayed implantation test and 25 times more potent in the deciduoma formation test [54]. On the other hand, 19-norprogesterone from silicone capsules was found to be 25 times more effective than subcutaneous injection of an oil solution formulation in inhibiting the growth of seminal vesicles in immature male rats (Table 1).

Androgenic acitvity of testosterone-releasing silicone capsules was evaluated by two biological assays. In the parabiotic rat assay, the silicone capsule which release 5 μg/day of testosterone was found to be sufficient to inhibit the secretion and/or release of pituitary gonadotropins and to stimulate the growth of ventral prostate and seminal vesicles in the castrated male rat. If administered by subcutaneous injection, a daily dose of 150 μg of testosterone was required to produce the same levels of suppression of ovarian growth and of stimulation of the growth of ventral prostate and seminal vesicles [56,57]. Apparently, both gonadotropin inhibition activity and androgenic activity of testosterone were enhanced by 30 times via the continuous subcutaneous administration at a controlled rate by silicone capsules (Table 1).

In castrated adult male rat, the silicone capsule which releases 40 μg/day of testosterone was able to maintain the growth of seminal vesicles, ventral prostate, and levator ani muscle during a 90-day observation. On the other hand, by subcutaneous injection a daily dose of 600–700 μg/day of testosterone was needed to achieve comparable biological activity [58]. The results suggested that the androgenic activity of testosterone is enhanced by approximately 15 times via the controlled administration by silicone capsules (Table 1).

The biological potency of norgestrel-releasing silicone capsules was also compared with a subcutaneous preparation of norgestrel using the delayed implantation test and the steroid-induced block of ovarian compensatory hypertrophy in hemicastrated rats [55]. The results of the delayed implantation test in rat indicated that blastocyst viability is fully preserved in all tested animals receiving a silicone capsule which releases a daily norgestrel dose of 8 μg/day. The average number of implantation sites (6.3 ± 0.3), however, was slightly less than that (9.0 ± 0.7) seen in the rats treated with daily injections of 160 μg of progesterone. By daily subcutaneous injection of 250 μg norgestrel, full activity of the norgestrel was achieved and all the animals treated had the average number of implantation sites (9.8 ± 0.6), similar to the progesterone-treated group. It was calculated that the relative potency of the norgestrel-releasing silicone capsule, in terms of the delayed implantation test, is 32 times that of the subcutaneous injection of norgestrel (Table 1).

The results of the compensatory ovarian hypertrophy test suggested that the hypertrophy observed in the remaining ovary as the result of removing one of the two ovaries could be blocked by a single, daily injection of 200 μg norgestrel. When norgestrel was

Table 2 Comparative Biological Activity and Toxicity of Atropine Base Administered by Silicone Capsules and Subcutaneous Injection

Dose (mg/rat)	Mydriasis duration (days)[a]		Mortality rate (%)	
	Capsule	Injection	Capsule	Injection
0	1	1	0	b
6.25	4	2	0	b
12.50	4	–	0	–
25.00	11	4	0	b
50.00	17	–	0	–
100.00	26	6	0	50
200.00	37	–	0	–
400.00	48	–	0	100

[a]The number of days each treatment group had a mean mydriatic response equal to or greater than +1 mydriasis (25% or more dilations over the control group).

[b]Severe necrosis is observed at the injection site.

Source: Compiled from data in Ref. 21.

administered continuously at a rate of 2 μg/day from silicone capsules, inhibition equivalent to that seen with a daily subcutaneous injection of 100 μg norgestrel was achieved. By statistical calculation, the norgestrel-releasing silicone capsule was found to be 41 times more effective than daily subcutaneous injection (Table 1). A similar response was also observed when the norgestrel-releasing silicone capsules were implanted in the intraperitoneal cavity. It appears that the norgestrel-releasing silicone capsule acts as an "artificial gland" at both sites of implantation.

The data summarized in Table 1 show that, for a specific biological response, a significantly smaller dose of steroids is needed if it is administered subcutaneously through the continuous-release mechanism from the silicone capsule as compared to the same steroid given by the conventional daily subcutaneous injection. The increase in biological potency for the steroids investigated ranges from a modest twofold increase in the uterotropic activity of estrone to the 41-fold increase in the steroid-induced blockade of ovarian compensatory hypertropy achieved by norgestrel. The variation in the degrees of increase in the effectiveness achieved by different steroids is attributable not only to the difference in the biological tests used, but to the difference in the biological half-lives among various steroids.

Controlled-release silicone capsules were also reported to extend the duration of mydriatic response produced by atropine base as well as to reduce its toxicity in rat [21]. When administered subcutaneously through controlled-release silicone capsules, atropine base was found to produce a dose-dependent mydriasis in rats: the higher the loading dose of atropine in the capsules, the longer the duration of mydriatic response produced (Table 2). It is interesting to note that the duration of mydriasis produced by the atropine-releasing silicone capsule was significantly longer than that produced by subcutaneous injection of the same atropine dose suspended in 1% aqueous methylcellulose solution. This prolongation in mydriatic response was observed to be dose-dependent. Additionally, the mortality rate and toxicity of the atropine base were markedly reduced by administering it in silicone capsules. This could be due to a more uniform tissue distribution of drug and its metabolites; silicone capsules prevent any abnormal accumulation of the drug or of its metabolites in any organs [59].

V. MEDICAL ASPECTS OF IMPLANTATION

A. The Environment of Living Tissues

Animal tissue contains approximately 70% body fluid. This fluid consists of two major compartments: intracellular fluid and extracellular fluid [60]. The extracellular fluid bathing all tissues is further subdivided into interstitial and intravascular (which includes plasma and lymph) fluid. The interstitial fluid, which the implants mostly encounter on the site of implantation, has the chemical composition shown in Table 3.

Oxygen is freely available and is readily replaced by complex biochemical processes and hemeostatic controls [61]. Carbon dioxide also exists. However, in certain tissues which have necrosed or are in various types of bacterial infections, an anaerobic condition may result. At cellular level, the pH value may be lower than the pH 7.4 measured in extracellular fluid.

Many enzymes, which are capable of oxidation, reduction or hydrolysis, are present in the environment of living tissues. Since many enzymatic reactions are characterized by various trace metals, thorough investigation is needed to search for early or long-term effects of chemicals or additives, that could leach out or result from the degradation of implanted polymeric materials.

Table 3 Chemical Composition of Interstitial Fluid (pH 7.4)

Cations		Anions	
Species	mEq/liter	Species	mEq/liter
Na^+	140	Cl^-	105
K^+	4	HCO_3^-	30
Ca^{2+}	5	HPO_4^{2-}	5
Mg^{2+}	3	SO_4^{2-}	3
		Organic acid	6
		Protein	3
	152		152

Source: Ref. 60.

B. Reactions of Host to Implant

Inflammation is the defensive reaction of the living body to any irritant, whether physical (e.g., burns), chemical (e.g., toxins), or bacterial [62]. Practically, any foreign agent can act as an irritant. The acute phase of the inflammatory reaction leads to the formation, at the affected site, of an exudate and fibrinous network. Vascular and lymphatic systems are activated. Leukocytes and mast cells accumulate and, with red blood cells, permeate the capillaries to the affected site.

The presence of a surgically implanted device calls for major adaptation by the host tissue unless the device is absorbable and replaceable, as is catgut ligature, for example. The polymeric device may remain as an incompletely covered foreign body with a barrier of connective tissue forming between it and the surface epithelium. Absorption and permeation of drugs may be effectively blocked [63–65]. Successful implantation may also be jeopardized by the immune response from the lymphatic system. Despite the availability of modern techniques to suppress this, natural tissues in the process of disrutpion and liquefaction may become antigenic, resulting in the rejection of the implants. In addition, the leaching out of any additives from the implants may also cause toxic reactions.

To minimize reaction, any polymeric device should have the minimum surface area by design and a very smooth surface finish. Ideally, such an implant should possess the same structural characteristics as the tissue in which it is embedded. A rigid plastic material inserted into soft tissues often becomes infected and rejected.

Little is known about the problems that arise when blood or other tissue fluids make contact with foreign surfaces. Electric phenomena occurring at the interface could, in certain situations, lead to thrombosis formation [66]. It was hoped that materials with a high negative zeta potential might resist this tendency. However, this negative potential was found to be immediately neutralized on contact with blood, plasma, albumin, fibrinogen, and γ-globulin [67]. To data, our knowledge suggests that to prevent thrombosis, the surface of vascular implants should be smooth and in contact only with an area of high velocity [61].

Folkman and Long [68] reported that any incision made in the myocardium healed by formation of a smooth envelope of fibrous tissue, which appeared to present a barrier to the permeation of the drug from the site of implantation. However, the amount of fibrosis in the myocardium was the same in areas in which only an incision and tunnel were made as it was in areas near silicone capsules containing either air or a drug [69]. On the other hand, subcutaneous and intraperitoneal implantations of silicone capsules resulted in only little foreign body reaction, and no formation of fibrous tissue could be noted [68]. Eleven-month subcutaneous implantation of silicone capsules in rats resulted in no evidence of local tumor formation, foreign body reaction, or signs of inflammation [70]. The implants were merely enclosed by a thin film of connective tissue. As previously mentioned [70], the inflammatory reaction, which was observed occasionally at the subcutaneous implantation site, was attributed to animal hair which had been brought inadvertenlty into the incision at the time of implantation.

The chemistry of polymer degradation in the human body is another area in which knowledge is scarce. Late degradation may lead to release of potential toxins or antigens and thence to failure and rejection of implants. For example, nylon can lose approximately 80% of its tensile strength in 3 years of implantation [61].

As an example, the effects on tissues after incorporation of additives, plasticizers, or catalysts used in fabrication of a plastic, high density polyethylene may be cited. A 2% phenolic antioxidant, if used, causes a marked inflammatory reaction of the guinea pig tissues to the polymer. A 2% amine antioxidant causes no such reaction. High concentration of catalyst residues in a Ziegler-type polyethylene can be similarly irritating [61].

More recent investigations revealed that the particle size of the foreign substances is most important in determining the extent of tissue reaction. The smaller the particle size of the foreign material, the greater the tissue reaction [71]. No direct correlation can be made between the tissue reaction and the surface area [72]. The particle size of fillers incorporated in polymers may also play a similar role should they move to the surface or even leach out of the polymeric device during implantation [73].

It become obvious that the form in which the polymeric device is implanted, the animal species used for investigation, and the duration of implantation all play an important part in deciding the degree of tissue reaction to a foreign material. These factors, as well as the aforementioned particle size, should all be considered when assessing the healing pattern of the tissues about an alloplastic material [74].

Any synthetic polymeric device from which potential toxins leach out, either as a result of faulty fabrication or breakdown during implantation, could lead, at any time, to immunological or allergic reaction, inflammation, and then rejection.

It was reported that approximately 20% of the users of conventional IUDs will expel the device within 5 months following the first insertion, although only 5% of the women will not ultimately retain some sort of IUD [75]. As expulsion is the result of uterine contractions, the expulsion rate may be reduced by delivering a continuous low dose of a progestational agent to decrease the uterine sensitivity and myometrium contractility [76,77].

Since the early 1920s, considerable controversy has existed as to the role that the cervicovaginal appendage or tail on the IUD plays in the development of bacterial infections of the upper genital tract [78–81]. The investigation conducted by Tatum et al. [82] has revealed that the tail of the Dalkon Shield is structurally and functionally different from the tails of the four other IUDs tested. The tail of the Dalkon Shield consists of a bundle of monofilaments enclosed freely within a thin plastic sheath. The unique construction of the Dalkon tail theoretically could provide a mechanism whereby pathogenic bacteria from the vagina enter the uterine cavity and cause sepsis.

C. Reactions of Implant to Host

After a period of time, no polymer is totally impermeable to the body fluids. Folkman et al. [83] reported that fat-soluble substances in the blood, such as cholesterol, testosterone, estradiol, and hydrocortisone, were absorbed by the lipophilic silicone elastomer. Most important in the clinical uses of polymeric devices are the effects of tissue enzymes and free radicals as well as hydrolysis caused by the absorption of body fluids.

Environmental stress cracking can happen in some implanted polymeric materials [84]. Changes in physical properties need not be related to chemical breakdown of the polymeric devices. Chemical breakdown will itself influence the mechanical strength of the implanted polymeric materials. Therefore, carbon-carbon bond cleavage may account for the loss of tensile strength in hydrophobic polymers, such as polyethylene. Heat, light, oxidation, moisture, and ionizing radiation can all be responsible for the degradation of polymeric materials.

The use of seemingly innocuous materials can be dangerous. Silicone oil used to coat tubing or oxygenator pumps in open heart surgery was reported to cause fatalities when subsequently released into the bloodstream [85]. Certain plastics may be affected by drugs used in association with chemotherapy [86]. Blood coagulation was observed with silicone shunts when anesthetic liquid was added to the chamber [83]. A tightly bonded heparin layer applied to the lumen of these shunts was reported to prevent clot formation, yet it did not cause systemic anticoagulation or interfere with anesthesia diffusion.

In conclusion, an ideal implantable therapeutic system should be biostable, biocompatible with minimal tissue-implant interactions, nontoxic, noncarcinogenic, removable if required, and should release the drug at a constant, programmed rate for a predetermined duration of medication.

REFERENCES

1. R. Deanesly and A. S. Parkes, Comparative Activities of compounds of the androsterone-testosterone series, *Biochem. J. 30*, 291 (1936).
2. R. Deanesly and A. S. Parkes, Factors influencing the effectiveness of administered hormones, *Proc. Roy. Soc. (London) S. B. 124*, 279 (1937).
3. B. E. Ballard and E. Nelson, Prolonged-action pharmaceuticals. In, *Remington's Pharmaceutical Sciences*, 15th ed. (A. Osol et al., Eds.), Mack, Easton, PA, 1975, Chap. 91.
4. M. B. Shimkin and J. White, Absorption rate of hormone-cholesterol pellets, *Endocrinology 29*, 1020 (1941).
5. F. Fuenzalida, Absorption of steroids from subcutaneously implanted tablets of the pure hormone and of the hormone mixed with cholesterol, *J. Clin. Endocrinol. 10*, 1511 (1950).
6. A. F. Pi, A. Oriol, L. H. Lasso, M. Maqueo, R. I. Dorfman, and F. A. Kincl, Inhibition of fertility in mice by steroid implants, *Acta Endocrinol. 48*, 602 (1965).
7. *Physicians' Desk Reference*, 33rd ed., Medical Economics Co., Oradell, NJ, 1979.

8. E. L. Way, H. H. Loh, and F. H. Shen, Simultaneous quantitative assessment of morphine tolerance and physical dependence, *J. Pharmacol. Exp. Ther. 167*, 1 (1969).
9. F. H. Shen, H. H. Loh, and E. L. Way, Brain serotonin turnover in morphine-tolerant and dependent mice, *J. Pharmacol. Exp. Ther. 175*, 427–434 (1970).
10. S. Algeri and E. Costa, Physical dependence on morphine fails to increase serotonin turnover rate in rat brain, *Biochem. Pharmac. 20*, 877 (1971).
11. I. Marshall and D. G. Grahame-Smith, Evidence against a role of brain 5-hydroxytryptamine in the development of physical dependence upon morphine in mice, *J. Pharmacol. Exp. Ther. 179*, 634–641 (1971).
12. J. Blasig, A. Herz, K. Reinhold, and S. Zieglgansberger, Development of physical dependence of morphine in respect to time and dosage and quantification of the precipitated withdrawal syndrome in rats, *Psychopharmacologia 33*, 19–38 (1973).
13. T. J. Cicero and E. R. Meyer, Morphine pellet implantation in rats: Quantitative assessment of tolerance and dependence, *J. Pharmacol. Exp. Ther. 184*, 404–408 (1973).
14. E. Wei, H. H. Loh, and E. L. Way, Quantitative aspects of precipated abstinence in morphine dependent rats, *J. Pharmacol. Exp. Ther. 184*, 398–403 (1973).
15. K. S. Hui and M. B. Roberts, An improved implantation pellet for rapid induction of morphine dependence in mice, *J. Pharm. Pharmacol. 27*, 569 (1975).
16. H. N. Bhargava, Rapid induction and quantitation of morphine dependence in the rat by pellet implantation, *Psychopharmacology 52*, 55–62 (1977).
17. H. N. Bhargava, Quantitation of morphine tolerance induced by pellet implantation in the rat, *J. Pharm. Pharmacol. 30*, 133 (1978).
18. J. Folkman, Controlled drug release from polymers, *Hosp. Practice 13*, 127–133 (1978).
19. J. Folkman and D. M. Long, Jr., The use of silicone rubber as a carrier for prolonged drug therapy, *J. Surg. Res. 4*, 139–142 (1964).
20. J. Folkman and D. M. Long, Jr., Drug pacemakers in the treatment of heart block, *Ann. NY Acad. Sci. 8*, 857 (1964).
21. P. Bass, R. A. Purdon, and J. N. Wiley, Prolonged administration of atropine or histamine in a silicone rubber implant, *Nature 208*, 591 (1965).
22. K. G. Powers, The use of silicone rubber implants for the sustained release of antimalarial and antischistosomal agents, *J Parasitology 51*, 53 (1965).
23. P. J. Dziuk and B. Cook, Passage of steroids through silicone rubber, *Endocrinology 78*, 208–211 (1966).

24. F. A. Kincl, G. Benagiano, and I. Anges, Sustained release hormonal preparations I. Diffusion of various steroids through polymer membranes, *Steroids 11*, 673 (1968).
25. C. M. Clifford, C. E. Yunker, and M. D. Corwin, Control of the louse *Polyplax serrata* with systemic insecticides administered in silastic rubber implants, *J. Econ. Entomol. 60*, 1210 (1967).
26. J. Folkman, W. Reiling, and G. Williams, Chronic analgesia by silicone rubber diffusion, *Surgery 66*, 194 (1969).
27. T. S. Gaginella and P. Bass, Nicotine: Release from silicone rubber implants *in vivo*, *Res. Commun. Chem. Pathol. Pharmacol. 7*, 213 (1974).
28. J. Folkman, D. M. Long, Jr., and R. Rosembaum, A new diffusion property useful for general anesthesia, *Science 154*, 148 (1966).
29. J. Folkman and V. H. Mark, Diffusion of anesthetics and other drugs through silicone rubber: Therapeutic implications, *Trans. NY Acad. Sci. 30*, 1187 (1968).
30. P. Siegel and J. R. Atkinson, *In vivo* chemode diffusion of *L*-dopa, *J. Appl. Physiol. 30*, 900 (1971).
31. Y. W. Chien, Intrauterine controlled-release drug administration. In, *Novel Drug Delivery Systems: Fundamentals, Development Concepts and Biomedical Assessments*, Marcel Dekker, Inc., New York, 1982, Chap. 4.
32. Y. W. Chien, Ocular controlled-release drug administration. In, *Novel Drug Delivery Systems: Fundamentals, Developmental Concepts and Biomedical Assessments*, Marcel Dekker, Inc., New York, 1982, Chap. 2.
33. Y. W. Chien, Intravaginal controlled-release drug administration. In, *Novel Drug Delivery Systems: Fundamentals, Developmental Concepts and Biomedical Assessments*, Marcel Dekker, Inc., New York, 1982, Chap. 3.
34. Y. W. Chien, Methods to achieve sustained drug delivery—The physical approach: Implants. In, *Sustained and Controlled Release Drug Delivery Systems* (J. R. Robinson, Ed.), Marcel Dekker, Inc., New York, 1978, Chap. 4.
35. Y. W. Chien, Controlled administration of estrus-synchronizing agents in livestock. In, *Novel Drug Delivery Systems: Fundamentals, Developmental Concepts and Biomedical Assessments*, Marcel Dekker, Inc., New York, 1982, Chap. 8.
36. D. S. T. Hsieh, N. Smith, and Y. W. Chien, Subcutaneous controlled administration of estradiol from compudose implants: *In vitro* and *in vivo* evaluations. In, *Proceeding of 11th International Symposium on Controlled Release of Bioactive Materials* (W. E. Meyers and R. L. Dunn, Eds.), The Controlled Release Society, Inc., Lincolnshire, IL, 1984, pp. 134–135.
37. Y. W. Chien and H. J. Lambert, Method for making a microsealed delivery device, U.S. patent 3,992,518 (Nov. 16, 1976).

38. Y. W. Chien and H. J. Lambert, Microsealed pharmaceutical delivery devices, U.S. patent 4,053,580 (Oct. 11, 1977).
39. Y. W. Chien, Microsealed drug delivery systems: Theoretical apsects and biomedical assessments. In, *Recent Advances in Drug Delivery Systems* (J. M. Anderson & S. W. Kim, Eds.), Plenum, New York, 1984, pp. 367–387.
40. Y. W. Chien, Fundamentals of controlled-release drug administration. In, *Novel Drug Delivery Systems: Fundamentals, Developmental Concepts, and Biomedical Assessments*, Marcel Dekker, Inc., New York, 1982, Chap. 9.
41. F. Theeuwes, Elementary osmotic pump, *J. Pharm. Sci. 64*, 1987 (1975).
42. F. Theeuwes and S. I. Yum, Principles of the design and operation of generic osmotic pumps for the delivery of semisolid or liquid drug formulations, *Ann. Biomed. Eng. 4*, 343 (1976).
43. Y. W. Chien, Implantable controlled-release drug delivery systems. In, *Novel Drug Delivery Systems: Fundamentals, Developmental Concepts, and Biomedical Assessments*, Marcel Dekker, Inc., New York, 1982, Chap. 7.
44. P. J. Blackshear, T. D. Rohde, J. D. Grotling, F. D. Dorman, P. R. Perkins, R. L. Varco, and H. Buchwald, Control of blood glucose in experimental diabetes by means of a totally implantable insulin infusion device, *Diabetes 28*, 634 (1979).
45. P. J. Blackshear, T. D. Rohde, R. L. Varco, and H. Buchwald, One year of continuous heparinization in the dog using a totally implantable infusion pump, *Surg. Gynecol. Obstet. 141*, 176 (1975).
46. Implantable pump for morphine, *Am. Pharmacy NS24* (8), 20 (1984).
47. D. S. T. Hsieh and R. Langer, Zero-order drug delivery systems with magnetic control. In, *Controlled Release Delivery Systems* (T. J. Roseman and S. Z. Mansdorf, Eds.), Marcel Dekker, Inc., New York, 1983, Chap. 7.
48. J. Kost, K. W. Leong, and R. Langer, Ultrasonic controlled polymeric delivery systems. In, *Proceedings of 11th International Symposium on "Controlled Release of Bioactive Materials"* (W. E. Meyers and R. L. Dunn, Eds.), The Controlled Release Society, Inc., Lincolnshire, IL, 1984, p. 84.
49. A. D. Schwope and D. L. Wise, Development of drug delivery systems for use in treatment of narcotic addiction. In, *Dynatech Quarterly Report (No. 1361) to NIDA* January 16, 1976.
50. D. L. Wise, T. D. Fellmann, J. E. Sanderson, and R. L. Wentworth, Lactic/glycolic and polymers. In, *Drug Carriers in Biology and Medicine* (G. Gregoriadis, Ed.), Academic Press, New York, 1979, Chap. 12.
51. J. Heller, Controlled drug release from poly (ortho esters). In, *Proceedings of 11th International Symposium on Controlled*

Release of Bioactive Materials (W. E. Meyers and R. L. Dunn, Eds.), The controlled Release Society, Inc., Lincolnshire, IL, 1984), p. 128.
52. C. C. Chang and F. A. Kincl, Sustained release hormonal preparations (3)-biologic effectiveness of 6-methyl-17α-acetoxypregna-4, 6-diene-3, 20-dione, *Steroids 12*, 689–696 (1968).
53. A. Cuadros, A. Brinson, and K. Sundaram, Progestational activity of megestrol acetate-polydimethylsiloxane (PDS) capsules in rhesus monkeys, *Contraception 2*, 29 (1970).
54. C. C. Chang and F. A. Kincl, Sustained release hormonal preparation: 4. Biologic effectiveness of steroid hormones, *Fertil. Steril. 21*, 134 (1970).
55. V. Zbuzkova and F. A. Kincl, Sustained release hormonal preparations: 11. Biological effectiveness, *Endocrinologia Experimentalis 4*, 215 (1970).
56. F. A. Kincl, H. J. Ringold, and R. J. Dorfman, Pituitary gonadotrophin inhibition by subcutaneously administered steroids, *Acta Endocrinol. 36*, 83 (1961).
57. F. A. Kincl and R. I. Dorfman, Pituitary gonadotrophin in inhibitory action of neutral steroids, *Acta Endocrinol. 46*, 300 (1964).
58. C. R. Moore and D. Price, Some effects of testosterone and testosterone propionate in the rat, *Anat. Rec. 71*, 59 (1938).
59. F. A. Kincl, I. Angee, C. C. Chang, and H. W. Rudel, Sustained release hormonal preparations: 9. Plasma levels and accumulation into various tissues of 6-methyl-17α-acetoxy-4,6-pregnadiene-3, 20-dione after oral administration or absorption from polydimethylsiloxane implants, *Acta. Endocrinol. 64*, 508 (1970).
60. G. H. Bell, J. N. Davidson, and H. Scarborough, *Textbook of Physiology and Biochemistry*, 5th ed., Livingston, London, Chap. 35.
61. B. Bloch and G. W. Hastings, *Plastics Materials in Surgery*, 2nd ed., Thomas, Springfield, IL, 1972, Chap. VI.
62. V. Menken, *Biochemical Mechanisms in Inflammation*, Thomas, Springfield, IL, 1956.
63. E. M. Coutinho, D. A. M. Ferreira, H. Prates, and F. A. Kincl, Excretion of [6-^{14}C] megestrol acetate (6-methyl-17-acetoxy-pregna-4, 6-diene-3, 20-dione) released from subcutaneous silastic implants in women, *J. Reprod. Fertil. 23*, 345 (1970).
64. G. Benagiano, M. Ermini, L. Carenza, and G. Rolfini, Studies on sustained contraceptive effects with subcutaneous polydimethylsiloxane implants. 1. Diffusion of megestrol acetate in humans, *Acta Endocrinol. 73*, 335 (1973).
65. G. Benagiano and M. Ermini, Continuous steroid treatment by subdermal polysiloxane implants, *Acta. Eur. Fertil. 3*, 119 (1972).

66. V. Mirkovitch, Bioelectric phenomena, thrombosis and plastics: A review of current knowledge, *Cleveland Clin. Q. 30*, 241 (1963).
67. V. Mirkovitch, R. E. Beck, and P. G. Andrus, The zeta potentials and blood compatibility characteristics of some selected solids, *J. Surg. Res. 4*, 395 (1964).
68. J. Folkman and D. M. Long, Jr., The use of silicone rubber as a carrier for prolonged drug therapy, *J. Surg. Res. 4*, 139 (1964).
69. J. Folkman and D. M. Long, Jr., Drug pacemakers in the treatment of heart block, *Ann. NY Acad. Sci. 111*, 857 (1963–1964).
70. R. Schuhman and H. D. Taubert, Long-term application of steroids enclosed in dimethyl-polysiloxane (Silastic): *In vitro* and *in vivo* experiments, *Acta Biol. Med. Germ. Band 24*, Seite 897 (1970).
71. R. H. Hall, Acute toxicity of inhaled beryllium: observations correlating toxicity with physiochemical properties of beryllium oxide dust, *Arch. Ind. Hyg. 2*, 25 (1950).
72. H. LeVeen and J. R. Barberio, Tissue reaction to plastics and in surgery with special reference to Teflon, *Ann. Surg. 12*, 974 (1949).
73. F. C. Usher and S. A. Wallace, Tissue reaction to plastics: A comparison of Nylon, Orlon, Dacron, Teflon and Marlex, *Am. Med. Assoc. Arch. Surg. 76*, 997 (1958).
74. N. E. Stinson, Tissue reaction induced in guinea pigs by particulate polymethylacrylate, polyethylene and nylon of the same size range, *Br. J. Exp. Pathol. 46*, 135 (1965).
75. C. Tietze, Evaluation of intrauterine devices, 9th Progress Report of the Cooperative Statistical Program, *Studies in Family Planning 55*, 1 (July 1970).
76. L. L. Doyle, Hormone-releasing silicone-rubber intrauterine contraceptive devices: Effect of incorporation of various compounds on intrauterine devices in rats, *Am. J. Obstet. Gynecol. 121*, 405 (1975).
77. L. L. Doyle and T. H. Clewe, Preliminary studies on the effect of hormone-releasing intrauterine devices, *Am. J. Obstet. Gynecol. 101*, 564 (1968).
78. C. C. Bollinger, Bacterial flora of the nonpregnant uterus: A new culture technique, *Obstet. Gynecol. 23*, 251 (1964).
79. M. I. Buchman, A study of the intrauterine contraceptive device with and without an extracervical appendage or tail, *Fertil. Steril. 21*, 348 (1970).
80. H. Lehfeldt, Intrauterine contraception: Tailed vs. tailless devices. In, *Extrail du Livre Jubilaire Offert au Dr. Jean Dalsace*, Masson et cie, Paris, 1966, pp. 199–213.
81. J. R. Wilson, C. C. Bollinger, and W. J. Ledger, The effect of an intrauterine contraceptive device on the bacterial flora

of the endometrial cavity, *Am. J. Obstet. Gynecol. 90*, 726 (1964).
82. H. J. Tatum, F. H. Schmidt, D. Phillips, M. McCarty, and W. M. O'Leary, The Dalkon Shield controversy: Structural and bacteriological studies of IUD tails, *JAMA 231*, 711 (1975).
83. J. Folkman, W. Reiling, and G. Williams, Chronic analgesia by silicone rubber diffusion, *Surgery 66*, 194 (1969).
84. B. S. Oppenheimer, Further studies of polymers as carcinogenic agents in animals, *Cancer Res. 15*, 333 (1955).
85. *Bull. Dow Corning Centre Med. Res. 5*, 7 (1963).
86. P. J. Dzuik and B. Cook, Passage of steroids through silicone rubber, *Endocrinology 78*, 208 (1966).

12

Transdermal Therapeutic Systems

YIE W. CHIEN / Rutgers–The State University of New Jersey, Piscataway, New Jersey

I. INTRODUCTION

Continuous intravenous infusion is recognized as a superior mode of drug administration not only to bypass hepatic "first-pass" metabolism, but also to maintain a constant and prolonged drug level in the body. A closely monitored intravenous infusion can provide the advantages of both direct entry of drug into the systemic circulation and control of circulating drug levels. However, such mode of drug administration entails certain risks and, therefore, necessitates hospitalization of the patients and close medical supervision of administration.

Recently, it is becoming evident that the benefits of intravenous drug infusion can be closely duplicated, without its hazards, by using the skin as the port of drug administration to provide continuous transdermal drug infusion into the systemic circulation [1].

To provide continuous drug infusion through an intact skin, several transdermal therapeutic systems have been developed for topical application onto the intact skin surface to control the delivery of drug and its subsequent permeation through the skin tissue. It is exemplified by the development and marketing of scopolamine-releasing transdermal therapeutic system for 72-hr prophylaxis or treatment of motion-induced nausea [2], of nitroglycerin and isosorbide dinitrate-releasing transdermal therapeutic systems for once-a-day medication of angina pectoris [3,4], and of clonidine-releasing transdermal therapeutic system for weekly treatment of hypertension [4]. The intesity of interests in the potential biomedical applications of transdermal controlled drug administration is demonstrated in the increasing research activities in a number of health care institutions in the development of various types of transdermal therapeutic systems for long-term continuous infusion of therapeutic agents, including antihypertensive, antianginal, anthistamine, antiinflammatory, analgesic, antiarthritic, steroidal, and contraceptive drugs.

This chapter intends to review fundamentals of skin permeation, approaches for transdermal controlled drug administration, *in vitro* and *in vivo* kinectic evaluations of transdermal therapeutic systems and their correlations, as well as formulation design and optimization.

II. SKIN AS A SITE FOR DRUG INFUSION

The skin of an average adult body covers around 2 m^2 of surface area and receives approximately one-third of all blood circulating through the body [5]. It is one of the most extensive and readily accessible organs on the human body. With a thickness of only a fraction of a millimeter, the skin separates the underlying blood circulation network from the outside environment and serves as a barrier against physical, chemical and microbial attacks, acts as a thermostat in maintaining body temperature, plays a role in the regulation of blood pressure, and protects against the penetration of ultraviolet rays.

The skin is a multilayered organ composed of many histological layers. It is generally described in terms of three major tissue layers: the epidermis, the dermis, and the hypodermis (Fig. 1). Microscopically, the epidermis is further divided into five anatomical layers with stratum corneum forming the outermost layer of the epidermis, exposing to the external environment.

The stratum corneum consists of many layers of compacted, flattened, dehydrated and keratinized cells. They are dead cells

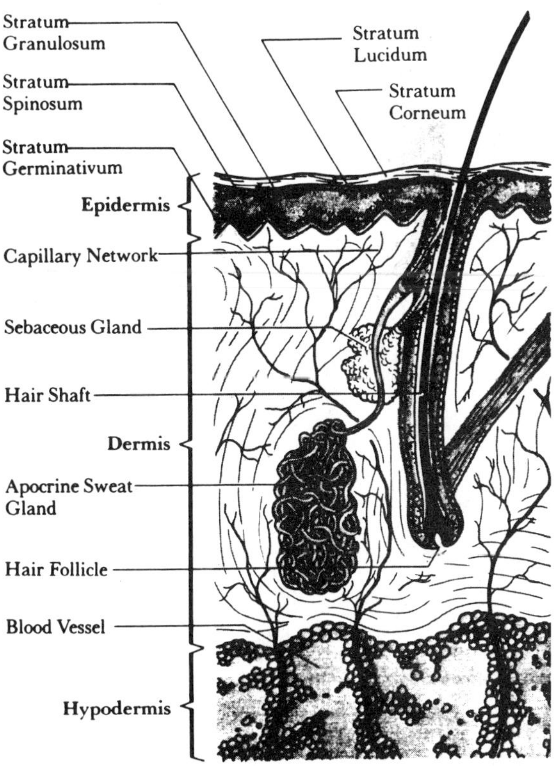

Fig. 1 A cross-section of human skin, showing various skin tissue layers and appendages. (Reproduced from Ref. 6.)

converted to protein and are continuously shed, requiring replacement from the underlying viable epidermal tissue [6]. The stratum corneum has a water content of only ∿20% as compared to the normal 70% in the physiologically active stratum germinativum (regenerative layer of the epidermis).

An average human skin surface is known to contain, on the average, 40–70 hair follicles and 200–250 sweat ducts on each square centimeter of skin area. These skin appendages, however, actually occupy, grossly, only 0.1% of the total human skin surface. Even though the foreign agents, especially the water-soluble ones, may be able to penetrate into the skin via these skin appendages at a rate which is faster than through the intact area of the stratum corneum, this trans-appendageal route of percutaneous absorption has, at steady-state, a very limited contribution to the overall kinetic profile of transdermal permeation. Therefore, the transdermal permeation of most neutral molecules can, thus, be considered as, primarily, a process of passive diffusion through the intact stratum corneum in the interfollicular region. So, for the sake of mechanistic analysis of transdermal drug infusion [7], the various skin tissue layers can be represented by a simplistic multilayer model as shown in Figure 2.

For many decades, the skin has been commonly used as the site for the administration of dermatological drugs to achieve a localized pharmacologic action in the skin tissues. In this case, the drug molecule is considered to diffuse to a target tissue in the proximity of drug application to produce its therapeutic effect before it is distributed to the blood circulation for elimination (Fig. 3). The use

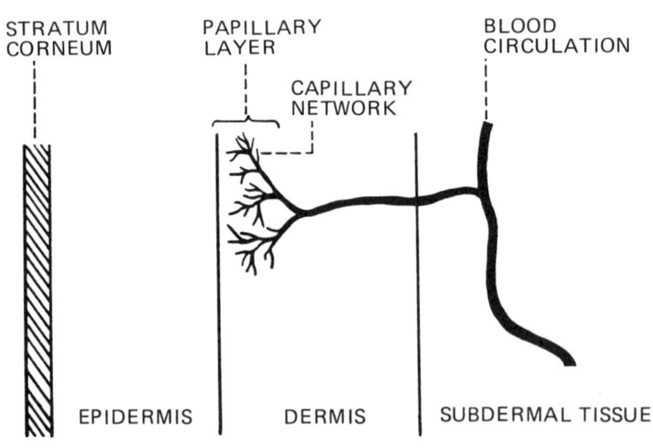

Fig. 2 Simplified model of the human skin for mechanistic analysis of skin permeation. (Reproduced from Ref. 7.)

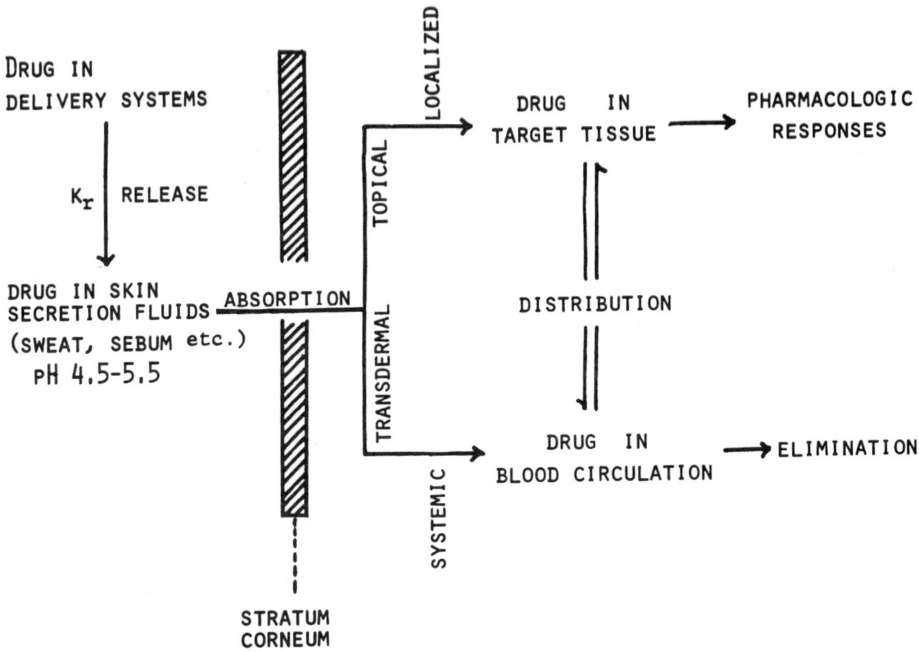

Fig. 3 Percutaneous absorption of drugs for localized therapeutic actions in the skin tissues or for systemic medications in the tissues remote from the site of topical drug application. (Reproduced from Ref. 7.)

of hydrocortisone for dermatitis, benzoyl peroxide for acne, and neomycin for superficial infection [8] are the few examples.

Most recently, there is an increasing recognition that the skin can also serve as the port of administration for systemically-active drugs (Fig. 3). In this case, the drug applied topically will be absorbed first into the blood circulation and then be transported to target tissues, which could be rather remote from the site of drug application, to achieve its therapeutic purposes. It is exemplified by the transdermal controlled administration of nitroglycerin for the treatment of angina pectoris, of scopolamine for the prevention of motion sickness, and of estradiol for the medication of postemenopause [9–11]. This chapter aims to provide a systematic overview on the development of transdermal thereapeutic systems for the transdermal controlled infusion of drugs for systemic medications.

III. FUNDAMENTALS OF SKIN PERMEATION

For a systemically-active drug to reach a target tissue remote from the site of drug administration on the skin surface, it has to possess some physicochemical properties which are capable of facilitating the sorption of drug by the stratum corneum, the penetration of drug through various skin tissues (Fig. 1), and also the uptake of the drug by the capillary network in the dermal papillary layer (Fig 2). The rate of permeation, dQ/dt, across a skin can be expressed, mathematically, by the following relationship [12]:

$$\frac{dQ}{dt} = P_s (C_d - C_r) \tag{1}$$

Where C_d and C_r are, respectively, the concentrations of a skin penetrant in the donor compartment, e.g., the drug concentration on the surface of stratum corneum, and in the receptor compartment, e.g., body; and P_s is the permeability coefficient of the skin as defined by:

$$P_s = \frac{K_s D_{ss}}{h_s} \tag{2}$$

Where K_s is the partition coefficient for the interfacial partitioning of the penetrant molecule from a transdermal therapeutic system onto the skin tissues; D_{ss} is the diffusivity for the steady-state diffusion of the penetrant molecule through the skin tissues; and h_s is the total thickness of the skin tissues. The permeability coefficient (P_s) for a skin penetrant can be considered as a constant since K_s, D_{ss} and h_s terms in Eq. (2) are essentially constant under a fixed condition.

Analysis of Eq. (1) suggests that in order to achieve a constant rate of drug permeation, it requires a condition being maintained that the drug concentration on the surface of stratum corneum (C_d) consistently and substantially greater than the drug concentration in the body (C_r), i.e., $C_d \gg C_r$; therefore, Eq. (1) can be reduced to:

$$\frac{dQ}{dt} = P_s C_d \tag{3}$$

and the rate of skin permeation (dQ/dt) becomes a constant, if the C_d value remains fairly constant throughout the course of skin permeation. To maintain the C_d at a constant value, it is critical to make the drug to be released at a rate (R_r) which is always greater than the rate of skin uptake (R_a), i.e., $R_r \gg R_a$ (Fig. 4). By

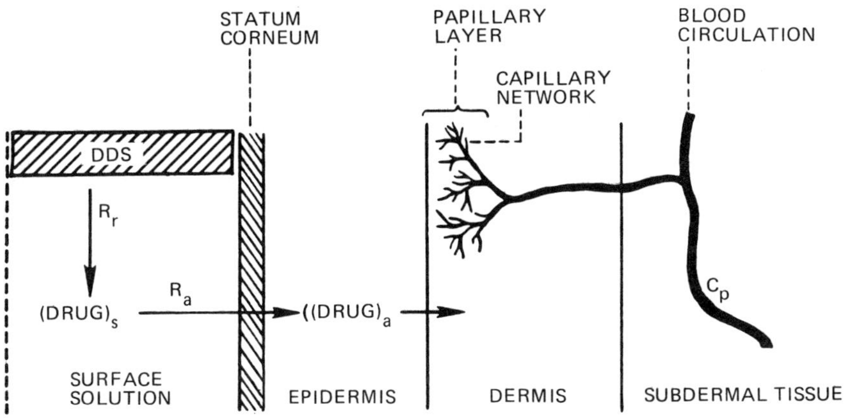

Fig. 4 Diagrammatic illustration of the relationship between the rate of drug release (R_r) from a transdermal drug delivery system (DDS) and the rate of drug uptake (R_a) by the skin.

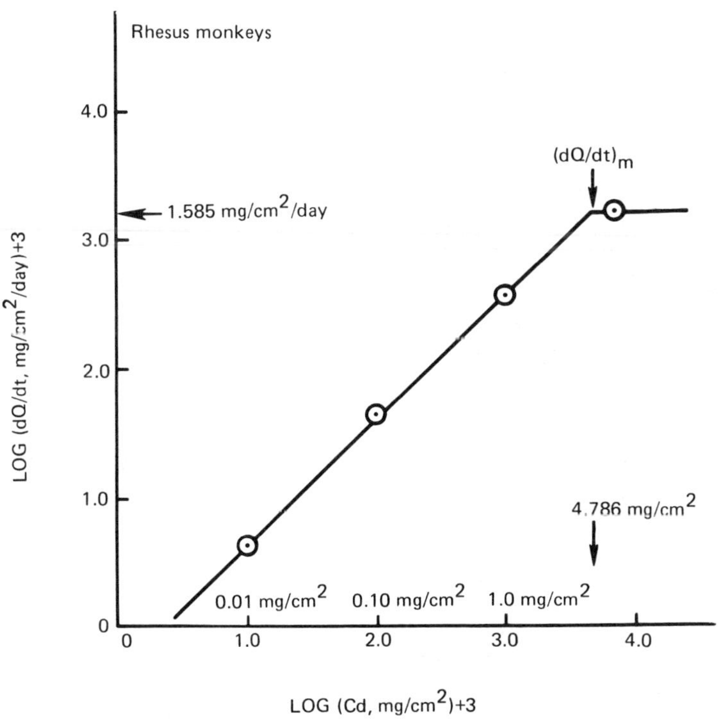

Fig. 5 Linear relationship between the rate of transdermal permeation of nitroglycerin (dQ/dt), determined from the daily urinary recovery data, and the nitroglycerin dose applied on the rhesus monkey skin (C_d) (plotted from the data in Ref. 13).

doing so, the drug concentration on the skin surface (C_d) is maintained at a level which is always greater than the equilibrium (or saturation) solubility of the drug in the stratum corneum (C_s^e), i.e., $C_d >> C_s^e$; and a maximum rate of skin permeation $(dQ/dt)_m$, as expressed by Equation (4), is thus reached:

$$\left(\frac{dQ}{dt}\right)_m = P_s C_s^e \tag{4}$$

Apparently, the magnitude of $(dQ/dt)_m$ is determined by the skin permeability coefficient (P_s) of the drug and its equilibrium solubility in the stratum corneum (C_s^e). This concept of stratum corneum-limited skin permeation was investigated by depositing various doses of pure, radiolabeled nitroglycerin, in a volatile organic solvent, onto a controlled skin surface area of rhesus monkeys [13]. Results from the urinary recovery data indicated that the rate of skin permeation (dQ/dt) increases as increasing the nitroglycerin dose (C_d) applied on a unity surface area of the skin (Fig. 5). It appears that a maximum rate of skin permeation (1.585 mg/cm^2/day) is achieved for nitroglycerin when the applied dose reaches the level at or greater than 4.786 mg/cm^2. It translates into a maximum transdermal bioavailability of 33.1%/day for nitroglycerin.

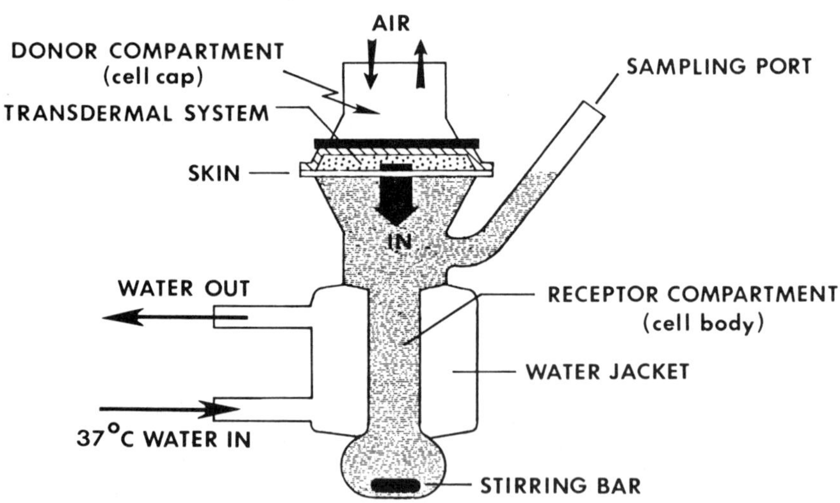

Fig. 6 Diagrammatic illustration of one unit of the commercially available 8-cell Franz diffusion apparatus. (From Crown Glass Co., Inc., Somerville, NJ.)

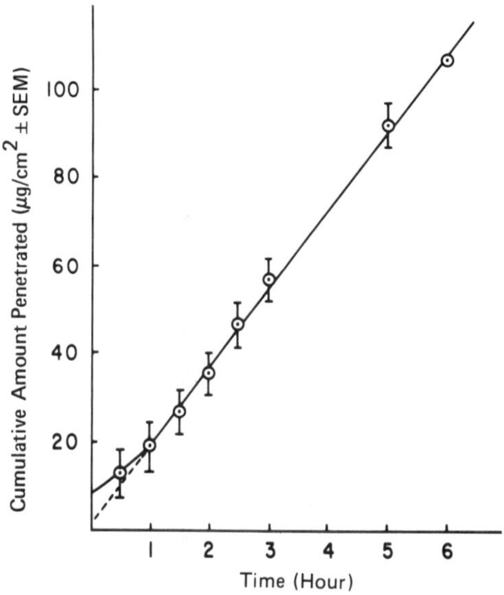

Fig. 7 Permeation profile of pure nitroglycerin across hairless mouse abdominal skin mounted on Franz diffusion apparatus at 37°. A constant skin permeation profile was obtained with a permeation rate of 19.85 (±1.71) $\mu g/cm^2/hr$. (From Ref. 14.)

The kinetics of skin permeation can be more precisely analyzed by studying the time course for the permeation of drug across a freshly excised skin mounted on a diffusion cell, such as the Franz diffusion cell (Fig. 6). A typical skin permeation kinetic profile is shown in Figure 7 for nitroglycerin. Results indicated that nitroglycerin penetrates through the freshly excised hairless mouse abdominal skin at a zero-order rate of 19.85 (±1.71) $\mu g/cm^2/hr$ [Eq. (4)]. Pure nitroglycerin (without the mediation of an organic solvent or drug delivery system) was used in this investigation [14]. Similar observations were made in a series of long-term skin permeation kinetic studies for estradiol [15], which provides a critical analysis on the relationships among skin permeation rate, permeability coefficient, partition coefficient, diffusivity, and solubility. The effects of skin uptake, binding, and metabolism kinetics on skin permeation profiles were also evaluated and demonstrated [16].

For thorough analysis of the fundamentals of skin permeation, interested readers are recommended to consult References 12, 15, and 16 for details.

IV. APPROACHES TO DEVELOPMENT OF TRANSDERMAL THERAPEUTIC SYSTEMS

Several technologies have been successfully developed to provide rate control over the release and the transdermal permeation of drugs. These technologies can be classified into four approaches as follows:

A. Membrane-Moderated Systems

In this system, the drug reservoir is totally encapsulated in a shallow compartment molded from a drug-impermeable metallic plastic laminate and a rate-controlling polymeric membrane (Fig. 8). The drug molecules are permitted to release only through the rate-controlling polymeric membrane. In the drug reservoir compartment, the drug solids are either dispersed in a solid polymer matrix or suspended in an unleachable, viscous liquid medium, e.g., silicone fluid to form a paste-like suspension. The rate-limiting membrane can be a microporous or a non-porous polymeric membrane, e.g., ethylene-vinyl acetate copolymer, with a defined drug permeability property. On the external surface of the polymeric membrane, a thin layer of drug-compatible, hypoallergenic adhesive polymer, e.g., silicone or polyacrylate adhesive, may be applied to achieve an intimate contact of the transdermal therapeutic system with the skin surface. The rate of drug release from this type of transdermal drug delivery system can be tailored by varying the polymer composition, permeability coefficient and/or thickness of the rate-limiting membrane and adhesive. Several transdermal therapeutic systems have been materialized from this technology and are best exemplified by the development and marketing of nitroglycerin-releasing transdermal therapeutic

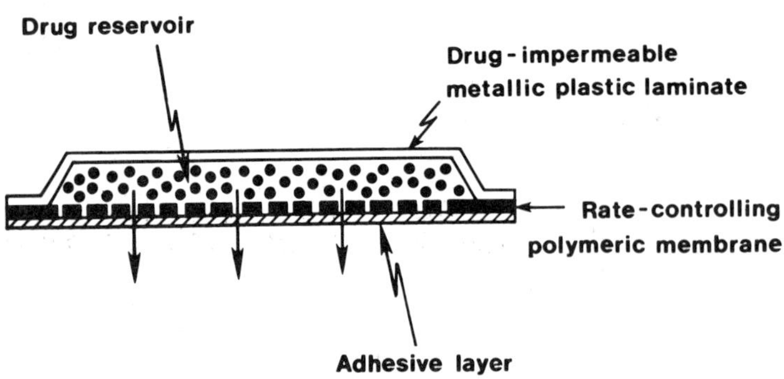

Fig. 8 The cross-sectional view of a membrane-moderated transdermal drug delivery system, showing various major structural components

system (Transderm-Nitro system/Ciba) for once-a-day medication of angina pectoris [17,18], of scopolamine-releasing transdermal therapeutic system (Transderm-Scop system/Ciba) for 3-day protection of motion sickness [2] and of clonidine-releasing transdermal therapeutic system (Catapres-TTS/Boehringer Ingelheim) for weekly treatment of hypertension [19–21].

The intrinsic rate of drug release from this type of drug delivery system is defined by:

$$\frac{dQ}{dt} = \frac{C_R}{\frac{1}{P_m} + \frac{1}{P_a}} \tag{5}$$

Where C_R is the drug concentration in the reservoir compartment; P_a and P_m are the permeability coefficients of the adhesive layer and the rate-controlling membrane, respectively. For a microporous membrane, P_m is the sum of permeability coefficients across the pores and the polymeric material [22]. P_m and P_a, respectively, are defined as follows:

$$P_m = \frac{K_{m/r} \cdot D_m}{\delta_a} \tag{6}$$

$$P_a = \frac{K_{a/m} \cdot D_a}{\delta_a} \tag{7}$$

where $K_{m/r}$ and $K_{a/m}$ are the partition coefficients for the interfacial partitioning of drug from the reservoir to the membrane and from the membrane to the adhesive, respectively; D_m and D_a are the diffusion coefficients in the rate-controlling membrane and adhesive layer, respectively; δ_m and δ_a are the thicknesses of the rate-controlling membrane and adhesive layer, respectively. In the case of microporous membrane, the porosity and tortuosity of the membrane should also be taken into consideration in the calculation of the D_m and δ_m values. Substituting Eq. (6) and (7) for P_m and P_a in Eq. (5) gives

$$\frac{dQ}{dt} = \frac{K_{m/r} K_{a/m} \cdot D_m \cdot D_a}{K_{m/r} D_m \delta_a + K_{a/m} D_a \delta_m} \cdot C_R \tag{8}$$

which defines the intrinsic rate of drug release from a membrane-moderated drug delivery system described here.

The membrane permeation-controlled transdermal drug delivery technology has also been applied to the development of transdermal therapeutic systems for the controlled percutaneous absorption of estradiol [23, 24] and prostaglandin derivative [25].

B. Adhesive Diffusion-Controlled Systems

This type of drug delivery system is a simplified version of the membrane-moderated drug delivery system outlined above. Instead of completely encapsulating the drug reservoir in a compartment fabricated from a drug-impermeable metallic plastic backing, in this system the drug reservoir is formulated by directly dispersing the drug in an adhesive polymer and then spreading the medicated adhesive, by solvent casting, onto a flat sheet of drug-impermeable metallic plastic backing to form a thin drug reservoir layer (Fig. 9). On the top of the drug reservoir layer, layers of non-medicated, rate-controlling adhesive polymer of constant thickness are applied to produce an adhesive diffusion-controlled drug delivery system. The rate of drug release is defined by:

$$\frac{dQ}{dt} = \frac{K_{a/r} \cdot D_a \cdot C_R}{\delta_a} \qquad (9)$$

where $K_{a/r}$ is the partition coefficient for the interfacial partitioning of drug from the reservoir layer to the adhesive layer.

This type of transdermal drug delivery system is best illustrated by the development and marketing of nitroglycerin-releasing transdermal therapeutic system (Deponit system/Pharma-Schwartz) in Europe and of isosorbide dinitrate-releasing transdermal therapeutic system (Frandol tape/Toaeiyo) in Japan for one-a-day medication of angina pectoris.

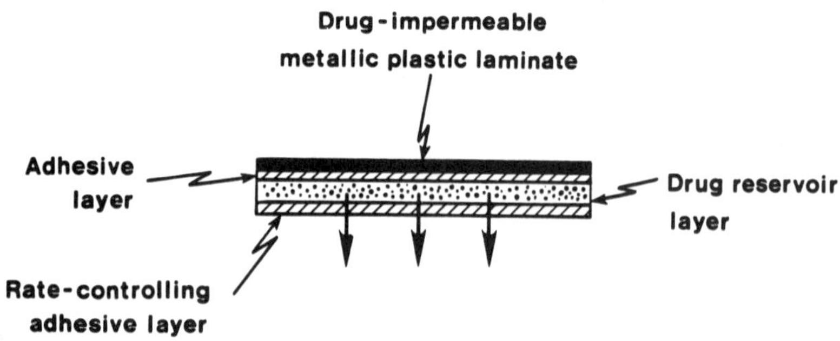

Fig. 9 The cross-sectional view of an adhesive diffusion-controlled transdermal drug delivery system, showing various major structural components.

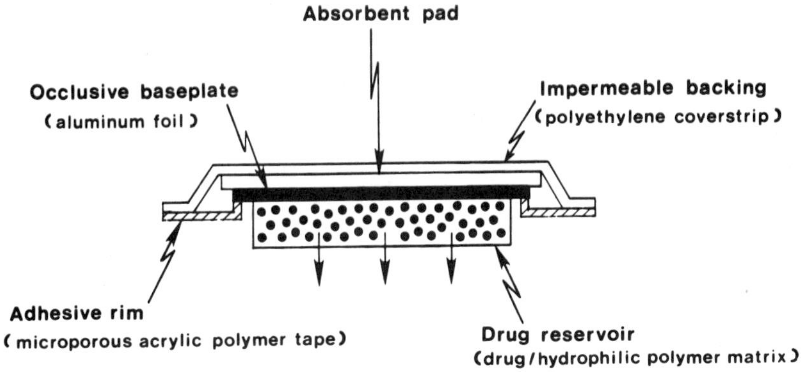

Fig. 10 The cross-sectional view of a matrix dispersion-type transdermal drug delivery system, showing various major structural components.

C. Matrix Dispersion-Type Systems

In this approach, the drug reservoir is formed by homogeneously dispersing the drug solids in a hydrophilic or lipophilic polymer matrix and the medicated polymer is then molded into medicated disc with a defined surface area and controlled thickness. This drug reservoir-containing polymer disc is then glued onto an occlusive baseplate in a compartment fabricated from a drug-impermeable plastic backing (Fig. 10). Instead of applying the adhesive polymer directly on the surface of the medicated disc as discussed earlier in the first two transdermal therapeutic systems, the adhesive polymer is spread along the circumference to form a strip of adhesive rim around the medicated disc. The rate of drug release from this matrix dispersion-type transdermal therapeutic system is defined as:

$$\frac{dQ}{dt} = \left(\frac{ACpDp}{2t}\right)^{\frac{1}{2}} \qquad (10)$$

where A is the initial drug loading dose dispersed in the polymer matrix; and Cp and Dp are the solubility and diffusivity of the drug in the polymer, respectively. In view of the fact that only the drug species dissolved in the polymer can release, so, practically Cp is equal to C_R.

At steady state, a Q *versus* $t^{\frac{1}{2}}$ drug release profile is obtained as defined [26] by:

$$\frac{Q}{t^{\frac{1}{2}}} = [(2A - Cp)CpDp]^{\frac{1}{2}} \qquad (11)$$

This type of transdermal drug delivery system is exemplified by the development and marketing of nitroglycerin-releasing transdermal therapeutic system (Nitro-Dur system/Key) which has been approved by FDA for once-a-day medication of angina pectoris [27]. Patent disclosures have also been filed for applying this drug delivery system for transdermal controlled administration of estradiol diacetate and verapamil.

D. Microreservoir Systems

This type of drug delivery system can be considered as a combination of the reservoir and matrix dispersion-type drug delivery systems. In this approach, the drug reservoir is formed by first suspending the drug solids in an aqueous solution of water-soluble polymer and then dispersing homogeneoulsy the drug suspension in a lipophilic polymer, by high-shear mechanical force, to form thousands of unleachable, microscopic spheres of drug reservoirs (Fig. 11). This thermodynamically unstable dispersion is quickly stabilized by immediately crosslinking the polymer chains *in situ*, which produces a medicated polymer disc with a constant surface area and a fixed thickness. A transdermal therapeutic system is produced, in which the medicated disc is positioned at the center and surrounded by an adhesive rim (Fig. 12). This technology has been successfully utilized in the development and marketing of nitroglycerin-releasing transdermal therapeutic system (Nitrodisc system/Searle) for once-a-day treatment of angina pectoris [13,28–32].

The rate of drug release from the microreservoir drug delivery system is defined [32] by:

$$\frac{dQ}{dt} = \frac{D_p D_s \alpha' K_p}{D_p \delta_d + D_s \delta_p \alpha' K_p}\left[\beta S_p - \frac{D_l S_l (1 - \beta)}{\delta_l}\left(\frac{1}{K_l} + \frac{1}{K_m}\right)\right] \qquad (12)$$

where $\alpha' = \partial'/\beta'$. ∂' is the ratio of the drug concentration in the bulk of elution solution over the drug solubility in the same medium and β' is the ratio of the drug concentration at the outer edge of the polymer coating membrane over the drug solubility in the same polymer composition; K_l, K_m, and K_p are the partition coefficients for the interfacial partitioning of drug from the liquid compartment to the polymer matrix, from the polymer matrix to the polymer coating membrane, and from the polymer coating membrane to the elution solution (or skin), respectively; D_l, D_p, and D_s are the drug diffusivities in the liquid compartment, polymer coating membrane, and elution solution (or skin), respectively: S_l and S_p are the solubilities of the drug in the liquid compartment and in the polymer matrix, respectively; δ_l, δ_p, and δ_d are the thicknesses of the liquid layer

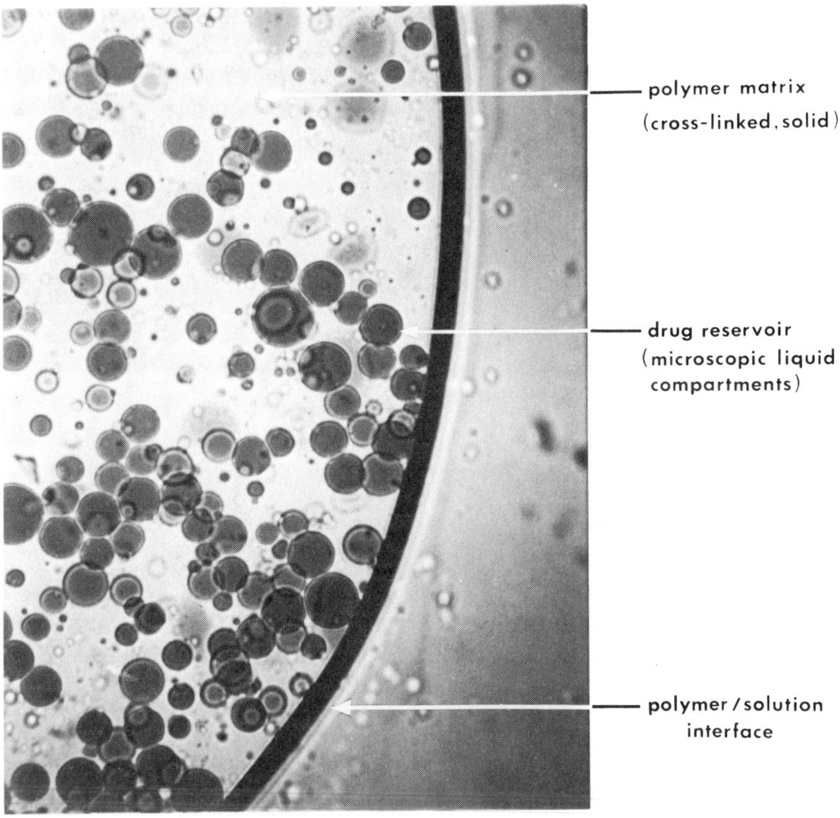

Fig. 11 Photomicrograph of a microreservoir-type drug delivery system, showing the microscopic structure of the system.

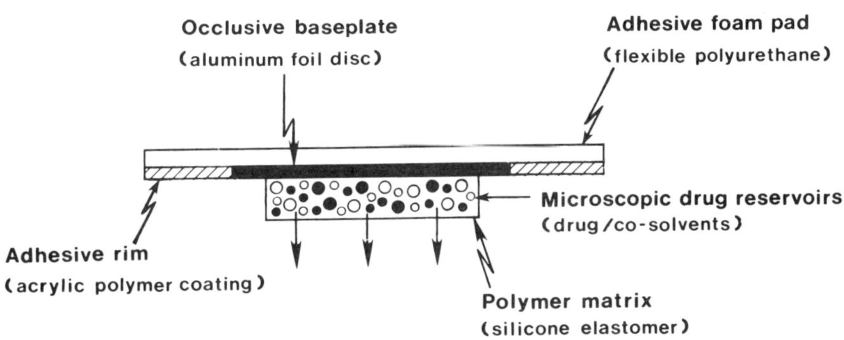

Fig. 12 The cross-sectional view of a microreservoir-type transdermal drug delivery system, showing various major structural components.

surrounding the drug particles, the polymer coating membrane around the polymer matrix, and the hydrodynamic diffusion layer surrounding the polymer coating membrane, respectively; β is the ratio of the drug concentration at the inner edge of the interfacial barrier over the drug solubility in the polymer matrix.

Release of drugs from the microreservoir-type drug delivery system can follow either a partition control- or matrix diffusion-control process depending upon the relative magnitude of S_l and S_p [32]. So, a Q *versus* t or Q *versus* $t^{\frac{1}{2}}$ release profile may result [14,33].

Development of other types of potential drug delivery systems are also undergoing for possible applications in the transdermal controlled infusion of drugs. It is exemplied by the development of poroplastic membrane [34] and hydrophilic polymeric reservoir [35]. Both of them are drug solution-saturated porous polymer matrix.

V. KINETIC EVALUATION OF TRANSDERMAL THERAPEUTIC SYSTEMS

The release and skin permeation kinetics of drug from these technologically- different transdermal therapeutic systems can be evaluated, using a two-compartment diffusion cell assembly, under identical conditions. It is carried out by mounting, individually, the full-thickness abdominal skin, which has been freshly excised from either human cadaver or hairless mouse [36], on an eight-cell Franz diffusion assembly (Fig. 6). The drug delivery systems are then applied with their drug-releasing surface in intimate contact with the stratum corneum surface of the skin [37]. The skin permeation profile of drug is followed by sampling the receptor solution at predetermined intervals for a duration of up to 30 hr and assaying drug concentrations in the samples by a sensitive analytical method, such as high performance liquid chromatographic (HPLC) method [14,37]. The release profiles of drug from these transdermal therapeutic systems can also be investigated using the same experimental setup without the skin [14].

In actual determination of drug release and skin permeation kinetics studies, the rate profiles obtained could well be below the intrinsic rates calculated from Eqs. (8), (9), (11), and (12) due to the existence of hydrodynamic diffusion layer on the surface of drug delivery system or dermis. The magnitude of reduction is related to the thickness of hydrodynamic diffusion layer and the physicochemical properties of the drugs [38]. It is rather important to take these factors into consideration in the determination of drug release and skin permeation rate profiles.

A. *In Vitro* Drug Release Kinetics

Using Franz diffusion cell assembly, the controlled release kinetics of drugs from these technologically-different transdermal therapeutic

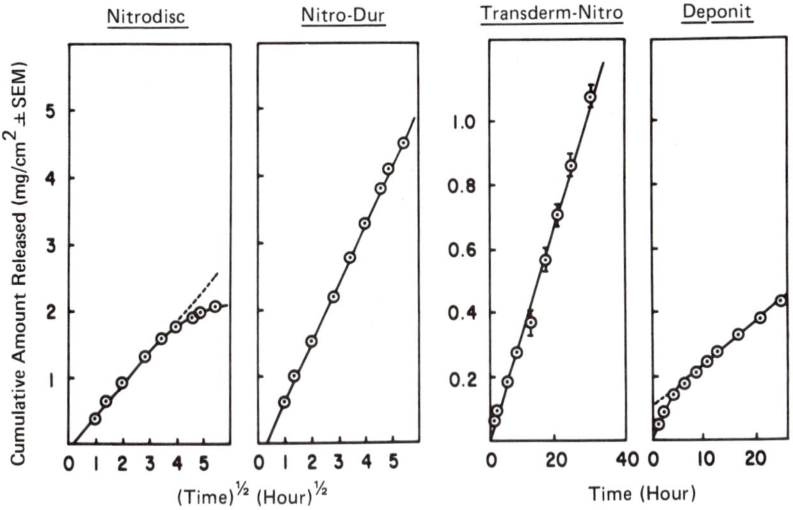

Fig. 13 Comparative release profiles of nitroglycerin from various transdermal drug delivery systems into saline solution containing 20% PEG 400 at 37°C. The release flux of nitroglycerin is: Nitrodisc system (2.443 ± 0.136 $mg/cm^2/day^{\frac{1}{2}}$), Nitro-Dur system (4.124 ± 0.047 $mg/cm^2/day^{\frac{1}{2}}$), Transderm-Nitro system (0.843 ± 0.035 $mg/cm^2/day$), Deponit system (0.324 ± 0.011 $mg/cm^2/day$). (From Ref. 14.)

system can be evaluated and compared [14]. The results indicated that nitroglycerin is released at a constant rate profile (Q *versus* t) from Transderm-Nitro system (a membrane-moderated transdermal therapeutic system) and Deponit system (an adhesive diffusion-controlled transdermal drug delivery system) (Fig. 13). The release rate of nitroglycerin from the Transderm-Nitro system (0.843 ± 0.035 $mg/cm^2/day$) is almost 3 times greater than that from the Deponit system (0.324 ± 0.011 $mg/cm^2/day$). It suggests that the rate-controlling adhesive layers in the Deponit system plays a greater rate-controlling role over the release of nitroglycerin than does the rate-controlling membrane in the Transderm-Nitro system.

On the other hand, the release profiles of nitroglycerin from Nitrodisc and Nitro-Dur systems are not constant, but are observed to follow a linear Q *versus* $t^{\frac{1}{2}}$ relationship as expected from the matrix diffusion-controlled drug release kinetics [35]. The release flux of nitroglycerin from the Nitro-Dur system (a matrix dispersion-type transdermal therapeutic system) is about twice greater than that from the Nitrodisc system (a microreservoir-type transdermal therapeutic system) (4.124 ± 0.047 versus 2.443 ± 0.136 $mg/cm^2/day^{\frac{1}{2}}$). Apparently, the mechanisms and rates of nitroglycerin release from these

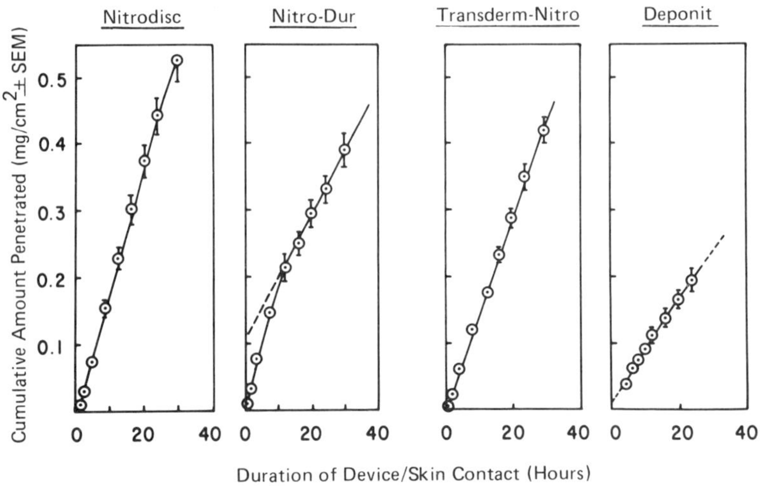

Fig. 14 Comparative permeation profiles of nitroglycerin from various transdermal drug delivery systems through the hairless mouse abdominal skin at 37°C. The rate of skin permeation is: Nitrodisc system (0.426 ± 0.024 $mg/cm^2/day$), Nitro-Dur system [0.408 ± 0.024 $mg/cm^2/day$ (<12 hr); 0.248 ± 0.018 $mg/cm^2/day$ (>12 hr)], Transderm-Nitro system (0.338 ± 0.017 $mg/cm^2/day$), Deponit system (0.175 ± 0.016 $mg/cm^2/day$). (From Ref. 14.)

4 transdermal therapeutic systems are quite different from one another, as expected from Eqs. (8), (9), (11), and (12).

B. *In Vitro* Skin Permeation Kinetics—Animal Model

Interestingly, the skin permeation studies suggested that all four transdermal therapeutic systems provide a constant rate of skin permeation as expected from Eq. (3) (Fig. 14). A highest rate of skin permeation was observed with Nitrodisc system (0.426 ± 0.024 $mg/cm^2/day$), which is statistically no different from the rate of skin permeation for pure nitroglycerin (0.476 ± 0.041 $mg/cm^2/day$, Fig. 7). For Nitro-Dur system, practically the same rate of skin permeation (0.408 ± 0.024 $mg/cm^2/day$) was observed initially and 12 hr later, the rate was slowed down to 0.248 (±0.018) $mg/cm^2/day$. On the other hand, the rate of skin permeation of nitroglycerin delivered by Transderm-Nitro system (0.338 ± 0.017 $mg/cm^2/day$) was found to be 30% lower than the rate achieved by pure nitroglycerin, (0.476 $mg/cm^2/day$), or 21% slower than that by Nitrodisc system (0.426 $mg/cm^2/day$). The lowest rate of skin permeation was observed with

Deponit system (0.175 ± 0.016 mg/cm²/day), which is only 37% of the skin permeation rate for pure nitroglycerine.

Comparing the rate of skin permeation with the rate of release indicated that, under the sink conditions, all transdermal therapeutic systems release nitroglycerin at a rate which is greater than the rate of uptake by the skin, i.e., $R_r >> R_a$ (Fig. 4). For example, nitroglycerin was released from Transderm-Nitro system, which is a membrane permeation-controlled drug delivery system, at a rate (0.843 mg/cm²/day) which is 2.5 times greater than the rate of uptake by the skin (0.338 mg/cm²/day). Likewise, the rate of release from the Deponit system, which is an adhesive diffusion-controlled drug

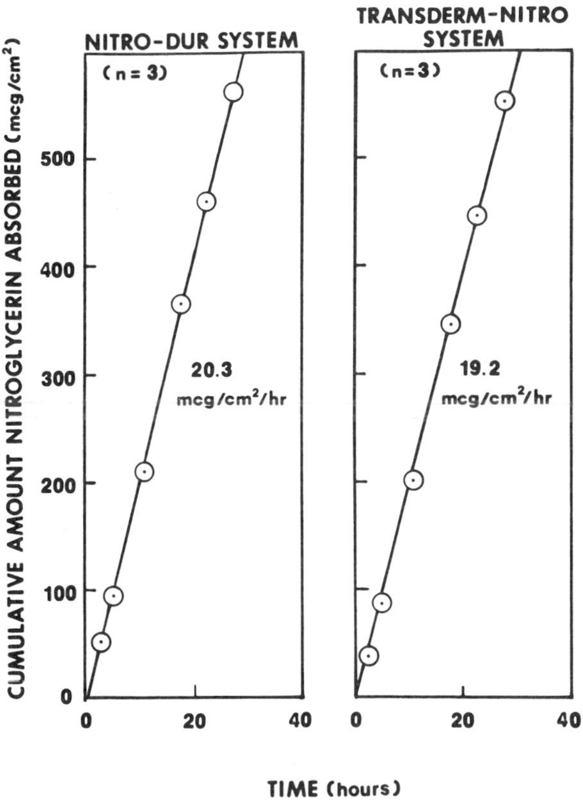

Fig. 15 Comparative permeation profiles of nitroglycerin from Nitro-Dur and Transderm-nitro systems across the human cadaver abdominal epidermis. The rate of skin permeation is: Nitro-Dur system (20.3 μg/cm²/hr) and Transderm-Nitro system (19.2 μg/cm²/hr) (plotted from data in Ref. 36).

delivery system and releases nitroglycerin at the slowest rate (Fig. 13), was also 1.9-fold faster than the rate of skin permeation (0.324 versus 0.175 mg/cm^2/day). The same observations were also true for Nitrodisc and Nitro-Dur systems. This phenomenon is indicative of the rate-limiting role of stratum corneum in the skin permeation of drugs as a result of its low permeability.

C. *In Vitro* Skin Permeation Kinetics—Human Cadaver

The permeation of nitroglycerin across the human cadaver skin was also investigated for Transderm-Nitro system, the membrane permeation-controlled transdermal therapeutic system, and for Nitro-Dur system, the matrix diffusion-controlled transdermal therapeutic system [39]. The results (Fig. 15) indicated that the skin permeation of nitroglycerin through the human cadaver abdominal epidermis also follows the same zero-order kinetic profile as observed with hairless mouse abdominal skin (Fig. 14). It is interesting to note that the rates of skin permeation generated from the excised skins of hairless mouse agree fairly well with the data obtained from human cadaver skin (Table 1), suggesting that hairless mouse skin could be an acceptable

Table 1 *In Vitro–In Vivo* Comparison on Skin Permeation Rates of Nitroglycerin

	Skin permeation rates (mg/cm^2/day)		
	In Vitro		
Delivery systems	Hairless mouse	Human cadaver	*In Vivo*[d]
Nitroglycerin alone	0.476[a]	0.312[b]	–
Nitrodisc	0.426	–	0.473
Nitro-Dur	0.408	0.487[c]	0.412
Transderm-Nitro	0.338	0.461[c]	0.428
Deponit	0.175	–	–

[a]Determined from skin permeation studies of pure nitroglycerin across full-thickness hairless mouse abdominal skin at 37°C.
[b]Determined from an aqueous solution of nitroglycerin at 30°C (Ref. 43).
[c]Determined from skin permeation studies at 37°C using the epidermis isolated from human cadaver abdominal skin (Ref. 39).
[d]Calculated from Eq. (13), in which k_e = 0.1575 min^{-1} and V_d = 179.6 liters (Ref. 42).

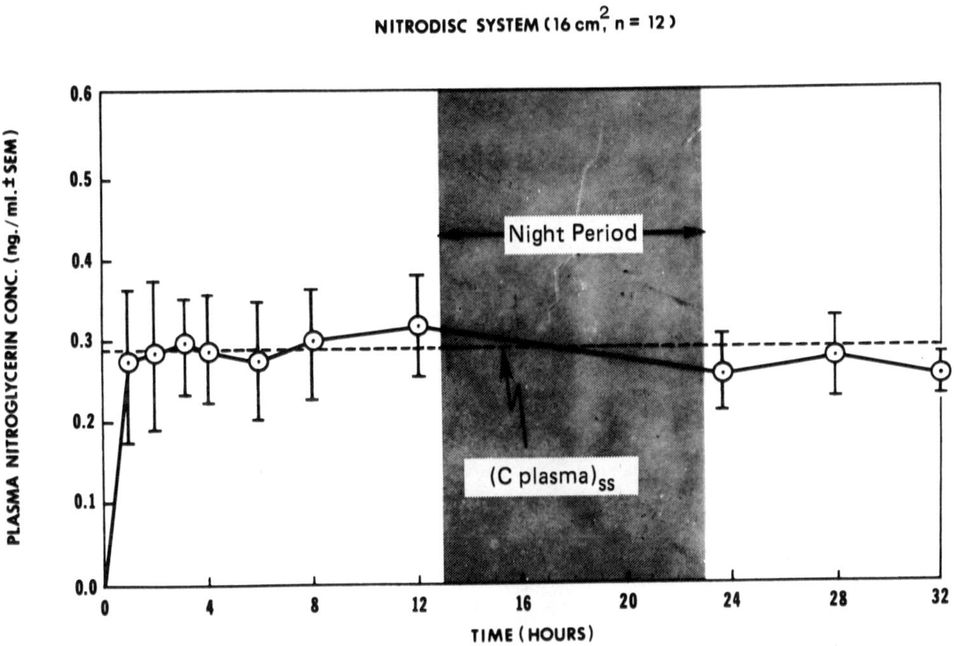

Fig. 16 Plasma profiles of nitroglycerin in 12 healthy male volunteers, each received a unit of Nitrodisc system (16 cm^2) on the chest for 32 hr. A steady-state plasma level, $(Cp)_{ss}$, of 280.6 ± 18.7 pg/ml was determined (plotted from the data in Ref. 28).

animal model for human skin in the skin permeation kinetics studies of nitroglycerin.

D. *In Vivo* Transdermal Bioavailability in Humans

The transdermal bioavailability of nitroglycerin resulted from the 24- to 32-hr topical applications of various transdermal therapeutic systems in human volunteers, as indicated by the plasma levels of nitroglycerin, is shown in Figures 16–18. Results suggested that a prolonged, steady-state plasma level of nitroglycerin is achieved within 1–2 hr and maintained for a duration of at least 24 hr as a result of continuous transdermal infusion of drug at controlled rate from the transdermal therapeutic systems.

The plasma level was found to be linearly proportional to the drug releasing surface of transdermal therapeutic systems in contact with the skin (Fig. 19). For every unit area (cm^2) of the drug releasing surface applied, a plasma level of 14 pg/ml was achieved.

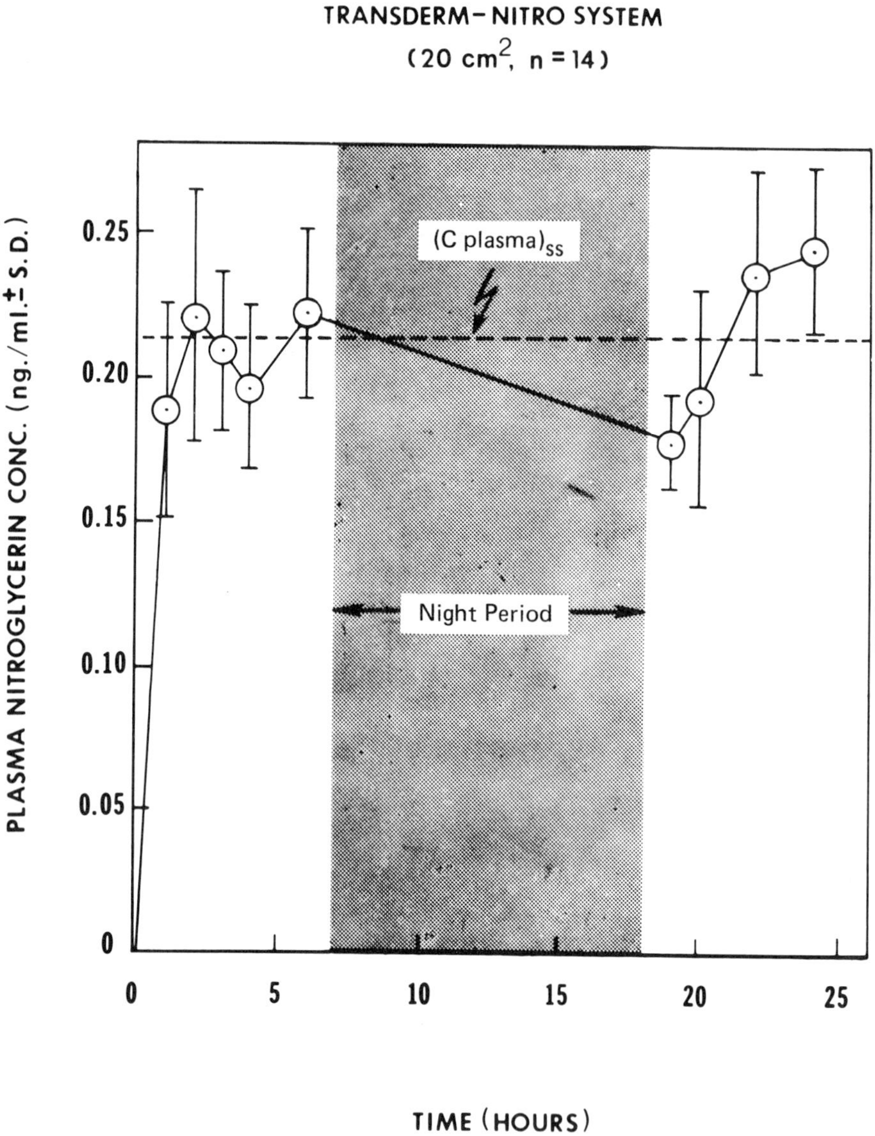

Fig. 17 Plasma profiles of nitroglycerin in 14 healthy human subjects, each received a unit of Transderm-Nitro system (20 cm^2) for 24 hr. A $(Cp)_{ss}$ value of 209.8 ± 22.8 pg/ml was determined (plotted from the data in Ref. 16).

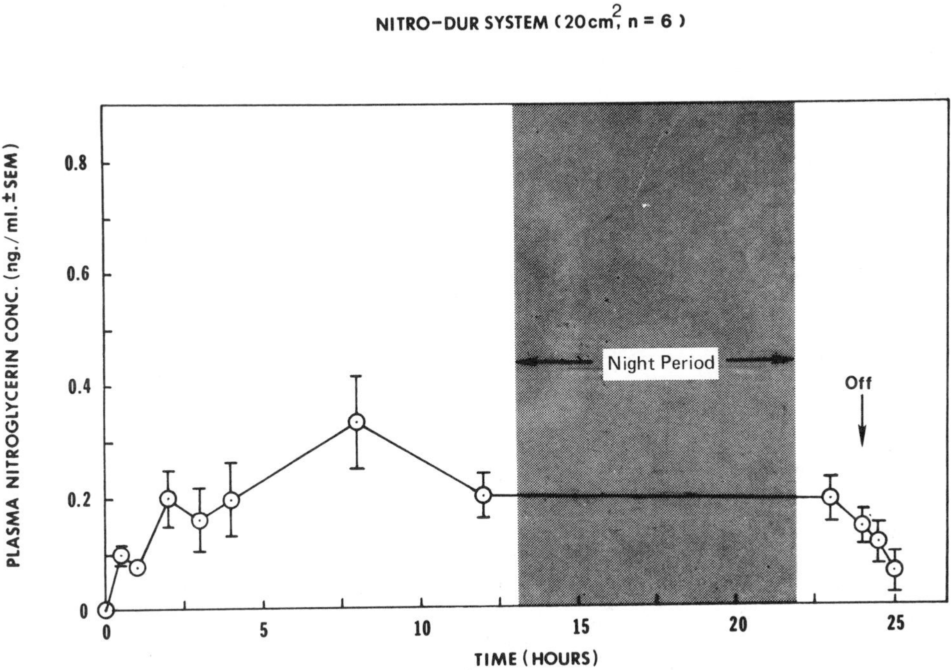

Fig. 18 Plasma profiles of nitroglycerin in 6 normal male volunteers, each received a unit of Nitro-Dur system (20 cm^2) over the chest for 24 hr. A (Cp)ss value of 201.4 ± 60.7 pg/ml was determined (plotted from the data in Ref. 44).

F. *In Vitro–In Vivo* Correlations

To further examine the feasibility of using freshly excised hairless mouse skin as the animal model for studying transdermal controlled permeation kinetics of drug across the human skin, the *in vivo* rate of skin permeation $(Q/t)_{i.v.}$ should be determined for comparison. It can be calculated from steady-state plasma level $(C_p)_{ss}$ data (Figs. 16–18), using the following relationship [40]:

$$\left(\frac{Q}{t}\right)_{i.v.} = (C_p)_{ss} \cdot k_e \cdot V_d \qquad (13)$$

where k_e is the first-order rate constant for elimination of drug and V_d is apparent volume of distribution of drug.

Results indicated that *in vivo* skin permeation rates calculated on the basis of Eq. (13) show a reasonably good agreement with the

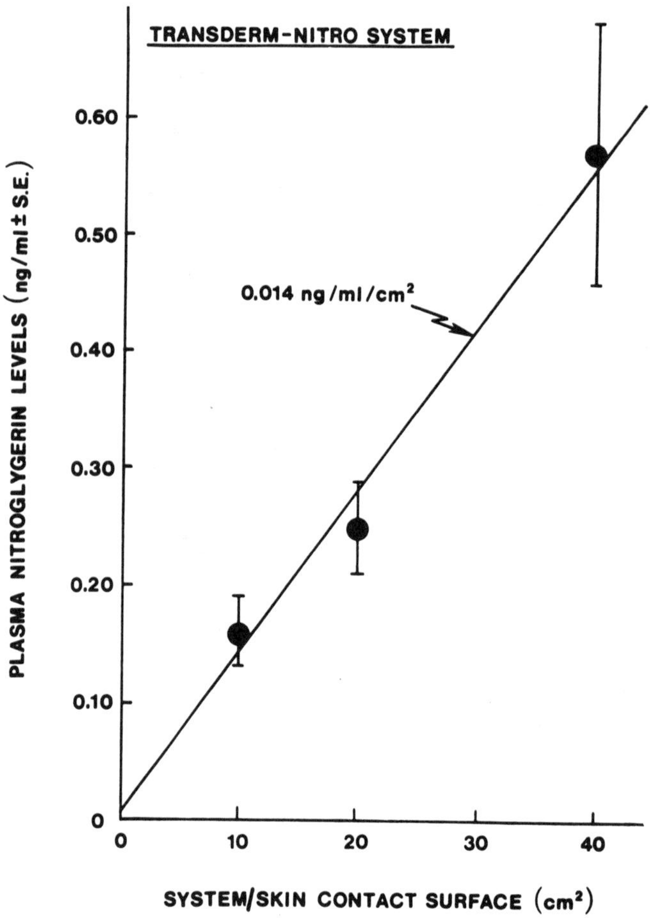

Fig. 19 Linear relationship between the steady-state plasma nitroglycerin levels in humans and the drug-releasing surface of Transderm-Nitro system in contact with the skin. A plasma nitroglycerin level of 14 pg/ml was achieved for every cm^2 of drug-releasing surface applied (plotted from the data in Ref. 15).

in vitro data determined from either human cadaver or hairless mouse skin (Table 1). This *in vivo–in vitro* agreement provides additional evidence that hairless mouse skin could be an acceptable animal model for studying skin permeation kinetics of systemically effective drugs, like nitroglycerin, in humans.

VI. FORMULATION DESIGN AND OPTIMIZATION

To formulate a transdermal therapeutic system one should take into consideration the relationship between rate of drug delivery to the skin surface and maximum achievable rate of drug absorption by the skin tissue. It is particularly important since the stratum corneum is known to be highly impermeable to many drugs. A properly designed transdermal therapeutic system should have a skin permeation rate that is determined by the actual rate of drug delivery to the skin surface, not by the skin permeability; so the transdermal bioavailability of a drug becomes independent of any possible intra- and/or interpatient variabilities in skin permeability.

The rate of skin permeation $(Q/t)_{ss}$ of a drug at steady state is related to the actual rate of drug delivery from a transdermal therapeutic system $(Q/t)_{tts}$ to the skin surface and the maximum achievable rate of skin absorption $(Q/t)_{m,s}$ as follows [41]:

$$\frac{1}{(Q/t)_{ss}} = \frac{1}{(Q/t)_{tts}} + \frac{1}{(Q/t)_{m,s}} \tag{14}$$

And, the actual rate of drug delivery from a transdermal therapeutic system to the skin surface (which acts as the receptor medium) can thus be determined from:

$$\frac{1}{(Q/t)_{tts}} = \frac{1}{(Q/t)_{ss}} - \frac{1}{(Q/t)_{m,s}} \tag{15}$$

Using the rate of skin permeation from the pure nitroglycerin as the value for $(Q/t)_{m,s}$, the actual delivery rate of nitroglycerin from various transdermal therapeutic systems can be calculated. Results (Table 2) indicated that the rates of delivery from Nitrodisc, Nitro-Dur and Transderm-Nitro systems are three- to ninefold greater than the maximum achievable rate of skin permeation (0.476 mg/cm^2/day) for nitroglycerin. On the other hand, the rate of delivery from Deponit system is only 58% of the maximum rate of skin permeation. The data suggested that the delivery rate of nitroglycerin from all four transdermal therapeutic systems has not been properly optimized.

Using a matrix diffusion-controlled transdermal therapeutic system, the relationship between the rate of drug delivery from the transdermal therapeutic system and the rate of skin permeation can be established. The skin permeation rate of a drug at steady state, $(Q/t)_{ss}$, is related to the drug delivery rate from the matrix-type transdermal therapeutic system, $(Q/t^{\frac{1}{2}})$, as follows [45]:

Table 2 Delivery Rate of Nitroglycerin from Various Transdermal Therapeutic Systems

Therapeutic systems	Delivery rate[a] (mg/cm^2/day)
Nitrodisc	4.058
Nitro-Dur	2.857
Transderm-Nitro	1.166
Deponit	0.277

[a]Calculated from the hairless mouse data in Table 1 using Eq. (15) and $(Q/t)_{ms}$ = 0.476 mg/cm^2/day.

$$(Q/t)_{ss} = \frac{\alpha' (Q/t^{1/2})^2}{1 + \beta' (Q/t^{1/2})^2} \qquad (16)$$

in which α' and β' are composite constants and defined as follows:

$$\alpha' = \frac{1}{2k}$$

$$\beta' = \frac{R_{sc}}{2K_1 k C_p}\left(1 + \frac{R_{vs}K_3 + R_{aq}}{K_2 K_3 R_{sc}}\right) \qquad (17)$$

where k is a constant; K_1, K_2, and K_3 are the partition coefficients for the interfacial partitioning between stratum corneum and polymer matrix, between viable skin and stratum corneum, and between aqueous layer and viable skin, respectively; C_p is the drug solubility in the polymer matrix; R_{sc}, R_{vs}, and R_{aq} are the diffusional resistances for stratum corneum, viable skin, and aqueous layer on the dermal surface, respectively.

As indicated by Eq. (16), a hyperbolic relationship exists between $(Q/t)_{ss}$ and $(Q/t^{\frac{1}{2}})^2$. When the rate of drug delivery from the transdermal therapeutic system is low, the skin permeation is controlled by the delivery system (Fig. 20). As increasing the rate of drug delivery, the rate of skin permeation increases, at hyperbolic fashion, and then reaches a plateau level, at which the rate of skin permeation becomes rate-controlled by the permeability of stratum corneum.

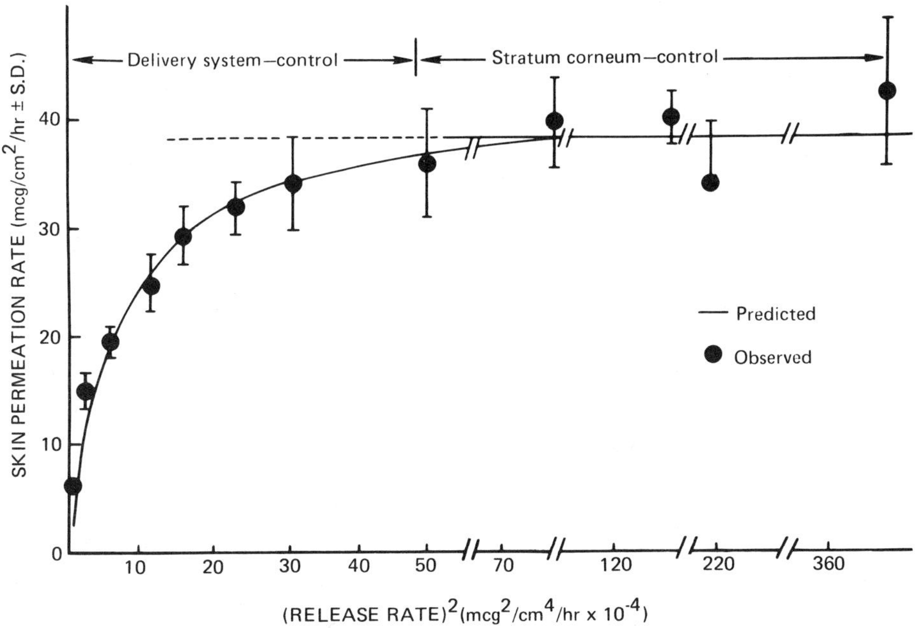

Fig. 20 Hyperbolic relationship between permeation rate across intact skin and the square of the release flux of nitroglycerin delivered by the matrix diffusion-controlled transdermal therapeutic system, as predicted from Equation 16. It was observed that when $(Q/t^{\frac{1}{2}})^2$ value is equal to or less than 48 $mcg^2/cm^4/hr$, the skin permeation rate of nitroglycerin is controlled by the delivery system; when the $(Q/t^{\frac{1}{2}})^2$ value is greater than 48 $mcg^2/cm^4/hr$, the skin permeation rate becomes limited by the stratum corneum. Each data point represents the mean value ± standard error of four determina tions. (Reproduced from Ref. 45.)

Using Eq. (16), one can optimize the formulation design of a transdermal therapeutic system with the rate of skin permeation controlled by the rate of drug delivery from the delivery system.

REFERENCES

1. J. E. Shaw, S. K. Chandrasekaran, and P. Campbell, Percutaneous absorption: Controlled drug delivery for topical or systemic therapy, *J. Invest. Dermatol. 67*, 677 (1976).
2. J. E. Shaw and S. K. Chandrasekaran, Controlled topical delivery of drugs for systemic action, *Drug Metab. Rev. 8*, 223 (1978).

3. 1982 Industrial Pharmaceutical R & D Symposium on *Transdermal Controlled Release Medication*, Rutgers' College of Pharmacy, Piscataway, NJ, January 14–15, 1982, *Drug Dev. Ind. Pharm.* *9* (4), 497–744 (1983).
4. World Congress of Clinical Pharmacology Symposium on *Transdermal Delivery of Cardiovascular Drugs*, Washington, D.C., August 5, 1983, *Am. Heart J. 108* (1), 195–236 (1984).
5. S. W. Jacob and C. A. Francone, *Structure and Function of Man*, 2nd ed., W. B. Saunders Co., Philadelphia, 1970, pp. 55–60.
6. P. Zanowiak and M. R. Jacobs, Topical anti-infective products. In, *Handbook of Nonprescription Drugs*, 7th ed. (S. C. Laitin, Ed.), American Pharmaceutical Association, Washington, DC, 1982, pp. 525–529.
7. Y. W. Chien, Logics of transdermal controlled drug administration, *Drug Dev. Ind. Pharm. 9*, 497 (1983).
8. E. K. Kastrup and J. R. Boyd, *Drug: Facts and Comparisons*, 1983 ed., J. B. Lippincott Co., St. Louis, 1983, pp. 1634–1708.
9. J. E. Shaw, W. Bayne, and L. Schmidt, Clinical pharmacology of scopolamine, *Clin. Pharmacol. Ther. 19*, 115 (1976).
10. P. W. Armstrong, J. A. Armstrong, and G. S. Marks; Pharmacokinetic-hemodynamic studies of nitroglycerin ointment in congestive heart failure, *Am. J. Cardiol. 46*, 670 (1980).
11. R. Sitruk-Ware, B. deLignieres, A. Basdevant, and P. Mauvais-Jarvis, Absorption of percutaneous oestradiol in postmenopausal women, *Maturitas 2*, 207 (1980).
12. Y. W. Chien, *Novel Drug Delivery Systems: Fundamentals, Developmental Concepts and Biomedical Assessments*, Marcel Dekker, Inc., New York, 1982, Chap. 5.
13. D. R. Sanvordeker, J. G. Cooney, and R. C. Wester, Transdermal nitroglycerin pad, U.S. patent #4,336,243 (June 22, 1982).
14. P. R. Keshary, Y. C. Huang, and Y. W. Chien, unpublished data, personal communication, 1984.
15. K. H. Valia and Y. W. Chien, Long-term skin permeation kinetics of estradiol: (I) Effect of drugs solubilizer-polyethylene glycol 400, *Drug Dev. Ind. Pharm. 10*, 951 (1984).
16. K. H. Valia and Y. W. Chien, Long-term skin permeation kinetics of estradiol: (II) Kinetics of skin uptake, binding and metabolism, *Drug Dev. Ind. Pharm. 10*, 991 (1984).
17. W. R. Good; Transderm-Nitro: Controlled delivery of nitroglycerin via the transdermal route, *Drug Dev. Ind. Pharm. 9*, 647 (1983).
18. A. Gerardin, J. Hirtz, P. Fankhauser, and J. Moppert, Achievement of sustained plasma concentrations of nitroglycerin (TNG) in man by a transdermal therapeutic system. In, *APhA/APS 31st National Meeting Abstracts, 11* (2), 84 (1981).

19. J. E. Shaw, Pharmacokinetics of nitroglycerin and clonidine delivered by the transdermal route, *Am. Heart J. 108*, 217 (1984).
20. M. A. Weber and J. I. M. Drayer, Clinical experience with rate-controlled delivery of antihypertensive therapy by a transdermal system, *Am. Heart J. 108*, 231 (1984).
21. D. Arndts and K. Arndts, Pharmacokinetics and pharmacodyamics of transdermally administered clonidine, *Eur. J. Clin. Pharmacol. 26*, 79 (1984).
22. S. Hwang, E. Owada, L. Suhardja, N. F. H. Ho, G. L. Flynn, and W. I. Higuchi, Systems approach to vaginal delivery of drugs V: *In situ* vaginal absorption of 1-alkanoic acids, *J. Pharm. Sci. 66*, 781 (1977).
23. L. Schenkel, J. Balestra, L. Schmitt, and J. Shaw, Transdermal oestrogen substitution in the menopause. In, *Second International Conference on Drug Absorption—Rate Control in Drug Therapy*, University of Edinburgh, Edinburgh, Scotland, September 21–23, 1983, p. 41.
24. L. R. Laufer, J. L. De Fazio, J. K. H. Lu, D. R. Meldrum, P. Eggena, M. P. Sambhi, J. M. Hershman, and H. L. Judd, Estrogen replacement therapy by transdermal estradiol administration, *Am. J. Obstet. Gyncol. 146*, 533 (1983).
25. T. J. Roseman, R. M. Bennett, J. J. Biermacher, M. E. Tuttle, and C. H. Spilman, Design criteria for carbopost methyl controlled release devices. In, *Proceedings of 11th International Symposium on Controlled Release of Bioactive Materials* (W. E. Meyers and R. L. Dunn, Eds.), Ft. Lauderdale, FL, 1984, p. 50.
26. Y. W. Chien, *Novel Drug Delivery Systems*, Marcel Dekker, Inc., New York, 1982, Chap. 9.
27. A. D. Keith, Polymer matrix considerations for transdermal devices, *Drug Dev. Ind. Pharm. 9*, 605 (1983).
28. Y. W. Chien and H. J. Lambert, Microsealed pharmaceutical delivery devices, U.S. patent #3,946,106 (March 23, 1976).
29. Y. W. Chien and H. J. Lambert, Method for making a microsealed delivery device, U.S. patent #3,992,518 (November 16, 1976).
30. Y. W. Chien and H. J. Lambert, Microsealed pharmaceutical delivery device, U.S. patent #4,053,580 (October 11, 1977).
31. A. Karim, Transdermal absorption: A unique opportunity for constant delivery of nitroglycerin, *Drug Dev. Ind. Pharm. 9*, 671 (1983).
32. Y. W. Chien, Microsealed drug delivery systems: Theoretical aspects and biomedical assessments. In, *International Symposium on Recent Advances in Drug Delivery Systems* (J. M. Anderson and S. W. Kim, Eds.), Plenum, New York, 1984, p. 367.
33. Y. W. Chien, Long-term controlled navel administration of testosterone, *J. Pharm. Sci. 73*, 1064 (1984).

34. S. J. Davidson, L. D. Nichols, A. S. Obermayer, M. B. Allen, E. J. Murphy, and R. N. Hurd, Developing a controlled release dual-antibiotic wound dressing. In, *Proceedings of 11th International Symposium on Controlled Release of Bioactive Materials* (W. E. Meyers and R. L. Dunn, Eds.), Ft. Lauderdale, FL, 1984, pp. 58, 60.
35. A. C. Humes, A hydrophilic polymeric reservoir for transdermal drug delivery. In, *APhA/APS Midwest Regional Meeting Abstract*, April 2, 1984, Chicago, IL, p. 4.
36. H. Durrheim, G. L. Flynn, W. I. Higuchi, and C. R. Behl, Permeation of hairless mouse skin I: Experimental methods and comparison with human epidermal permeation by alkanols, *J. Pharm. Sci. 69*, 781 (1980).
37. Y. W. Chien, P. R. Keshary, Y. C. Huang, and P. P. Sarpotdar, Comparative controlled skin permeation of nitroglycerin from marketed transdermal delivery systems, *J. Pharm. Sci. 72*, 968 (1983).
38. K. Tojo, M. Ghannam, Y. Sun, and Y. W. Chien, Intrinsic rates of permeation and release through polymeric drug delivery systems. In, *APS/APhA 37th National Meeting Abstracts*, vol. 14, No. 2, 1984, p. 193.
39. D. E. Magnuson, personal communication, 1983.
40. Y. W. Chien, Pharmaceutical considerations of transdermal nitroglycerin delivery: The various approaches, *Am. Heart J. 108*, 207 (1984).
41. J. E. Shaw, S. K. Chandrasekaran, A. S. Michaels, and L. Taskovich, Controlled transdermal delivery, *in vitro* and *in vivo*. In, *Animal Models in Dermatology* (H. Maibach, Ed.), Churchill Livingston, Edinburgh, 1975, Chap. 14.
42. P. W. Armstrong, J. A. Armstrong, and G. S. Marks, Blood levels after sublingual nitroglycerin, *Circulation 59*, 585 (1979).
43. A. S. Michaels, S. K. Chandrasekaran, and J. E. Shaw, Drug permeation through human skin: Theory and *in vitro* experimental measurement, *AICHE J.*, *21*, 985 (1975).
44. Dr. A. D. Keith, personal communication 1983.
45. P. R. Keshary, Y. C. Huang, and Y. W. Chien, Mechanism of transdermal controlled nitroglycerin administration: (III) Control of skin permeation rate and optimization, *Drug Dev. Ind. Pharm.*, *11*, 1213 (1985).

III

Biochemical and Molecular Biology Approaches to Controlled Drug Delivery

13

Microparticulate Drug Carriers: Liposomes, Microspheres, and Cells

RUDY L. JULIANO / University of Texas Medical School, Houston, Texas

I. INTRODUCTION

The behavior of drugs *in vivo* can often be changed in dramatic fashion by coupling the drug to a carrier moiety. The plasma clearance kinetics, tissue distribution, metabolism and cellular interactions of the drug will be dictated, or at least strongly influenced, by the behavior of the carrier. In some cases, judicious exploitation of these changes in pharmacodynamic behavior can lead to an enhanced therapeutic index for the drug. However, an intelligent approach to therapeutics using drug-carrier technology requires a detailed understanding of the interaction of the carrier with critical cellular and organ systems.

A variety of agents have been used as drug carriers. These include immunoglobulins [1,2], serum proteins [3], synthetic polymers [4,5], lipid vesicles [6], microspheres composed of proteins, polysaccharides, or other macromolecules [7], and even cells, most commonly the erythrocyte [8]. In this chapter we will exclude consideration of drug-antibody conjugates and of drugs coupled to macromolecules or small polymers [9,10]. This topic has been extensively reviewed elsewhere [11] and is the subject of Chapter 15. Thus, we are excluding from consideration drug carriers of molecular weight less than about 1,000,000 daltons. We are also excluding consideration of what is often termed "microcapsules" or "microparticles" in the pharmaceutical literature (see 12 for example); these particles, which are mainly for oral controlled release preparations or for *ex vivo* use, are usually many tens to hundreds of microns in diameter and are thus not "micro" in terms of this review. Rather we will concentrate on several types of drug carriers including liposomes, protein microspheres and cells, which are used systemically and which range in diameter from about 250 angstroms (25 nm) to 10 microns (10,000 nm). As we will see, despite their diverse chemical and physical characteristics, these microparticulate drug carriers shown very similar *in vivo* behavior and are acted upon by the same biological constraints. Thus, in considering the development of microparticulate drug-carrier systems, it is necessary to explore in detail not only the chemical and physical characteristics of the carrier, but its biological behavior as well.

II. PREPARATION OF DRUG CONTAINING MICROPARTICULATES

A. Liposomes

When phospholipids are dispersed in water they spontaneously form closed structures with internal aqueous compartments bounded by phospholipid bilayer membranes [14]; these structures are called liposomes. A large variety of amphiphilic compounds can be used in conjunction with glycerophospholipids to make liposomes, including sterols (e.g. cholesterol), sphingolipids, glycolipids, long-chain fatty acids and even membrane proteins [6,15]. Lyso-phospholipids and even detergents can be accomodated in small quantities, but larger amounts will disrupt the liposome structure. Recently, a number of workers have prepared phospholipid analogs capable of undergoing polymerization reactions [16], which can be used to form liposomes and which provide some unusual properties [17]. Nonphospholipid compounds including sterol esters and even certain amphililic polymers [18] can form vesicle structures which resemble phospholipid liposomes. Thus, a wide variety of amphiphilic substances can be used in the formulation of liposomes. The choice of chemical constitutents will, of course, influence the charge, stability, chemical reactivity and biological properties of the liposomal preparation.

The simplest technique for preparing drug containing liposomes involves drying a solution of lipids in an organic solvent on to the wall of a flask or tube; the lipid is then hydrated and dispersed by adding buffer and vortexing. Drug to be incorporated into the liposomes can be included in the buffer if it is water soluble, or included in the organic solvent if it is hydrophobic. A fraction of the water soluble drug will be trapped in the internal aqueous compartment of the liposome; hydrophobic drugs dissolve in the lipid phase and actually become part of the liposome membrane [19]. Free and liposome bound drug can then be separated by gel filtration chromatography (e.g., a short column of Sephadex G50). The liposomes formed in this manner are heterogeneous in size (about 0.1–3 microns) and have several concentric layers of membranes (and are thus called MLVs-multi-lamellar vesicles). Liposomes of this type entrap or encapsulate only a small fraction (up to 5%) of the available aqueous volume and thus of the available water soluble drug. The amount of lipid soluble (hydrophobic) drug entrapped depends only on the amount of lipid and on the degree of drug induced destabilization of the liposome which can be tolerated—a practical upper limit is usually about 10 mol% drug [19,20]. A large variety of drugs have been successfully incorporated into liposomes (see 15 for a comprehensive review); antitumor drugs, polyene antibiotics, antibacterial drugs and antiparasitic agents have all been studied in the liposomal format.

Over the last ten years a large number of refinements of the basic technique of liposome preparation have been introduced (for review see Refs. 21,22). Most of these refinements have had one of two goals: either to increase the size uniformity of the liposome preparation, or to increase the fraction of drug which is entrapped in the liposomes. Thus some workers have used sonication or solvent dilution techniques to prepare SUVs (small unilamellar vesicles) with diameters in the 300–500-angstrom range which are very uniform in size. Unfortunately these preparations are very inefficient in trapping water soluble compounds. Other groups have prepared LUVs (large unilamellar vesicles) of about 1 micron diameter using reverse emulsion techniques or other approaches; these vesicles are extremely efficient in terms of trapping water soluble drug (up to 40–60% entrapment) but seem to be somewhat less stable than other vesicle types. A simple method for increasing the size homogeneity of liposomes involves passing them through straight-channel polycarbonate filters; this process produces a population of vesicles whose mean diameter centers around the channel diameter. Thus a variety of vesicle preparation technologies are available and different approaches may be suitable for different applications.

There has been considerable concern about the problem of lack of stability of drug containing liposomes during prolonged storage *in vitro* [23]. However, the problem of liposome stability seems to have been solved to a fair degree. For example, in our hands a liposomal preparation of amphotericin B (a lipophilic drug) retained its physical, chemical and therapeutic properties during 9 months of storage at 4°. Liposomes containing water-soluble drugs have also proven stable during prolonged (1 yr) periods of storage at refrigerator temperatures (M. Ostro, personal communication). In general, liposomes containing cholesterol and/or composed of long chain saturated lipids are highly stable, while use of sphingomyelin rather than phosphatidylcholine has also been reported to increase stability [24]. Details of liposome preparations and their physical and chemical properties can be found in several excellent reviews of these topics [15,21,22,24].

B. Microspheres

There has been considerable interest of late in using protein or polymer based microspheres as drug carriers (for reviews see Refs. 7, 26). We shall consider particles ranging between 100 nm and a micron or so as microspheres (the smaller ones are also sometimes termed "nanoparticles"). Two basic methods of microsphere preparation have been described. One approach involves coacervation of a protein solution and subsequent desolvation and hardening of the colloidal particles formed [25]. A more widely used approach involves a phase separation emulsion technique. Here a protein or polymer in water is emulsified by sonication into an organic phase. The polymeric particles are chemically crosslinked or hardened by heat treatment and the residual organic phase is removed. Water soluble drug molecules can be incorporated into the microspheres by including them in the polymer solution. Up to 10% w/w drug can sometimes be trapped in the microparticles in this way [7,26]. This general approach has been used to make albumin or gelatin microspheres [27], protein microspheres coated with polymers [28], acrylic microspheres containing immobilized protein [29,30], magnetically "steerable" protein microspheres containing magnetite [31], and even hemoglobin microspheres which retain useful oxygen transport characteristics [32]. In contrast to the case of liposomes, there has been little concern about the *in vitro* stability properties of protein or polymer microspheres; they can be dried or lyophilized and thus should be reasonably stable during prolonged storage. Microspheres can also be made from substances which undergo controlled bioerosion and thus have sustained release capability [33].

C. Cells

A decade ago Ihler et al. [34] and Zimmermann [35] independently suggested that resealed erythrocytes might be used as drug carriers. There are several intriguing potential advantages in using one of the body's own cell types as a drug delivery system. Thus, autologous red cells are non-immunogenic and fully biocompatible. Carefully prepared resealed erythrocyte preparations can have long circulation times (days) [36,37] and thus serve as circulating drug depots. Finally, the relatively large internal volume of red cells, compared to other microparticulate carriers, can allow large amounts of drug to be carried. Recent work on the use of resealed erythrocytes as carriers has been ably reviewed by Dale [38], by Humphreys and Ihler [39], and by Ihler [8].

There are two basic procedures for loading of drugs into red cells. One approach, developed by Zimmerman, involves the lysis of the cells by an intense electric field [40], followed by resealing of the membrane by incubation at 37°. When this is done in the presence of drug, a fraction of the drug becomes entrapped within the cells. Recently, a machine for cell lysis based on the Zimmerman effect has become available commercially. The other major procedure involves exposure of the cells to hypotonic buffers; the cells then swell until they reach approximately 1.6 times their original volume. At this point, pores or channels of about 2–500 Å diameter appear in the membrane, thus allowing equilibration of intracellular and extracellular spaces [41]. Upon restoration of isotonicity and incubation at 37° in the presence of divalent cation, the pores reseal

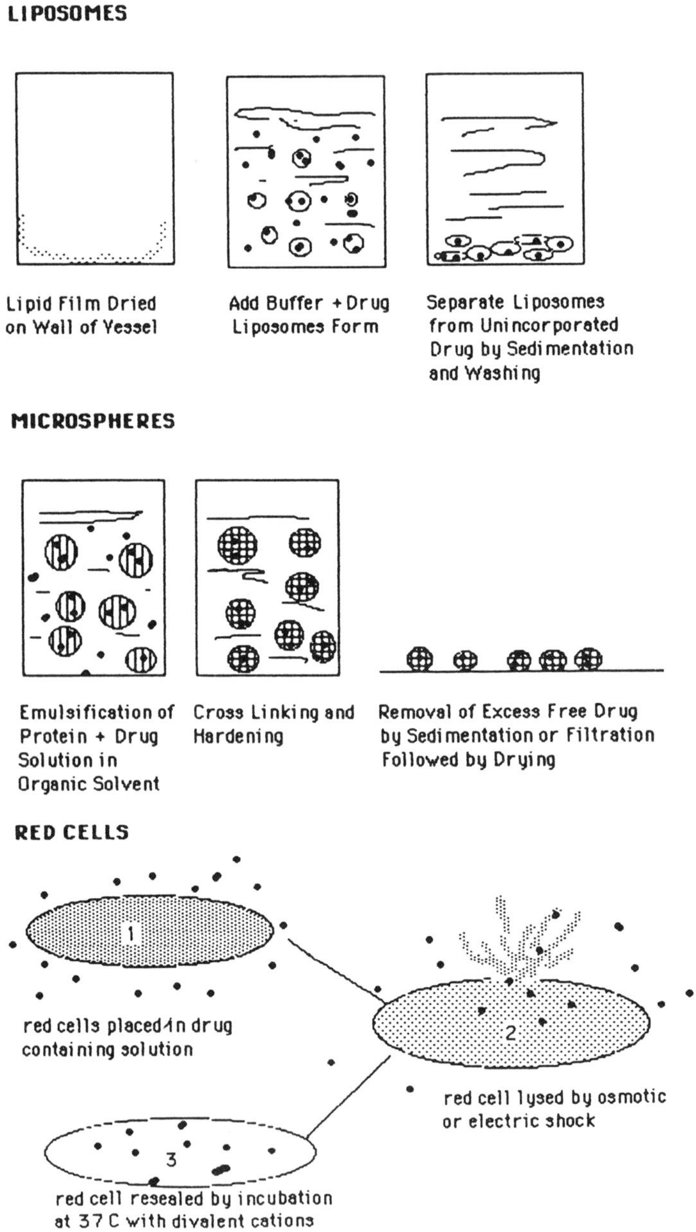

Fig. 1 Strategies for preparing various microparticulate drug carriers.

leaving a portion of the external solute (e.g. drug molecules) trapped within the red cell. Various types of hypotonic lysis procedures have been analysed in detail by Fiddler et al. [42]. Both drugs and macromolecules such as enzymes and DNA have been entrapped in red cells by these procedures.

The biological characteristics of resealed erythrocyte carriers are very sensitive to the method and degree of care in the preparation procedure. Small changes in red cell biochemistry such as cleavage of a few sialic acid residues from cell surface glycoproteins [43], increased membrane rigidity [44], oxidation of membrane sulfhydryl groups [45], or exposure of cryptic phosphatidylserine residues [46], can reduce the circulation lifetime of resealed red cells from days to minutes. Another problem with this approach to drug carrier technology is that erythrocytes are inherently unstable *in vitro* even under the best conditions, such as those used in blood banking. Thus, the normal storage time for red cells used for transfusion is about three weeks; partially damaged resealed erythrocytes would probably have a much shorter shelf life.

Strategies for preparing various microparticulate drug carriers are summarized in Figure 1.

III. *IN VIVO* BARRIERS TO MICROPARTICULATE DISTRIBUTION

The ultimate pharmacological target of a drug containing microparticulate preparation will be a receptor, enzyme, or other macromolecule in a cell which in turn lies within a tissue. Generally, microparticulate drug carriers are injected into the systemic circulation (although other routes are sometimes used) and must find their way from the bloodstream to the target site. There are a number of barriers which constrain the *in vivo* distribution and kinetic behavior of injected microparticles. Generally, these barriers are the same or at least similar for liposomes, protein microparticles, and modified cells. In order for a therapeutic strategy which utilizes microparticulate carriers to be successful, it must take into account the existence of these various barriers. Avoiding or overcoming these barriers is, as we shall see, a rather daunting problem at present; thus only therapeutic approaches which are consistent with the constraints imposed by these *in vivo* barriers will have a high probability of success. We will discuss in turn three of the major barriers or restraints on the *in vivo* distribution of drug bearing microparticulates. These are (a) the endothelial barrier of the vasculature; (b) the phagocytic cells of the reticuloendothelial system, and finally (c) the barrier represented by the complex compartmentalized organization of cells themselves.

A. The Endothelial Barrier

The lumen of the vasculature is circumscribed by a layer of endothelial cells which demarcate the vascular and extravascular (tissue) compartments and which regulate the flow of solutes, including macromolecules and microparticles, between these compartments. Most solute exchange takes place at the capillary endothelium, rather than in the larger blood vessels. The surface area of the systemic capillary bed is enormous; for example, in man it has been estimated to be about 60 M^2 [47]. The nature of the capillary endothelium differs in different tissues. In liver and spleen sinusoidal vessels, both the endothelial cell layer and the underlying basement membrane are "fenestrated" in that they have small gaps or openings [48]. An endothelium of this type will thus allow the egress of small microparticles (diameter 1000 Å) into the tissue spaces of these organs. Another type of capillary endothelium is found in the renal glomerulus and in some glandular tissues. Here a thin cellular layer is penetrated by transverse openings of about 600–800 Å with an underlying continuous basement membrane. The most common capillary barrier (found in skeletal and cardiac muscle and in a variety of other tissues) is a continuous endothelium where the cells closely abut one upon another, are joined by tight occluding junctions and are subtended by a continuous basement membrane of 200–500 Å thickness.

Although the cellular lining of a continuous type capillary will clearly prevent the egress of particles with a diameter in excess of 1000 Å, it is also clear that macromolecules of more modest dimensions can cross this barrier. For a number of years a debate has proceeded between proponents of the "pore" theory of transcapillary transport and proponents of the "plasmalemmal vesicle" theory [48–50]. Most recent evidence supports the view that macromolecules cross the capillary endothelial cell layer by riding in a system of vesicles which engulf fluid and solutes on the intimal side of the capillary and release their contents on the tissue side [47]. Using electron microscopic tracer techniques, investigators have shown that macromolecules ranging in size from cytochrome C (30 Å) to ferritin or glycogen (300 Å) cross the endothelial cell enclosed within endosomal vesicles via a process that has been called "transcytosis." One should also keep in mind the fact that macromolecules which have moved across the endothelial cell will still have restricted diffusion because of the presence of the basement membrane layer which subtends these cells [51].

In summary then, while macromolecules up to a diameter of several hundred angstoms can cross the capillary endothelial barrier by "transcytosis", larger particles such as liposomes, most microspheres, and drug laden cells will be excluded from the trancytosis vesicles. Thus these microparticulate carriers will either remain impacted upon the luminal side of the capillary endothelium, or may exit from the circulation in specialized (fenestrated) sites such as the sinusoidal vessels of liver and spleen. The relationship between molecular or particle size and the permeation characteristics of the circulatory vessels has been nicely summarized by Poste and Kirsh [52].

B. The Reticuloendothelial (RE) System Barrier

The RE system is comprised of a set of mononuclear phagocytic cells. These cells originate from precursors in bone marrow, enter the blood stream as monocytes and then pass into various tissues where they differentiate into macrophages [53]. The macrophages are an essential part of the defense functions of the body. Thus they are involved in antibody production via antigen processing and presentation to T lymphocytes [54]. They are also responsible for secreting certain factors (lymphokines) which regulate the functions of lymphoid cells. Finally, macrophages are themselves effector cells for host defense since, under certain circumstances, they can acquire the ability to attack and destroy both pathogens and tumor cells [55].

A primitive but crucial function of the macrophages of the RE system is to monitor the bloodstream and to remove and engulf circulating pathogens, tissue debris and damaged macromolecules [56]. Likewise the RE system cells will very effectively capture microparticulate drug carriers and clear them from the circulation. The cells most involved with particle clearance are the macrophage-like Kupffer cells of the liver and the macrophages which border the splenic sinusoidal vessels. Scanning EM studies have revealed that the Kupffer cells actually sit astride the channels of the liver sinusoidal vessels, ideally positioned to intercept circulating particles [57].

The nonspecific phagocytic capabilities of macrophages are highly developed and these cells readily take up a variety of microparticles including liposomes [58,59], microspheres [7,30], as well as other colliodal particles [56]. In addition, macrophages possess specific, receptor mediated endocytotic mechanisms of truly awesome efficiency. Thus, most macrophages express surface receptors for the Fc domain of IgG [60,61], for complement components [62], for mannosyl/fucosyl terminated glycoproteins [63], and for fibronectin [59]. Particle uptake via these specific systems can often exceed basal uptake by a factor of 100 or more. These specific receptor mediated endocytotic systems may sometimes come into play in the clearance of circulating microparticulate drug carriers. For instance, repeated use of a drug coupled to a protein microcarrier may elecit an immune response. The antibodies formed would then bind to the microparticle and promote rapid uptake via the Fc receptor of macrophages. Highly charged anionic particles can trigger the alternate pathway of complement activation [64,65], thereby causing complement components to bind to the particle and hastening its uptake via macrophage C3 receptors. Alternatively, microparticulates may simply adsorb certain serum proteins, such as fibronectin, which can interact with macrophage receptors and thus promote particle clearance.

Red cells would seem ideal as long-lived circulating drug carriers since normal erythrocytes seem able to evade the grasp of RE system cells and remain in the circulation for long periods (120 days in man). However, slight perturbations of the red cell membrane can reduce the half-time of red cell clearance from weeks to minutes [66]. Protocols used for incorporating drugs into red cells usually involve some type of hemolysis and resealing procedure [39], which can lead to changes in membrane ridigity, loss of cell surface sialic acid residues, or exposure of cryptic surface antigens. All of these changes can lead to a marked increase in red cell uptake by macrophages and thus to a reduced circulating lifetime. Nonetheless, some of the better preparations of drug or enzyme loaded red cell carriers have circulating times similar to normal red cells [37].

In summary, an understanding of the cells of the RE system seems a prerequisite to the intelligent design of macroparticulate drug carriers. This is because the fate of such carriers will largely be determined by the phagocytic activities of the RE system cells.

C. Cellular Barriers

Drugs act at specific sites or "receptors" within cells. The task of a drug delivery system then is not so much to get a drug to a given tissue or cell type but rather to get the drug to the appropriate receptor. Recent advances in cell biology show that cells are highly organized entities, with receptors located in specific subcellular compartments, so that the cell itself represents a further barrier to controlled drug delivery. At this juncture it would not be appropriate to attempt to review the vast and rapidly growing literature on the mechanisms underlying the complex traffic of large and small molecules which occurs within cells. Some of this information and its implications for controlled drug delivery are considered elsewhere [11]. Here a few examples should suffice to illustrate the problem.

The simple fact that a drug carrier entity binds to a particular cell does not ensure that the drug will have an effect on that cell. For example, Leserman's group [67,68] has recently used monoclonal antibodies to bind liposomes containing a cytotoxic drug specifically to lymphoid tumor cells. When the antibodies were directed against certain cell surface antigens, the liposomes were internalized and the drug was able to exert its effect on the cell. On the other hand, with antibodies directed against other determinants, the liposomes were bound to the cells but not internalized and thus the drug was without effect.

Another example of this type stems from our own work with liposomal amphotericin B (AMB). This drug is ordinarily very toxic to mammalian cells because it interacts with cholesterol in the plasma membrane to form pores or channels which then leads to osmotic lysis of the cell. We have found that when AMB is incorporated in liposomes it is much less toxic to mammalian cells, even when the cells take up large quantities of liposomal drug. Thus, macrophages can internalize substantial amounts of liposomal AMB, presumably into an endosome compartment, without any appreciable cytotoxicity. The drug is within the cell but not at the critical place for an effect to occur [69].

D. Factors Affecting the Clearance and Distribution of Microparticulate Carriers

The chemical and physical characteristics of the carrier which affect its behavior *in vivo* have been studied in most detail for liposomes. It has been known for many years that both particle size and charge can affect liposome clearance kinetics. Thus, large liposomes are cleared more rapidly than small ones and negatively charged vesicles are cleared more far rapidly than neutral or positive ones [70]. The chemical composition of the liposomes, particularly with respect to stabilization of the membrane against the disrupting effects of serum lipoproteins is also an important aspect of liposome behavior [71–73]. Another important consideration is the dose or load of liposomes administered [58]. It has been known for many years that the particle clearance rate of the reticuloendothelial system is inversely related to the load of particles [56]. Thus, the fractional rate of clearance of a large dose of liposomes (or other microparticulate) is slower than for a smaller dose. One must also keep in mind changes in clearance due to possible toxicities of liposomes and other microparticles to the reticuloendothelial system, although, except for the case of sphingomyelin liposomes, the toxicities reported thus far have been rather minimal [74,75]. There have been a number of studies of the kinetic behavior of liposomes in humans; a good recent one is that of Lopez-Berestein et al. [76], which in turn references earlier studies. Other aspects of the *in vivo* behavior of liposomes have been reviewed elsewhere [11,24,77].

The literature on factors controlling the *in vivo* behavior of drug containing microspheres is currently somewhat limited, although some analyses are beginning to appear [30]. Earlier literature on particle clearance is referenced in Altura and Saba [56]. An interesting recent development is the observation that coating microspheres with certain detergents can result in a markedly prolonged circulation lifetime [78]. Nonetheless, one must keep in mind possible detergent toxicities to the reticuloendothelial system. The factors controlling the circulation lifetime of red cell carriers have been discussed in Sec. II above.

Thus, a variety of physical factors including particle size, surface charge, surface chemistry and the "load" of particle will all affect the particle clearance rate. Nonetheless, the structure of the capillary endothelium and the phagocytic capabilities of the RE cells will tend to eventually cause the accumulation of most microparticles in organs such as liver and spleen where the endothelium is fenestrated and macrophages are abundant.

IV. SELECTED EXAMPLES OF DRUG DELIVERY WITH MICROPARTICULATE CARRIERS

Liposomes, microspheres, and red cells have been used to carry a wide variety of pharmaceutical agents in a number of different therapeutic situations; thus the literature on these topics is a rather vast and oftentimes a confusing one. We will confine ourselves to a discussion of certain applications where the characteristics of the carrier system seem very well matched to the intended therapeutic application. Some likely applications of microparticulate drug carriers are summarized in Table 1.

A. Liposomal Immunomodulators

As mentioned above, lipid vesicles are avidly taken up by macrophages and consequently are an excellent means for the relatively selective delivery of drug to these cells [6,79,80]. The macrophage is a multifunctional cell with many important roles in the host-defense system [54,55]. Among these functions is the ability, upon appropriate stimulation, to attack and destroy tumor cells. This aspect of macrophage behavior seems to be vital to the control of metastatic spread of tumors [81]. Macrophages can be stimulated *in vitro* to tumoricidal competence by a variety of immunomodulating factors including lymphokines such as MAF, double stranded polynucleotides, and by products or analogs of bacterial cell wall structures, such as lipopolysaccharide (LPS) and muramyl dipeptide (MDP). All of these agents, however, have proven to be unsuitable for *in vivo* stimulation of macrophage function either because of inherent toxicities or because of low potency due to rapid degradation and/or excretion.

Recognizing these problems, Fidler, Poste, and their colleagues began to explore the use of liposome encapsulated immunomodulators, both *in vitro* and *in vivo* [82–84]. Among the highlights of these studies are the following observations: (a) incorporation of lymphokines or of MDP into liposomes can increase the potency of the agent in stimulating macrophage tumoricidal function *in vitro* by 2–4 orders of magnitude; (b) liposomal MDP and lymphokines seem to act synergistically when used together; (c) administration of liposomal MDP or

Table 1 Likely Applications of Microparticulate Drug Carriers

Type of Carrier	Therapeutic problem	Ref.
Liposomes	Control of tumor metastases by immuno stimulation	83,84,89,90
Liposomes	Reduction of toxicity of anti tumor drugs	99–101,104
Liposomes	Therapy of intracellular pathogens	108–110,113,114
Liposomes	Therapy of systemic fungal infections	115,116
Microspheres	Localized therapy of tumors	123,7
Microspheres	Systemic therapy of tumors	120
Red cells	Enzyme replacement therapy of genetic disease	128

lymphokine can protect mice against the metastatic spread of tumors such as B16 melanoma; and (d) the therapeutic effects seem to be largely due to actions mediated via macrophages, rather than via other cells of the immune system [81].

Recently, a number of other workers have extended these studies in various directions. For example, the effects of liposomal MDP on the activation of various biochemical parameters correlated with macrophage cytotoxic functions have been studied [85,86]. Other agents such as poly I:C [87] and C-reactive protein [88] have also been shown to cause macrophage activation when incorporated into liposomes. Liposomes containing the C-reactive protein have also been able to inhibit the spread of metastatic disease in murine fibrosarcomas and adenocarcinomas [89,90]. Finally, the strategy of liposomal activation of macrophage function has also been applied to the problem of macrophage defenses against herpes virus infection [91].

Based on this rapidly growing assemblage of observations, it seems clear that liposomes can provide a useful means of delivering immunomodulating agents to macrophages. This will certainly have many important ramifications in enhancing host responses to neoplastic and viral diseases.

B. Reduction of Toxicity of Antitumor Drugs Using Liposomes

Some years ago, liposomes were hailed as a major new opportunity for refining cancer chemotherapy. This enthusiasm was generated primarily by the notion that one might be able to use liposomes to "target" drugs to tumors. Although some success has been claimed in certain specialized instances, such as blood borne neoplasms [92], the overall history of liposome enhanced therapy of solid tumors has been rather dismal [93,94]. Part of this is due to the fact that most early investigators had little appreciation of the multiple barriers lying between a drug-liposome complex in the circulation and the ultimate site of action of that complex in a solid neoplasm. As discussed earlier, the functions of the capillary endothelium and the reticuloendothelial system, as well as the properties of most tumor cells, which are nonphagocytic, would tend to prevent selective delivery of liposomal drugs to solid neoplasms, irrespective of whether one uses conventional liposomes or liposomes coupled with the most exquistely precise monoclonal antibody.

This does not imply that the use of lipid vesicles in tumor therapy is a senseless undertaking, only that the attainable goals may be somewhat more limited than once anticipated. For example, a modest but quite valuable application of lipid vesicle technology in the chemotherapy arena concerns the use of liposomes to reduce the toxicity of a number of lipophilic antitumor drugs. Several workers have experimented with use of hydrophobic drugs in liposomes, including alkylating agents [95–97], anti-mitotic agents [98] and, most importantly, anthracyclines such as doxorubicin [99–101].

Quite compelling evidence has now accumulated showing that liposomal encapsulation of doxorubicin can reduce its dose-limiting toxicity to the myocardium without loss of antitumor potency [100,102]. Reduced toxicity to the skin has also been reported [103]. The mechanisms underlying these results are somewhat obscure; low uptake of the drug by the myocardium may be involved [101,104]. However, a number of other changes may also be implicated, including a reduction in immunosuppressive actions [105] and enhanced tumoricidal effects in certain organs such as the liver [106]. Another possibility is an enhancement of the membrane directed actions of doxorubicin [107]. In any case, the considerable improvement in the therapeutic index of this important drug deserves further study and development, and may serve as a model for use of other amphipathic antitumor drugs in a liposomal format.

C. Liposomes in the Therapy of Obligate and Facultative Intracellular Pathogens

A number of important pathogens including *Brucella, Salmonella,* mycobacteria, *Rickettsia, Chlamydia*, various fungi, and many protozooans, spend at least part of their time within the intracellular environment, oftentimes within macrophages [80]. Many commonly used antimicrobial drugs are rather effectively excluded from mamalian cells (e.g., aminoglycosides), complicating the treatment of intracellular pathogens. Therefore, the idea of using liposomes to convey antimicrobial agents to the intracellular (endosomal) compartment of macrophages is a sensible and natural outgrowth of our understanding of liposome behavior *in vivo*.

This was first done, almost simultaneously by three laboratories, in connection with therapy of leishmaniasis, an obligate intracellular protozoan parasitic disease common in subtropical areas [108–110]. The results were quite impressive in terms of a marked enhancement in the potency of the antimonial drugs used to treat this condition. Similar effects have also been seen with other antileishmanial agents entrapped in liposomes [111,112].

Recently, liposome encapsulated antibiotics, either used singly or in combination, have shown considerable promise as highly efficacious therapy of salmonellosis [113,114] and of brucellosis.

A somewhat similar approach, although one in which the therapeutic effects cannot be ascribed entirely to "targeting" of the drug to macrophages, concerns the use of liposomal antifungal agents, particularly amphotercin B. Systemic fungal infections are a severe problem in immunocompromised individuals, especially cancer patients. For many years, the mainstay for therapy in these cases has been the polyene antibiotic amphotericin B, a potent yet extremely toxic agent. The multiple adverse effects of amphotericin B prominently include severe nephrotoxicity as well as toxicities to the cardiovascular and central nervous systems.

Recently, it has been shown that both for cryptococcosis [115] and for candida infection [116], incorporation of amphotericin B in liposomes results in a marked reduction in toxicity with no loss of antifungal potency. These effects seem to be based primarily on a rather fundamental change in the action of amphotericin B at the cellular level. Thus, while free amphotericin B is toxic to both fungal and mammalian cells, the liposomal drug remains toxic to fungi but is no longer toxic to mammalian erythrocytes or other mammalian cells [117,118]. Interestingly, the antifungal effects of liposomal amphotericin B persist in neutropenic animals [119], indicating that a normal complement of monocytes and macrophages is not essential to the therapeutic effect. This drug-liposome combination seems highly promising and is now being pursued at the preclinical and clinical levels.

Thus the use of liposomes in the therapy of infectious diseases, especially those caused by intracellular pathogens, seems a promising area. This subject has been further reviewed by Richardson [120].

D. Antitumor Drugs in Microspheres

The use of antitumor drugs in protein or polymer microspheres affords some of the same opportunities and is restricted by the some of the same limitations as for liposomal carriers. Basically, two distinct approaches have been used in this area. In the first instance, the microspheres are injected into the general circulation and thus may be expected to behave in the same way as other circulating microparticulates; in the second instance the microspheres are administered directly to the tumorous organ by means of local intraarterial injection.

Edman and colleageus [29,120] have studied the effects of the antineoplastic enzyme asparaginase when incorporated into polyacrylamide microspheres. When given either systemically or by an intramuscular route, these preparations reduced blood asparagine levels significantly more effectively than did free asparaginase.

Kato and colleagues [121–123] have used catheterization to deliver mitomycin C containing ethylcellulose microspheres to specific organs, in particular, kidney carcinoma. The microspheres employed were rather large (200 microns) and contained up to 80% drug. Good localization of drug in the target organ was found for up to 6 hr, with relatively low systemic drug levels or systemic toxicity. This approach is apparently undergoing large-scale clinical evaluation in Japan [11].

Magnetic microspheres have also been used for antineoplastic therapy [7,26]. Use of intraarterial infusion combined with high external magnetic fields has achieved impressive levels of drug localization, and effective therapy of the Yoshida rat tumor has been obtained in this way. An obvious limitation with this approach is that it is only applicable to relatively large, easily accessible tumors that can be catheterized and subjected to localized magnetic fields. Thus, it really does not address the prime problem of antinoeplastic chemotherapy, which is the treatment of multiple occult metastases.

Tökés and colleagues have explored the use of anthracycline drugs coupled to polygluteraldehyde microspheres [124–126]. Most of this work has been with neoplastic cells in tissue culture rather than *in vivo* and thus some of the "barriers" to this type of therapy have not yet been addressed. Nonetheless, this group has reported some interesting *in vitro* effects including the ability of the conjugated drug to overcome anthracycline resistance, and perhaps most importantly, the conversion of an inactive derivative to an active agent by coupling to the microsphere carrier [126]. Presumably, the multiple repetative interactions of the drug-polymer conjugate with the cell surface produces novel opportunities for cytotoxicity.

Microspheres have not been studied as extensively as liposomes in terms of tumor therapy. Hopefully the workers in this area will learn from the early mistakes of people in the liposome field and develop a realistic assessment of the opportunties and limits of their technology.

E. Red Cells as Enzyme Carriers

Although cells have been used to carry drugs, the prime application of erythrocyte carriers has been in the area of enzyme therapy of genetic defects [8]. In particular, the therapy of storage diseases of RE system cells (e.g., Gaucher's disease) by this approach seems quite sensible. As discussed above, large quantities of enzyme can be loaded into the red cells and the cells, slightly damaged by osmotic or electric lysis, will be taken up by the RE system thus conveying enzyme to the target site. This approach and its clinical application has been discussed at length by Beutler et al. [128]. Unfortunately, the sites of pathogenesis in many other enzyme deficiency diseases are not accessible to red cells or other microparticulates. For example, in sphinogolipidoses such as Tay-Sachs disease, GMl gangliosidosis and Sandhoff disease, lipid accumulation in CNS cells is a major problem and is thus not accessible to microparticulate therapy. Thus, at the present time, at least from this reviewer's perspective, the indications for therapy with red cell carriers seem rather limited and one would suspect that carriers which are more manageable in a pharmaceutic sense, such as microparticles or liposomes, would find broader application.

V. SUMMARY

The inclusion of drugs in microparticulate carriers clearly holds significant promise for improvements in the therapy of several disease categories. One must keep in mind, however, that the behavior of all microparticulate carriers, be they liposomes, microspheres, or modified cells, will be constrained by the same set of biological barriers, the most important of these being the impermeant walls of the microvasculature and the avid phagocytic cells of the RE system. With a clear understanding of the factors which regulate the clearance, disposition and degradation of microparticulates *in vivo* , one can then begin to select appropriate disease categories and appropriate strategies for therapy. Presently, we are rapidly learning about the chemistry and biology of microparticulate carriers, and we can begin to devise some general rules. There are hints that a drug carrier complex is more than the sum of its parts and that, in some cases, novel therapeutic mechanisms may be produced by joining the drug to the carrier moiety [117,126]. This reviewer is confident that microparticle technology will take its place, along with other drug delivery technologies, in enhancing the effectiveness, convenience and general utility of new and existing drugs.

REFERENCES

1. E. S. Vitetta, K. A. Krolick, M. Miyama-lanab, W. Cushley, and J. W. Uhr, Immunotoxins: A new approach to cancer therapy, *Science 219*, 644–650 (1983).
2. D. C. Edwards, P. E. Thorpe, and A. J. S. Davies, Antibody-toxin conjugates as potential therapeutic agents, In, *Targeting of Drugs* (G. Gregoriadis, J. Senior, and A. Trouet, eds.), Plenum Press, New York, 1982, pp. 83–96.
3. M. J. Poznansky and L. G. Cleveland, Biological macromolecules as carriers of drugs and enzymes, In, *Drug Delivery Systems* (R. Juliano, ed.), Oxford University Press, New York, 1980, pp. 253–315.
4. Langer, R., Implantable controlled release eystems, *Pharm. Ther. 21*, 35–52 (1983).
5. Y. W. Chien, Controlled drug release from polymeric delivery system, In, *Drug Delivery Systems* (R. Juliano, ed.), Oxford Press, New York, 1980, pp. 11–63.
6. R. L. Juliano and D. Layton, Liposomes as a drug delivery system, In, *Drug Delivery Systems* (R. L. Juliano, ed.), Oxford University Press, New York, 1980, pp. 189–236.
7. K. J. Widder and A. E. Senyei, Magnetic microspheres: A vehicle for selective targeting of drugs, *Pharm. Ther. 20*:377–396 (1983).
8. G. M. Ihler, Erythrocyte carriers, *Pharm. Ther. 20*:151–170 (1983).
9. A. Abuchowski and F. F. Davies, Soluble polymer-enzyme adducts, In, *Enzymes as Drugs* (J. Holcenberg and R. Roberts, ed.), Wiley, New York, 1981, pp. 367–384.
10. L. Gros, H. Ringsdorf, and H. Schupp, Polymer antitumor agents on a molecular and on a cellular level, *Angew. Chem. Int. Ed. Engl. 20*:305–325 (1981).
11. M. S. Poznansky and R. L. Juliano, Biological approaches to the controlled delivery of drugs: A critical review, *Pharm. Rev. 36*:277–336 (1984).
12. P. Rambourg, J. Levy, and M. C. Levy, Preparation of invertase microcapsules, *J. Pharm. Sci. 71*:753–60 (1982).
13. T. M. S. Chang and N. Malave, The development and first clinical use of semipermeable microcapsules (artificial cells) as a compact artificial kidney, *Trans. Am. Soc. Artif. Intern. Organs 16*:141–148 (1970).
14. A. D. Bangham, Liposomes, *Ann. Rev. Biochem. 41*:753 (1972).
15. R. L. Juliano, Interactions of proteins and drugs with liposomes, In, *Liposomes*, (M. Ostro, ed.), Marcel Dekker, New York, 1983, pp. 53–86.
16. S. L. Regen, Polymerizable lipids, *Ann. NY Acad. Sci.* (in press).

17. R. L. Juliano, S. L. Regen, M. Singh, M. J. Hsu, and A. Singh, Stability properties of photopolymerized liposomes, *Biotechnology 1*:882–885 (1983).
18. J. Fendler and H. Tundo, Polymerized surfactants, *Acc. Chem. Res. 17*:3 (1984).
19. R. L. Juliano and D. Stamp, Interactions of drugs with lipid membranes, *Biochim. Biophys. Acta 586*:137–145 (1979).
20. A. G. Lee, Effects of charged drugs on the phase transition temperature of phospholipid bilayers, *Biochim. Biophys. Acta 514*:95–104 (1978).
21. F. Szoka, Jr. and D. Papahadjopoulos, Comparative properties and methods in preparation of lipid vesicles (liposomes), *Ann. Rev. Biophys. Bioeng. 9*:467–508 (1980).
22. D. W. Deamer and P. S. Uster, Liposome preparation: Methods and mechanism, In, *Liposomes* (M. Ostro, ed.), Marcel Dekker, New York, 1982, pp. 27–51.
23. F. J. T. Fildes, Liposomes, the industrial viewpoint, In, *Liposomes: Physical Structure to Therapeutic Applications* (G. Knight, ed.), Elsevier, Amsterdam, 1981, pp. 465–485.
24. G. Gregoriadis, C. Kirby, and J. Senior, Optimization of liposome behavior *in vivo*, *Biol. Cell 47*:11–18 (1983).
25. R. C. Oppenheim, Nanoparticles, in *Drug Delivery Systems* (R. Juliano, ed.), Oxford University Press, New York, 1980, pp. 177–188.
26. K. J. Widder, A. E. Senyei, and B. Sears, Experimental methods in cancer therapeutics, *J. Pharm. Sci. 71*:379–387 (1982).
27. P. A. Kramer, Albumin microspheres are vehicles for achieving specificity in drug deliveries, *J. Pharm. Sci. 63*:646–647 (1974).
28. W. E. Long, H. Iwata, T. A. Lindheimer, and E. P. Goldberg, Preparation of hydrophilic albumin microspheres using polymeric dispersing agents, *J. Pharm. Sci. 71*:1323–1328 (1982).
29. P. Edman and I. Sjoholm, Acrylic microspheres *in vivo*. VI: Antitumor effect of microparticles with immobilized *L-asparaginase* against 6C3HED lymphoma, *J. Pharm. Sci. 72*:654–658 (1983).
30. P. Arturson, T. Laskso, and P. Edman, Acrylic microspheres *In vivo*. IX: Blood elimination kinetics and organ distribution of microparticles with different surface characteristics, *J. Pharm. Sci. 72*:1415–1420 (1983).
31. K. Widder, G. Floret, C., and A. Senyei, A.: Magnetic microspheres: synthesis of a novel parenteral drug carrier, *J. Pharm. Sci. 68*:79–83 (1979).
32. M. C., Levy, P. Rambourg, J. Levy, and G. Ptron, Microencapsulation. IV: cross-linked hemoglobin microcapsules, *J. Pharm. Sci. 71*:759–762 (1982).
33. J. Heller, R. F. Helwing, R. W. Baker, and M. E. Tuttle, Controlled release of water-soluble macromolecules from bioerodible hydrogels, *Biomaterials 4*:262–266 (1983).

34. G. Ihler, R. H. Glen, and F. W. Schnure, Enzyme loading of erythrocytes, *Proc. Natl. Acad. Sci. USA 70*:2663–2666 (1973).
35. U. Zimmermann, *Jahresbericht der Kernforschungsanlage*, Julich GmbH, 1973, pp. 55–58.
36. S. J. Updike, R. T. Wakamija, and E. N. Lightfoot, Asparaginase entrapped in red blood cells: Action and survival, *Science 193*:681–683 (1976).
37. K. Kinosita and T. Y. Tsung, Survival of sucrose loaded erythrocytes in the circulation, *Nature 272*:258–260 (1978).
38. G. Dale, Resealed erythrocytes as drug carriers, In, *Drug Delivery Systems* (R. Juliano, ed.), Oxford University Press, New York, 1980, pp. 237–252.
39. J. D. Humphreys and G. M. Ihler, Encapsulation of drugs, enzymes and DNA within human and mouse erythrocytes, In, *Optimization of Drug Delivery*, Alfred Benzon Symposium 17 (H. Bundgaard, A. B. Hansen, and H. Kofod, eds.), Munksgaard, Copenhagen, 1982, pp. 270–284.
40. U. Zimmerman, G. Pilwat, and B. Esser, The effect of encapsulation in red blood cells on the distribution of methotrexate in mice, *J. Clin. Chem. Clin. Biochem. 16*:135–147 (1978).
41. P. Seeman, Transient holes in the erythrocyte membrane during hypotonic hemolysis and stable holes in the membrane after lysis by saponin and lysolecithin, *J. Cell Biol. 32*:55–70 (1967).
42. M. B. Fiddler, L. D. S. Hudson, J. G. White, and R. J. Desnick, Comparison of methods for enzyme entrapment in human erythrocytes, *J. Clin. Lab Med. 96*:307–317 (1980).
43. J. P. Durocher, R. D. Payne, and M. E. Conrad, Role of sialic acid in erythrocyte survival, *Blood 45*:11–20 (1975).
44. F. Kirkpatrick, Spectrin: Current understanding of its physical, biochemical and functional properties, *Life Sci. 19*:1–18 (1976).
45. C. W. M. Haest, G. Plasa, D. Kamp, and B. Deuticke, Intra and intermolecular crosslinking of membrane proteins in intact erythrocytes and ghosts by SH-oxidizing agents, *Biochim. Biophys. Acta 469*:226–230 (1977).
46. A. J. Schroit and I. J. Fidler, Effects of liposome structure and lipid composition on the activation of the tumoricidal properties of macrophages, *Cancer Res. 42*:161–167 (1982).
47. N. Simionescu and M. Simionescu, The cardiovascular system, In, *Histology* (L. Weiss, ed.), Elsevier, New York, 1983, pp. 371–433.
48. N. Freudenberg, K. H. Riese, and M. A. Freudenberg, *The Vascular Endothelial System*, Gustav Fisher, Stuttgart, 1983.
49. M. Bundgaard, Transport pathways in capillaries. In search of pores, *Ann. Rev. Physiol. 42*:325–335 (1980).
50. C. C. Michel, Filtration coefficients and osmotic reflection coefficients of the walls of single mesenteric capillaries, *J. Physiol. 309*:341–355 (1980).

51. A. Martinez-Hernandez, The basement membrane in the microvasculature, In, *Microcirculation* (R. Effros, H. Schmid-Shonben, and J. Ditzel, eds.), Academic Press, New York, 1981, pp. 125–146.
52. G. Poste and R. Kirsh, Site specific drug delivery in cancer therapy, *Biotechnology 1*:869–878 (1983).
53. C. Meuret, Kinetics of mononuclear phagocytes in man, *Hematol. Bluttransfus. 27*:11–122 (1981).
54. E. Unanue, Regulatory role of macrophages in antigenic stimulation, *Adv. Immunol. 31*:1–121 (1981).
55. D. O. Adams, Macrophage activation and secretion, *Fed. Proc. 41*:2193–2197 (1982).
56. B. M. Altura and T. M. Saba, *Pathophysiology of the Reticuloendothelial System*, Raven Press, New York, 1981.
57. D. L. Knook and E. Wisse, *Sinusoidal Liver Cells*, Elsevier, Amsterdam 1982.
58. Y. J. Kao and R. L. Juliano, Interaction of liposomes with the reticuloendothelial system: Effects of blockade on the clearance of large unilamellar vesicles, *Biochim. Biophys. Acta 677*:453–461 (1981).
59. M. J. Hsu and R. L. Juliano, Interaction of liposomes with the reticuloendothelial system II. Non specific and receptor mediated uptake of liposomes by mouse peritoneal macrophages, *Biochim. Biophys. Acta 720*:411–419 (1982).
60. S. C. Silverstein, R. M. Steinman, and Z. A. Cohn, Endocytosis, *Ann. Rev. Biochem. 46*:669–722 (1977).
61. R. M. Steinman, I. S. Mellman, W. A. Muller, and Z. A. Cohn, Endocytosis and the recycling of plasma membrane, *J. Cell Biol. 96*:1–27 (1983).
62. J. D. Lambris and C. D. Ross, Assay of membrane complement receptors with C3b and C3d coated fluorescent microspheres, *J. Immunol. 128*:186–191, 1982.
63. P. Stahl and S. Gordon, Expression of mannosyl fucosyl receptor function for endocytosis in cultured primary macrophages and their hybirds, *J. Cell Biol. 93*:49–54 (1982).
64. C. M. Cunningham, M, Kingzette, R. L. Richards, C. R. Alving, T. F. Lint, and H. Gewurz, Activation of human complement by liposomes: A model for membrane activation of the alternative pathway, *Immunology 122*:1237–1242 (1979).
65. A. Allison, Macrophage activation and non specific immunity, *Int. Rev. Exp. Pathol. 18*:303–346 (1978).
66. J. W. Harris and R. W. Kellermeyer, *The Red Cell*, Harvard University Press, Cambridge, MA, 1970.
67. P. Machy, J. Barbet, and L. D. Leserman, Differential endocytosis of T and B lymphocyte surface molecules evaluated with antibody-bearing fluorescent liposomes containing methotrexate, *Proc. Natl. Acad. Sci. USA 79*:4148–4152 (1982).

68. P. Machy, M. Pierres, J. Barbet, and L. D. Leserman, Drug transfer into lymphoblasts mediated by liposomes bound to distinct sites on H-2 encoded I-A, I-E, and K molecules, *J. Immunol.* *129*:2098–2101 (1982).
69. R. L. Juliano, G. Lopez-Berestein, R. Hopfer, R. Mehta, K. Mehta, and K. Mills, Selective toxicity of and enhanced therapeutic efficacy of liposomal amphotericin B, *Ann. NY Acad. Sci.* *446*:390–402 (1985).
70. R. L. Juliano and D. Stamp, Effects of particle size and charge on the clearance rates of liposomes and liposome encapsulated drugs, *Biochem. Biophys. Res. Commun.* *63*:651–658 (1975).
71. G. Gregoriadis, L. D. Kirby, P. Large, A. Meehan, and J. Senior, Targeting of liposomes: Study of influencing factors, In, *Targeting of Drugs* (C. Gregoriadis, J. Senior, and A. Trouet, eds.), Plenum Publishing Corp., New York, 1982, pp. 155–184.
72. C. F. Gotfredsen, S. Frokjaer, E. L. Hjorth, K. D. Jorgensen, and M. C. Debroux-Guisset, Disposition of intact liposomes of different compositions and of liposomal degradation products, *Biochem. Pharmacol.* *32*:3381–3387 (1983).
73. F. Roerdink, J. Regts, B. Van Leeuwen, and G. Scherphof, Intrahepatic uptake and processing of intravenously injected small unilamellar phospholipid vesicles in rats, *Biochim. Biophys. Acta* *770*:195–202 (1984).
74. I. R. Hart, W. E. Fogler, G. Poste, and I. J. Fidler, Toxicity studies of liposome encapsulated immunomodulators administered intravenously to dogs and mice, *Cancer Immunol. Immunother.* *10*:57–196 (1981).
75. T. M. Allen, L. Murray, S. MacKeigan, and M. Shah, Chronic liposome administration in mice: Effects on reticuloendothelial function and tissue distribution, *J. Pharmacol. Exp. Ther.* *229*:267–275 (1984).
76. G. Lopez-Berestein, L. Kasi, M. G. Rosenblum, T. Haynie, M. Jahns, H. Glenn, R. Mehta, G. M. Mavligit, and E. M. Hersh, Clinical pharmacology of 99mTc-labeled liposomes in patients with cancer, *Cancer Res.* *44*:375–378 (1984).
77. G. Poste, Liposome targeting *in vivo*: Problems and opportunities, *Biol. Cell* *47*:19–37 (1983).
78. L. Illum and S. S. Davies, The organ uptake of intravenously administered colloidal particles can be altered using a non-ionic surfactant (Poloxamer 388), *FEBS Lett.* *167*:79–82 (1984).
79. R. L. Juliano, Interaction of liposomes with the reticuloendothelial system: Implications for the controlled delivery of drugs, In, *Optimization of Drug Delivery* (H. Bundgaard, A. B. Hansen, and H. Kofod, eds.), Munskgaard, Copenhagen, 1981, pp. 405–415.

80. C. R. Alving, Delivery of liposome-encapsulated drugs to macrophages, *Pharmacol. Ther.* *22*:407–424 (1983).
81. I. J. Fidler and G. Poste, Macrophage-mediated destruction of malignant tumor cells and new strategies for the therapy of metastatic disease, *Spring Sem. Immunopathol.* 5:161–174 (1982).
82. G. Poste, R. Kirsh, W. E. Fogler, and I. J. Fidler, Activation of tumoricidal properties in mouse macrophages by lymphokines encapsulated in liposomes, *Cancer Res.* *39*:881–892 (1979).
83. I. J. Fidler, Therapy of spontaneous metastases by intravenous injection of liposomes containing lymphokines, *Science* *208*:1469–1471 (1980).
84. I. J. Fidler, S. Sone, W. E. Fogler, and Z. L. Barnes, Eradication of spontaneous metastases and activation of alveolar macrophages by intravenous injection of liposomes containing muramyl dipeptide, *Proc. Natl. Acad. Sci. USA* *78*:1680–1684 (1981).
84. K. Mehta, R. L. Juliano, and G. Lopez-Berestein, Stimulation of macrophage protease secretion via liposomal delivery of muramyl dipeptide derivatives to intracellular sites, *Immunology* *51*:517–527 (1984).
86. G. Lopez-Berestein, K. Mehta, R. Mehta, R. L. Juliano, and E. M. Hersh, Activation of human monocytes by liposome encapsulated muramyl dipeptide analogs, *J. Immunol.* *130*:1500–1502 (1983).
87. C. Pidgeon, R. D. Schreiber, and R. M. Schultz, Macrophage activation: Synergism between hybridoma MAF and poly I-poly C delivered by liposomes, *J. Immunol.* *131*:311–314 (1983).
88. S. D. Deodhar, S. Gautam, B. Yen Lieberman, and D. Roberts, Macrophage activation and generation of tumoricidal activity by liposome-associated human C-reactive protein, *Cancer Res.* *44*:305–310 (1984).
89. S. D. Deodhar, K. James, T. Chiang, M. Edinger, and B. P. Barna, Inhibition of lung metastases in mice bearing a malignant fibrosarcoma by treatment with liposomes containing human C-reactive protein, *Cancer Res.* *4*:5084–5088 (1982).
90. P. S. Thombre and S. D. Deodhar, Inhibition of liver metastases in murine colon adenocarcinoma by liposomes containing human C-reactive protein or crude lymphokine, *Cancer Immunol. Immunother.* *16*:145–150 (1984).
91. W. C. Koff, S. D. Showlater, D. A. Seniff, and B. Hampar, Lysis of herpes virus-infected cells by macrophages activated with free or liposome-encapsulated lymphokine produced by a murine T cell hybridoma, *Infect. Immunol.* *42*:1067–1072 (1983).
92. Y. Hashimoto, M. Sugawara, T. Musakuo, and H. Hojo, Antitumor effect of actinomycin D entrapped in liposomes bearing subunits of tumor-specific monoclonal immunoglobulin M antibody, *Cancer Res.* *43*:5328–5334 (1983).

93. S. B. Kaye, Liposomes-problems and promise as selective drug carriers, *Cancer Treat. Rev.* *8*:27–150 (1981).
94. J. N. Weinstein, Liposomes as drug carriers in cancer therapy, *Cancer Treat. Rep.* *68*:127–135 (1984).
95. J. Khato, A. A. del Campo, and S. M. Sieber, Carrier activity of sonicated small liposomes containing melphalan to regional lymph nodes of rats, *Pharmacology 26*:23–40 (1983).
96. J. W. Babbage and M. C. Berenbaum, Increased therapeutic efficiency of a lipid-soluble alkylating agent incorporated in liposomes, *Br. J. Cancer 45*:830–834 (1982).
97. P. Large and G. Gregoriadis, Phospholipid composition of small unilamellar liposomes containing melphalan influences drug action in mice bearing PC6 tumors, *Biochem. Pharmacol.* *32*:1315–1318 (1983).
97. J. Hildebrand, J. M. Ruysschaert, and C. Laduron, Antitumor activity of a water-insoluble compound entrapped in liposomes on L1210 leukemia in mice, *J. Natl. Cancer Inst.* *70*:1081–1086 (1983).
99. A. Rahman, A. Kessler, N. More, B. Sikic, G. Rowden, P. Woolley, and P. S. Schein, Liposomal protection of adriamycin-induced cardiotoxicity in mice, *Cancer Res.* *40*:1532–1537 (1980).
100. E. A. Forssen and Z. A. Tökés, Use of anionic liposomes for the reduction of chronic doxorubicin-induced cardiotoxicity, *Proc. Natl. Acad. Sci. USA 78*:1873–1877 (1981).
101. A. Gabizon, A. Dagan, D. Goren, Y. Barenholz, and Z. Fuks, Liposomes as *in vivo* carriers of adriamycin: Reduced cardiac uptake and preserved antitumor activity in mice, *Cancer Res.* *42*:4734–4739 (1982).
102. E. H. Herman, A. Rahman, V. J. Ferrans, J. A. Vick, and P. S. Schein, Prevention of chronic doxorubicin cardiotoxicity in beagles by liposomal encapsulation, *Cancer Res.* *43*:5427–5432 (1983).
103. E. A. Forssen and Z. A. Tökés, Attenuation of dermal toxicity of doxorubicin by liposome encapsulation, *Cancer Treat. Rep.* *67*:481–484 (1983).
104. R. Olson, E. Mayhew, D. Maslow, Y. Rustum, and F. Szoka, Characterization, toxicity and therapeutic efficacy of adriamycin encapsulated in liposomes, *Eur. J. Cancer Clin. Oncol.* *18*:167–176 (1982).
105. E. A. Forssen and Z. A. Tökés, Improved therapeutic benefits of doxorubicin by entrapment in anionic liposomes, *Cancer Res.* *43*:546–550 (1983).
106. A. Gabizon, D. Goren, Z. Ruks, Y. Barenholz, A. Dagan, and A. Meshorer, Enhancement of adriamycin delivery to liver metastatic cells with increased tumoricidal effect using liposomes as drug carriers, *Cancer Res.* *43*:4730–4735 (1983).

107. T. R. Tritton and G. Yee, The anticancer agent adriamycin can be actively cytotoxic without entering cells, *Science 217*: 248–250 (1982).
108. C. R. Alving, E. A. Steck, W. L. Chapman, V. B. Waits, L. D. Hendricks, G. M. Swartz, and W. L. Hanson, Therapy of leishmaniasis: superior efficacies of liposome encapsulated drugs, *Proc. Natl. Acad. Sci. USA 75*:2959–2963 (1978).
109. C. D. V. Black, C. J. Watson, and R. J. Ward, Use of pentostam liposomes in the chemotherapy of experimental leishmaniasis, *Trans. Roy. Soc. Trop. Med. Hyg. 71*:550–552 (1977).
110. R. R. C. New, M. L. Chance, S. C. Thomas, and W. Peters, Antileishmanial activity in antimonials entrapped in liposomes, *Nature 272*:55–56 (1978).
111. C. R. Alving, E. A. Steck, W. L. Chapman, Jr., V. B. Waits, L. D. Hendricks, G. M. Swartz, Jr., and W. L. Hanson, Liposomes in leishmaniasis: therapeutic effects of antimonial drugs, 8-aminoquinolines, and tetracycline, *Life Sci. 26*:2231–2238 (1980).
112. R. R. C. New, M. L. Chance, and S. Heath, Antileishmanial activity of amphotericin and other antifungal agents entrapped in liposomes, *J. Antimicrob. Chemother. 8*:371–381 (1981).
113. J. V. Desiderio and S. G. Campbell, Liposome-encapsulated cephalothin in the treatment of experimental murine salmonellosis, *J. Reticuloendothel. Soc. 34*:279–287 (1983).
114. J. V. Desiderio and S. G. Campbell, Intraphagocutic killing of *Salmonella typhimurium* by liposome-encapsulated cephalothin, *J. Infect. Dis. 148*:563–570 (1983).
115. J. R. Graybill, P. C. Craven, R. L. Taylor, D. M. Williams, and W. E. Magee, Treatment of murine cryptococcosis with liposome-associated amphotericin B, *J. Infect. Dis. 145*:748–752 (1982).
116. G. Lopez-Berestein, R. Mehta, R. L. Hopfer, K. Mills, L. Kasi, K. Mehta, V. Fainstein, M. Luna, E. M. Hersh, and R. Juliano, Treatment and prophylaxis of disseminated infection due to *Candida albicans* in mice with liposome-encapsulated amphotericin B, *J. Infect. Dis. 147*:939–945 (1983).
117. R. Mehta, G. Lopez-Berestein, R. Hopfer, K. Mills, and R. L. Juliano, Liposomal amphotericin B is toxic to fungal cells but not to mammalian cells, *Biochim. Biophys. Acta 77*:230–234 (1984).
118. R. L. Hopfer, K. Mills, R. Mehta, G. Lopez-Berestein, V. Fainstein, and R. L. Juliano, *In vitro* antifungal activities of amphotericin B and liposome encapsulated amphotericin B, *Antimicrob. Agents Chemother. 24*:387–389 (1984).
119. G. Lopez-Berestein, R. L. Hopfer, R. Mehta, K. Mehta, E. N. Hersh, and R. L. Juliano, Prophylaxis of Candida albicans

infections in neutropenic mice with liposome encapsulated amphotericin B, *Antimicrob. Agents Chemother.* *25*:366–367 (1984).
120. P. D. Edman and I. Sjoholm, Prolongation of effect and asparaginase by implantation in polyacrylaride in rats, *J. Pharm. Sci.* *70*:684–685 (1981).
121. T. Kato, R. Nemoto, H. Mori, K. Iwata, S. Sato, K. Unno, A. Goto, M. Harada, M. Homma, M. Okada, and T. Minowa, An approach to magnetically controlled cancer chemotherapy. III. Magnetic control of ferromagnetic mitomycin C microcapsules in the artery, *J. Jpn. Soc. Cancer Ther.* *15*:28–32 (1980).
122. T. Kato, R. Nemoto, H. Mori, and I. Kumagai, Sustained-release properties, of microencapsulated mitomycin C with ethylcellulose infused into the renal artery of the dog, *Cancer* *46*:14–21 (1980).
123. T. Kato, R. Nemoto, H. Mori, M. Takahashi, and Y. Tamakawa, Transcatheter arterial chemoembolization of renal cell carcinoma with microencapsulated Mitomycin C, *J. Urol.* *125*:19–24 (1981).
124. K. E. Rogers, B. I. Carr, and Z. A. Tökés, Cell surface-mediated cytotoxicity of polymer-bound adriamycin against drug-resistant hepatocytes, *Cancer Res.* *43*:2741–2748 (1983).
125. K. E. Rogers and Z. A. Tökés, Novel mode of cytotoxicity obtained by coupling inactive anthracycline to a polymer, *Biochem. Pharmacol.* *33*:605–608 (1984).
126. Z. A. Tökés, K. E. Rogers, and A. Rembaum, Synthesis of adrimaycin-coupled polyglutaraldehyde microspheres and evaluation of their cytostatic activity, *Proc. Natl. Acad. Sci. USA* *79*:2026–2030 (1982).
127. E. Beutler, G. L. Dale and W. L. Kull, Replacement therapy in Gaucher's disease, In, *Therapy in Genetic Diseases* (R. Desnick, ed.) Alan Liss, New York, 1980, pp. 369–381.

14

Selective Endocytosis of Macromolecular Drug Carriers

RUTH DUNCAN / University of Keele, Keele, Staffordshire, England

I. INTRODUCTION

Use of endocytic capture of macromolecules to achieve selective delivery of macromolecular drugs or drug conjugates is not new. It has been 10 years since DeDuve and colleagues [1] first coined the phase "lysosomotropic agents" to describe compounds that accumulate in the lysosomes of cells. Since then, there have been numerous attempts to devise clinically useful drug delivery systems to utilize cell-specific endocytic mechanisms for drug targeting. Although there have not yet been any significant clinical developments, considerable progress has been made in terms of a technology to produce tailor-made drug delivery systems.

Attachment of low molecular weight drugs to macromolecular carriers, as well as entrapment of drugs within vesicular carriers, automatically limits cellular capture of drug-carriers to the endocytic route. Drug pharmacokinetics is inevitably altered, and the possibility to limit the body distribution of drug and perhaps even achieve targeting arises. In this chapter the basic principles of selective endocytosis will be defined and discussed, and recent attempts to develop macromolecular drug-carriers for targeted drug delivery will be reviewed. In many respects, the use of soluble macromolecules as drug-carriers relates closely to the use of liposomes and other vesicular carriers. These aspects have been discussed in Chapter 13.

A. Definition of Endocytosis

To understand the reasons for using a macromolecular drug-carrier, it is important to consider the usual routes of entry of compounds into cells. Many pharmacological agents, particularly low molecular weight derivatives, pass readily into cells across the plasma membrane using either passive processes or carrier-mediated transport mechanisms. As such, unless they have inherent specificity of action, they are likely to produce unwanted side effects in cells remote from the site of action. Anticancer agents provide one obvious example where lack of specificity gives a poor therapeutic index. In contrast, macromolecules normally do not pass across the plasma membrane and their capture by cells is restricted to a mechanism called endocytosis.

Endocytosis is defined as the internalization of plasma membrane with concomitant engulfment of extracellular material and extracellular fluid. As discussed elsewhere [2–7], endocytosis can be divided into two types: phagocytosis and pinocytosis. Phagocytosis involves the internalization of particulate matter such as bacteria, erythrocytes, latex beads, and liposomes. It is only carried out by a few specialized cell types called phagocytes. Uptake of particulate matter is initiated by attachment of the particle to the cell surface with subsequent movement of plasma membrane over the particle surface eventually leading to formation of a phagocytic vacuole which is then internalized (Fig. 1). Multiple attachment of particle-associated ligands with membrane receptors is an essential stimulus for phagocytic capture of particles, and this particle/membrane interaction has been termed "zippering" [8].

In contrast, pinocytosis or "cell drinking" is an ubiquitous process common to most, if not all, cell types [9,10]. It involves continuous internalization of small droplets of extracellular fluid. Unlike phagocytosis, which is substrate-triggered, pinocytic membrane infolding appears to be a continual process. The newly formed pinocytic vesicles pinching off from the cell surface are generally smaller [0.1–0.2 μm in diameter) than larger phagocytic vacuoles whose size is governed by the dimensions of the engulfed particle (generally in the order of 1 μm in diameter). Other differences in the metabolic and cytoskeletal requirements of pinocytosis have been reviewed [9].

During pinocytic uptake, macromolecules are captured simply as solutes in the extracellular fluid, a process called fluid-phase pinocytosis [10]. Their rate of capture is relatively slow, being directly proportional to the concentration of macromolecules in the extracellular fluid. Table 1 shows some examples of molecules reported to be internalized by cells via fluid-phase pinocytosis. These molecules display considerable chemical diversity, including low molecular weight species [^{14}C]sucrose), proteins (horseradish peroxidase), and synthetic polymers ^{125}I-labeled poly (vinylpyrrolidone).

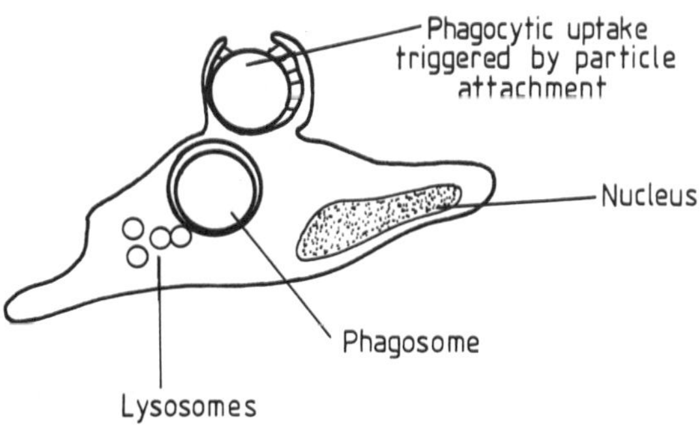

Fig. 1 Phagocytic uptake of particles. The few cell types able to phagocytize materials have been called 'professional phagocytes'. Particle attachment to the cell surface triggers the membrane to move outwards, covering the particle surface and eventually engulfing it. The internalized phagosome eventually fuses with intracellular lysosomes.

Table 1 Comparison of Rates of Uptake of Molecules Captured by Fluid-Phase or Adsorptive Pinocytosis

Pinocytic substrate	Cell types	Rate of pinocytic uptake (μl/mg protein/hr)	Ref.
Fluid-phase pinocytosis			
^{125}I-PVP	Rat yolk sac	1.71	11
^{125}I-HPMA copolymers	Rat yolk sac	2–4	12,13
[^{14}C] Sucrose	Rat yolk sac	2.04	14
^{125}I-PVP	Adult rat jejunum	1.48	15
^{125}I-PVP	Rat peritoneal macrophages	0.43	16
Horseradish peroxidase	Mouse peritoneal macrophages	0.56	17,18
Adsorptive pinocytosis			
^{125}I-PHEA tyramine	Rat yolk sac	86.99	19
^{125}I-HPMA tyrosinamide	Rat yolk sac	30–40	13

^{125}I-BSA (modified)	Rat yolk sac	8–74	20,21
Receptor mediated pinocytosis			
Asialoglycoproteins	Hepatocytes	3.7×10^{-3}/sec[a]	22
^{125}I-asialoorosomucoid	Human hepatoma cell line	475	23
^{125}I-asialofetuin	Hepatocytes	700	24
Lysosomal enzymes/neoglycoproteins	Macrophages	2×10^{-6}/hr[b]	25
β-glucuronidase	Normal human skin	5.8/27	25
N-acetylglucosaminidase	Fibroblasts		
N-acetylglucosaminidase	Nonparenchymal liver cells	470	27
^{125}I-mannoseBSA	Simulated peritoneal macrophages	130	28

[a]First-order rate constant for receptor-bound ligand.

[b]Rate of uptake of receptors per hour.

Capture of macromolecules adherent to the infolding surface membrane is termed adsorptive pinocytosis [10]. This is a more efficient mechanism of capture, in that the rate of uptake is higher than that measured for fluid-phase pinocytosis. The magnitude of the rate of capture and its cell specificity relate to the nature of substrate-membrane interaction.

Adsorptive pinocytosis can be subdivided into two categories. If the substrate-membrane interaction is a non-cell-specific phenomenon involving binding of substrate to a general membrane binding site, uptake is usually classified simply as adsorptive pinocytosis or non-specific adsorptive pinocytosis [29]. However, if the substrate binds to a distinct membrane receptor (usually with limited cellular distribution), uptake is usually termed receptor-mediated pinocytosis. Some examples of macromolecules captured by adsorptive and receptor-mediated pinocytosis are given in Table 1.

Soluble macromolecules are taken into cells by the pinocytic instead of phagocytic mechanism (so the remainder of this discussion will be limited to events that accompany and follow pinocytic internalization of materials). These events are shown schematically in Figure 2. (Intracellular processing of phagocytosed material is very similar.) Prior to membrane internalization the macromolecules adherent to membrane receptors often patch into domains or areas of the membrane called "coated pits" [30]. From these regions, the pinocytic vesicles form. Pinocytic vesicles pinch off from the plasma membrane and migrate into the cell, fusing with other incoming vesicles or vesicles of intracellular origin. The first intracellular compartment encountered by pinocytosed materials, called the endosome or receptosome [31,32], is still being characterized. This is an intracellular organelle with an acidic interior, buoyant density of 1.02–1.12 g/cc (i.e., less dense than lysosomes) and, unlike the lysosome, probably contains little enzyme activity. It has been suggested that this organelle serves as a sorting station [33] to route internalized ligands to their appropriate intracellular location. Recent work on liver hepatocytes has shown differential processing of IgA [34], transferrin, [35], and asialoglycoproteins [36]. In most cell types it would appear that macromolecules internalized are usually transferred directly from the endosome to the secondary lysosomal compartment of the cell. Lysosomes are vesicles of intracellular origin that have an internal acid pH [37] and contain a large number of hydrolytic enzymes capable of degrading all naturally occurring macromolecules they encounter, including proteins, carbohydrates, and lipids [29,38]. After fusion with incoming vesicles, the lysosome is termed a secondary lysosome. It is here that internalized macromolecules first encounter the battery of lysosomal enzymes. If biodegradable, the pinocytosed materials are digested to their monomeric constituents, which can then pass across the lysosomal membrane for either reutilization in the cell or excretion from the cell. Nondegradable materials

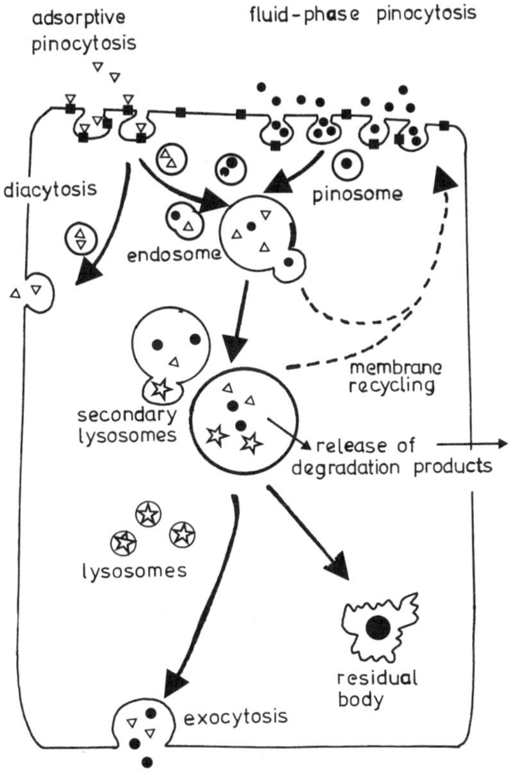

Fig. 2 Schematic representation of pinocytosis. Substrates captured by adsorptive pinocytosis (▽) and fluid-phase pinocytosis (●) are shown. Both enter the cell in pinocytic vesicles which rapidly join the endosomal compartment of the cell before moving on to fuse with lysosomes which contain many lysosomal enzymes (☆). In some cells the secondary lysosome then regresses to form a residual body which stores any non-degraded material (•). In others there is fusion of lysosome with the cell membrane leading to loss or exocytosis of its contents. Specialized cells such as the endothelium can transport materials rapidly across, probably without passage through lysosomes and this process has been termed diacytosis. To compensate for the vast amounts of surface membrane internalized there is an obvious need for rapid membrane recycling.

are sequestered in the secondary lysosome until they are released by exocytosis or cell death.

Three lysosomal properties are of particular importance to selective drug delivery. First, the lysosomal interior has a pH of approximately 4.5–5.5, which is maintained by the lysosomal proton pump [40]. Although this can be used to advantage in the design of labile drug-carrier linkages or when using any prodrug activated by an acidic environment, it restricts drug delivery to compounds stable at acidic pH. Second, the lysosomal membrane, like the plasma membrane, is highly selective in terms of the molecules capable of traversing it. Transport is clearly related to molecular weight (molecules greater than 220–240 in molecular weight are unable to pass across), and passive [41] and active transport processes [42] have been described. Unless they are specifically designed to act within the lysosome, lysosomotropic drug delivery systems must liberate, intralysosomally, drug which is both pharmacologically active and capable of passing across the lysosomal membrane to its intracellular site of action (receptor). Finally, the lysosomal enzyme contribution must be considered. The enzymes can be used to advantage to liberate drug from drug-carrier facilitating intracellular delivery. However, drugs susceptible to inactivation by lysosomal enzymatic hydrolysis should not be delivered via the lysosomal route.

B. Quantitation of Endocytosis

A variety of different techniques have been used to quantitate endocytosis [10]. Morphological methods in which the number of particles or vesicles visible within a cell or the number of cells taking up a substrate have been used as a measure of endocytic activity. More direct methods using radioisotopes as tracers, fluorescent labels, or macromolecules which can be detected chemically [43] have also been used. Nondegradable pinocytic substrates such as ^{125}I-labeled (polyvinylpyrrolidone) (PVP) and ^{125}I-labeled *N*-(2-hydroxypropyl) methacrylamide (HPMA) copolymers have been shown to be captured linearly with time by rat yolk sacs cultured *in vitro* [11,12]. Results from typical uptake experiments are shown in Figure 3. As these molecules are released slowly by the tissue, the rate of accumulation of radioactivity truly represents the rate of pinocytic capture.

The pattern of tissue accumulation of a pinocytic substrate degraded in the lysosomes is somewhat different. For example, the tissue association of ^{125}I-labeled bovine serum albumin (BSA) by rat yolk sacs cultured *in vitro* was found to plateau after 1–2 hr of incubation [43] and similar results were obtained with ^{125}I-labeled HPMA copolymers, whose radiolabel was attached to tyrosine residues in degradable oligopeptide side chains [13]. (For typical experiments see Fig. 4.) The observed plateau in level of tissue-associated

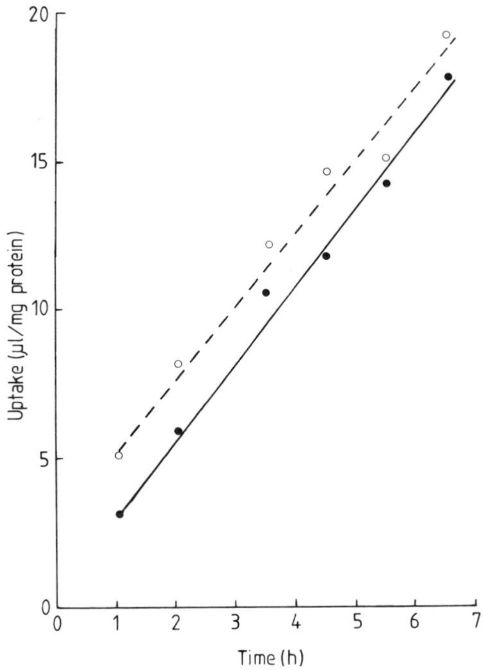

Fig. 3 Pinocytic uptake of nondegradable macromolecules by rat visceral yolk sacs. Uptake of ^{125}I-labeled poly(vinylpyrrolidone) (●) and ^{125}I-labeled *N*-(2-hydroxypropyl)methacrylamide (○) by rat visceral yolk sacs cultured *in vitro*. Uptake is expressed as a clearance, the volume of culture medium (μL) whose contained substrate is captured per mg yolk sac protein. (R. Duncan, unpublished results, for methods see Refs. 11–13.)

radioactivity is due to intralysosomal degradation of macromolecule to low molecular weight products (in these cases, [^{125}I]iodo-*L*-tyrosine) [45], which can escape from the lysosome and subsequently the cell. Depending on the degradation rate, a steady state arises in which the rate of pinocytic capture of radioactivity is balanced by the loss of radioactively labelled degradation product from the cell. Release of low molecular weight species from the cell can be confirmed by either trichloroacetic acid precipitation of the incubation medium (for proteins [44]) or Sephadex column chromotography (for polymers [13] and proteins [44]). When quantitating the rate of pinocytic capture of a biodegradable molecule it is essential that both rates of tissue accumulation and rates of intracellular degradation are taken into account.

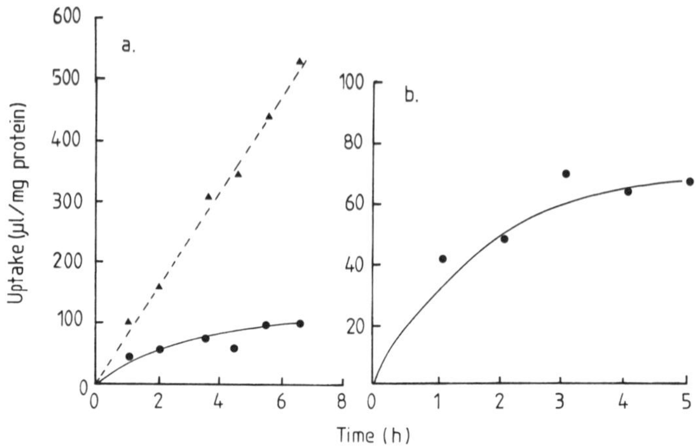

Fig. 4 Pinocytic uptake of degradable macromolecules by rat visceral yolk sacs. (a) Accumulation of radioactivity (●) and radioactivity released in the form of TCA soluble degradation products (▲) during incubation of rat yolk sacs with ^{125}I-labeled formaldehyde denatured bovine serum albumin. (b) Accumulation of ^{125}I-labeled *N*-(2-hydroxypropyl)methacrylamide copolymer during incubation with rat visceral yolk sacs. This copolymer bears diglycyltyrosinamide side chains to which the ^{125}I is bound (tyrosinamide). These side chains are degraded by lysosomal enzymes [12]. (R. Duncan, unpublished results, for experimental details see Refs. 12 and 44.)

Some molecules display high rates of release, or exocytosis, from cells. Besterman et al. [46] examined the accumulation and release [^{14}C]sucrose by pulmonary alveolar macrophages and fetal lung fibroblasts cultured *in vitro*. The kinetics of exocytosis was such that the actual pinocytic rate was some 50% greater than that measured form a linear initial rate of accumulation by the cells. Similarly, Weisbecker et al. [47] showed that rat yolk sacs loaded with ^{125}I-labeled rat immunoglobulin G, washed and placed in substrate-free medium, released more than 50% of tissue-associated radiolabel within 2–3 hr. Therefore, before quantitating absolute rates of pinocytic uptake, it is also essential to account for any subsequent loss of material from the cell.

The highly sophisticated techniques developed over the last decade for the analysis of endocytic phenomena have made it possible to describe accurately the specific uptake mechanisms that are discussed in Section II.

C. Design of Drug-Carriers for Drug Delivery via Selective Endocytosis

A variety of macromolecules, as shown in Table 2, have been proposed and investigated as drug-carriers (reviewed in [48–51]). Both natural macromolecules and synthetic polymers have been used. The design of macromolecular drug-carriers has been discussed at length elsewhere [6,7,84–87]. In essence, the drug-carrier must serve the following functions: (a) it should be water soluble for ease of administration and to facilitate access to the target cell; (b) it should be amenable to covalent conjugation with pharmacological agents (with optimal drug loading) such that the drug-carrier linkage is stable during transport to the target cell, but hydrolyzable within the cell; (c) it should be a candidate for pinocytic capture by cells (ideally the carrier would include inherent properties to enable it to target to particular cell types or, alternatively, be suitable for chemical modification to facilitate targeting); (d) it should have good biocompatibility, being nonimmunogenic, noncarcinogenic, or displaying general cytotoxic properties; and (e) it must be either metabolizable or have a route of removal from the organism once fulfilling its drug delivery function. A schematic diagram of an idealized drug-carrier is shown in Figure 5.

The relationship between the drug-carrier and its pinocytic capture will be discussed at length in the following section so discussion here is restricted to the carrier-drug linkage, and aspects of biocompatibility. Non-covalent attachment of a drug to a carrier is a major disadvantage due to lack of stability of the carrier complex *in vivo*. Although DNA-anthracycline complexes can be easily prepared and were found to cause no obvious DNA-induced toxic effects in the treatment of 700 patients [86], they were not very stable in blood. More recently, Trouet and colleagues [52,88,89] have conjugated daunorubicin (DNR) to succinylated serum albumin using covalent linkages. Drug linked to serum albumin directly, or via one amino acid, was inactive against L1210 leukemia *in vivo*. However, conjugates with a dipeptide spacer, albumin-Ala-Leu-DNR, a tripeptide spacer, albumin-Leu-Ala-Leu-DNR, or a tetrapeptide spacer, albumin-Ala-Leu-Ala-Leu-DNR, displayed marked therapeutic effects. The tri- and tetra-peptide spacers seemed particularly valuable as they were shown to be stable in serum, but released DNR on incubation with lysosomal enzymes *in vitro*.

The possibility of using oligopeptide side chains in *N*-(2-hydroxypropyl)methacrylamide (HPMA) copolymers as polymer-drug linkages has been explored at length in our own laboratory, a collaborative study with Dr. J. Kopecek and colleagues, Institute of Macromolecular Chemistry, Prague [90–93]. Kopecek et al. [94] showed that

Table 2 Macromolecules Used as Drug Carriers[a]

Drug-carrier	Pharmacological agent carried	Ref.
Proteins		
Human serum albumin	Daunorubicin	52
	Primaquine	53
	Methotrexate	54
Bovine serum albumin	Methotrexate	55
Bovine fibrinogen	Methotrexate	56
Glycoproteins	Adenine arabinoside	57
Nucleic acids		
DNA	Daunorubicin	58–60
Antibodies		
Immunoglobulin fraction	Daunomycin/ Adriamycin	61
H59 hybridoma antibody	Ricin A-chain	62
Anti-CEA[b]—antibodies	Vindesine	63
Hormones		
Insulin	Enzymes/Drugs	64
Melanotropin	Daunorubicin	65
Lectins		
Concanavalin A	*L*-Asparaginase	66
	Daunorubicin	67
Polysaccharides		
Dextran/inulin	Procainamide	68,69
Dextran	Interferon	70
Dextran	Daunomycin	71
Carboxymethyldextran and carboxymethylcellulose	Daunomycin	72

Table 2 (Continued)

Drug-carrier	Pharmacological agent carried	Ref.
Soluble synthetic polymers		
Poly(*L*-lysine)	Methotrexate	73,74
Poly(*L*-aspartic acid)	Daunorubicin	75,76
Poly-(2-hydroxyethyl)-*D,L*-asparagine	Trypsin-kallikrein Inhibitor	77
Divinylether maleic anhydride	Cyclophosphamide/ methotrexate	78,79
N-(2-hydroxypropyl) methacrylamide copolymers	Various drug models	80
Poly(vinylpyrrolidone)	Trypsin	81
Poly(*N*-vinyl-2-pyrrolidone-covinylamine)	Chlorambucil	82
Poly(1-vinyl-2-pyrrolidone-comaleic anhydride)	Quinine	83

[a]The examples given include both covalent and noncovalent binding of drug to carrier.

[b]Carcinoembryonic antigen, a specific tumor-associated antigen.

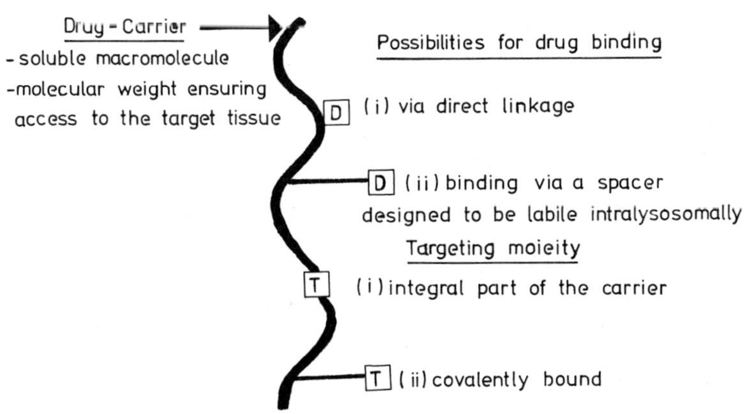

Fig. 5 Essential characteristics of a macromolecular drug-carrier.

oligopeptide sequences in HPMA copolymers were degraded by chymotrypsin, the rate of hydrolysis being dependent on amino acid composition of the side chain and the number of amino acid residues (two to four) in the oligopeptide sequences. Longer spacers showed an increase in the rate of cleavage of terminal moieties. More recent experiments have confirmed the suitability of such sequences as potential polymer-drug linkages. While they are not hydrolyzed in plasma and serum [95], they effectively release a terminal residue (a) on incubation with a mixture of purified rat liver lysosomal enzymes [96–98], (b) during incubation with cathepsins B, H, and L (purified lysosomal-proteinases) [99,100], and (c) following pinocytic capture by cells cultured *in vitro* [12]. Formation of an enzyme-substrate complex is a prerequisite for enzymatically catalyzed hydrolysis [92]. However, as yet, there is no definitive knowledge of the amino acid sequences required for substrate interaction with the lysosomal thiol-proteinases. Nonetheless, it appears that hydrophobic amino acids (such as phenylalanine, tyrosine, and alanine) in the P_1, P_2, and P_3 positions relative to the terminal bond in any combination ensure hydrolytic cleavage of a terminal residue by lysosomal enzymes. See Ref. 101 for nomenclature.

Drug-carrier linkages hydrolyzed by chemical means have also been developed. Shen and Ryser prepared a *N*-*cis*-aconityl derivative of daunorubicin which was conjugated to either Affi-gel 701 (aminoethyl poly-acrylamide beads) or poly(*D*-lysine) [102].

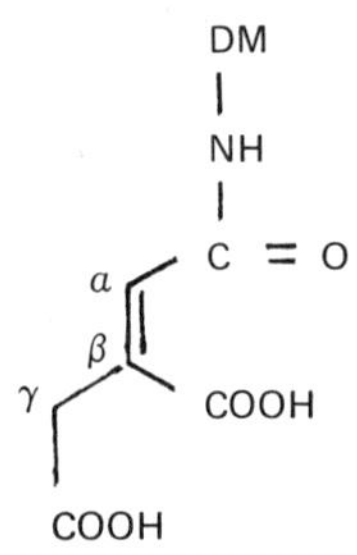

N-*Cis*-Aconityl Daunorubicin

The *cis*-aconityl linkage between drug and Affi-Gel 701 was hydrolyzed at pH 4 (half-life 3 hr), but not appreciably at pH 6 (half-life 96 hr). Moreover, these conjugates were found to be nontoxic to WEH 1-5 cells cultured *in vitro*. In contrast, poly(*D*-lysine) conjugates caused 90% inhibition of growth of the same cell line. Unlike the polyacrylamide bead conjugates, poly(*D*-lysine) conjugates were able to enter cells by pinocytosis and, on reaching the lysosomal compartment, liberate daunorubicin. As poly(*D*-lysine) is not biodegradable, drug release must be due to pH sensitivity of the *cis*-aconityl linkage. A similar *cis*-aconityl linkage has recently been used [103] to bind daunorubicin to anti-Stage-Specific-Embryonic-Antigen 1 (SSEA 1). SSEA-1 is found on the surface of MH-15 mouse tumor and can be used as a model system to study antibody-mediated drug-targeting. Preliminary experiments showed that tumor retention of ^{125}I-daunomycin-antibody alone was comparable to that of ^{125}I-antibody and that conjugates killed antigen-bearing cells (*in vitro*) specifically.

It is important to consider carefully the fate of the drug-carrier in the body. If the carrier induces unwanted side effects, its usefulness will obviously be severely limited. Systemic effects of biomaterials in the body has recently been reviewed [104]. The types of effects recognized include; carcinogenic, metabolic, immunological and bacteriological effects. The particularly important effects are immunogenicity of the drug-carrier and biodegradability. Both natural and synthetic carriers have been reported to show little or no immunogenicity. Daunorubicin-DNA complexes administered intravenously to patients produced no allergic anaphylatic reactions or anti-DNA antibodies [59]. *N*-(2-hydroxypropyl)methacrylamide (HPMA) copolymers bearing oligopeptide side chains and synthesized as drug-carriers produced little or no antibody response after repeated intraperitoneal administration to mice [105]. Moreover, it was later demonstrated [106] that what little antibody was formed was predominantly directed against the oligopeptide side chains. Immunogenicity of polymers has been reviewed at length elsewhere [43,87,107] and polymers, particularly synthetic polypeptides have provided much information about the chemical basis of immunogenicity [108,109].

Drug-carriers which are not biodegradable will persist in the cell following pinocytic capture, unless the cell displays high rates of exocytosis. This is exemplified by storage of poly(vinylpyrrolidone) following administration as a plasma expander [110]. Prolonged accumulation is more likely to cause long term alterations in metabolism [111], while rapid degradation may liberate residues capable of inducing unwanted effects. Cross-linking HPMA copolymers with diamine-containing peptidyl sequences has proved itself useful in conferring limited degradability to a non-degradable polymer system. The oligopeptidyl cross-links of the soluble HPMA copolymers were found to be cleaved by trypsin [112], chymotrypsin [113], papain [114], cathespin B [99] as well as after incubation with cells *in vitro* [115]. Moreover, following intravenous administration to rats, such cross-linked HPMA copolymers were degraded to yield lower molecular weight polymer chains which were excreted in the urine [116]. This would be a novel, if somewhat complicated, method to rid the body of nondegradable drug-carrier.

II. MECHANISMS FOR ACHIEVING SELECTIVE CAPTURE

The phrase "drug targeting" is very fashionable, but unfortunately often used out of context. All the drug delivery regimes currently under investigation, including both macromolecular and vesicular drug-carriers, simply alter normal body distribution of free drug. Often the modified body distribution shows predominant deposition of drug-carrier in the cells of the reticuloendothelial system and this is particularly true when liposomes are used as drug-carriers [117].

It should be stressed that the mechanisms described below, which aid selective direction of soluble macromolecular drug-carriers, are still somewhat limited. They hopefully divert the carrier towards the target cell and their success should be measured in terms of the percentage of the administered dose which arrives at the target tissue.

A. Selection According to Substrate Size

The pinocytic uptake of macromolecules by different cell types is a size-dependent phenomenon. Pinocytosis of ^{125}I-labeled poly(vinyl pyrrolidone) (PVP) by rat visceral yolk sacs and rat peritoneal macrophages cultured *in vitro* was shown to be dependent on the mean molecular weight of the ^{125}I-labeled PVP fraction used [118]. Yolk sac cells which have a highly organized, microvillous surface captured the lowest molecular weight fraction (M_w 50,000) much faster than the highest molecular weight fraction (M_w 700,000), indicating that the cell surface limits access of large molecules to the newly forming pinocytic vesicles at the cell surface. In contrast, macrophages captured all ^{125}I-labeled PVP fractions at the same rate, with the exception of the highest molecular weight species (M_w 7,000,000), which seemed to trigger phagocytosis.

Substrate selection according to size by the yolk sac has been confirmed using molecular weight fractions of ^{125}I-labeled *N*-(2-hydroxypropyl)methacrylamide (HPMA) copolymers [115,119]. These data illustrate the need to select carefully the molecular weight of the drug-carrier in order to permit pinocytic capture by the target cell.

As described above macrophages engulf very large polymers more avidly, probably by phagocytosis. Results obtained with smaller macromolecules show that other cell types also pinocytose more efficiently as substrate molecular weight rises. Cartlidge et al. [119] found that different molecular weight fractions (M_w 34,000–400,000) of ^{125}I-labeled HPMA copolymers were pinocytosed by rat intestine cultured *in vitro* and uptake increased with increasing molecular weight. Similarly, Vince and Dean [120] showed that kidney tubule cells cultured *in vitro* take up large plasma proteins more efficiently than smaller ones (the plasma proteins were previously separated into fractions by gel filtration and then radioiodinated). As the rate of capture of all fluid-phase pinocytic substrates is the same for any one cell type the examples reported above suggest that adsorptive pinocytosis increases with increasing substrate size, but as yet experimental data have not been reported which describe the number of binding sites and their specificity.

In conclusion, drug-carrier size (molecular weight and molecular configuration) is vital to its functional design. Carriers destined to reach reticuloendothelial cells should be of high molecular weight, but limitation of molecular weight to a minimum ($M_W < 100,000$) is crucial if the desire is to gain access to cells like the rat visceral yolk sac. Size is also an important factor governing movement of carrier from one body compartment to another (reviewed in Ref. 7). This is of particular importance if the carrier is destined for the kidney tubule cells. The glomerular filter is an effective barrier retaining molecules of molecular weight 30,000–60,000 (depending on their configuration), so lower molecular weight carriers must be chosen for delivery to the kidney. It should be noted that synthetic polymeric carriers have certain advantages over natural macromolecules in respect of drug-carrier size. Synthetic polymers can, within the limits of synthetic chemistry, be tailor-made to produce the optimum molecular weight for any carrier function.

B. Nonspecific Determinants Regulating Membrane Interactions

Nonspecific adsorptive pinocytosis has recently been discussed with special reference to pinocytosis in macrophages [121] and rat visceral yolk sacs [29]. Charge and hydrophobicity of the pinocytic substrate appear to be two important factors which govern nonspecific affinity for cell surfaces. Polycations such as poly(*L*-ornithine) have been shown to increase the rate of pinocytic uptake of colloidal ^{198}Au by rat yolk sacs and rat peritoneal macrophages cultured *in vitro* [122]. However, their mechanism of action was not by stimulation of the rate of pinocytic vesicle formation at the cell surface [123]. DEAE-dextran and poly(amino acid) stimulation of albumin uptake by tumor cells *in vitro* was shown to increase as the molecular weight of the stimulator increased [4000–200,000], suggesting that multiple attachment of the macromolecule was necessary to optimize biological function [124].

Kooistra and colleagues have examined the effect of size and charge on endocytosis of proteins *in vivo* and *in vitro*. Monomer, dimer, and polymer fractions of lysozyme were injected intravenously into nephrectomised rats and the blood clearance and uptake by the liver and spleen was measured [125]. After 15 min, 8%, 37%, and 89% of the monomer, dimer, and polymer, respectively, were recovered in the liver. Autoradiography and cell isolation showed the protein to be taken up by the sinusoidal cells of the liver. Experiments with acetylated and succinylated lysozyme confirmed that positively charged groups contributed to the adsorptive pinocytic capture of lysozyme.

Isoenzymes (M4 and H4) of lactate dehydrogenase were also found to be cleared from rat plasma at very different rates, about 75% of M4 and 8% of H4 being cleared from the bloodstream 1 hr after intravenous administration [126]. As these two proteins are identical in three dimensional structure, it was concluded that these dramatic differences in pinocytic uptake (by the liver) must be due to differences in their amino acid composition (approximately 25% of the amino acid residues of the two proteins are different). Specifically, M4 is positively charged at neutral pH. Studies on the pinocytosis of lactate dehydrogenase H4, M4, and bovine serum albumin by rat yolk sacs and rat peritoneal macrophages cultured *in vitro* confirmed that positive charge of the substrate is the major characteristic responsible for adsorptive pinocytosis in the macrophage [127].

Yolk sacs cultured *in vitro* have been used as a model system to study adsorptive pinocytosis. Analysis of the uptake of several simple proteins, such as calcitonin, insulin, ribonuclease, lysozyme, albumin, and formaldehyde denatured albumin, showed that they were all captured by an adsorptive mechanism, but that they formed two distinct subgroups [128]. These include those that are captured by binding to negatively charged residues on the membrane and those that adhere to hydrophobic sites. Hydrophobic interactions of pinocytic substrates have been investigated further using modified HPMA copolymers [13] and poly(α,β-(2-hydroxyethyl)-*DL*-aspartamides (PHEA) [19,129]. Substitution of these polymers with tyrosinamide (HPMA copolymers) or tyramine (PHEA) increased the affinity of polymer for the yolk sac membrane, the enhancement pinocytic uptake being most marked above levels of 10 mol% substitution [13, 129]. *In vivo* studies with polyaspartamides have shown that, following intravenous administration, a PHEA-tyramine derivative was captured more avidly than the parent compound by kidney tubule cells [130]. The efficiency of tubular uptake of PHEA-tyramine gave a similar correlation with tyramine content (mol%) [131] as that described with the yolk sac [129].

Denatured, and chemically modified, proteins injected intravenously are cleared rapidly from the bloodstream [132,133] and are taken up quickly by cells cultured *in vitro* [20]. The hepatic receptors that mediate pinocytosis of these proteins *in vivo*, called scavenger receptors, are located on the liver macrophages. Increased negative charge on ligands, such as that induced by formaldehyde treatment, may direct the ligands to this binding site. There is certainly evidence that rat peritoneal macrophages have high affinity for negatively charged molecules as they rapidly accumulate divinyl ether-maleic anhydride (DIVEMA) [134] and gelatin stabilized (^{198}Au) colloidal gold [16] when cultured with these substrates *in vitro*.

Techniques other than those used to monitor pinocytic rate can give an indication of membrane-substrate interactions. With particular reference to the development of novel bioadhesive materials, Robinson and colleagues [135,136] have examined polymer interactions with cell surface glycoproteins. The fluorescent probe pyrene was used to study polymer interactions with Chang conjunctival cells grown in monolayer. It was found that polyacrylic acid, carboxymethycellulose, hyaluronic acid and gelatin bind strongly to the cell surface. Tirrell and Boyd [137] used differential scanning calorimetry (DSC) to study interaction of polymers with human red blood cells and erythrocyte ghosts. Neutral polymers such as poly *N*-(2-hydroxypropyl)methacrylamide and poly(vinylpyrrolidone) caused no perturbation in the heat capacity profile, whereas the polycation polybrene, poly(dimethyliminotrimethylenedimethyliminohexamethylene dibromide), strongly interacted with negatively charged spectrin molecules in the erythrocyte membrane.

Each cell type has an array of binding sites with their own specificity. Should appropriate ligand, cation or anion, appear, they will bind it without obvious substrate discrimination. Therefore, utilization of nonspecific binding for targeted drug delivery has its limitations. However, this cellular property should prove useful for development of bioadhesives [136]. Nonspecific binding is an important phenomenon which must be overcome if a drug-carrier is to concentrate efficiently in the target tissue. Ideally, the carrier should be captured by fluid-phase pinocytosis only by the target cell. High loading of carrier with ionic residues or hydrophobic drugs can initiate non-specific adherance of the conjugate to all cell surfaces encountered en route to the target tissue. A relationship between procainamide substitution of a procainamide-dextran conjugate and its adsorptive pinocytosis *in vitro* and *in vivo* has been reported [68, 138].

C. Cell-Specific Recognition Systems

Identification of cell-specific recognition systems leading to receptor-mediated endocytic capture of drug-carriers is the goal of all scientists working on lysosomotropic drug delivery. Although several "cell-specific" systems have been proposed, evaluation of the pinocytic properties of a wide range of cell types has shown that some receptors are present on more than one cell type. There is no doubt that the ligand-specificity of these receptors is such that they facilitate receptor-mediated endocytosis.

In recent years there has been a considerable review literature on the carbohydrate-specific receptor systems [22,139–142]. Receptors present on the surface of some cells appear to recognize, and bind, certain carbohydrate moieties on glycoproteins (see Table 3 for examples). One of the earliest described was the capture of asialoglycoproteins by liver hepatocytes [22,139,143]. Fully sialylated glycoproteins have a half-life in the bloodstream of several days, but enzymatic removal of the terminal sialic acid residues resulted in clearance within minutes. Chemical modification of the galactose moieities exposed by desialyation again prolonged survival time of the glycoprotein [144], indicating the importance of galactose residues in receptor-mediated pinocytosis. Since these early observations, there have been numerous investigations to identify the cell type responsible for asialoglycoprotein capture, kinetics of pinocytic capture, intracellular fate of pinocytosed ligand, nature of the membrane receptor, and synthesis and recycling of membrane receptors. Some of the relevant features are discussed below.

Desialyated glycoproteins injected intravenously are rapidly cleared from circulation. They are captured specifically by the parenchymal liver cells [145]. The rat liver receptor that binds desialylated glycoproteins was originally isolated by affinity chromatography [145] and more recently its molecular size has been determined *in situ* by radiation inactivation [147].

Table 3 Receptor-Mediated Pinocytosis Based on Carbohydrate Recognition Systems

Residue on macromolecule recognized by cell-surface receptor	Cells bearing the receptor	Ref.
Galactose	Hepatocytes	22,145
	Hepatoma	23
Galactose attached to a particle	Kupffer cells	160,161
Mannose/*N*-acetylglucosamine/fucose	Macrophages	25,163 169
Fucose	Hepatocytes	175
Mannose-6-phosphate	Fibroblasts	176,178
	Liver cells	179
Glucose	Lewis lung carcinoma	182

The molecular weight of the rat liver receptor has been reported as 30,000–150,000. The kinetics of pinocytic capture of galactose-containing ligands has been investigated *in vivo* [148,149] and with isolated hepatocytes cultured *in vitro* [24,150,151]. It was estimated that the exterior surface of liver cells can bind a maximal amount of 32 μg of asialo-orosomucoid per 10^8 cells [149]. This compares reasonably well with the value of 8 μg/10^8 cells reported for *in vitro* binding [152]. It is likely that the enzymatic treatment used for hepatocyte isolation results in partial loss of receptor sites, since uptake of asialofetuin by hepatocytes *in vitro* is less than that measured *in vivo* [24]. Using galacytosylated bovine serum albumin coupled to colloidal gold as an electron dense probe, the uptake pathway has been characterized at the ultrastructural level [151]. Binding to the membrane receptors of cultured hepatocytes was followed by internalization in coated vesicles, passage into tubular structures, multivesicular bodies (endosomes), with final accumulation in lysosomes. A number of studies have suggested that the asialoglycoprotein ligand normally dissociates from its receptor prior to degradation [153] or, for that matter, entry into the lysosome [154]. This process would seem to take place within the acidic milieu of the endosome and facilitate receptor recycling back to the cell surface to enable continuing capture. Obviously, ligand that does not dissociate from its receptor in the endosome would be in danger of routing back to the cell surface along with the receptor, thereby escaping the lysosomal compartment of the cell. This possibility has obvious implications if the drug-carrier requires lysosomal activation.

The asialoglycoprotein receptor has been used as a target for a number of different drug delivery systems. Diphtheria toxin fragment A (DTA) is highly cytotoxic and has been used in many studies to evaluate the possibility of producing receptor-specific cytotoxic agents. Linkage of DTA to asialofetuin by a disulphide bond produced a conjugate that was highly toxic to primary rat hepatocytes cultures, in fact some 1800 times more toxic than DTA alone [155]. Experiments performed *in vivo* have shown that lactosaminated human serum albumin coupled with adenine-9-β-D-arabinofuranoside (ara-A) is taken up by the mouse asialoglycoprotein hepatic receptor after intravenous administration [156]. Infusion of ara-A is used to treat patients having chronic hepatitis B. Using a mouse model system to study the therapeutic potential of the ara-A conjugate, it was found that the conjugate was effective at a 10-fold lower concentration [156]. Pepstatin, an inhibitor of the lysosomal enzyme cathepsin D, when linked through a carboxyl group to asialofetuin, was effectively delivered to the lysosomes of rat hepatocytes following intravenous injection [157]. Moreover, N-(2-hydroxypropyl)methacrylamide copolymers can be modified by incorporation of galactosamine residues to bring about efficient deposition in the liver [158]. Synthesis of polymers containing 1–11 mol% galactosamine showed that blood clearance increased with increasing sugar content and with optimal targeting more than 80% of the injected dose was taken into the liver just 10 min after intravenous administration [159].

Galactose-specific receptors are found not only on hepatocytes but on Kupffer cells as well. Recent studies have shown that rat Kupffer cells *in vitro* strongly bind neuraminidase-treated rat erthrocytes [160], a process that is specifically inhibited by *D*-galactose and related sugars. The major difference between the Kupffer cell receptor and the hepatocyte receptor is that the former does not seem to mediate pinocytosis of soluble macromolecules. It probably serves the physiological function of removing aging (desialylated) red blood cells. Quantitative analysis of lectin-dependent particle endocytosis by Kupffer cells was studied using a conjugate of asialofetuin and colloidal gold (17 nm particles). Freshly isolated cells ingested these particles at a rate of 4200 particles/cell/min [161].

Better known receptors are Macrophage receptors which recognize mannose and *N*-acetylglucosamine [25,139] residues on glycoproteins. Many workers, including Stahl and colleagues, have studied these receptors, which were discovered from the observation that lysosomal enzyme β-glucuronidase was, like asialoglycoproteins, cleared rapidly from rat plasma [162,163]. Clearance was inhibited by agalactoorosomucoid (which has a terminal *N*-acetylglucosamine residue) [163] and by yeast mannan [164]. Using immunohistochemical techniques, human β-glucoronidase was shown to localize specifically in the non-parenchymal cells of the liver [165]. Incubation of isolated rat alveolar macrophages with synthetic conjugates of bovine serum albumin (BSA), so-called neoglycoproteins [166,167], confirmed unequivocally the existence of a mannose/*N*-acetyl glucosamine recognition system on macrophages [168]. Shepherd et al. [169] showed that mannose-BSA and *L*-fucose-BSA were the most potent inhibitors of ^{125}I-labeled-β-glucuronidase uptake. *N*-acetyl-glucosamine-BASA was also an active inhibitor. There are approximately 50,000–150,000 receptor sites per cell [170,171], and pinocytic uptake of mannose-BSA by alveolar macrophages is linear with time over several hours [170].

Several attempts have been made to isolate and characterize the mannose/*N*-acetylglucosamine/fucose receptor from rat [172–174] and human liver [174]. The receptor appears to be a binding protein of molecular weight 30,000–225,000, consisting of several subunits. Much of the experimental work on mannose-recognition systems has been carried out using mammalian systems, therefore the isolation of a mannose-binding protein from human liver [174] is particularly important as it confirms the potential of mannose-mediated endocytosis for clinical use.

Although a fucose-recognizing receptor has been described on the macrophage surface [169], there is evidence that fucose-bearing glycoproteins are rapidly cleared from the circulation and concentrated in the liver hepatocytes after administration to mice [175]. Binding of fucose to glycoprotein via a 1,3-linkage to *N*-acetylglucosamine was an essential requirement for receptor-glycoprotein interaction, and attachment of fucose to asialotransferrin via such a linkage produced a derivative that was rapidly cleared [22]. The rat liver fucose receptor has been isolated and characterized by Lehrman and Hill [22]. SDS gel electrophoresis showed it to have a molecular weight of 67,000–73,000.

In the mid seventies it became apparent from the work of Neufeld and colleagues that human fibroblasts have a receptor-mediated system for the pinocytic capture of lysosomal hydrolases [176]. Kaplan et al. [177] showed that (a) uptake of β-glucuronidase by fibroblasts *in vitro* was inhibited by mannose-6-phosphate and (b) the rates of uptake were decreased if the enzyme was pretreated by phosphatase. These and later observations cofirmed the importance of mannose-6-phosphate residues on the enzyme for receptor-mediated pinocytic capture. The mechanism of uptake and transport of lysosomal enzymes have been comprehensively reviewed by Sly [178]. Ullrich et al. [179] showed that a receptor with similar specificity was located on rat liver cells cultured *in vitro* and Fischer et al. [180] found activity in other rat organs. Mannose-6-phosphate receptor binding may therefore be a universal component of all cell membranes thus of limited potential for cell-specific targeting.

Glycoproteins and glycolipids are integral components of mammalian cell membranes. Studies have shown that differences exist between these glycoconjugates of normal and malignant cells [141,181]. Sugar binding proteins or endogenous lectins found on tumor cells have been comprehensively reviewed by Monsigny et al. [141]. The galactose-recognizing binding protein is found to be retained on the surface of hepatoma [23]. Attempts have been made to utilize these recognition systems to deliver drugs to tumor cells. Roche et al. [182] have shown that Lewis lung carcinoma binds neoglycoproteins containing α-*D*-glucose residues and internalizes them by receptor-mediated pinocytosis. Attachment of the toxin gelonin to the glucose-containing-neoglycoprotein produced a conjugate that was some hundred times more toxic than the free drug.

In constrast, receptor-mediated pinocytic capture of low density lipoprotein (LDL) by fibroblasts does not depend on a carbohydrate recognition system [183]. Binding of ^{125}I-labeled human LDL to its receptor on fibroblasts involves ionic interaction, in that positive residues of the apoprotein B component of LDL interact with negatively charged groups on the LDL receptor. Most studies of LDL pinocytosis have been carried out in human fibroblasts, although some studies used aortic smooth muscle cells [184,185], hepatoma [186], and human leukocytes [187]. This apparent lack of cell specificity of the LDL receptor indicates limitations in the usefulness of these receptors for selective targeting, but it should be remembered that the number of binding sites and their LDL affinities have been only rigorously examined in human fibroblasts.

Table 3 gives a summary of some of the receptor-mediated pinocytic systems that have been described in this section.

III. USE OF SELECTIVE ENDOCYTOSIS FOR DRUG TARGETING

Many macromolecular conjugates have been synthesized to improve the therapeutic index of certain drugs. Some were completely inactive, others were effective only in *in vitro* test systems and a few have shown potential *in vivo*. As yet, there are very few reports of clinical trials. The concept of drug targeting has been described by the phrase "old drugs in new clothing" [188]. In this context it is the new clothing that must provide the address system for selective capture by the target cell.

Pharmacological studies of macromolecular conjugates based on soluble synthetic polymers have been reviewed at length elsewhere [6,7]. Table 4 shows a number of different drug-conjugate treatments which have been tested against model disease situations in animals. Several examples are selected for discussion.

Many of the recessively inherited inborn errors of metabolism have been linked with specific enzyme defects. For example, in lysosomal storage diseases, absence of a single enzyme leads to excessive accumulation of substrate intralysosomally. Pompe's disease or type II glycogenosis is a deficiency in the lysosomal enzyme α-1,4-glucosidase, leading to glycogen accumulation in lysosomes, particularly of the liver and cardiac muscle, and eventually to infantile death due to cardio-respiratory failure. The notion of therapy by replacement of the missing enzyme is not new [189]. Recently, attempts have been made to improve enzyme replacement therapy using liposomes [190] and enzyme conjugates [181]. Pozansky and Bhardwaj [191] synthesized a conjugate using three components; antibody (IgG raised against isolated rat hepatocytes), homologous albumin, and α-1,4-glucosidase. Following intravenous administration to rats the conjugate localized preferentially in hepatocytes. Studies carried out *in vitro* showed the conjugate to have increased resistance to heat denaturation and proteolytic inactivation [192]. Since simple introduction of foreign enzymes can lead to immunological reactions, accompanied by minimal enzyme activity at the desired site of action, use of enzyme conjugates is an interesting prospect.

Trouet and colleagues have undertaken many investigations to evaluate the antitumoral activity of drugs linked to proteins. More recently, they reported the synthesis of carrier-bound antiprotozoal

Table 4 Treatment of Diseases with Drug Conjugates

Disease	Treatment	Drug-carriers	Ref.
Cancers (various)	Chemotherapy (various agents)	Proteins, polyaminoacids, acids, DIVEMA, antibodies	54,55,62 73,75,78 86
	Immunopotentiation	Liposomes	117,193
	L-Asparaginase	Albumin	195
Enzyme deficiencies (lysosomal storage diseases)	α-1,4-Glucosidase	Albumin-antibody	191,192
	α-1,4-Glucosidase	Albumin-insulin	64
Parasitic infections			
Liver stages of *Plasmodium*	Primaquine	Asialofetuin	53,194
Leishmaniasis	Primaquine	Liposomes	196
Hepatitis B infection	Adenine-9-β-*D*-arabinofuranoside	Lactosaminated albumin	57,156

drugs [53]. Primaquine is a widely used antimalarial agent which acts predominantly on the hepatic stages of malaria. These can be particularly troublesome as the protozoa remains dormant in the liver hepatocytes. Use of primaquine is limited by its toxicity, so an attempt was made to reduce primiquine toxicity by linking it to asialofetuin, a glycoprotein captured by the galactose-dependent pinocytic uptake system of hepatocytes. When tested against an experimental murine malaria (*Plasmodium berghei*), the asialofetuin-primaquine conjugate was more active than free drug, most probably due to a higher hepatic concentration [53].

Hepatocyte receptor-mediated endocytosis has also been used to deliver adenine-9-*L*-*D*-arabinofuranoside (ara-A) to liver infected with chronic hepatitis B [57,166]. Ten times less ara-A is required to inhibit virus DNA synthesis in mice if the drug is infused as a conjugate with lactosaminated human serum albumin. Therefore, provided human hepatocytes have the same capacity to capture the drug-glycoconjugate, this new treatment for chronic hepatitis B may overcome some of the dose-dependent side-effects associated with the administration of ara-A.

Shepherd et al. [107] recently showed that β-glucoronidase is taken up by bone marrow macrophages and accumulates intracellularly in vacuoles harboring the parasite *Leishmaniamexicana amazonesis*, thus confirming the potential of mannosylated macromolecules for delivery of leishmanicidal drugs to parasite-containing vacuoles of infected macrophages.

IV. CONCLUSIONS

Since 1974 several carbohydrate-specific endocytic recognition systems have been discovered and characterized, and cell-specific antigenicity has come to the forefront and monoclonal antibody technology is proceeding by leaps and bounds. Each in its own way provides hope of providing the key component to selective drug delivery, i.e., targeting. As yet pharmacological products proven in the clinics have not emerged, but it is surely only a matter of time as many experimental studies give cause for optimism. If, during the next decade, new selective endocytic mechanisms can be identified and characterized, it is likely that the necessary cell-specific uptake mechanisms will emerge.

ACKNOWLEDGMENTS

I thank the British Cancer Research Campaign for funding my research and the British Council and Royal Society for supporting collaborative projects.

REFERENCES

1. C. DeDuve, T. DeBarsy, B. Poole, A. Trouet, P. Tulkens, and F. Van Hoof, Lysosomotropic agents, *Biochem. Pharmacol. 23*, 2495 (1974).
2. T. P. Stossel, Endocytosis. In, *Receptors and Recognition* Series A, Vol. 4 (P. Cuatrecasas and M. F. Greaves, Eds.), Chapman and Hall, London, 1977, pp. 105–141.
3. S. C. Silverstein, R. M. Steinman, and Z. A. Cohn, Endocytosis, *Annu. Rev. Biochem. 46*, 669 (1977).
4. J. M. Besterman and R. B. Low, Endocytosis: A review of mechanism and plasma membrane dynamics, *Biochem. J. 210*, 1 (1983).
5. R. M. Steinman, I. S. Mellman, W. A. Muller, and Z. A. Cohn, Endocytosis and recycling of plasma membrane, *J. Cell Biol. 96*, 1 (1983).
6. R. Duncan and J. Kopecek, Soluble synthetic polymers as potential drug carriers, *Ad. Polymer Sci. 57*, 51 (1984).
7. R. Duncan, Biological effects of soluble synthetic polymers as drug carriers, *CRC Crit. Rev. Ther. Drug Carrier Systems 1*, 281 (1985).
8. F. M. Griffin Jr., J. A. Griffin, J. E. Leider, and S. C. Silverstein, Studies on the mechanism of phagocytosis. 1. Requirements for circumferential attachment of particle-bound ligands to specific receptors on the macrophage plasma membrane, *J. Exp. Med. 142*, 1263 (1975).
9. A. C. Allison and P. Davies, Mechanisms of endocytosis and exocytosis. In, *Transport at the Cellular Level* (M. A. Sleigh and D. H. Jennings, Eds.), Society for Experimental Biology, Symp. 28, Cambridge University Press, Cambridge, 1974, pp. 419–446.
10. M. K. Pratten, R. Duncan, and J. B. Lloyd, Adsorptive and passive pinocytic uptake. In, *Coated Vesicles* (C. J. Ockleford and A. Whyte, Eds.), Cambridge University Press, Cambridge, 1980, pp. 179–218.
11. K. E. Williams, E. M. Kidston, F. Beck, and J. B. Lloyd, Quantitative studies of pinocytosis 1. Kinetics of uptake of [^{125}I]polyvinylpyrrolidone by rat yolk sac cultured *in vitro*, *J. Cell Biol. 64*, 113 (1975).
12. R. Duncan, P. Rejamanova, J. Kopecek, and J. B. Lloyd, Pinocytic uptake and intracellular degradation of *N*-(2-hydroxypropyl)methacrylamide copolymers. A potential drug delivery system, *Biochim. Biophys. Acta 678*, 143 (1981).
13. R. Duncan, H. C. Cable, P. Rejmanova, and J. Kopecek, Tyrosinamide residues enhance pinocytic capture of *N*-(2-hydroxypropyl)methacrylamide copolymers, *Biochim. Biophys. Acta 799*, 1 (1984).

14. A. V. S. Roberts, K. E. Williams, and J. B. Lloyd, The pinocytosis of ^{125}I-labelled poly(vinylpyrrolidone) [^{14}C] sucrose and colloidal [^{198}Au] by rat yolk sac cultured *in vitro, Biochem. J. 168*, 239 (1977).
15. J. F. Bridges and J. F. Woodley, The uptake of [^{125}I]polyvinylpyrrolidone by adult rat gut *in vitro*. In, *Maternofoetal Transmission*, Vo. 2 (W. A. Hemmings, Ed.), Elsevier, Amsterdam, 1979, pp. 249–257.
16. M. K. Pratten, K. E. Williams, and J. B. Lloyd. A quantitative study of pinocytosis and intracellular proteolysis in rat peritoneal macrophages, *Biochem. J. 168*, 365 (1977).
17. R. M. Steinman and Z. A. Cohn, The interaction of soluble horseradish peroxidase with mouse peritoneal macrophages *in vitro, J. Cell Biol. 55*, 186 (1972).
18. P. J. Edelson, R. Zweibel, and Z. A. Cohn, The pinocytic rate of activated macrophages, *J. Exp. Med. 126*, 941 (1975).
19. R. Duncan, D. Starling, F. Rypacek, J. Drobnik, and J. B. Lloyd, Pinocytosis of poly(α,β-(N-2-hydroxyethyl)-*DL*-aspartamide and a tyramine derivative by rat visceral yolk sacs cultured *in vitro, Biochim. Biophys. Acta 717*, 248 (1982).
20. A. T. Moore, K. E. Williams, and J. B. Lloyd, The effect of chemical treatments of albumin and orosomucoid on rate of clearance from the rat bloodstream and rate of pinocytic capture by rat yolk sac cultured *in vitro, Biochem. J. 164*, 607 (1977).
21. G. E. Ibbotson and K. E. Williams, Rate of pinocytic capture of macromolecular substrates by rat yolk sac incubated in serum-free culture medium, *Biochem. J. 178*, 785 (1979).
22. G. Ashwell and J. Harford, Carbohydrate specific receptors of the liver, *Annu. Ref. Biochem. 51*, 531 (1982).
23. A. L. Schwartz, S. E. Fridovich, and H. F. Lodish, Kinetics of internalization and recycling of the asialoglycoprotein receptor in a hepatoma cell line, *J. Biol. Chem. 257*, 4230 (1982).
24. H. Tolleshaug, T. Berg, M. Nilsson, and K. R. Norum, Uptake and degradation of ^{125}I-labeled asialofetuin by isolated rat hepatocytes, *Biochim. Biophys. Acta, 499*, 73 (1977).
25. P. Stahl, Lysosomes and mononuclear phagocytes. In, *Receptors and Recognition* Series B, Vol. 15 (P. Cuatrecasas and T. Roth, Eds.), Chapman and Hall, London, 1983, pp. 141–165.
26. K. Von Figura, H. Kresse, U. Meinhard, and D. Holtfrerich, Studies on secretion and endocytosis of macromolecules by cultivated skin fibroblasts, *Biochem. J. 170*, 313 (1978).
27. K. Ullrich and K. Von Figura, Endocytosis of β-N-acetylglucosaminidase from secretions of mucolipidosis-II and -III fibroblasts by non-parenchymal rat liver cells, *Biochem. J. 182*, 245 (1979).
28. P. Stahl and S. Gordon, Expression of a mannosyl-fucosyl receptor for endocytosis on cultured primary macrophages and their hybrids, *J. Cell Biol. 93*, 49 (1982).

29. J. B. Lloyd and K. E. Williams, Non-specific adsorptive pinocytosis, *Biochem. Soc. Trans. 12,* 527 (1984).
30. B. M. F. Pearse and M. S. Bretscher, Membrane recycling by coated vesicles. *Annu. Rev. Biochem. 50,* 85 (1981).
31. A. Helenius, J. Mellman, D. Wall and A. Hubbard, Endosomes, *Trends in Biochem. Sci. July,* 245 (1983).
32. I. Pastan and M. C. Willingham, Receptor-mediated endocytosis: coated pits, receptosomes and Golgi, *Trends in Biochem. Sci. July,* 250 (1983).
33. C. R. Hopkins, The importance of the endosome in intracellular traffic, *Nature 305,* 684 (1983).
34. J. N. Limet, Y-J. Schneider, J-P. Vaerman, and A. Trouet, Binding, uptake and intracellular processing of polymeric rat immunoglobulin A by cultured rat hepatocytes, *Eur. J. Biochem. 125,* 437 (1982).
35. J-C. Sibile, J-N. Octave, Y-J. Schneider, A. Trouet, and R. R. Crichton, Transferrin protein and iron uptake by cultured hepatocytes, *FEBS Lett. 150,* 365 (1982).
36. P. L. Zeitlin and A. L. Hubbard, Cell surface distribution and intracellular fate of asialoglycoproteins. A morphological and biochemical study of isolated rat hepatocytes and monolayer cultures, *J. Cell Ciol. 92,* 634 (1982).
37. J. P. Reeves, The mechanism of lysosomal acidification. In, *Lysosomes,* Vol. 7 (J. T. Dingle, R. T. Dean, and W. Sly, Eds.), Elsevier, Amsterdam, 1984, pp. 175–200.
38. R. T. Dean, *Lysosomes,* Edward Arnold (Publishers) Ltd., London, 1977.
39. J. T. Dingle (Ed.), *Lysosomes: A Laboratory Handbook,* 2nd ed. North Holland Publishing Company, Amsterdam, 1977.
40. M. Geisow, Lysosome proton pump identified, *Nature 298,* 515 (1982).
41. J. B. Lloyd, A study of permeability of lysosomes to amino acids and small peptides, *Biochem. J. 121,* 245 (1971).
42. C. N. Hales, K. Docherty, and G. A. Maguire, Sugar transport in lysosomes. In, *Lysosomes in Biology and Pathology,* Vol. 7, (J. T. Dingle, R. T. Dean, and W. Sly, Eds.), Elsevier Science Publishers B.V., Amsterdam, 1984, pp. 165–174.
43. J. Drobnik and F. Rypacek, Soluble synthetic polymers in biological systems, *Adv. Polymer Sci. 57,* 1 (1984).
44. K. E. Williams, E. M. Kidston, F. Beck, and J. B. Lloyd. Quantitative studies of pinocytosis, II. Kinetics of protein uptake and digestion by rat yolk sac cultured *in vitro, J. Cell Biol. 64,* 123 (1975).
45. G. Livesey and K. E. Williams, Hydrolysis of an exogenous ^{125}I-labeled protein by rat yolk sacs, *Biochem. J. 184,* 519 (1979).

46. J. M. Besterman, J. A. Airhart, R. C. Woodworth, and R. B. Low, Exocytosis of pinocytosed fluid in cultured cells: Kinetic evidence for rapid turnover and compartmentation, *J. Cell Biol. 91*, 716 (1981).
47. U. Weisbecker, G. E. Ibbotson, G. Livesey, and K. E. Williams, The fate of homologuos ^{125}I-labelled immunoglobulin G within rat visceral yolk sacs incubated *in vitro, Biochem. J. 214*, 815 (1983).
48. G. Gregoriadis, Ed., *Drug Carriers in Biology and Medicine*, Academic Press, London, 1979.
49. G. Gregoriadis, J. Senior, and A. Trouet, Eds., *Targeting of Drugs*, Plenum Press, New York, 1982.
50. G. Gregoriadis and J. Senior, Eds., *Receptor-Mediated Targeting of Drugs*, Plenum Press, New York, 1984.
51. H. Bundgaard, A. B. Hansen, and H. Kofod, Eds., *Optimization of Drug Delivery*, Munksgaard, Copenhagen, 1982.
52. R. Baurain, M. Masquelier, D. Deprez-De Campeneere, and A. Trouet, Targeting of daunorubicin by covalent and reversible linkage to carrier proteins, lysosomal hydrolysis and antitumoral activity of conjugates prepared with peptidic spacer arms, *Drugs Exp. Clin. Res. 9*, 303 (1983).
53. A. Trouet, R. Baurain, D. Deprez-De Campaneere, M. Masquelier, and P. Pirson, Targeting of antitumoral antiprotozoal drugs by covalent linkage to protein carriers. In, *Targeting of Drugs* (G. Gregoriadis, J. Senior, and A. Trouet, Eds.), Plenum press, New York, 1982, pp. 19–30.
54. M. C. Garnett, M. J. Embleton, E. Jacobs, and R. W. Baldwin, Preparation and properties of a drug-carrier-antibody conjugate showing selective antibody-directed cytotoxicity *in vitro, Int. J. Cancer 31*, 661 (1983).
55. B. C. F. Chu and J. M. Whiteley, Control of solid tumor metastases with a high molecular weight derivative of methotrexate, *J. Natl. Cancer Inst. 62*, 79 (1979).
56. K. Motycka, K. Slavik, J. E. Dyr, A. Balcarova, and Z. Vodrazka, The chemotherapy of C-3H mice bearing Gardner lymphosarcoma with bovine fibrinogen methotrexate derivative, *Neoplasma 28*, 3 (1981).
57. L. Fiume, C. Busi, and A. Matlioli, Targeting of antiviral drugs by coupling with protein carriers, *FEBS Lett. 153*, 6 (1983).
58. A. Trouet, D. Deprez-De Campeneere, and C. De Duve, Chemotherapy through lysosomes, with a DNA-daunorubicin complex, *Nature 239*, 110 (1972).
59. A. Trouet and G. Sokal, Clinical studies with daunorubicin-DNA and adriamycin DNA complexes: A review, *Cancer Treat Rep. 63*, 895 (1979).
60. R. Hulhoven and C. Harvengt, Distribution of daunorubicin intravenously injected or intravenously infused as free drug and as a complex with DNA in rabbits, *Pharmacology 24*, 253 (1982).

61. R. Arnon, E. Hurwitz, and M. Sela, Antibodies as carriers for oncostatic materials, *Rec. Res. Cancer Res. 75*, 236 (1980).
62. K. A. Krolick, D. Yuan, and E. S. Vitetta, Specific killing of a human breast carcinoma cell line by a monoclonal antibody coupled to the A-chain of ricin, *Cancer Immunol. Immunother. 12*, 39 (1981).
63. C. H. J. Ford, C. E. Newman, J. R. Johnson, C. S. Woodhouse, T. A. Reeder, G. F. Rowland, and R. G. Simmonds, Localization and toxicity study of a vindesine-anti-CEA conjugate in patients with advanced cancer, *Br. J. Cancer. 47*, 35 (1983).
64. M. J. Poznanzky, R. Singh, and B. Singh, Insulin: Carrier potential for enzyme and drug therapy, *Science 223*, 1304 (1984).
65. J. M. Varga, N. Asato, S. Lande, and A. B. Lerner, Melanotropin-daunomycin conjugate shows receptor-mediated cytotoxicty in cultured murine melanoma cells, *Nature 267*, 56 (1977).
66. W. T. Shier, Lectins as drug carriers. In, *Drug Carriers in Biology and Medicine* (G. Gregoriadis, Ed.), Academic Press Inc., New York, 1979, pp. 44–70.
67. T. Kitao and K. Hatto, Concanavalin A as a carrier of daunomycin, *Nature 265*, 81 (1977).
68. J. P. Remon, R. Duncan, and E. Schacht, Polymer-drug combinations: Pinocytic uptake of modified polysaccharides containing procainamide moieties by rat visceral yolk sacs cultured *in vitro*, *J. Controlled Release 1*, 47 (1984).
69. E. Schacht, Use of polysaccharides as drug carriers, *Ann. Natl. Acad. Sci.* (in press).
70. M. Konieczny, D. Charytonowicz, and A. D. Inglot, Search for carriers for non-covalent binding of interferon among 1,3,5 triazine derivatives of dextran, *Arch. Immunol. Ther. Exp. 30*, 1 (1982).
71. A. Bernstein, E. Hurwitz, R. Maron, R. Arnon, M. Sela, and M. Wilchek, Higher antitumor efficacy of daunomycin when linked to dextran, *in vivo* and *in vitro* studies, *J. Natl. Cancer Inst. 60*, 379 (1978).
72. E. Hurwitz, M. Wilchek, and J. Pitha, Soluble macromolecules as carriers of daunomycin, *J. Appl. Biochem. 2*, 25 (1980).
73. H. J-P. Ryser and W-C. Shen, Conjugation of methotrexate to poly(L-lysine) increases drug transport and overcomes drug resistance in cultured cells, *Proc. Natl. Acad. Sci. USA 75*, 3867 (1978).
74. B. C. F. Chu and S. B. Howell, Pharmacological and therapeutic properties of carrier bound methotrexate against tumor confined to a third space body compartment, *J. Pharmacol. Exp. Ther. 219*, 389 (1981).
75. F. Zunino, F. Giulliani, G. Savi, T. Dasdia, and R. Gambetta, Anti-tumor activity of daunorubicin linked to poly-*L*-aspartic acid, *Int. J. Cancer. 30*, 465 (1982).

76. F. Zunino, G. Savi, F. Giuliani, R. Gambetta, R. Supino, S. Tinelli, and G. Pezzoni, Comparison of antitumor effects of daunorubicin covalently linked to poly-L-amino acid carriers, *Eur. J. Cancer Clin. Oncol. 20*, 421 (1984).
77. M. Havranova, D. Cechova, V. Saudek, M. Metalova, and J. Drobnik, A high molecular mass derivative of trypsin-kallikrein inhibitor for potential medical use, *Hoppe-Seyler's Z. Physiol. Chem. 363*, 295 (1982).
78. T. Hirano, H. Ringsdorf, and D. S. Zaharko, Antitumor activity of monomeric and polymeric cyclophosphamide derivatives compared with *in vitro* hydrolysis, *Cancer Res. 40*, 2263 (1980).
79. M. Przybylski, E. Fell, H. Ringsdorf, and D. Z. Zaharko, Pharmacologically active polymers, 17. Synthesis and Characterization of polymeric derivatives of the antitumor agent methotrexate, *Makromol. Chem. 179*, 1719 (1978).
80. J. Kopecek, P. Rejmanova, R. Duncan, and J. B. Lloyd, Controlled release of drug model from *N*-(2-hydroxypropyl)methacrylamide copolymers, *Ann. NY Acad. Sci. 446*, 93 (1985).
81. B-U. Von Specht, H. Sainfeld, and W. Brendel, Polyvinylpyrrolidone as a soluble carrier of proteins, *Hoppe-Seyler's Z. Physiol. Chem. 354*, 1659 (1973).
82. J-C. Soutif, F. Mouity-Moussounda, and J.-C. Brosse, Polymeric carriers of glycerol derivatives, 2. Chlorambucil derivatives, *Makromol. Chem. 4*, 61 (1983).
83. J. Pato, M. Azori, and F. Tudos, Polymeric prodrugs. 2. Synthesis by coupling of drugs via spacer group, *Makromol. Chem. Rapit Commun. 4*, 25 (1983).
84. H. Ringsdorf, Structure and properties of pharmacologically active polymers, *J. Polymer Sci. Polymer Symp. 51*, 135 (1975).
85. J. Kopecek, Synthesis of tailor-made soluble polymeric drug carriers. In, *Recent Advances in Drug Delivery Systems* (S. W. Kim and J. M. Anderson, Eds.), Plenum Press, New York, 1984 pp. 41–62.
86. A. Trouet, R. Baurain, D. Deprez-De Campeneere, D. Layton, and M. Masquelier, DNA, Liposomes and proteins as carriers for antitumoral drugs. In, *Recent Results in Cancer Research*, Vol. 75 (G. Mathe and F. M. Muggia, Eds.), Springer-Verlag, Berlin, 1980, pp. 229–235.
87. L. Gros, Biological activity of polymers. In, *Encyclopedia of Polymer Science* (J. I. Kroschwitz, Ed.), John Wiley & Sons Inc., New York, 1984 (in press).
88. M. Masquelier, R. Baurain, D. Deprez-De Campeneere, and A. Trouet, Antitumor activity of daunorubicin linked to proteins: Biological and antitumor properties of peptidic derivatives of daunorubicin used as intermediates. In, *Current Chemotherapy and Immunotherapy*, Proceedings of the 12th International Congress of Chemotherapy, Florence, Italy, 19–24 July 1981, p. 1428.

89. A. Trouet, M. Masquelier, R. Baurain, and D. Deprez-De Campeneere, A covalent linkage between daunorubicin and proteins that is stable in serum and reversible by lysosomal hydrolyses, as required for a lysosomotropic drug-carrier conjugate: *In vitro* and *in vivo* studies, *Proc. Natl. Acad. Sci. USA 79*, 626 (1982).
90. R. Duncan, J. Kopecek, and J. B. Lloyd, Development of *N*-(2-hydroxypropyl)-methacrylamide copolymers as carriers of therapeutic agents. In, *Polymers in Medicine: Biomedical and Pharmacological Applications* (E. Chiellini and P. Guisti, Eds.), Plenum Press, New York, 1983, pp. 97–114.
91. J. Kopecek, Biodegradation of polymers of biomedical use. In, *IUPAC Macromolecules* (H. Benoit and P. Rempp, Eds.), Pergamon Press, New York, 1982, pp. 305–320.
92. J. Kopecek and P. Rejmanova, Enzymatically degradable bonds in synthetic polymers. In, *Controlled Drug Delivery* Vol. 1 (S. D. Bruck, Ed.), CRC Press, Boca Raton, FL, 1983, pp. 81–124.
93. J. Kopecek, Controlled biodegradability of polymers—A key to drug delivery systems, *Biomaterials 5*, 19 (1984).
94. J. Kopecek, P. Rejmanova, and V. Chytry, Polymers containing enzymatically degradable bonds, 1. Chymotrypsin catalyzed hydrolysis of *p*-nitroanilides of phenylalanine and tyrosine attached to side-chains of copolymers of *N*-(2-hydroxypropyl)-methacrylamide, *Makromol. Chem. 182*, 799 (1981).
95. P. Rejamnova, J. Kopecek, R. Duncan, and J. B. Lloyd, Susceptibility of oligopeptide sequences in *N*-(2-hydroxypropyl)-methacrylamide copolymers to degradation by rat plasma and serum, *Biomaterials 6*, 45 (1985).
96. R. Duncan, J. B. Lloyd, and J. Kopecek, Degradation of side chains of *N*-(2-hydroxypropyl)methacrylamide copolymers by lysosomal enzymes, *Biochem. Biophys. Res. Commun. 94*, 824 (1980).
97. R. Duncan, H. C. Cable, J. B. Lloyd, P. Rejmanova, and J. Kopecek, Degradation of side-chains of *N*-(2-hydroxypropyl)-methacrylamide copolymers by lysosomal thiol-proteinases, *Biosci. Rep. 2*, 1041 (1982).
98. R. Duncan, H. C. Cable, J. B. Lloyd, P. Rejmanova, and J. Kopecek, Polymers containing enzymatically degradable bonds, 7. Design of oligopeptide side-chains in poly *N*-2(hydroxypropyl)methacrylamide copolymers to promote efficient degradation by lysosomal enzymes, *Makromol. Chem. 184*, 1997 (1983).
99. P. Rejmanova, J. Pohl, M. Baudys, M. Kostka, J. Kostka, and J. Kopecek, Degradation of oligopeptide sequences in *N*-(2-hydroxypropyl)methacrylamide copolymers by bovine spleen cathepsin B, *Makromol. Chem. 184*, 2009 (1983).

100. P. Rejmanova, J. Pohl, V. Subr, M. Baudys, V. Kostka, and J. Kopecek, (unpublished results).
101. I. Schechter and A. Berger, On the size of active site in proteases. 1 Papain, *Biochem. Biophys. Res. Commun. 27,* 157 (1967).
102. W-C. Shen and H.J-P. Ryser, Cis-aconityl spacer between daunomycin and macromolecular carriers: A model of pH-sensitive linkage releasing drug from a lysosomotropic conjugate, *Biochem. Biophys. Res. Commun. 102,* 1048 (1981).
103. B. Ballou, R. J. Taylor, W-C. Shen, M. Liebert, H. J-P. Ryser, D. Solter, and T. R. Hakala, Daunomycin targeting to the MH-15 teratocarcinoma using anti SSEA-1., *Fed. Proc. 42,* 685 (1983).
104. J. Black, Systemic effects of biomaterials, *Biomaterials 5,* 11 (1984).
105. B. Rihova, K. Ulbrich, J. Kopecek, and P. Mancal, Immunogenicity of *N*-(2-hydroxypropyl)methacrylamide copolymers—Potential hapten or drug carriers, *Folia Microbiol. 28,* 217 (1983).
106. B. Rihova, J. Kopecek, K. Ulbrich, M. Pospisil, and P. Mancal, Effect of chemical structure of *N*-(2-hydroxypropyl)methacrylamide copolymers on the immune response of inbred strains of mice, *Biomaterials* (in press).
107. B. Rihova and I. Riha, Immunological problems of polymer-bound drug, *CRC Crit. Rev. Ther. Drug Carrier Systems 1,* 311 (1985).
108. T. J. Gill III and W. Kunz, The immunogenicity of vinyl polymers, *Proc. Natl. Acad. Sci. USA 61,* 490 (1968).
109. M. Sela, S. Fuchs, and R. Arnon, Studies on the chemical basis of the antigenicity of proteins. 5. Synthesis, characterization and immunogenicity of some multichain and linear polypeptides containing tyrosine, *Biochem. J. 85,* 223 (1962).
110. E. Reske-Nielsen, M. Bojsen-Moller, M. Vetner, and J. C. Hansen, Polyvinylpyrrolidone-storage disease, *Acta Path. Microbiol. Scand. Sect. A. 8,* 397 (1976).
111. A. E. F. H. Meijer and R. G. J. Willinghagen, The activity of glucose-6-phosphatase, adenosine triphosphatase, succinic dehydrogenase, and acid phosphatase after dextran or polyvinylpyrrolidone uptake by the liver *in vivo, Biochem. Pharmacol. 12,* 973 (1963).
112. K. Ulbrich, J. Strohalm, and J. Kopecek, Polymers containing enzymatically bonds. 3. Poly *N*-(2-hydroxypropyl)methacrylamide chains connected by oligopeptide sequences cleavable by trypsin, *Makromol. Chem. 182,* 1917 (1981).
113. P. Rejmanova, B. Obereigner, and J. Kopecek, Polymers containing enzymatically degradable bonds. 2. Poly *N*-(2-hydroxypropyl)methacrylamide chains connected by oligopeptide sequences cleavable by chymotrypsin, *Makromol. Chem. 182,* 1899 (1981).

114. K. Ulbrich, E. I. Zacharieva, B. Obereigner, and J. Kopecek, Polymers containing enzymatically degradable bonds. V. Hydrophilic polymers degradable by papain, *Biomaterials 1*, 199 (1980).
115. S. A. Cartlidge, R. Duncan, J. B. Lloyd, P. Rejmanova, and J. Kopecek, Pinocytic capture and intracellular degradation of poly *N*-(2-hydroxypropyl)methacrylamide chains connected by oligopeptide sequences. Abstract from the International Conference on Biomedical Polymers, Durham, U.K., July, 1982.
116. J. Kopecek, I. Cifkova, P. Rejmanova, J. Strohalm, B. Obereigner, and K. Ulbrich, Polymers containing enzymatically degradable bonds. 4. Preliminary experiments *in vivo, Makromol. Chem. 182*, 2941 (1981).
117. G. Poste, Liposome targeting *in vivo*: Problems and opportunities, *Biol. Cell 47*, 19 (1983).
118. R. Duncan, M. K. Pratten, H. C. Cable, H. Ringsdorf, and J. B. Lloyd, Effect of molecular size of ^{125}I-labelled poly(vinylpyrrolidone) on its pinocytosis by rat visceral yolk sacs and rat peritoneal macrophages, *Biochem. J. 196*, 49 (1981).
119. S. A. Cartlidge, R. Duncan, P. Rejmanova, J. Kopecek, and J. B. Lloyd, Pinocytosis of soluble crosslinked *N*-(2-hydroxypropyl)methacrylamide copolymers by rat visceral yolk sacs and rat intestine cultured *in vitro*, Effect of molecular weight on uptake and intracellular degradation, *J. Controlled Release 3*, 55 (1986).
120. G. S. Vince and R. T. Dean, Comparative studies on the endocytosis of proteins in kidney tubule cells, *Biochem. Soc. Trans.* (in press).
121. R. Duncan and M. K. Pratten, Pinocytosis: Mechanism and regulation. In *Mononuclear Phagocytes: Physiology and Pathology* (R. T. Dean and W. Jessup, Eds.), Elsevier Biomedical Press, Amsterdam 1985, pp. 27–51.
122. M. K. Pratten, R. Duncan, and J. B. Lloyd, A comparative study of the effects of polyamino acids and dextran derivatives on pinocytosis in the rat yolk sac and the rat peritoneal macrophage, *Biochim. Biophys. Acta 540*, 455 (1978).
123. R. Duncan, M. K. Pratten, and J. B. Lloyd, Mechanism of polycation stimulation of pinocytosis, *Biochim. Biophys. Acta, 587*, 463 (1979).
124. H. J-P. Ryser, A membrane effect of basic polymers dependent on molecular size, *Nature 215*, 934 (1967).
125. T. Kooistra, A Duursma, J. M. W. Bouma, and M. Gruber, Effect of size and charge on endocytosis of lysozyme derivatives by sinusoidal rat liver cells *in vivo, Biochem. Biophys. Acta 631*, 439 (1980).
126. J. Sinke, J. M. W. Bouma, T. Kooistra, and M. Gruber, Endocytosis and breakdown of ^{125}I-labelled lactate dehydrogenase

isoenzyme M4 by rat liver and spleen *in vivo*, *Biochem. J. 180*, 1 (1979).
127. T. Kooistra, M. K. Pratten, and K. E. Williams, Endocytosis of simple proteins by rat yolk sacs and by rat peritoneal macrophages incubated *in vitro*, *Acta Biol. Med. Germ. 40*, 1637 (1981).
128. G. Livesey and K. E. Williams, Heterogenicity of binding sites for adsorptive pinocytosis of simple proteins by rat yolk sacs, *Eur. J. Biochem. 122*, 147 (1982).
129. R. Duncan, H. C. Cable, F. Rypacek, J. Drobnik, and J. B. Lloyd, Enhancement of adsorptive pinocytosis of a polyaspartamide by incorporation of tyramine residues, *Biochem. Soc. Trans. 12*, 1064 (1984).
130. F. Rypacek, J. Drobnik, V. Chmelar, and J. Kalal, The renal excretion and retention of macromolecules. The chemical structure effect, *Pflügers Arch. 392*, 211 (1982).
131. F. Rypacek, J. Drobnik, and J. Kalal, Progess in model studies in cellular uptake, *Ann. NY Acad. Sci.* (in press).
132. C. H. C. M. Buys, A. S. H. De Jong, J. M. W. Bouma, and M. Gruber, Rapid uptake by liver sinusoidal cells of serum albumin modified with retention of its compact conformation, *Biochim. Biophys. Acta 392*, 95 (1975).
133. R. Blomhoff, W. Eskild, and T. Ber, Endocytosis of formaldehyde-treated serum albumin via scavenger pathway in liver endothelial cells, *Biochem. J. 218*, 81 (1984).
134. M. K. Pratten, R. Duncan, H. C. Cable, R. Schnee, H. Ringsdorf, and J. B. Lloyd, Pinocytic uptake of divinylether-maleic anhydride (pyran copolymer) and its failure to stimulate pinocytosis, *Chem. Biol. Interact. 35*, 319 (1981).
135. K. Park and J. R. Robinson, Polymer binding to epithelial cells. In, *Optimization of Drug Delivery* (H. Bundgaard, A. B. Hansen, and H. Kofod, Eds.), Munksgaard, Cophenhagen, 1982, pp. 35–52.
136. K. Park, H. S. Ch'ng, and J. R. Robinson, Alternative approaches to oral controlled drug delivery: bioadhesives and *in-situ* systems. In, *Recent Advances in Drug Delivery Systems* (S. W. Kim and J. M. Anderson, Eds.), Plenum Press, New York, 1984.
137. D. A. Tirrell and P. M. Boyd, Interaction of synthetic polymers with cell membranes and model membrane systems, 1. Differential scanning calorimetry, *Makromol. Chem. Rabid Commun. 2*, 193 (1981).
138. J. Vermeersch, L. Ruys, E. Schacht, J. P. Remon, and R. Duncan, Synthesis and biological evaluation of procainamide containing polysaccharides, Abstract from the 26th Microsymposium on Macromolecules on Polymers in Medicine and Biology, Prague, July 9–12, 1984, pp. S4-1 to S4-4.

139. E. F. Neufeld and G. Ashwell, Carbohydrate recognition systems for receptor-mediated pinocytosis. In, *The Biochemistry of Glycoproteins and Proteoglycans* (W. J. Lennarz, Ed.), Plenum Press, New York, 1980, Chap. 6.
140. P. Cuatrecasas and T. Roth, Eds., Receptors and Recognition Series B, Vol. 15, *Receptor-Mediated Endocytosis*, Chapman and Hall, London, 1983.
141. M. Monsigny, C. Kieda, and A-C. Roche, Membrane glycoproteins, glycolipids and membrane lectins as recognition signals in normal and malignant cells, *Biol. Cell. 47*, 95 (1983).
142. M. I. Horowitz, Ed., *The Glycoconjugates*, Vol. IV. *Glycoproteins, Glycolipids and Proteoglycans*, Part B, Academic Press, New York, 1982.
143. G. Ashwell and A. G. Morell, The role of surface carbohydrates in the hepatic recognition and transport of circulating glycoproteins, *Adv. Enzymol. 41*, 99 (1974).
144. A. G. Morell, R. A. Irvine, I. Sternlieb, I. M. Scheinberg, and G. Ashwell, Physical and Chemical studies on ceruloplasmin V. Metabolic studies on sialic acid-free ceruloplasmin *in vivo*, *J. Biol. Chem. 243*, 155 (1968).
145. A. L. Hubbard, G. Wilson, G. Ashwell, and H. Stukenbrok, An electron microscope autoradiographic study of the carbohydrate recognition systems in the rat liver. I. Distribution of ^{125}I-ligands among the liver cell types, *J. Cell. Biol. 83*, 47 (1979).
146. T. Tanabe, W. E. Pricer, Jr., and G. Ashwell, Subcellular membrane topology and turnover of rat hepatic binding protein specific for asialoglycoproteins, *J. Biol. Chem. 254*, 1038 (1979).
147. C. J. Steer, E. S. Kempner, and G. Ashwell, Molecular size of the hepatic receptor for asialoglycoproteins determined in situ by radiation inactivation, *J. Biol. Chem. 256*, 5851 (1981).
148. H. B. Haimes, R. J. Stockert, A. G. Morell, and A. B. Novikoff, Carbohydrate-specified endocytosis: Localization of ligand in the lysosomal compartment, *Proc. Natl. Acad. Sci. USA 78*, 6936 (1981).
149. W. M. Partridge, A. J. Vantlerle, R. T. Naruse, G. Fierar, and A. Costin, *In vivo* quantification of receptor mediated uptake of asialoglycoproteins by rat liver, *J. Biol. Chem. 258*, 990 (1983).
150. K. Kawaguchi, M. Kuhlenschmidt, S. Roseman, and J. C. Lee, Differential uptake of *D*-galactosyl- and *D*-glucosyl-neoglycoproteins by isolated rat hepatocytes, *J. Biol. Chem. 256*, 2230 (1981).
151. M. Deschuyteneer, J-P. Pricels, and R. Mosselmans, Galactose-specific adsorptive endocytosis: An ultrastructural qualitative and quantitative study in cultured rat hepatocytes, *Biol. Cell. 50*, 17 (1984).

152. C. J. Steer and G. Ashwell, Studies on a mammalian hepatic binding protein specific for asialoglycoproteins, *J. Biol. Chem. 255*, 3008 (1980).
153. K. Bridges, J. Harford, G. Ashwell, and R. D. Klausner, Fate of receptor and ligand during endocytosis of asialoglycoproteins by isolated hepatocytes, *Proc. Natl. Acad. Sci. USA 79*, 350 (1982).
154. J. U. Baenziger and D. Fiete, Recycling of the hepatocyte asialoglycoprotein receptor does not require delivery of ligand to lysosomes, *J. Biol. Chem. 257*, 6007 (1982).
155. D. B. Cawley, D. L. Simpson, and H. R. Herschman, Asialoglycoprotein receptor mediates the toxic effects of an asialofetulin diptheria toxin fragment A conjugate on cultured rat hepatocytes, *Proc. Natl. Acad. Sci. USA 78*, 3383 (1981).
156. L. Fiume, C. Busi, and A. Matlioli, Lactosaminated human serum albumin as hepatotropic drug carrier. Rate of uptake by mouse liver, *FEBS Lett. 146*, 42 (1982).
157. K. Furnuno, N. Miwa, and K. Kato, Receptor-mediated introduction of pepstatin-asialofetuin conjugate into liposomes of rat hepatocytes, *J. Biochem. 93*, 249 (1983).
158. R. Duncan, J. Kopecek, P. Rejmanova, and J. B. Lloyd, Targeting of *N*-(2-hydroxypropyl)methacrylamide copolymers to liver incorporation of galactose residues, *Biochim. Biophys. Acta 755*, 518 (1983).
159. R. Duncan, J. B. Lloyd, P. Rejmanova, and J. Kopecek, Methods of targeting *N*-(2-hydroxypropyl)methacrylamide copolymers to particular cell types, *Makromol. Chem. Suppl. 9*, 3 (1985).
160. H. Kolb and V. Kolb-Bachafen, A lectin-like receptor on mammalian macrophages, *Biochem. Biophys. Res. Commun. 85*, 678 (1978).
161. R. Teradaira, V. Kolb-Bachofen, J. Schlepper-Schafer, and H. Kolb, Galactose-particle receptor on liver macrophages. Quantitation of particle uptake, *Biochim. Biophys. Acta 759*, 306 (1983).
162. P. Stahl, P. H. Schlesinger, J. Rodman, and T. Doebber, Recognition of lysosomal glycosidases *in vivo* inhibited by modified glycoproteins, *Nature 264*, 86 (1976).
163. P. Stahl, H. Siz, J. S. Rodman, P. Schlesinger, D. R. P. Tulsiani, and O. Touster, Evidence for specific recognition sites mediating clearance of lysosomal enzymes *in vivo, Proc. Natl. Acad. Sci. USA 73*, 4045 (1976).
164. D. T. Achord, F. E. Brot, and W. S. Sly, Inhibition of the rat clearance system for agalacto-orosomucoid by yeast mannans and by mannose, *Biochem. Biophys. Res. Commun. 77*, 409 (1977).
165. D. T. Achord, F. E. Brot, C. E. Bell, and W. S. Sly, Human B-glucuronidase: *In vivo* clearance and *in vitro* uptake by a

glycoprotein recognition system on reticuloendothelial cells, *Cell 15*, 269 (1978).
166. Y. C. Lee, C. P. Stowell, and M. K. Krantz, 2-Imino-2-methoxyethyl-*L*-thioglycosides: New reagents for attaching sugars to proteins, *Biochemistry 15*, 3956 (1976).
167. R. T. Lee and Y. C. Lee, Preparation and some biochemical properties of neoglycoproteins produced by reductive amination of thioglycosides containing co-aldehydoaglycan, *Biochemistry 19*, 156.
168. P. D. Stahl, J. S. Rodman, J. M. Miller, and P. H. Schlesinger, Evidence for receptor-mediated binding of glycoproteins, glycon-jugates and lysosomal glycosidases by alveolar macrophages, *Proc. Natl. Acad. Sci. USA 75*, 1399 (1978).
169. V. Shepherd, J. C. Lee, P. H. Schlesinger, and P. Stahl, *L*-Fucose-terminated glycoconjugates are recognized by pinocytosis receptors on macrophages, *Proc. Natl. Acad. Sci. USA 78*, 1019 (1981).
170. P. Stahl, P. Schlesinger, E. Sigardson, J. S. Rodman, and Y. C. Lee, Receptor-mediated pinocytosis of mannose glycon-jugates by macrophages: characterization and evidence for receptor recycling, *Cell 19*, 207 (1980).
171. Y. Maynard and J. U. Baenziger, Oligosaccharide specific endocytosis by isolated rat hepatic reticuloendothelial cells, *J. Biol. Chem. 256*, 8063 (1981).
172. Y. Mizuno, Y. Kozutsumi, T. Kowasaki, and I. Yamashina, Isolation and characterization of a mannan-binding protein from rat liver, *J. Biol. Chem. 256*, 4247 (1981).
173. R. Townsend and P. Stahl, Isolation and characterization of a mannose/*N*-acetylglucosamine/fucose-binding protein from rat liver, *Biochem. J. 194*, 209 (1981).
174. J. Wild, D. Robinson, and B. Winchester, Isolation of mannose-binding proteins from human and rat liver, *Biochem. J. 210*, 167 (1983).
175. J-P. Prieels, S. V. Pizzo, L. R. Glasgow, J. C. Paulson, and R. L. Hill, Hepatic receptor that specifically binds oligosaccharides containing fucosyl α-1-3-N-acetyl glucosamine linkages, *Proc. Natl. Acad. Sci. USA 75*, 2215 (1978).
176. E. F. Neufeld, T. W. Lim, and L. J. Shapiro, Inherited disorders of lysosomal metabolism, *Annu. Rev. Biochem. 44*, 357 (1975).
177. A. Kaplan, D. T. Achord, and W. S. Sly, Phosphohexoxyl components of a lysosomal enzyme are recognized by pinocytosis receptors on human fibroblasts, *Proc. Natl. Acad. Sci. USA 74*, 2026 (1977).
178. W. S. Sly, The uptake and transport of lysosomal enzymes. In, *The Glycoconjugates*, Vol. IV (M. I. Horowitz, Ed.), Academic Press, New York, 1982, pp. 3–25.

179. K. Ullrich, G. Mersmann, M. Fleischer, and K. Von Figura, Epithelial rat liver cells have cell surface receptors recognizing a phosphorylated carbohydrate on lysosomal enzymes, *Hoppe-Seyler's Z. Physiol. Chem. 359*, 1591 (1978).
180. H. D. Fischer, A. Gonzalez-Noriega, W. S. Sly, and D. J. Morre, Phosphomannosylenzyme receptors in rat liver, *J. Biol. Chem. 255*, 9608 (1980).
181. T. Feizi, Monoclonal antibodies reveal saccharide structures of glycoproteins and glycolipids as differentiation and tumor-associated antigens, *Biochem. Soc. Trans. 12*, 545 (1984).
182. A. C. Roche, M. Barzilay, P. Midoux, S. Junqua, N. Sharon, and M. Monsigny, Sugar-specific endocytosis of glycoproteins by Lewis lung carcinoma cells, *J. Cell Biochem. 22*, 131 (1983).
183. J. L. Goldstein and M. S. Brown, The low density lipoprotein pathway and its relation to atherosclerosis, *Annu. Rev. Biochem. 46*, 897 (1977).
184. E. L. Biermann and J. J. Albers, Lipoprotein uptake by cultured human arterial smooth muscle cells, *Biochim. Biophys. Acta 388*, 198 (1975).
185. D. B. Weisnstein, T. E. Carew, and D. Steinberg, Uptake and degradation of low density lipoprotein by swine arterial smooth muscle cells with inhibition of cholesterol biosynthesis, *Biochim. Biophys. Acta 424*, 404 (1976).
186. E. A. Kirsten and J. A. Watson, Regulation of 3-hydroxy-3-methylglutaryl coenzyme A reductase in hepatoma tissue culture cells by serum lipoproteins, *J. Biol. Chem. 249*, 6104 (1974).
187. A. M. Fogelman, J. Edmond, J. Seager, and G. Popjak, Abnormal induction of 3-hydroxy-3-methylgutamyl coenzyme A reductase in leukocytes from subjects with heterozygous hypercholesterolemia, *J. Biol. Chem. 250*, 2045 (1975).
188. G. Gregoriadis, Old drugs in new clothing, *Nature 310*, 186 (1984).
189. R. J. Desnick, S. R. Thorpe, and M. B. Fiddler, Toward enzyme therapy for lysosomal storage diseases, *Physiol. Rev. 56*, 57 (1976).
190. G. Gregoriadis, Liposomes in the therapy of lysosomal storage diseases, *Nature 275*, 695 (1978).
191. M. J. Poznansky and D. Bhardwaj, Antibody-mediated targeting of α-1,4-glucosidase-albumin polymers to rat hepatocytes. A model for enzyme therapy, *Biochem. J. 196*, 89 (1981).
192. M. J. Poznansky and D. Bhardwaj, 1,4-Glucosidase-albumin polymers: *In vitro* properties and advantages for enzyme replacement therapy, *Can. J. Physiol. Pharmacol. 58*, 322 (1980).
193. G. Poste and I. J. Fidler, Stimulation of macrophage mediated destruction of lung metastases by administration of immunomodulators encapsulated in liposomes. In, *Liposomes, Drugs and*

Immunocompetent Cell Functions (C. Nicolau and A. Paraf, Eds.), Academic Press, New York, 1981, pp. 147–162.

194. P. Pirson, R. F. Steiger, R. Baurain, M. Masquelier, and A. Trouet, Antimalarial activity of liposomal primaquine and peptidic derivatives of primaquine. In, *The Host Invader Interplay* (H. Van den Bossche, Ed.), Elsevier/North-Holland Biomedical Press, Amsterdam, 1980, pp. 663–667.
195. M. J. Poznansky, M. Shandling, M. A. Salkie, J. Elliott, and E. Lau, Advantages in the use of L-asparaginase-albumin polymer as an antitumor agent, *Cancer Res. 42*, 1020 (1982).
196. R. R. C. New, M. L. Chance, and S. Heath, Liposome therapy for experimental cutaneous and visceral leishmaniasis, *Biol. Cell 47*, 59 (1983).
197. V. L. Shepherd, P. D. Stahl, P. Bernol, and M. Rabinovitch, Receptor mediated entry of beta glucoronidase into the parasitophorus vacuoles of macrophages infected with Leishmania-mexicana-amozonesis, *J. Exp. Med. 157*, 147 (1983).

15

Antibodies for Drug Delivery

KARL ERIK HELLSTRÖM and INGEGERD HELLSTRÖM / ONCOGEN, Seattle, Washington

GARY E. GOODMAN / Tumor Institute, Swedish Hospital Medical Center, Seattle, Washington

I. INTRODUCTION

While cancer chemotherapy has had remarkable success for certain tumors, e.g., childhood leukemia, choriocarcinoma, and testicular carcinoma [1], it has been relatively ineffective for many of the more common tumors, e.g., lung cancer and colon cancer. Its effectiveness also against these tumors may increase, if one could find drugs that are more specific, or if one could selectively concentrate ("target") the available drugs to tumors. For those tumors which are confined to a certain site, e.g., to an extremity or a specific organ, local perfusion with a chemotherapeutic agent may achieve such targeting [2]. However, this approach is unfortunately not feasible in disseminated cancer.

Antibodies may be used for concentrating drugs to tumor and obtain the degree of selectivity needed to achieve a therapeutic effect. This concept, which goes back to Paul Ehrlich's postulated "magic bullets" [3], received an experimental basis from the demonstration that there are antigens with some degree of tumor specificity [4–9], and that antibodies to such antigens can be made, for example, by immunizing a different species [7]. Antisera of the latter type have been conjugated with anti-cancer drugs, such as methotrexate [10], chlorambucil [11], adriamycin [12], and platinum [13]. It is very difficult, however, to develop a standardized therapeutic protocol with antisera since their specificity is often hard to determine.

The monoclonal antibody technique [14] should be helpful in this context, since it makes it possible to obtain large amounts of antibodies of uniform specificity and affinity. Using this technique, several antigens in human tumors have been identified and characterized [15]. Those antigens which both have a high degree of tumor-association and are strongly expressed at the cell surface are of the greatest interest for tumor targeting. There is already evidence that both radiolabeled [16] and unlabeled [17–19] antibodies to such antigens can localize in tumors when infused into patients.

This chapter summarizes work on monoclonal antibody-defined human tumor antigens with an eye towards therapy with antibody-drug conjugates, and it discusses some present and potential uses of such conjugates. It does not include work with antibodies that have been labeled with radioisotopes or coupled with toxins, nor does it cover the use of antibodies which, by themselves, have an antitumor effect. For this, we refer to recent review articles [20–22].

II. TUMOR ANTIGENS DEFINED BY MONOCOLONAL ANTIBODIES

A. General Aspects

1. *Nature of the Antibodies*

Most of the available monoclonal antitumor antibodies have been obtained by immunizing mice with human tumor cells, hybridizing their spleen cells with drug-marked mouse myeloma cells [14,23], and screening the hybridomas for the formation of antibodies that can bind to cells from the immunizing tumor but not to a panel of normal cells [24,25]. Antibodies have been obtained representing different classes and isotypes and are often available to several different epitopes on the same antigen molecule. For targeting we need affinity of $10^8 M^{-1}$ or better. Furthermore, IgG antibodies appear to be preferable to IgM, since they are easier to work with and may localize better to tumor because of their smaller molecular size. There are at least two ways to obtain an IgG-producing hybridoma when starting with a hybridoma making an IgM of the desired specificity. First, one can perform "class-switching" [26], and, second, it is a fairly straightforward procedure to obtain new hybridomas, producing a specific antibody isotype when the antigen is already defined [27,28]. For therapeutic purposes one also needs hybridomas that can produce the large amounts of antibodies likely to be required for clinical trials (see further below).

It is hard to predict whether whole antibodies or antibody fragments, such as Fab and $F(26')_2$, are preferable for tumor targeting, and there will probably be different needs under different circumstances. An advantage of the fragments is that they are less immunogenic than whole antibodies by lacking the Fc part of the molecule, and their smaller size may facilitate penetration into tumor tissue [16]. Fab fragments have less affinity than whole antibodies and $F(26')_2$ fragments. It may, therefore, not be practical to work with Fab, unless an antibody has an avidity better than $10^8 M^{-1}$.

It is, in principle, advantageous to have human rather than mouse antibodies for therapeutic purposes, since they are less foreign to patients and thus less prone to induce antibodies to themselves and since they may have a stronger antitumor activity on their own. The goal of obtaining human monoclonal antibodies is being approached from several directions. These include hybridizing lymphocytes obtained from cancer patients with human [29,30] or mouse [31] myeloma cells or transforming them with the EBV virus [32]. Using the former approach, antibodies with some tumor specificity have been obtained [31, 33–35]. However, many of these antibodies are less tumor specific than the best ones of mouse origin, perhaps because of a lack of immunogenicity of many tumor antigens in the host. This should not be taken as a reason for not trying to obtain human antibodies, but as a suggestion to try alternative strategies for generating them. These include the use of mouse antibodies to first isolate an antigen followed by *in vitro* sensitization of human lymphocytes to it. Starting with a mouse hybridoma, it may also become feasible to splice the mouse gene coding for the antigen binding site onto a human gene coding for the constant region [36]. Human genes coding for some desirable biological qualities, such as activation of complement and/or of macrophages, and mediation of antibody-dependent cellular cytotoxicity [37], may be the ones of choice for combination with mouse genes determining a desirable antibody specificity.

Although human antibodies have the advantage of lacking immunogenic determinants of mouse origin, they will still elicit immune responses when repeatedly injected into patients, since they have both allotypic and idiotypic antigenic determinants. Although the latter responses are likely to be weaker and need a longer period of exposure than those against mouse antibodies, some procedures for "tolerizing" human patients may have to be worked out. There is then, of course, the possibility that these procedures may be sufficiently effective to allow also the repeated infusion of mouse antibodies. It is encouraging that many cancer patients who have received large doses of mouse immunoglobulin (up to 420 mg) have not formed detectable levels of anti-mouse antibodies until after several weeks [19].

2. *Antigen Specificity*

The modern era of tumor immunology started when it was found that inbred mice could be rendered immune to syngeneic tumor transplants. This immunity was detected by the ability of the mice to reject a small number of cells derived from the immunizing tumor and, sometimes, from certain other tumors with cross-reacting antigens [4–6, 38]. Tumors induced by large doses of chemical carcinogens were found to have individually unique antigens, and those induced by viruses to have antigens that are shared by most tumors associated with the same virus. Since none of these different antigens was detected in normal tissues [6], the findings were taken as evidence for tumor specificity.

It has not been possible to prove the existence of any similar, truly tumor specific antigens in human neoplasms by using monoclonal mouse antibodies. Rather, the tumor antigens detected have been found also in normal tissues, although commonly only in trace amounts [22,39]. When considering these data one needs to realize that the techniques used to analyze the specificity of monoclonal antibodies are many times more sensitive than those employed in the early days of tumor immunology. Although this may account for the differences observed; there may, of course, be human antigens that are tumor specific but not yet identified.

The demonstration that most (all?) monoclonal antibody-defined human tumor antigens have relative rather than absolute specificity can be illustrated by our own studies on the melanoma-associated glycoprotein p97, which is one of the antigens that has been investigated the most. Approximately 50% of melanomas have ⩾50,000 molecules of p97 (with values up to 400,000 molecules) per cell and a few other tumors have intermediary p97 levels (10,000–50,000 molecules/cell) [40,41]. Normal adult tissues, on the other hand, express less than about 8000 p97 molecules per cell, and generally only a few hundred molecules/cell. Thus, about half of all melanomas have approximately a 10-fold greater amount of p97 than the most positive normal cells, and some 100 times more p97 than normal cells in organs such as blood, bone marrow, kidney, gut and brain. It is interesting to note that the difference in expression of oncogene products, between neoplastic and normal cells, is also quantitative and of a similar magnitude [42,43].

It has been argued that since mouse antibodies initially failed to detect much of the fine specificity of HLA antigens, as this can be defined by using human antisera, immunization of mice with human tumors induces antibodies to "framework" determinants of antigen molecules rather than to any determinants that are unique to tumor, and that unique antigens may have been detected had they been searched for in other ways. Although this argument cannot be dismissed, it does not negate two facts. First, the specificity obtained with most of the monoclonal human antitumor antibodies so far available appears worse than that seen with the best mouse antibodies. Second, it has not been possible to obtain antibodies to any truly specific tumor antigens in mice by immunizing syngeneic, allogeneic, or xenogeneic hosts [44,45]. Some of the most tumor-specific antibodies to mouse neoplasms have, as a matter of fact, been obtained by immunizing rats rather than mice [45]. Furthermore, recent work has shown that highly specific mouse antibodies to HLA determinants can, indeed, be obtained, making the argument invalid that the mouse only recognizes framework determinants.

When considering an antigen as a target for therapy, the number of antigen molecules per tumor cell may be as important as the degree of antigen specificity, since it will determine how many antibody molecules can bind to each tumor cell. An entirely tumor-specific antigen would be useless for targeting, if its expression at the cell surface would not allow the binding of the number of molecules of antibody (conjugate) needed to achieve a therapeutic effect; the number of such molecules needed may, however, be low if the antigen is intimately connected with the neoplastic transformation. It is noteworthy that the procedures presently used to obtain monoclonal mouse antibodies to human tumors seem to favor the generation of antibodies to antigens that are expressed at high levels by tumor cells.

3. *Localization of Antibodies to Tumor*

An antibody to be considered for targeting must be able to localize into tumor tissue. An obvious prerequisite for this is that it is targeted to an antigen that is expressed *in vivo* and not just on cultured cells. Furthermore, normal tissues should bind very little, if any, of the antibody. Immunohistological techniques applied to frozen sections are useful to assess this [46,47]. Antigen expression *in vivo* can also be measured by performing binding assays with cell membrane preparations from tumors and normal tissues [40]. The former approach is better by showing which cells express a given antigen, although it does not, like the binding assays, give quantitative information.

After having identified an antigen as expressed *in vivo*, experiments are commonly performed in nude mice which have been transplanted with an appropriate human tumor. The mice are injected simultaneously with specific and control antibodies (or antibody fragments) which have been labelled with different isotopes, and the ratios of the uptake of the two in tumor is calculated [48,49].

If an antibody can specifically localize to tumors in nude mice, a logical next step is to investigate its localization in man. Such studies, using labelled whole antibodies as well as Fab fragments, have been done for several types of neoplasms. These include colon carcinoma [50–53] and melanoma [54–56].

A key question is whether the localization of injected antibody has specificity for tumor antigens. It was answered affirmatively in an investigation [16,54], in which melanoma patients were injected with Fab fragments specific for the melanoma-associated antigen p97. Anti-p97 and control Fab fragments were labelled with ^{125}I and ^{131}I, respectively, and given together, after which the binding of the two preparations was measured in tumors versus normal tissues. While the binding to normal tissues was approximately the same, the anti-p97 fragments localized 3–8 (mean 3.7) times better in tumor than did the controls. Further evidence of specificity came from experiments in which the same patient was injected, on different occasions, with ^{131}I-labeled anti-p97 or control Fab fragments, after which the localization of the labeled material was established by "imaging" with a gamma camera; only the anti-p97 fragments localized into tumor [16].

Although the extent of tumor uptake of specific versus nonspecific Fab fragments was much less than that expected from data on antibody binding *in vitro*, it may be sufficient to achieve a therapeutically useful degree of tumor selectivity. Pilot studies have, therefore, been initiated, in which a large ^{131}I dose (400–800 mCi) of radiolabeled Fab fragments was injected into patients with metastatic melanoma. Some beneficial effects were observed in the form of arrested tumor growth and partial regression [57,58]. Pioneering therapeutic work with whole radiolabeled polyclonal (but not yet monoclonal) antibodies have been done by Order's group [59] and given some promising results. It is, however, premature to draw any conclusions about either the therapeutic efficiacy of radiolabeled antibodies or their mechanisms of action.

Evidence that injected anti-tumor antibodies actually bind to individual tumor cells has come from studies in which large doses of unlabelled anti-melanoma antibodies, specific for a melanoma-associated proteoglycan antigen or for p97, were infused into patients with metastatic melanoma [18,19]. These studies are discussed in Section III.G.

B. Antigens Defined by Monoclonal Antibodies in Some Human Cancers

1. *Types of Antigens Observed*

Many monoclonal antibodies have been made to antigens that are strongest expressed by human tumors. Most of these antigens are differentiation ("oncofetal") antigens, which are shared by tumors and fetal tissues, or clone specific, that is, unique to the clone of cells forming a tumor.

The oncofetal antigens were first described in the middle of the 1960s when Abelev et al. [8] and Gold and Freedman [7] discovered alfafetroprotein (AFP) and carcinoembryonic antigen (CEA), respectively. Shortly afterwards, tumor-type specific antigens, at least some of which were oncofetal [60], were implicated as targets for anti-tumor immune responses which were observed in cancer patients and found to be mediated by both serum antibodies [61,62] and lymphocytes [62]. A recent article reviews some of the latter work in the light of present understanding [63].

The most definitive studies on oncofetal antigens have been performed with the monoclonal antibody technique [14]. Some of these antigens have been identified in many types of tumors, while others are expressed most strongly in tumors of one type [22]. The tumor-type specificity of the latter antigens is far from absolute, however. This can be illustrated by findings on three melanoma-associated antigens, p97, a proteoglycan, and a GD3 ganglioside. Most melanomas have large amounts of all three antigens and most other tumors have very little of each. Nevertheless, there are some non-melanoma tumors which express one of the antigens in the "melanoma range," and 15% of these tumors (as compared to 96% of melanomas) express two of the three antigens. The situation is analogous for other neoplasms. For example, Bast et al. [64] have described an antigen which is most commonly seen in ovarian carcinomas, but which is also present in many carcinomas of breast and colon. The lack of absolute tumor-type specificity does not detract from the usefulness of an antigen as a therapeutic target. It rather widens the number of tumors against which an antibody may be used.

Clone-specific antigens have been demonstrated as idiotypic determinants in B-cell leukemias and are, operationally, highly specific for the given neoplasm. Antibodies to these antigens have been utilized therapeutically with at least one patient achieving a complete remission [65]. Individually unique ("Class I") tumor antigens have been detected also in some solid tumors by studying antibodies in patient sera [66]. They may fall into the category of clone-specific antigen. The problem with using any individually unique tumor antigens as therapeutic targets is, of course, that the antibodies will have to be tailor-made for each patient.

Virus-associated cell surface antigens would be expected to have high degree of specificity for all tumors associated with the same virus [6]. The best examples of this are the membrane antigens of Burkitt lymphoma cells [67]. However, few monoclonal antibodies to such antigens are available for targeting purposes.

A short status report on monoclonal antibodies to some different human cancers will now follow in order to exemplify what antigens have been identified. We make no attempt to cover the vast literature and expect that for the tumors discussed, many additional antigens will have been identified before this Chapter appears in print. As a complement to the examples given, we recommend four recent books reviewing the area [68–71].

2. *Leukemias*

Monoclonal antibodies have been made to idiotype-specific antigens on B cell lymphoma and to various differentiation antigens. As already mentioned, the former distinguish the clone of B cells from which the lymphoma originated from the patient's normal cells [65].

The differentiation antigens comprise markers of distinct subpopulations of hematopoietic cells. Their expression can have prognostic significance by showing from what lineage of normal cells a given leukemia is derived as well as its level of differentiation [72]. Some of these antigens may be used for targeting, since they are most strongly expressed by neoplastic (e.g. *B. lymphoma*) cells and their normal counterparts (e.g., B cells), and not by hematopoietic skin cells. One of the most studied differentiation antigens is CALLA (common acute lymphatic leukemia antigen). It was so named since it was first detected in cells from such tumors [73–75]. It can, however, be also detected in certain normal tissues, including kidney epithelium. Antibodies to CALLA have been conjugated with ricin A chain to produce immunotoxins [76]. CALLA-positive cells lose their antigen ("modulate") in the presence of anti-CALLA antibody [77].

Many leukemias have high levels of an antigen which has been identified as the transferrin receptor [78]. It is strongly expressed in rapidly proliferating cells, neoplastic as well as normal, and serves a crucial function in the uptake of iron coupled to transferrin. Like transferrin, it is coded for by a gene on chromosome 3 [79]. Antibodies to the transferrin receptor have an antitumor affect *in vitro* [80] and might be considered for therapeutic trials.

One of the anti-lymphoma antibodies most studied is T101, an IgG2a specific for a 65,000 dalton glycoprotein (T65) present on normal mature T cells and on most T-cell neoplasms [81]. Injection of T101 has produced regression of cutaneous tumor infiltrates in some patients with mycosis fungoides [82]. Analogous findings have been made in mice by Bernstein et al. [83], who found an antitumor effect against transplanted and spontaneous mouse T cell lymphomas after treatment with monoclonal antibodies to Thy-1, an antigen shared by normal and neoplastic T cells. Antibody T101 has recently been used for imaging of cutaneous lymphoma in man [84].

3. *Melanomas*

Melanomas have been studied intensely with the monoclonal antibody technology. Since they may serve as prototypes for other solid tumors, we discuss them in more detail than is justified by their clinical prevalence. Antibodies have been made to many cell surface antigens of melanoma, a few of which stand out as particularly interesting. We have recently reviewed this work [22,25,85] and confine our discussion to the following points.

The melanoma antigen studied the most is p97, a phosphorylated sialoglycoprotein of approximately 97,000 molecular weight, which is strongly expressed by approximately 50% of melanomas [40,86], present in only trace amounts in normal adult cells. Some 15 anti-97 antibodies, of different isotypes, have been obtained, defining 5 antigenic determinants [41]. This makes it possible to combine several antibodies for targeting a greater amount of an agent to the tumor cell surface. For example, by combining antibodies to two different epitopes of p97, a synergistic increase of complement-mediated killing of p97-positive melanoma cells was achieved [87]. Anti-idiotypic antisera, using a p97 antibody as the immunogen have been made in rabbits and have been used to induce immunity to p97 in mice [88]. More recently, monoclonal anti-idiotypic antibodies have been made in mice (Hellström and Kahn, unpublished observations).

The p97 antigen has substantial homology to transferrin, a known growth factor, and it can bind iron [89]. Like transferrin and the transferrin receptor, it is coded for by a gene on chromosome 3 [90]. cDNA sequences [91] and recently the gene [912] coding for p97 have been cloned. This should make it possible to analyze the structure and function of the antigen in depth, to transfect mouse tumor cells to establish models in which to study various aspects of passive and active immunity to tumors expressing p97, and even better, to establish models in which a mouse homologue as p97, and even better, to establish models in which a mouse homologue as p97 is the target. One may, for example, be able to test in such models the antitumor activity of an immune response induced by using synthetic peptides [92] or anti-idiotypic antibodies [88], as well as the effect of various antibody-drug conjugates specific for a human tumor marker.

One of the most melanoma specific antigens identified is a proteoglycan. It was first described by Reisfeld's and Ferrone's groups [93,94], followed by ourselves [95] and others [96]. It is strongly expressed by most melanomas, but is also present in a few carcinomas and, at low levels, in some endothelial cells. Some antiproteoglycan antibodies of the IgG2a give antibody-dependent cellular cytotoxicity (ADCC) to target cells expressing the proteoglycan [97].

A third antigen of interest is a GD3 ganglioside. It was first defined by antibody R_{24} from Old's group (98,99) and subsequently by antibodies made by ourselves [100] and others. It differs from the GD3 of normal brain by having a longer ceramid portion [101]. Several IgG3 antibodies to the antigen mediate strong ADCC, and one of two such antibodies tested was found to be tumor inhibitory in nude mice [37]. Another IgG3 antibody MG-21, is cytotoxic to melanoma cells in the presence of human serum as a source of complement and mediates ADCC [37]; it has not yet been tested in nude mice.

Recent studies [102] have shown that an antibody [103] raised against a neuroectoderm antigen of fetal rats is specific for an o-acetylated GD3, which as far as has been tested, appears to be entirely tumor-specific [104]. The authors speculate that this antigen was generated by a combination of two events, namely, the synthesis of GD3 and the presence of an o-acetyltransferase capable of acetylating the 9-hydroxyl position of the terminal sialic acid residue. This may be the most tumor-specific oncofetal antigen so far identified.

4. *Colon Carcinomas*

Colon carcinomas have been much studied by the monoclonal antibody technique [105,106]. Both protein and glycolipid [107] antigens have been demonstrated which are strongly expressed by most carcinomas of the colon, pancreas, and stomach. They are present in much smaller amounts on normal tissues and hence are relatively specific for tumor. One of the glycolipid antigens occurs at increased levels in sera from patients with carcinomas of the colon, stomach or pancreas, as compared to patients with other diseases [105,106] and is possibly a better diagnostic marker than CEA.

A protein antigen defined by an antibody called 9.25 is a promising target for *in vivo* diagnosis and therapy, since this antibody can localize to tumor *in vivo* [53], has an antitumor effect in nude mice, and possibly in humans [108]. Some patients responding to such infusion have antibodies to idiotypic determinants on 9.25 [109]. Conjugates between antibody 9.25 and the ricin A chain have been found to be selectively cytotoxic to colon carcinoma cells *in vitro* [110].

Monoclonal anti-CEA antibodies have been employed for tumor localization both in nude mice [49] and in human patients [51,52]. Such antibodies have also been conjugated with vindesine and found to subsequently have antitumor effects [111] (see below).

5. *Ovarian Carcinoma*

Bast et al. [64] immunized mice with cultured human ovarian carcinoma cells and obtained a monoclonal antibody, which according to immunohistological staining, reacts with ovarian carcinomas and some other adenocarcinomas but not with normal tissues. The antigen which it defines is expressed at the cell surface and is a potential target for therapy. It is also a promising diagnostic marker, since sera from patients with ovarian carcinoma, as well as from some patients with other carcinomas, have increased level of the antigen [64].

6. *Breast Carcinoma*

Schlom et al. [31], Colcher et al. [33], Braban et al. [112], and others have generated antibodies which bind to cells from human breast carcinoma. Some of these antibodies react with normal breast epithelium, while others do not. One of the antibodies of Colcher et al. [33] localizes to both breast carcinoma and colon carcinoma tissue in nude mice. It may be useful for targeting, since it remains for several days at the cell surface following antibody injection.

7. *Lung Carcinoma*

There are antibodies to antigens that are strongly expressed by small cell lung cancer [113–115]. The most interesting of these binds to bombesin, a molecule associated with small cell lung carcinomas. This antibody has strong inhibitory activity against small cell lung cancer xenografts in nude mice (Minna, personal communication). There are also antibodies that bind to non-small lung carcinomas and certain other tumors but not to small cell lung carcinomas [116,117a,b].

III. DRUG-ANTIBODY CONJUGATES

Many drug antibody conjugates are being developed and some are undergoing preclinical testing. In this section, we discuss some questions of principal nature including questions to be posed when the conjugates enter clinical trials, including potential problems. The development of procedures to conjugate anti-cancer drugs with antibodies is beyond our scope. Since the field is rapidly changing, the reader is referred to the current literature for updates.

A. When Is Targeting Needed?

If a therapeutic agent could be found which either kills tumor cells selectively or induces them to differentiate into their normal counterparts, and if this agent could reach all tumor cells and stay there for the period of time needed to be effective, there would be no need for "targeting." This holds true whether the hypothetical agent acts directly on the neoplastic cells or in an indirect way.

Some of the agents that may ultimately provide the degree of selectivity needed are naturally occuring tumor inhibitors which selectively inhibit the growth of cancer cells [118], molecules which induce differentiation [119], and immunomodulators which activate macrophages, NK cells and other lymphoid cells with antitumor activity [120]. Some of these "biological response modifiers" are presently undergoing Phase I/II evaluation in cancer patients. Of these, interferon has already proven clinically useful for certain types of tumors [121]. Likewise, inducers of differentiation, particularly retinoids, have given promising results in a limited group of neoplasms [122, 123]. Preclinical studies in mice have shown that activation of macrophages can induce regression of small established tumors in organs rich in macrophages [120], setting the stage for similar studies in the clinic. Some of the biological response modifiers may need to be present at the tumor site for several days to cause tumor cell death. Conjugation with antibodies has a theoretical advantage also for these agents, therefore, since it may concentrate them in the area of neoplastic cells and prolong the duration of contact.

The cytotoxic effect of presently available chemotherapeutic drugs is not specific to the cancer cells, but is directed against any rapidly proliferating cell population. Nevertheless, such drugs can be very effective against rapidly growing tumors [1]. Since they commonly kill a fraction of all neoplastic cells rather than a defined, limited number (first-order kinetics), they can be used to induce regression of even large tumors. Because of their non-specificity, the agents have a low therapeutic index, that is doses that induce an antitumor response are often toxic to normal tissues and, for many tumors, no clinically useful drugs are available. A method of targeting drugs to neoplastic tissues which could increase their concentration there may improve the therapeutic index. Conjugation of drugs to antibodies should be viewed in this context as an approach for delivering high doses of drug specifically to antigen-positive tumor cells while sparing antigen-negative normal cells. For those tumors lacking clinically useful drugs, the situation may improve if one, as a result of targeting, could utilize drugs whose overall toxicity makes them useless for conventional systemic therapy.

We conclude that targeting with monoclonal antibodies has theoretical advantages for both currently available nonselective agents and for potential, more specific agents.

B. Choice of Target Antigen

Since most drugs must enter neoplastic cells to exert an effect, the degree to which a drug-antibody conjugate is taken up by the cells is important; alternatively, active drug must be released from the conjugate at the tumor site. Uptake generally occurs by endocytosis, and thus procedures facilitating endocytosis may play a role when using drug conjugates. There is experimental evidence that some drug-antibody conjugates are endocytosed [124,125]. Since the degree of endocytosis may vary between different antigens, conjugates that are specific to some antigens may be more effective for delivery a drug intracellularly. It is not clear whether protein and glycolipid antigens differ in this respect. It also needs to be investigated what factors determine the degree of endocytosis of an antigen-antibody complex, the kinetics of endocytosis, and the extent of regeneration of surface antigens.

C. Choice of Drugs

It would be rational to perform the initial conjugate Phase I trials with drugs whose antitumor activity and toxicity are known, since the toxicity results can then be compared with the known toxicity of equal molar doses of free drug. Subsequent Phase II trials can then compare the therapeutic effect of a drug conjugate with an equally toxic dose of free drug. If the conjugate has a higher therapeutic index than the free drug, one can assume that there has been some degree of targeting. For this reason, one may want to start by developing conjugates for neoplasms for which relatively effective chemotherapy exists, for example, for leukemia, breast cancer, small-cell lung cancer and ovarian cancer [1]. There may be less need for randomized trials in this case, since the anti-cancer effect of many single drugs is known and since it is likely that many patients treated with conjugates have already shown tumor progression when treated with maximally-tolerated levels of the free drug. If one, instead, selects presently drug-refractory tumors for the initial work, one risks concluding that targeting of conjugates has no therapeutic benefit when, in fact, targeting occurs but because of drug resistance treatment is ineffective even when high intracellular concentrations are reached. Nevertheless, we realize that the ultimate goal is to develop successful therapy for just such tumors, since the therapeutic needs are the greatest for them.

The choice of the drug to be conjugated with antibody should be based on its defined mechanism of action and pharmacokinetic properties. Because most antibodies are specific for cell surface antigens, a surface-active cytotoxic drug would be predicted to be most effective. Few of the currently available drugs express their cytotoxic effect via cell surface mechanisms, however. Most of them act via intracellular mechanisms, affecting DNA or protein synthesis, the formation and function of the spindle apparatus, etc. [126]. For these agents to be active, we *a priori* assume that endocytosis of the drug-antibody complex must occur. Once intracellular, the ideal drug-antibody complex would exert a cytotoxic effect even if the drug remains covalently bound to antibody. Drugs, such as the anthracyclines, which require an intimate interaction with DNA [126] may be inactive, unless they are cleaved from the antibody molecule to release free drug. Anti-metabolites may also be inactive when covalently bound to antibody, since steric interference may prevent them from interacting with the target enzyme. Alkylating agents on the other hand, may be effective as intact complexes. If these drugs maintain their active bifunctional alkylating capacity, they may be capable of not only cross-linking DNA and other cellular constituents but also of covalently binding the antibody to cellular components and thereby further interfere with normal functions. The intracellular metabolism/deconjugation of drug-antibody conjugates needs investigation before a rational choice can be made on which drugs would be best to conjugate with antibody. From the practical standpoint, however, clinical trials may determine therapeutic efficiacy before the details of intracellular antibody conjugate deposition is defined.

Another point to consider is the molar ratio of conjugated drug to antibody. One would predict that an antibody with multiple conjugated drug molecules would be more effective than an antibody with only one molecule of drug conjugated. Obviously, the chemistry of synthesizing drug-antibody-conjugates which retain active antigenic combining sites will be the limiting factor in determining molar ratios.

Based on our knowledge about the number of antigenic sites at the tumor cell surface, one can roughly estimate the maximum number of drug-antibody conjugates that can be bound per cell. Assuming that each antibody complex is endocytosed, and that only one episode of binding and endocytosis per antigenic site occurs, one can try to estimate the maximal number of drug-antibody-antigen complexes taken up per cell. We use, as an example, a conjugate specific for the p97 melanoma antigen, which is expressed in 50% of melanoma cells at a level of at least 50,000 molecules/cell. If one assumes a cell volume of 100 pL and an antibody to drug ratio of 1:1, one can calculate the intracellular volume and the intracellular molarity of a specific drug. With p97 as target, one can estimate an intracellular drug concentration approaching 10^{-6} molar. For drugs like vinca alkaloids, this is in excess of that likely to be achieved by intravenous drug treatment (peak plasma concentraton 0.4 mM [126]) and suggests that high intracellular drug concentrations are possible by using antibody for targeting. Because of the theoretical limit of the intracellular drug concentration that can be achieved, it seems advantageous to choose a drug with a high molar activity, for example, actinomycin-D or vinca alkaloids.

Conjugates that are not directly taken up by cells may also be useful, if they can increase local extracellular concentration of free drug. The extent to which this occurs may vary depending on the strength of the covalent bond between drug and antibody. Deconjugation via a chemical or enzymatic process at the cell surface would result in a locally higher extracellular drug concentration, hence higher drug uptake by cells, than can be achieved by intravenous administration of free drug at a dose with acceptable systemic toxicity.

Two important questions to be asked about drug conjugates can be answered by available technology: can they selectively kill antigen-positive cells *in vitro* and can they localize to tumor *in vivo*? The first question can be approached by measuring the effects of conjugates, versus free drug, free antibody, and mixtures, on tumor cell colony formation in soft agar [127], using tumor lines whose degree of expression of a given antigen is known (as the number of antigen molecules per cell). The second question can be answered by transplanting similar cell lines into nude mice, labeling the conjugates with a radioisotope, and measuring the degree of localization into tumor [48,49].

D. Impact of Tumor Cell Heterogeneity

Approaches to treatment of cancer must take into account the fact that tumor cell populations are heterogeneous with respect to a large variety of characteristics [128–130]. These include sensitivity to chemotherapeutic drugs and expression of tumor antigens [131, 132].

The therapeutic problems caused by cellular heterogeneity in drug sensitivity can be approached by conjugating multiple drugs to the same antibody and treating with combinations of the conjugates. Variability in antigen expression, on the other hand, calls for a mixture of different antibodies each specific for a different tumor antigen, since each antigen is expressed independently [131,132]. Conjugating mixtures of antibodies may also be advantageous in view of the fact that those normal cells which express significant amounts of a given antigen are commonly different for each antigen. This can be illustrated for the melanoma-associated p97, proteoglycan, and GD3 antigens. Whereas all three antigens are expressed by most melanomas, the normal adult cells which have most are smooth muscle cells, endothelial cells, and brain cells, respectively. By combining antibodies to the three antigens, it may become possible to treat patients with antibody concentrations that are too low to seriously affect the three types of normal cells (in the example given) but sufficient to damage tumor cells, most of which express high amounts of two or three of the antigens.

The combination of antibodies to multiple antigens of the same tumor may not be sufficient to prevent the rapid selection of antigen-negative cells upon treatment with conjugates. One should, therefore, consider therapies that can destroy not only those cells that attract a given conjugate but also neighboring, antigen-negative tumor cells. This will be discussed under Section III.F.

E. Existing Conjugates Between Monoclonal Antibodies and Chemotherapeutic Agents

A number of conjugates with antitumor activity have been made, using drugs such as methotrexate [10], chlorambucil [11,133], adriamycin [12], melphalan [134], and platinum [13]. Unfortunately, most of them have not been tested for either antitumor effect or toxicity *in vivo* nor have they been compared with unconjugated antibodies, free drug or a combination of the two.

A study by Sela's group [135] represents one of the few exceptions. It was carried out by preparing conjugates between daunomycin and antibodies to alfafetoprotein (AFP) and testing for therapeutic effects *in vivo* against a mouse hepatoma expressing AFP. Antibodies alone, drug alone, and mixtures of the two were included among the controls, as were conjugates between daunomycin and antibodies to an irrelevant antigen. When the specific conjugate was injected intravenously, a significant fraction of the mice with established tumors was cured, while no complete responses were seen in any of the control groups, including the group given free drug.

Rowland's group has also performed well-controlled studies in this area [111,136–138]. Monoclonal antibodies to several different human tumor antigens were conjugated with the synthetic vinca alkaloid vindesine. Their effects were first tested *in vitro* by measuring inhibition of DNA synthesis and/or of colony formation by plated tumor cells. Free vindesine inhibited all tumor lines tested while unconjugated antibodies were not inhibitory. The conjugates, on the other hand, inhibited only those cells that could bind a certain minimum number of molecules of unconjugated antibody (and, presumably, of conjugates). For conjugates with an antibody to p97, approximately 50,000 molecules/cell needed to be bound. This was encouraging, since approximately 50% of all melanomas express that much p97 per cell, while the highest concentration of p97 observed on any normal adult cell is about 5 times less. Tests were also performed in nude mice with xenotransplanted human tumors. The mice were injected with conjugates, antibodies alone or drug alone, starting on the day of transplantation and followed by four to six repeated injections at 3-day intervals. A tumor-inhibitory effect of the conjugates was observed, which was always greater than that produced by the respective antibodies given alone, some of which had no antitumor activity at all. Although vindesine alone was also inhibitory, the conjugates had an improved therapeutic index, to the extent tested, since they gave the same or better tumor inhibition at a lower level of toxicity.

F. Future Perspectives

There are two major problems (disregarding the chemistry of conjugation) which need to be solved for conjugate-based therapy to be practical: few if any of the antibodies are truly specific for tumor, and tumors are heterogeneous in terms of antigen expression. The ideal solution to these problems would be the finding of an antibody to a molecule that is intimately associated with the neoplastic phenotype so that a cell lacking the molecule would no longer be neoplastic, for example an antibody to an essential tumor growth factor. Intense efforts are given to find molecules of that uniqueness to cancer.

Although therapeutic modalities that are not truly tumor-specific are compromises, pragmatic approaches based on presently available monoclonal antibodies to human tumor antigens deserve to be pursued. Beyond using combinations of conjugates involving multiple antibodies to the same tumor and multiple drugs, as discussed above, additional approaches are needed. A few will be suggested in this section.

Different cell surface antigens that are strongly expressed by the same tumor are unequally distributed among different normal tissues. It should be possible, therefore, to select antibodies to two antigens that are both shared by most cells within a tumor but where the normal cells, at most, express significant amounts of one of the antigens. Using these two antibodies, conjugates would then be prepared in such a way that the first conjugate produces a cytotoxic compound when it comes in contact with the second conjugate at the tumor cell surface. This would not happen for normal cells which, at most, would bind one of the conjugates. An increased degree of tumor specificity would thus be created.

Most available conjugates used for targeting drugs to tumors probably kill only those tumor cells that express antigen and bind the particular conjugates (although this has not been properly tested); all conjugates with toxins would be expected to act this way. A problem using any of these conjugates is that variants lacking the target antigen will be selected for and may, therefore, emerge as a dominant population. One approach to prevent this from happening may be to develop a conjugate that localizes to the antigen-positive cells but destroys not only these but also any surrounding, potentially antigen-negative tumor cells. There may be several ways toward this goal. One possibility is to develop a conjugate that releases free drug when it is bound to a tumor cell, as a result of the microenvironment of the tumor. Drugs which would be non-toxic until "activated" by an agent (e.g., an enzyme) localized to tumor may be considered as another approach to the same end. Active drug would then diffuse locally, establishing a higher extracellular drug concentration in the tumor than in the rest of the organism and be taken up by and destroy both antigen-positive and antigen-negative cells. Normal stroma cells in the tumor area would be affected as well but this may constitute an acceptable degree of toxicity.

Also to be considered is to develop conjugates between an antitumor antibody and a hapten in order to carry the hapten to the tumor site. This could be used to induce delayed-type hypersensitivity (DTH) reactions in the tumor area, which may be a desirable goal, since neoplastic cells are much more sensitive than their normal counterparts to such reactions [120,139]. Antibodies coupled to chemoattractants and activators of macrophages, T cells and/or K cells may serve the same purpose. Likewise, a therapeutic effect may occur, if anti-tumor antibodies can be used to attract to tumor activated macrophages, natural killer cells, or other lymphoid cells with antitumor activity [140]. An advantage of this approach is that it is likely to have fewer side-effects on normal tissues. The use of antibodies to concentrate to tumors, tumor inhibitors such as Oncostatin [118], also appears attractive.

Finally, one should consider antibodies (or fragments) labeled with radiosotopes emitting α or β particles, since labeled antibodies may be destructive to adjacent, antigen-negative tumor cells, in spite of the fact that the destructive effect would be directed also against normal stroma cells. A discussion of radiolabeled antibodies is, however, beyond the scope of this chapter.

G. Current Planned Phase I–Phase II Trials with Monoclonal Antibody Conjugates

There are several ongoing, pilot studies [17–19,65], which probably will be expanded into formal Phase I trials to further define the pharmacokinetic parameters of whole unconjugated murine antibodies. These trials will form a basis for work with conjugates in that the antibody half-life in plasma, as well as the degree of binding to tumor *in vivo* and the half-life of this binding can all be determined. Many of the parameters need to be defined before clinical trials with drug conjugates can be initiated.

We have completed a pilot study of two murine monoclonal antibodies in treatment of patients with metastatic melanoma [19]. One antibody, 96.5, is directed against the p97 antigen, and the other one, 48.7, is against a proteoglycan antigen. Five patients with multiple skin metastases from antigen-positive melanoma were studied. Antibodies were administered as a 4–6-hr intravenous infusion in 250–500 ml of 5% albumin and 0.9% NaCl daily for 10 days. One patient received 4 mg of antibody 96.5 on day 1, 20 mg on day 2, and 50 mg on each of days 3 through 10 for a total antibody dose of 424 mg. Each of four other patients received the same total immunoglobulin dose but equally divided between antibody 96.5 and 48.7. Plasma pharmacokinetics was determined at the end of the antibody infusion as summarized in Table 1. Mouse antibody half-life in plasma varied between 21 and 53 hr. This suggests that the administration of antibody as a loading dose followed by maintenance doses every 48–72 hr may be sufficient to maintain detectable antibody levels in plasma.

Biopsies of tumor nodules were taken at the end of the infusion and at varying intervals over the subsequent 10 days. Tumor nodules biopsied within 24 hr after the end of treatment showed extensive *in vivo* binding of mouse antibodies to surface antigen. This

Table 1 Summary of Pharmacokinetic Parameters of Monoclonal Antibodies 96.5 and 48.7.

Patient no.	MAb given	Dose (mg)	Peak MAb plasma conc. (μg/ml)	MAb $t_{1/2}$
1	96.5	212	62[a]	21.2 hr[a]
	48.7	212		
2	96.5	424	38	53.0 hr
4	96.5	212		
			24	44.2 hr
	48.7	212		
5	96.5	212		
			34	36.7 hr
	48.7	212		

[a]Patient 1 had human antimouse antibodies (HAMA) present at time of treatment. This likely accounts for the rapid elimination $t_{1/2}$. HAMA present in plasma at the time of treatment and interference with the assay for murine MAb may also account for the calculated high plasma concentrations of MAb.

was observed across the diameter of the tumor nodules and suggested that the dose and schedule at which the antibodies were given led to detectable binding by essentially all tumor cells. Studies on biopsies taken post treatment showed that the antibody binding persisted for 3–5 days after the last infusion, while biopsies from two patients failed to demonstrate residual antibody binding, when taken 10 days after the last infusion. Hence, it appears that once there is *in vivo* binding to the majority of tumor cells, it may be maintained by administering antibodies every 3 days. This information should have an impact on trials with drug-antibody conjugates and also for trials using conjugates with biological response modifiers or radiolabeled antibodies.

IV. CONCLUSIONS

Monoclonal antibodies to tumor-associated cell surface antigens should be useful for targeting a variety of agents which directly, or indirectly, have anti-cancer activity. Although most antigens detected in human neoplasms have relative rather than absolute specificity for tumor, there are several antigens which are expressed at high concentrations in tumor cells and only a trace amounts in normal cells and therefore logical choices as therapeutic targets.

Therapeutic modalities must take into account that tumor cell populations are heterogeneous in terms of antigen expression. Combinations of antibodies to multiple antigens expressed by the same tumor are likely to be needed to decrease the possibility that antigen-negative cell variants are selected. One should also consider conjugates capable of causing the destruction of antigen-negative neoplastic cells, as long as these are surrounded by antigen-positive cells. Antibody-drug conjugates which release free drug upon binding to tumor cells may meet this need, as may conjugates between antibodies and certain biological modifiers and antibodies labeled with proper radioisotopes.

The pharmacology of intact murine monoclonal antibodies is still unclear, and the human pharmacology on antibody-drug conjugates has not been studied at all. Carefully planned clinical trials are needed to learn how to best administer drug-antibody conjugates with the goal to improve the therapeutic index over that which can be reached by using free drugs.

REFERENCES

1. V. T. DeVita and R. S. Hellman, Eds., *Cancer, Principles and Practice of Oncology*, J. B. Lippincott & Co., Philadelphia, 1982.
2. W. Ensminger, J. Niederhuber, S. Dakhil, J. Thrall, and R. Wheeler, Totally implanted drug delivery system for hepatic arterial chemotherapy, *Cancer Treat. Rep. 65*, 393 (1981).
3. B. Himmelweit, Ed. *The Selected Papers of Paul Ehrlich*, Pergamon Press, Oxford, 1957.
4. E. J. Foley, Antigenic properties of methylcholanthrene-induced tumors in mice of the strain origin, *Cancer Res. 13*, 835 (1953).
5. R. Prehn and D. Main, Immunity to methylcholanthrene induced sarcomas, *J. Natl. Cancer Inst. 18*, 768 (1957).
6. H. O. Sjögren, Transplantation methods as a tool for detection of tumor specific antigens, *Prog. Exp. Tumor Res. 6*, 289 (1965).
7. T. P. Gold and S. Freedman, Demonstration of tumor-specific antigens in human colonic carcinoma by immunological tolerance and absorption techniques, *J. Exp. Med. 121*, 439 (1965).
8. G. I. Abelev, S. D. Perova, A. P. Khramkova, Z. A. Postnihova, and I. S. Irtin, Production of embyronal α-globulin by transplantable mouse hepatomas, *Transplantation 1*, 174 (1963).
9. K. E. Hellström and I. Hellström, Cellular immunity against tumor specific antigens, *Adv. Cancer Res. 12*, 167 (1969).

10. G. Mathe, T. B. Loc, and J. Bernard, Medecine experimentale—Effet sur la leucemie 1210 de la Souris d'une combinaison par diazotation d'A-methopterine et de γ-globulines de hamsters porteurs de celle leucemia par heterogreffe, *Acad. Sc. C. R. 246,* 1626 (1958).
11. T. Ghose, S. T. Novell, A. Guclu, D. Cameron, A. Bodurtha, and A. S. MacDonald, Immunochemotherapy of cancer with chlorambucil-carrying antibody, *Br. Med. J. 3,* 495 (1972).
12. F. Hurwitz, R. Levy, R. Maron, M. Wilchek, R. Arnon, and M. Sela, The covalent binding of daunomycin and adriamycin to antibodies, *Cancer Res. 35,* 1175 (1975).
13. F. Hurwitz, R. Kashi, and M. Wilcheck, Platinum-complexed anti-tumor immunoglobulins that specifically inhibit DNA synthesis of mouse tumor cells, *J. Natl. Cancer Inst. 69,* 47 (1982).
14. G. Köhler and C. Milstein, Continuous culture of fused cells secreting antibodies of predefined specificity, *Nature 256,* 495 (1975).
15. K. E. Hellström, I. Hellström, and J. P. Brown, Human tumor-associated antigens identified by monoclonal antibodies. In, *Springer Seminars in Immunopathology Series, Mechanisms of Host Resistance in Cancer,* Vol. 5 (R. W. Baldwin, ed.), Springer-Verlag, New York, 1982, p. 127.
16. S. M. Larson, J. A. Carrasquillo, K. A. Krohn, J. P. Brown, R. W. McGuffin, J. M. Ferens, M. M. Graham, L. D. Hill, P. L. Beaumier, K. E. Hellström, and I. Hellström, Localization of p97 specific Fab fragments in human melanoma as a basis for radiotherapy, *J. Clin. Invest. 72,* 2101 (1983).
17. H. F. Sears, J. Mattis, and D. Herlyn, Phase I clinical trial with monoclonal antibody in the treatment of gastrointestinal tumors, *Lancet 1,* 762 (1982).
18. R. K. Oldham, K. A. Foon, A. C. Morgan, C. S. Woodhouse, R. W. Schraff, P. G. Abrams, M. Fer, C. S. Schoenberger, M. Farrell, E. Kimball, and S. A. Sherwin, Monoclonal antibody therapy of malignant melanoma: *In vivo* localization in cutaneous metastasis after intravenous administration, *J. Clin. Oncol. 2,* 1235 (1984).
19. G. E. Goodman, P. L. Beaumier, I. Hellström, B. Fernyhough, and K. E. Hellström, Phase I trial of murine monoclonal antibodies in patients with advance melanoma, *J. Clin. Onocol. 3,* 340 (1984).
20. F. K. Jansen, H. E. Blythman, D. Carriere, P. Casellas, P. Gros, O. Gros, J. C. Laurent, F. Paloucci, B. Pau, P. Poncelet, G. Richer, H. Vidal, and G. A. Voisin, Immunotoxins: Hybrid molecules combining high specificity and potent cytotoxicity, *Immunol. Rev. 62,* 185 (1982).
21. Vitetta and J. W. Uhr, The potential use of immunotoxins in transplantation, cancer therapy, and immunoregulation, *Transplant 37,* 535 (1984).

22. K. E. Hellström and I. Hellström, Monoclonal anti-melanoma antibodies and their possible clinical use. In, *Monoclonal Antibodies for Cancer Detection and Therapy* (R. W. Baldwin, Ed.), Academic Press, New York, 1984 p. 17.
23. G. Galfre, S. C. Howe, C. Milstein, G. W. Butcher, and J. C. Howard, Antibodies to major histocompatability antigens produced by hybrid cell lines, *Nature 266*, 550 (1977).
24. H. Koprowski and Z. Steplewski, Human solid tumor antigens defined by monoclonal antibodies. In, *Monoclonal Antibodies and T-Cell Hybridomas* (G. J. Hammerling, U. Hammerling, and J. F. Kearney, Eds.), Elsevier, North-Holland, 1981, p. 161.
25. K. E. Hellström, J. P. Brown, and I. Hellström, Monoclonal antibodies to tumor antigens. In, *Contemporary Topics in Immunobiology*, Vol. II (N. L. Warner, Ed.), Plenum Press, New York, 1980, p. 117.
26. P. Thammana and M. D. Scharff, Immunoglobulin heavy chain class switch from IgM to IgG in a hybridoma, *Eur. J. Immunol. 13*, 614 (1983).
27. J. P. Brown, P. W. Wright, C. E. Hart, R. G. Woodbury, K. E. Hellström, and I. Hellström, Protein antigens of normal and malignant human cells identified by immunoprecipitation with monoclonal antibodies, *J. Biol. Chem. 255*, 4980 (1980).
28. T. Brodin, I. Hellström, K. E. Hellström, K. A. Karlsson, H. O. Sjögren, N. Stromberg, and J. Thurin, Mouse monoclonal antibodies with specificity for the melanoma-associated ganglioside disialyllactosylceramide (GD3) also react with the structural analogue disialylparagloboside. *Biochim. Biophys. Acta 837*, 349 (1985).
29. L. Olsson and H. S. Kaplan, Human-human hybridomas producing monoclonal antibodies of predefined antigenic specificity, *Proc. Natl. Acad. Sci. USA 77*, 5429 (1980).
30. C. Croce, A. Linnenbach, W. Wall, Z. Steplewski, and H. Koprowski, Production of human hybridomas secreting antibodies to measles virus, *Nature 288*, 488 (1980).
31. J. Schlom, D. Wunderlich, and Y. A. Teramoto, Generation of human monoclonal antibodies reactive with human mammary carcinoma cells, *Proc. Natl. Acad. Sci. USA 77*, 6841 (1980).
32. A. W. Siadak and M. E. Lostrom, Cell-driven viral transformation, in Human Hybridomas and Monoclonal Antibodies (E. G. Engleman, S. K. H. Foung, J. Larrick, and A. Raubitschek, eds.), Plenum Publishing, 1985, p. 167.
33. D. Colcher, P. Horan Hand, M. Nuti, and J. Schlom, A spectrum of monoclonal antibodies reactive with human mammary tumor cells, *Proc. Natl. Acad. Sci. USA 78*, 3199 (1981).
34. R. J. Cote, D. M. Morrissey, A. N. Houghton, E. J. Beattie, and H. F. Oettgen, Generation of human monoclonal antibodies reactive with cellular antigens, *Proc. Natl. Acad. Sci. USA 80*, 2026 (1983).

35. T. Tai, L. D. Cahan, J. C. Paulson, R. E. Saxton, and R. F. Irie, Human monoclonal antibody against ganglioside G_{D2}: Use in development of enzyme-linked immunosorbent assay for the monitoring of anti-G_{D2} in cancer patients, *J. Natl. Cancer Inst. 73*, 627 (1984).
36. S. L. Morrison, M. J. Johnson, L. A. Herzenberg, and V. T. Oi, Chimeric human antibody molecules: Mouse antigen-binding domains with human constant region domains, *Proc. Natl. Acad. Sci. USA 81*, 6851 (1984).
37. I. Hellström, V. Brankovan, and K. E. Hellström, An IgGl antibody to a human melanoma-associated antigen has strong antitumor effects *in vitro* and *in vivo*, *Proc. Natl. Acad. Sci. 82*, 1499 (1985).
38. G. Klein, H. O. Sjögren, E. Klein, and K. E. Hellström, Demonstration of resistance against methylcholanthrene-induced sarcomas in the primary autochthonous host, *Cancer Res. 20*, 1561 (1960).
39. K. D. Bageshaw, Third Gordon Hamilton-Fairley Memorial Lecture. Tumour markers—Where do we go from here? *Br. J. Cancer 48*, 167 (1983).
40. J. P. Brown, R. G. Woodbury, C. E. Hart, I. Hellström, and K. E. Hellström, Quantitative analysis of melanoma-associated antigen p97 in normal and neoplastic tissues, *Proc. Natl. Acad. Sci. USA 78*, 539 (1981).
41. J. P. Brown, K. Nishiyama, I. Hellström, and K. E. Hellström, Structural characterization of human melanoma-associated antigen p97 using monoclonal antibodies, *J. Immunol. 127*, 539 (1981).
42. D. J. Slamon, J. B. DeKernion, I. M. Verma, and M. J. Cline, Expression of cellular oncogenes in human maligancies, *Science 224*, 256 (1984).
43. R. T. Schimke, Gene amplification, drug resistance and cancer, *Cancer Res. 44*, 1735 (1984).
44. J. M. Klitzman, J. P. Brown, K. E. Hellström, and I. Hellström, Antibodies to murine leukemia virus gp70 and p15(E) in sera of BALB/c mice immunized with syngeneic chemically induced sarcomas, *J. Immunol. 124*, 2552 (1980).
45. I. Hellström, K. E. Hellström, N. Rollins, V. K. Lee, and G. T. Nepom, Monoclonal antibodies to cell surface antigens shared by chemically induced mouse bladder carcinomas *Cancer Res.*, *45*, 2210 (1985).
46. L. A. Sternberger, The unlabelled antibody peroxidase-antiperoxidase (PAP) method. In, *Immunocytochemistry*, John Wiley & Sons, Inc., New York, 1979, p. 104.
47. H. J. Garrigues, W. Tilgen, I. Hellström, W. Ranke, and K. E. Hellström, Detection of a human melanoma-associated antigen, p97, in histological sections of primary human melanomas, *Int. J. Cancer 29*, 511 (1982).

48. P. L. Beaumier, K. A. Krohn, J. A. Carrasquillo, J. Eary, I. Hellström, K. E. Hellström, W. B. Nelp, and S. M. Larson, Melanoma localization in nude mice with monoclonal Fab against p97 *J. Nucl. Med. 26*, 1172 (1985).
49. F. Buchegger, C. M. Haskell, M. Schreyer, B. R. Scazziga, S. Randin, S. Carrel, and J-P. Mach, Radiolabelled fragments of monoclonal antibodies against carcinoembryonic antigen for localization of human colon carcinoma grafted into nude mice, *J. Exp. Med. 158*, 413 (1983).
50. D. Herlyn, J. Powe, A. Alavi, J. A. Mattis, M. Herlyn, C. Ernst, R. Vaum, and H. Koprowski, Radioimmunodetection of human tumor xenografts by monoclonal antibodies, *Cancer Res. 43*, 2731 (1983).
51. M. O. Nelson, F. H. DeLand, D. Shocat, S. J. Bennett, and D. M. Goldenberg, External imaging of gastric-cancer metastases with radiolabelled CEA and CSAp antibodies, *N. Engl. J. Med. 7*, 309 (1983).
52. J-P. Mach, F. Buchegger, M. Forni, J. Ritschard, C. Berche, J-L. Schreyer, C. Giradrdet, R. S. Accolla, and S. Carrel, Use of radiolabelled monoclonal anti-CEA antibodies for the detection of human carcinomas by external photoscanning and tomoscintigraphy, *Immunol. Today 2*, 239 (1981).
53. J. F. Chatal, J. C. Saccavini, P. Fumoleau, J. Y. Douillard, C. Curtet, M. Kremer, B. Le Mevel, and H. Koprowski, Immunoscintigraphy of colon carcinoma, *J. Nucl. Med. 25*, 307 (1984).
54. S. M. Larson, J. P. Brown, P. W. Wright, J. A. Carrasquillo, I. Hellström, and K. E. Hellström, Imaging of melanoma with ^{131}I-labelled monoclonal antibodies, *J. Nucl. Med. 24*, 123, (1983).
55. S. M. Larson, J. A. Carrasquillo, K. A. Krohn, R. W. McGuffin, I. Hellström, K. E. Hellström, and D. Lyster, Diagnostic imaging of malignant melanoma with radiolabeled anti-tumor antibodies, *JAMA 249*, 811 (1983).
56. S. Ferrone, S. P. Giacomini, P. G. Natali, D. Ruiter, G. Buraggi, L. Callegaro, and U. Rosa, A high molecular weight-melanoma associated antigen (HWM-MAA) defined by monoclonal antibodies: A useful marker to radioimage tumor lesions in patients with melanoma. In, *Proceedings of the First International Symposium on Neutron Capture Therapy, Brookhaven National Laboratories* (R. G. Fairchild and G. L. Brownell, Eds.), 1983, pp. 174–183.
57. J. A. Carrasquillo, K. A. Krohn, P. Beaumier, R. W. McGuffin, J. P. Brown, K. E. Hellström, and I. Hellström, Diagnosis and therapy of solid tumors tumors with radiolabelled Fab, *Cancer Treat. Rep. 68*, 317 (1984).

58. S. M. Larson, J. A. Carrasquillo, R. W. McGuffin, K. A. Krohn, J. M. Ferens, L. D. Hill, P. L. Beaumier, K. E. Hellström, and I. Hellström, Use of I^{131}-labelled, murine Fab against a high molecular weight antigen of human melanoma: Preliminary experience. *Radiology 155*, 487 (1985).
59. D. S. Ettinger, S. E. Order, M. D. Wharam, M. K. Parker, J. L. Klein, and P. K. Leichner, Phase-II study of isotoic immunoglobulin therapy for primary liver cancer, *Cancer Treat. Rep. 66*, 289 (1982).
60. I. Hellström, K. E. Hellström, and T. H. Shepherd, Cell-mediated immunity against antigens common to human colonic carcinomas and fetal gut epithelium, *Int. J. Cancer 6*, 346 (1970).
61. D. L. Morton, R. A. Malmgren, E. C. Holmes, and A. S. Ketcham, Demonstration of antibodies against human malignant melanoma by immunofluorescence. *Surgery 64*, 233 (1968).
62. I. Hellström, K. E. Hellström, G. E. Pierce, and J. P. S. Yang, Cellular and humoral immunity to different types of human neoplasms, *Nature 220*, 1352 (1968).
63. I. Hellström and K. E. Hellström, Cell-mediated reactivity to human tumor-type associated antigens: Does it exist? *J. Biol. Response Modifiers*, *2*, 310, 1983.
64. R. C. Bast, Jr., T. L. Klug, E. St. John, E. Jenison, J. M. Niloff, H. Lazarus, R. S. Berkowitz, C. T. Griffiths, L. Parker, V. R. Zurawski, and R. C. Knapp, A radioimmunoassay using a monoclonal antibody to monitor the course of epithelial ovarian cancer, *N. Engl. J. Med. 309*, 883 (1983).
65. R. A. Miller, D. G. Maloney, R. Warnke, and R. Levy, Treatment of B-cell lymphoma with monoclonal anti-idiotypic antibody, *N. Engl. J. Med. 306*, 517 (1981).
66. H. Shiku, T. Takahashi, H. F. Oettgen, and L. J. Old, Cell surface antigens of human malignant melanoma: II. Serological typing with immune adherence assays and definition of two new surface antigens, *J. Exp. Med. 144*, 873 (1976).
67. G. Klein, P. Clifford, E. Klein, and E. Stjernswärd, Search for tumor-specific immune reactions in Burkitt's lymphoma patients by the immunofluorescence reaction, *Proc. Natl. Acad. Sci. USA 55*, 1628 (1966).
68. R. W. Baldwin, Ed., *Springer Seminars in Immunopathology Series, Mechanisms of Host Resistance in Cancer* Springer-Verlag, New York, 1982
69. R. W. Baldwin, Ed., *Monoclonal Antibodies for Cancer Detection and Therapy*, Academic Press, New York (1985).
70. R. A. Reisfeld and S. Ferrone, Eds., *Melanoma Antigens and Antibodies*, Plenum Press, New York, 1982.

71. G. Reithmüm, H. Koprowski, S. von Kleist, and K. Munk, Eds., *Contribution to Oncology*, Genes and Antigens in Cancer Cells, Karger/Basel, Vol. 19, 1984.
72. M. F. Greaves, Analysis of the clinical and biological significance of lymphoid phenotypes in acute leukemia, *Cancer Res. 42*, 4752 (1981).
73. J. Ritz, J. M. Pesando, J. Notis-McConarty, H. Lazarus, and S. F. Schlossman, A monoclonal antibody to human acute lymphoblastic leukemia antigen, *Nature 283*, 583 (1980).
74. J. Ritz, J. M. Pesando, J. Notis-McConarty, J. Clavell, L. A. Sallan, and S. F. Schlossman, Use of monoclonal antibodies as diagnostic and therapeutic reagents in acute lymphoblastic leukemia, *Cancer Res. 41*, 4771 (1981).
75. S. E. Sallen, J. Ritz, J. Pesando, R. Gelbar, C. O'Brien, S. Hitchcock, F. Coral, and S. F. Schlossman, Cell surface antigens; prognostic implications in childhood acute lymphoblastic leukemia, *Blood 55*, 395 (1980).
76. V. Raso, J. Ritz, M. Basala, and S. F. Schlossman, Monoclonal antibody-ricin A chain conjugate selectively cytotoxic for cells bearing the common acute lymphoblastic leukemia antigen, *Cancer Res. 42*, 457 (1982).
77. J. Ritz, J. M. Pesando, J. Notis-McConarty, and S. F. Schlossman, Modulation of human acute lymphoblastic leukemia antigen induced by monoclonal antibody *in vitro*. *J. Immunol. 125*, 1506 (1980).
78. R. Sutherland, D. Delia, C. Schnieder, R. Newman, J. Kemshead, and M. Greaves, Ubiquitous cell surface glycoprotein on tumor cells is proliferation-associated receptor for transferrin, *Proc. Natl. Acad. Sci. USA 78*, 4515 (1981).
79. P. J. McAlpine and D. Bootsma, Report of the committee on the genetic constitution of chromosomes, 2, 3, 4, and 6. Oslo Conference (1981): Sixth International Workshop on Human Gene Mapping, *Cytogenet. Cell Genet. 32*, 121 (1982).
80. I. S. Trowbridge and F. Lopez, Monoclonal antibody to transferrin receptor blocks transferrin binding and inhibits human tumor cell growth, *Proc. Natl. Acad. Sci. USA 79*, 1175 (1982).
81. I. Royston, J. A. Majda, S. M. Baird, B. L. Meserve, and J. C. Griffiths, Human T cell antigens defined by monoclonal antibodies: the 65,000 dalton antigen of T cells (T65) is also found on chronic lymphocytic leukemia cells bearing surface immunoglobulin, *J. Immunol. 125*, 725 (1980).
82. R. A. Miller and R. Levy, Response of cutaneous T cell lymphoma to therapy with hybridoma monoclonal antibody, *Lancet 2*, 8240 (1981).
83. I. D. Bernstein, R. C. Nowinski, M. R. Tam, B. McMaster, L. L. Houston, and E. A. Clark, Monoclonal antibody therapy of mouse leukemia. In, *Monoclonal Antibodies* (R. H. Kennett, T. G. McKearn, and K. B. Bechtol, Eds.), Plenum Press, New York, 1980, pp. 275.

84. P. A. Bunn, Jr., J. A. Carrasquillo, A. M. Keenan, R. W. Schroff, K. A. Foon, S. M. Hsu, A. F. Gazdar, J. C. Reynolds, P. Perentesis, and S. M. Larson, Imaging of T-cell lymphoma by radiolabeled monoclonal antibody, *Lancet, 2*, 1219, (1984).
85. K. E. Hellström, I. Hellström, and J. P. Brown, Monoclonal antibodies to melanoma-associated antigens. In, *Monoclonal Antibodies and Cancer* (G. L. Wright, Ed.), Marcel Dekker, Inc., New York, 1984, pp. 31–47.
86. R. G. Woodbury, J. P. Brown, S. M. Loop, K. E. Hellström, and I. Hellström, Analysis of normal and neoplastic human tissues for the tumor-associated protein p97, *Int. J. Cancer 27*, 145 (1981).
87. I. Hellström, J. P. Brown, and K. E. Hellström, Monoclonal antibodies to two determinants of melanoma-antigen p97 act synergistically in complement-dependent cytotoxicity, *J. Immunol. 127*, 157 (1981).
88. G. T. Nepom, K. A. Nelson, S. L. Holbeck, I. Hellström, and K. E. Hellström, Induction of immunity to a human tumor marker by *in vivo* administration of anti-idiotypic antibodies in mice, *Proc. Natl. Acad. Sci. USA 81*, 2864 (1984).
89. J. P. Brown, R. M. Hewick, I. Hellström, K. E. Hellström, R. F. Doolittle, and W. J. Dreyer, Human melanoma-associated antigen p97 is structurally and functionally related to transferrin, *Nature 296*, 171 (1982).
90. G. Plowman, J. P. Brown, C. A. Enns, J. Schröder, B. Nikinmaa, H. H. Sussman, K. E. Hellström, and I. Hellström, Assignment of the gene for human melanoma-associated antigen p97 to chromosome 3, *Nature 303*, 70 (1983).
91. J. P. Brown, T. M. Rose, J. W. Forstrom, I. Hellström, and K. E. Hellström, Isolation of a cDNA clone for human melanoma-associated antigen p97. In, *Molecular Biology of Tumor Cells, 1984*, (B. Wahren, ed.), Raven Press, New York 1985, p. 157.
91a. T. M. Rose, G. D. Plowman, D. B. Teplow, W. J. Dreyer, K. E. Hellström, and J. P. Brown, Primary structure of the human melanoma-antigen p97 (melanotransferrin) deduced from the mRNA sequence, *Proc. Natl. Acad. Sci. USA, 83*, 1261 (1986).
92. M. J. Atassi, Precise determination of the entire antigenic structure of lysozyme: molecular features of protein antigenic structures and potential of surface stimulation synthesis—A powerful new concept for protein binding sites, *Immunochemistry 15*, 909 (1978).
93. T. F. Bumol and R. A. Reisfeld, Unique glycoprotein-proteoglycan complex defined by monoclonal antibody on human melanoma cells, *Proc. Natl. Acad. Sci. USA 79*, 1245 (1982).
94. K. Imai, B. S. Wilson, A. Bigotti, P. G. Natali, and S. Ferrone, J., A 94,000-dalton glycoprotein expressed by human melanoma and carcinoma cells, *J. Natl. Cancer Inst. 69*, 761, 1982.

95. I. Hellström, H. J. Garrigues, L. Cabasco, G. H. Mosely, J. P. Brown, and K. E. Hellström, Studies of a high molecular weight human melanoma-assocated antigen, *J. Immunol. 130*, 1467 (1983).
96. A. H. Ross, M. Herlyn, C. S. Ernst, D. Guerry, J. Bennicell, B. F. D. Ghrist, B. Atkinson, and H. Koprowski, Immunoassay for melanoma-associated proteoglycan in the sera of patients using monoclonal and polyclonal antibodies, *Cancer Res. 44*, 4642 (1984).
97. G. Schultz, T. F. Bumol, and R. A. Reisfeld, Monoclonal-directed effector cells selectively lyse human melanoma cells *in vitro* and *in vivo*, *Proc. Natl. Acad. Sci. USA 80*, 5407 (1983).
98. W. G. Dippold, K. O. Lloyd, L. T. C. Li, H. Ikeda, H. F. Oettgen, and L. J. Old, Cell surface antigens of human malignant melanoma: Definition of six antigenic systems with mouse monoclonal antibodies, *Proc. Natl. Acad. Sci. USA 77*, 6114 (1980).
99. K. O. Pukel, L. R. Lloyd, W. G. Trabassos, W. G. Dippold, H. F. Oettgen, and L. J. Old, GD3, a prominent ganglioside of human melanoma. Detection and characterization by mouse monoclonal antibody, *J. Exp. Med. 155*, 1133 (1982).
100. M-Y. Yeh, I. Hellström, J. P. Brown, G. A. Warner, J. A. Hansen, and K. E. Hellström, Cell surface antigens of human melanoma identified by monoclonal antibody, *Proc. Natl. Acad. Sci. USA 76*, 2927 (1979).
101. E. Nudelman, S. Hakomori, R. Kannagi, S. Levery, M-Y. Yeh, K. E. Hellström, and I. Hellström, Characterization of a human melanoma-associated ganglioside antigen defined by a monoclonal antibody, 4.2, *J. Biol. Chem. 257*, 12752 (1982).
102. D. A. Cheresh, R. A. Reisfeld, and A. P. Varki, O-Acetylation of disialoganglioside GD3 by human melanoma cells creates a unique antigenic determinant, *Science 225*, 846 (1984).
103. J. M. Levine, L. Beasley, and W. B. Stallcup, The D.1.1 antigen: A cell surface marker for germinal cells of the central nervous system, *J. Neurosci. 4*, 831 (1984).
104. D. A. Cheresh, A. P. Varki, N. M. Varki, W. B. Stallcup, J. Levine, and R. A. Reisfeld, A monoclonal antibody recognizes an O-acylated sialic acid in a human melanoma-associated ganglioside, *J. Biol. Chem. 259*, 259 7453 (1984).
105. H. Koprowski, M. Herlyn, Z. Steplewski, and H. F. Sears, Specific antigen in serum of patients with colon carcinoma, *Science 212*, 53 (1981).
106. M. Herlyn, M. Blaszczyk, and H. Koprowski, Immunodiagnosis of human solid tumours, *Contr. Oncol. 19*, 160 (1984).

107. V. Ginsburg, P. Fredman, and J. L. Magnani, Cancer-associated carbohydrate antigens detected by monoclonal antibodies, *Contr. Oncol. 19*, 44 (1984).

108. H. F. Sears, D. Heryln, H. Koprowski, and J. Wen Shen, Immunotherapy of gastrointestinal malignancies with a murine IgG2a antibody, *Contr. Oncol. 19*, 180 (1984).

109. H. Koprowski, D. Herlyn, M. Lubeck, E. DeFreitas, and H. F. Sears, Human anti-idiotype antibodies in cancer patients: Is the modulation of the immune response beneficial for the patient? *Proc. Natl. Acad. Sci. USA 81*, 216 (1984).

110. D. G. Gilliland, Z. Steplewski, R. J. Collier, K. F. Mitchell, T. H. Chang, and H. Koprowski, Antibody-directed cytotoxic agents: Use of monoclonal antibody to direct the action of toxin A chains to colorectal carcinoma cells, *Proc. Natl. Acad. Sci. USA 77*:4539 (1980).

111. G. F. Rowland, C. A., Axton, R. W. Baldwin, J. P. Brown, J. R. F. Corvalan, M. J. Embleton, V. A. Gore, I. Hellström, K. E. Hellström, E. Jacobs, C. H. Marsden, M. V. Pimm, R. G. Simmonds, and W. Smith, Anti-tumor properties of vindesine-monocolonal antibody conjugates *Cancer Immunol. Immunothera., 19*, 1 (1985).

112. A. C. Braban, J. F. Williams, and R. D. Cardiff, A monoclonal antibody to a human breast tumor protein released in response to estrogen, *Cancer Res. 44*, 2704 (1984).

113. S. B. Baylin, A. F. Gazdar, J. D. Minna, S. D. Bernal, and J. H. Shaper, A unique cell-surface protein phenotype distinguishes human small-cell from non-small-cell lung cancer, *Proc. Natl. Acad. Sci. USA 79*, 4650 (1982).

114. L. C. Huang, M. Brockhaus, J. L. Magnani, F. Cuttitta, S. Rosen, J. D. Minna, and V. Ginsburg, Many monoclonal antibodies with an apparent specificity for certain lung cancers are directed against a sugar sequence found in lacto-N-fucopentaose III, *Arch. Biochem. Biophys. 220*, 318 (1983).

115. S. T. Rosen, J. L. Mulsine, F. Cuttitta, J. Fedorko, D. N. Carney, A. F. Gazdar, and J. D. Minna, Analysis of human small cell lung cancer differentiation antigens using a panel of rat monoclonal antibodies, *Cancer Res. 44*, 2052 (1984).

116. M. M. Varki, R. A. Reisfeld, and L. E. Walker, Antigens associated with a human lung adenocarcinoma defined by monoclonal antibodies, *Cancer Res. 44*, 681 (1984).

117a. I. Hellström, D. Horn, P. Linsley, J. P. Brown, V. Brankovan, and K. E. Hellström, Monoclonal mouse atibodies raised against human lung carcinoma, *Cancer Res., 46*, 3917 (1986).

117b. I. Hellström, P. L. Beaumier, and K. E. Hellström, Antitumor effects of L6, an IgG2a antibody reacting with most human carcinomas, *Proc. Natl. Acad. Sci. USA, 83,* 7059 (1986).

118. G. J. Todaro, H. Marquardt, D. R. Twardzik, P. A. Johnson, C. M. Fryling, and J. E. DeLarco, Transforming growth factors produced by tumor cells. In, *Tumor Cell Heterogeneity, Origins and Implications*, Vol. 4, Academic Press, New York, 1982, p. 205.

119. L. Sachs, Control of growth and normal differentiation in leukemic cells: Regulation of the developmental program and restoration of the normal phenotype in myeloid leukemia, *J. Cell. Physiol. Suppl. 1,* 151 (1982).

120. I. J. Fidler and G. Poste, Macrophage-mediated destruction of malignant tumor cells and new strategies for the therapy of metastatic diseases, *Springer Emin. Immunopathol.* 5, 161 (1982).

121. J. Gutterman and J. Quesda, Clinical investigation of partially pure and recombinant DNA derived leukocyte interferon in human cancer, *Tex. Rep. Biol. Med. 41,* 626 (1981–1982).

122. F. L. Meyskens, Jr., E. Gilmartin, D. S. Alberts, N. S. Levine, R. Brooks, S. E. Salmon, and E. A. Surwit, Activity of isoretinoin against squamous cell cancers and pre-neoplastic lesions, *Cancer Treat. Rep. 66,* 1315 (1982).

123. G. E. Goodman, D. S. Alberts, D. L. Ernest, and F. L. Meyskens, Trial of retinol in cancer patients, *J. Clin. Oncol. 1,* 394 (1983).

124. R. Arnon and E. Hurwitz, Antibody-and polymer-drug conjugates, In, *Durable Resistance in Crops* (F. Lamberti, J. M. Waller, and N. A. Van der Graff, Eds.), Plenum Press, New York, 1983, p. 23.

125. M. Sela, E. Hurwitz, and R. Maron, Use of antibodies for delivery of chemotherapeutic drugs. In, *Non-specific Immunity in the Prevention and Treatment of Cancer*, Vol. 43, Pontificia Academia Scientiarvm, 1979, p. 481.

126. B. A. Chabner and C. E. Myers. In, *Cancer, Principles and Practice of Oncology* (V. T. DeVita and R. S. Hellman, Eds.), J. B. Lippincott & Co., Philadelphia, 1982, p. 156.

127. S. E. Salmon, A. W. Hamberger, B. Soehlen, G. G. Durie, D. S. Alberts, and T. E. Moon, Quantitation of differential sensitivity of human tumor stem cells to anti-cancer drugs, *N. Engl. J. Med. 298,* 1321 (1978).

128. L. Foulds, The experimental study of tumor progression: A review, *Cancer Res. 14,* 327 (1954).

129. I. R. Hart and I. J. Fidler, The implications of tumor hetergeneity for studies on the biology of cancer metastasis, *Biochim. Biphys. Acta 651,* 37 (1981).

130. G. L. Nicolson and G. Poste, Tumor cell diversity and host responses in cancer metastasis. Part I. Properties of metastatic cells, *Curr. Probl. Cancer* 7, 1 (1982).

131. M-Y. Yeh, I. Hellström, and K. E. Hellström, Clonal variation in expression of a human melanoma antigen defined by a monoclonal antibody, *J. Immunol. 126*, 1312 (1981).
132. K. Albino, O. Lloyd, A. N. Houghton, H. F. Oettgen, and L. J. Old, Heterogeneity in surface antigen and glycoprotein expression of cell lines derived from different melanoma metastases of the same patient. Implications for the study of tumor antigens, *J. Exp. Med. 154*, 1764 (1981).
133. T. Ghose and A. H. Blair, Antibody-limited cytotoxic agents in the treatment of cancer, *J. Natl. Cancer Inst. 61*, 657 (1978).
134. J. D. Everall, P. Dowd, D. A. L. Davies, G. J. O'Neill, and G. F. Rowland, Treatment of melanoma by passive humoral immunotherapy using antibody drug synergism, *Lancet 1*, 1105 (1977).
135. I. Tsukada, W. K. Bishop, N. Hibe, H. Hirai, E. Hurwitz, and M. Sela, Effect of conjugates of daunomycin and antibodies to rat alphafetoprotein-producing tumor cells, *Proc. Natl. Acad. Sci. USA 79*, 621 (1982).
136. G. F. Rowland, R. G. Simmonds, J. R. F. Corvalan, R. W. Baldwin, J. P. Brown, M. J. Embleton, C. H. J. Ford, K. E. Hellström, I. Hellström, J. T. Kemshead, C. E. Newman, and C. S. Woodhouse, Monoclonal antibodies for targeted therapy with vindesine. In, *Protides of the Biological Fluids, Proceedings of Colloquium 30* (H. Peeters, Ed.), Pergamon Press, New York, 1983, pp. 375–379.
137. M. J. Embleton, G. F. Rowland, R. G. Simmonds, E. Jacobs, C. H. Marsden, and R. W. Baldwin, Selective cytotoxicity against human tumour cells by a vindesine-monoclonal antibody conjugate, *Br. J. Cancer 47*, 43 (1983).
138. G. F. Rowland and R. G. Simmonds, Effects of monoclonal antibodies-drug conjugates on human tumour cell cultures and xenografts. In, *Monoclonal Antibodies for Cancer Detection and Therapy* (R. W. Baldwin, Ed.), Academic Press, New York 1985, p. 345,
139. E. Klein, Tumors of the skin X. Immunotherapy of cutaneous and mucosal neoplasms, *NY State J. Med. 68*, 900 (1968).
140. J. J. Mule', S. Shu, S. L. Schwartz, and S. A. Rosenberg, Adoptive immunotherapy of established pulmonary metastases with LAK cells and recombinant Interleukin-2, *Science 225*, 1487 (1984).

Author Index

Numbers in brackets are reference numbers and indicate that an author's work is referred to although his name is not cited in the text. Underlined numbers give the page on which the complete reference is listed.

B

C

E

F

G

H

K

O

P

Q

R

S

T

W

Y

Subject Index

B

E

F

1987